BIOMECHANICS
Principles and Practices

BIOMECHANICS
Principles and Practices

Edited by

Donald R. Peterson
Professor of Engineering
Dean of the College of Science, Technology, Engineering,
Mathematics, and Nursing
Texas A&M University – Texarkana
Texarkana, Texas, U.S.A.

Joseph D. Bronzino
Founder and President
Biomedical Engineering Alliance and Consortium (BEACON)
Hartford, Connecticut, U.S.A.

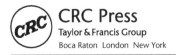

CRC Press
Taylor & Francis Group
Boca Raton London New York

CRC Press is an imprint of the
Taylor & Francis Group, an **informa** business

CRC Press
Taylor & Francis Group
6000 Broken Sound Parkway NW, Suite 300
Boca Raton, FL 33487-2742

First issued in paperback 2017

ISBN-13: 978-1-4398-7098-3 (hbk)
ISBN-13: 978-1-138-74804-0 (pbk)

Library of Congress Cataloging-in-Publication Data

Biomechanics (Peterson)
    Biomechanics : principles and practices / edited by Donald R. Peterson and Joseph D. Bronzino.
    p. ; cm.
    Includes bibliographical references and index.
    ISBN 978-1-4398-7098-3 (hardcover : alk. paper)
    I. Peterson, Donald R., editor. II. Bronzino, Joseph D., 1937- editor. III. Title.
    [DNLM: 1. Biomechanical Phenomena. 2. Musculoskeletal Physiological Phenomena. 3. Cardiovascular Physiological Phenomena. WE 103]

QP303
610.28--dc23   2014037516

Visit the Taylor & Francis Web site at
http://www.taylorandfrancis.com

and the CRC Press Web site at
http://www.crcpress.com

Contents

Preface

Biomechanics is deeply rooted throughout scientific history and has been influenced by the research work of early mathematicians, engineers, physicists, biologists, and physicians. Not one of these disciplines can claim the sole responsibility for maturing biomechanics to its current state; rather, it has been a conglomeration and integration of these disciplines, involving the application of mathematics, physical principles, and engineering methodologies that have been responsible for its advancement. Several examinations exist that offer a historical perspective on biomechanics in dedicated chapters within a variety of biomechanics textbooks. For this reason, a historical perspective is not presented within this brief introduction, and it is left to the reader to discover the material within one of these textbooks. As an example, Fung (1993) provides a reasonably detailed synopsis of those who were influential to the progress of biomechanical understanding. A review of this material and similar material from other authors commonly shows that biomechanics has occupied the thoughts of some of the most conscientious minds involved in a variety of the sciences.

The study of biomechanics, or biological mechanics, employs the principles of mechanics, which is a branch of the physical sciences that investigates the effects of energy and forces on matter or material systems. Biomechanics often embraces a broad range of subject matter that may include aspects of classical mechanics, material science, fluid mechanics, heat transfer, and thermodynamics in an attempt to model and predict the mechanical behaviors of living systems.

The contemporary approach to solving problems in biomechanics typically follows a sequence of fundamental steps that are commonly defined as observation, experimentation, theorization, validation, and application. These steps are the basis of the engineering methodologies, and their significance is emphasized within a formal education of the engineering sciences, especially biomedical engineering. Each step is considered to be equally important, and an iterative relationship between steps, with mathematics serving as the common link, is often necessary to converge on a practical understanding of the system in question. An engineering education that ignores these interrelated fundamentals may produce engineers who are ignorant of the ways in which real-world phenomena differ from mathematical models. Since most biomechanical systems are inherently complex and cannot be adequately defined using only theory and mathematics, biomechanics should be considered as a discipline whose progress relies heavily on research and the careful implementation of this approach. When a precise solution is not obtainable, utilizing this approach will assist in identifying critical physical phenomena and obtaining approximate solutions that may provide a deeper understanding as well as improvements to the investigative strategy. Not surprisingly, the need to identify critical phenomena and obtain approximate solutions seems to be more significant in biomedical engineering than in any other engineering discipline, which is primarily due to the complex biological processes involved.

Applications of biomechanics have traditionally focused on modeling the system-level aspects of the human body, such as the musculoskeletal system, the respiratory system, and the cardiovascular and cardiopulmonary systems. Technologically, the most progress has been made on system-level device development and implementation, with obvious implications on athletic performance, work–environment interaction, clinical rehabilitation, orthotics, prosthetics, and orthopedic surgery. However, more recent biomechanics initiatives are now focusing on the mechanical behaviors of the biological subsystems, such as tissues, cells, and molecules, to relate subsystem functions across all levels by showing how mechanical function is closely associated with certain cellular and molecular processes. These initiatives have a direct impact on the development of biological nano- and microtechnologies involving polymer dynamics, biomembranes, and molecular motors. The integration of system and subsystem models will enhance our overall understanding of human function and performance and advance the principles of biomechanics. Even still, our modern understanding about certain biomechanical processes is limited, but through ongoing biomechanics research, new information that influences the way we think about biomechanics is generated and important applications that are essential to the betterment of human existence are discovered. As a result, our limitations are reduced and our understanding becomes more refined. Recent advances in biomechanics can also be attributed to advances in experimental methods and instrumentation, such as computational and imaging capabilities, which are also subject to constant progress. Therefore, the need to revise and add to the current selections presented within this section becomes obvious, ensuring the presentation of modern viewpoints and developments. The fourth edition of this section presents a total of 20 chapters, 15 of which have been substantially updated and revised to meet this criterion. These 20 selections present material from respected scientists with diverse backgrounds in biomechanics research and application, and the presentation of the chapters has been organized in an attempt to present the material in a systematic manner. The first group of chapters is related to musculoskeletal mechanics and includes hard- and soft-tissue mechanics, joint mechanics, and applications related to human function. The next group of chapters covers several aspects of biofluid mechanics and includes a wide range of circulatory dynamics, such as blood vessel and blood cell mechanics, and transport. It is followed by cellular mechanics, which introduces current methods and strategies for modeling cellular mechanics. The next group consists of two chapters introducing the mechanical functions and significance of the human ear, including a new chapter on inner ear hair cell mechanics. Finally, the remaining two chapters introduce performance characteristics of the human body system during exercise and exertion.

It is the overall intention of this section to serve as a reference to the skilled professional as well as an introduction to the novice or student of biomechanics. Throughout all the editions of the biomechanics section, an attempt was made to incorporate material that covers a bulk of the biomechanics field; however, as biomechanics continues to grow, some topics may be inadvertently omitted, causing a disproportionate presentation of the material. Suggestions and comments from readers are welcomed on subject matter that may be considered for future editions.

Donald R. Peterson

Reference

Fung, Y.C. 1993. *Biomechanics: Mechanical Properties of Living Tissues*. 2nd ed. New York, Springer-Verlag.

Editors

Donald R. Peterson is a professor of engineering and the dean of the College of Science, Technology, Engineering, Mathematics, and Nursing at Texas A&M University in Texarkana, Texas, and holds a joint appointment in the Department of Biomedical Engineering (BME) at Texas A&M University in College Station, Texas. He was recently an associate professor of medicine and the director of the Biodynamics Laboratory in the School of Medicine at the University of Connecticut (UConn) and served as chair of the BME Program in the School of Engineering at UConn as well as the director of the BME Graduate and Undergraduate Programs. Dr. Peterson earned a BS in aerospace engineering and a BS in biomechanical engineering from Worcester Polytechnic Institute, in Worcester, Massachusetts, in 1992, an MS in mechanical engineering from the UConn, in Storrs, Connecticut, in 1995, and a PhD in biomedical engineering from UConn in 1999. He has 17 years of experience in BME education and has offered graduate-level and undergraduate-level courses in the areas of biomechanics, biodynamics, biofluid mechanics, BME communication, BME senior design, and ergonomics, and has taught subjects such as gross anatomy, occupational biomechanics, and occupational exposure and response in the School of Medicine. Dr. Peterson was also recently the co-executive director of the Biomedical Engineering Alliance and Consortium (BEACON), which is a nonprofit organization dedicated to the promotion of collaborative research, translation, and partnership among academic, medical, and industry people in the field of biomedical engineering to develop new medical technologies and devices.

Dr. Peterson has over 21 years of experience in devices and systems and in engineering and medical research, and his work on human–device interaction has led to applications on the design and development of several medical devices and tools. Other recent translations of his research include the development of devices such as robotic assist devices and prosthetics, long-duration biosensor monitoring systems, surgical and dental instruments, patient care medical devices, spacesuits and space tools for NASA, powered and non-powered hand tools, musical instruments, sports equipment, computer input devices, and so on. Other overlapping research initiatives focus on the development of computational models and simulations of biofluid dynamics and biomechanical performance, cell mechanics and cellular responses to fluid shear stress, human exposure and response to vibration, and the acoustics of hearing protection and communication. He has also been involved clinically with the Occupational and Environmental Medicine group at the UConn Health Center, where his work has been directed toward the objective engineering analysis of the anatomic and physiological processes involved in the onset of musculoskeletal and neuromuscular diseases, including strategies of disease mitigation.

Dr. Peterson's scholarly activities include over 50 published journal articles, 2 textbook chapters, 2 textbook sections, and 12 textbooks, including his new appointment as co-editor-in-chief for *The Biomedical Engineering Handbook* by CRC Press.

Joseph D. Bronzino is currently the president of the Biomedical Engineering Alliance and Consortium (BEACON; www.beaconalliance.org), which is a nonprofit organization dedicated to the promotion of collaborative research, translation, and partnership among academic, medical, and industry people in the field of biomedical engineering to develop new medical technologies and devices. To accomplish this goal, Dr. Bronzino and BEACON facilitate collaborative research, industrial partnering, and the development of emerging companies. Dr. Bronzino earned a BSEE from Worcester Polytechnic Institute, Worcester, Massachusetts, in 1959, an MSEE from the Naval Postgraduate School, Monterey, California, in 1961, and a PhD in electrical engineering from Worcester Polytechnic Institute in 1968. He was recently the Vernon Roosa Professor of Applied Science and endowed chair at Trinity College, Hartford, Connecticut.

Dr. Bronzino is the author of over 200 journal articles and 15 books, including *Technology for Patient Care* (C.V. Mosby, 1977), *Computer Applications for Patient Care* (Addison-Wesley, 1982), *Biomedical Engineering: Basic Concepts and Instrumentation* (PWS Publishing Co., 1986), *Expert Systems: Basic Concepts* (Research Foundation of State University of New York, 1989), *Medical Technology and Society: An Interdisciplinary Perspective* (MIT Press and McGraw-Hill, 1990), *Management of Medical Technology* (Butterworth/Heinemann, 1992), *The Biomedical Engineering Handbook* (CRC Press, 1st Edition, 1995; 2nd Edition, 2000; 3rd Edition, 2006), *Introduction to Biomedical Engineering* (Academic Press, 1st Edition, 1999; 2nd Edition, 2005; 3rd Edition, 2011), *Biomechanics: Principles and Applications* (CRC Press, 2002), *Biomaterials: Principles and Applications* (CRC Press, 2002), *Tissue Engineering* (CRC Press, 2002), and *Biomedical Imaging* (CRC Press, 2002).

Dr. Bronzino is a fellow of IEEE and the American Institute of Medical and Biological Engineering (AIMBE), an honorary member of the Italian Society of Experimental Biology, past chairman of the Biomedical Engineering Division of the American Society for Engineering Education (ASEE), a charter member of the Connecticut Academy of Science and Engineering (CASE), a charter member of the American College of Clinical Engineering (ACCE), a member of the Association for the Advancement of Medical Instrumentation (AAMI), past president of the IEEE-Engineering in Medicine and Biology Society (EMBS), past chairman of the IEEE Health Care Engineering Policy Committee (HCEPC), and past chairman of the IEEE Technical Policy Council in Washington, DC. He is a member of Eta Kappa Nu, Sigma Xi, and Tau Beta Pi. He is also a recipient of the IEEE Millennium Medal for "his contributions to biomedical engineering research and education" and the Goddard Award from WPI for Outstanding Professional Achievement in 2005. He is presently editor-in-chief of the Academic Press/Elsevier BME Book Series.

Contributors

Kai-Nan An
Mayo Clinic
Rochester, Minnesota

Thomas J. Burkholder
School of Applied Physiology
Georgia Institute of Technology
Atlanta, Georgia

Thomas R. Canfield
Argonne National Laboratory
Argonne, Illinois

Roy B. Davis III
Motion Analysis Laboratory
Shriners Hospitals for Children
Greenville, South Carolina

Peter A. DeLuca
Center for Motion Analysis
Connecticut Children's Medical Center
Farmington, Connecticut

Philip B. Dobrin
Hines VA Hospital
Hines, Illinois

and

Loyola University Medical Center
Maywood, Illinois

Cathryn R. Dooly
Department of Physical Education
Lander University
Greenwood, South Carolina

Michael J. Furey
Department of Mechanical Engineering
Virginia Polytechnic Institute and State
    University
Blacksburg, Virginia

Wally Grant
Department of Biomedical Engineering
and
Department of Engineering Science and
    Mechanics
College of Engineering
Virginia Polytechnic Institute and State
    University
Blacksburg, Virginia

Alan R. Hargens
Department of Orthopaedic Surgery
UCSD Medical Center
University of California, San Diego
San Diego, California

Robert M. Hochmuth
Department of Mechanical Engineering and
    Materials Science
Duke University
Durham, North Carolina

Ben F. Hurley
University of Maryland
Baltimore, Maryland

Arthur T. Johnson
University of Maryland
Baltimore, Maryland

J. Lawrence Katz (deceased)
Department of Biomedical Engineering
Case School of Engineering and School of
    Medicine
and
Department of Oral and Maxillofacial Surgery
School of Dental Medicine
Case Western Reserve University
Cleveland, Ohio

and

Department of Mechanical Engineering and
    Surgery, Orthopedics
Schools of Engineering and Medicine
University of Kansas
Lawrence, Kansas

Kenton R. Kaufman
Mayo Clinic
Rochester, Minnesota

Roy C. P. Kerckhoffs
School of Bioengineering
Institute of Engineering in Medicine
University of California, San Diego
La Jolla, California

Albert I. King
Wayne State University
Detroit, Michigan

Baruch B. Lieber
Department of Neurosurgery
State University of New York at Stony Brook
Stony Brook, New York

Richard L. Lieber
Departments of Orthopaedics, Radiology and
    Bioengineering
Biomedical Sciences Graduate Group
University of California, San Diego
and
Veterans Administration Medical Centers
La Jolla, California

Orestes Marangos
Bioengineering Research Center
School of Engineering
University of Kansas
Lawrence, Kansas

Andrew D. McCulloch
School of Bioengineering
Institute of Engineering in Medicine
University of California, San Diego
La Jolla, California

Anil Misra
Bioengineering Research Center
School of Engineering
University of Kansas
Lawrence, Kansas

Jong-Hoon Nam
Department of Biomedical Engineering
and
Department of Mechanical Engineering
Hajim School of Engineering and Applied
    Sciences
University of Rochester
Rochester, New York

Sylvia Õunpuu
Center for Motion Analysis
Connecticut Children's Medical Center
Farmington, Connecticut

Muralidhar Padala
Division of Cardiothoracic Surgery
Emory University School of Medicine
Atlanta, Georgia

Roland N. Pittman
Department of Physiology and Biophysics
Medical College of Virginia Campus
Virginia Commonwealth University
Richmond, Virginia

Aleksander S. Popel
Department of Biomedical Engineering
School of Medicine
Johns Hopkins University
Baltimore, Maryland

Sunil Puria
Department of Mechanical Engineering
and
Department of Otolaryngology-HNS
Stanford University
Stanford, California

Carl F. Rothe
Department of Cellular and Integrative
    Physiology
School of Medicine
Indiana University
Indianapolis, Indiana

Geert W. Schmid-Schönbein
Department of Bioengineering
University of California, San Diego
La Jolla, California

Artin A. Shoukas
Department of Biomedical Engineering
School of Medicine
Johns Hopkins University
Baltimore, Maryland

Alexander A. Spector
Department of Biomedical Engineering
School of Medicine
Johns Hopkins University
Baltimore, Maryland

Paulette Spencer
Department of Mechanical Engineering
Bioengineering Research Center
School of Engineering
University of Kansas
Lawrence, Kansas

Erin Spinner
School of Biomedical Engineering
Georgia Institute of Technology
Atlanta, Georgia

Charles R. Steele
Department of Mechanical Engineering
Stanford University
Stanford, California

Roger Tran-Son-Tay
University of Florida
Gainesville, Florida

David C. Viano
Wayne State University
Detroit, Michigan

Samuel R. Ward
Departments of Orthopaedics, Radiology and
    Bioengineering
Biomedical Sciences Graduate Group
University of California, San Diego
and
Veterans Administration Medical Centers
La Jolla, California

Richard E. Waugh
Department of Biomedical Engineering
University of Rochester
Rochester, New York

Choon Hwai Yap
School of Biomedical Engineering
Georgia Institute of Technology
Atlanta, Georgia

Qiang Ye
Bioengineering Research Center
School of Engineering
University of Kansas
Lawrence, Kansas

Ajit P. Yoganathan
School of Biomedical Engineering
Georgia Institute of Technology
Atlanta, Georgia

1

Mechanics of Hard Tissue

J. Lawrence Katz
Case Western Reserve University
University of Kansas

Anil Misra
University of Kansas

Orestes Marangos
University of Kansas

Qiang Ye
University of Kansas

Paulette Spencer
University of Kansas

1.1 Introduction

Hard tissue, mineralized tissue, and calcified tissue are often used as synonyms for bone when describing the structure and properties of bone or tooth. The hard is self-evident in comparison with all other mammalian tissues, which often are referred to as soft tissues. The use of the terms mineralized and calcified arises from the fact that, in addition to the principle protein, collagen, and other proteins, glycoproteins, and protein-polysaccharides, comprising about 50% of the volume, the major constituent of bone is a calcium phosphate (thus the term calcified). The calcium phosphate occurs in the form of a crystalline carbonate apatite (similar to naturally occurring minerals, thus the term mineralized). Irrespective of its biological function, bone is one of the most interesting materials known in terms of structure–property relationships. Bone is an anisotropic, heterogeneous, inhomogeneous, nonlinear, thermorheologically complex viscoelastic material. It exhibits electromechanical effects, presumed to be due to streaming potentials, both *in vivo* and *in vitro* when wet. In the dry state, bone exhibits piezoelectric properties. Because of the complexity of the structure–property relationships in bone, and the space limitation for this chapter, it is necessary to concentrate on one aspect of the mechanics. Currey (1984, p. 43) states unequivocally that he thinks, "the most important feature of bone material is its stiffness." This is, of course, the premiere consideration for the weight-bearing long bones. Thus, this chapter will concentrate on the elastic and viscoelastic properties of compact cortical bone and the elastic properties of trabecular bone as exemplar of mineralized tissue mechanics.

1.2 Structure of Bone

The complexity of bone's properties arises from the complexity in its structure. Thus it is important to have an understanding of the structure of mammalian bone in order to appreciate the related properties. Figure 1.1 is a diagram showing the structure of a human femur at different levels (Park, 1979). For convenience, the structures shown in Figure 1.1 are grouped into four levels. A further subdivision of structural organization of mammalian bone is shown in Figure 1.2 (Wainwright et al., 1982). The individual figures within this diagram can be sorted into one of the appropriate levels of structure shown in Figure 1.1 and are described as follows in hierarchical order. At the smallest unit of structure we have the tropocollagen molecule and the associated apatite crystallites (abbreviated Ap). The former is approximately 1.5 × 280 nm, made up of three individual left-handed helical polypeptide (alpha) chains coiled into a right-handed triple helix. Ap crystallites have been found to be carbonate-substituted hydroxyapatite, generally thought to be nonstoichiometric. The crystallites appear to be about 4 × 20 × 60 nm in size. This is denoted at the molecular level. Next is the ultrastructural level. Here, the collagen and Ap are intimately associated and assembled into a microfibrillar composite, several of which are then assembled into fibers from approximately 3 to 5 mm thickness. At the next level, the microstructural, these fibers are either randomly arranged (woven bone) or organized into concentric lamellar groups (osteons) or linear lamellar groups (plexiform bone). This is the level of structure we usually mean when we talk about bone tissue properties. In addition to the differences in lamellar organization at this level, there are also two different types of architectural structure. The dense type of bone found, for example, in the shafts of long bone is known as compact or cortical bone. A more porous or spongy type of bone is found, for example, at the articulating ends of long bones. This is called cancellous bone. It is important to note that the material and structural organization of collagen–Ap making up osteonic or Haversian bone and plexiform bone are the same as the material comprising cancellous bone.

Finally, we have the whole bone itself constructed of osteons and portions of older, partially destroyed osteons (called interstitial lamellae) in the case of humans or of osteons and/or plexiform bone in the case of mammals. This we denote as the macrostructural level. The elastic properties of the whole bone results from the hierarchical contribution of each of these levels.

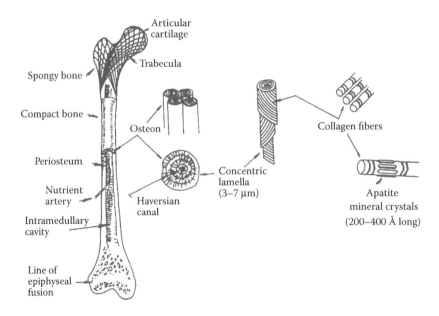

FIGURE 1.1 Hierarchical levels of structure in a human femur. (From Park JB. *Biomaterials: An Introduction.* New York: Plenum, 1979. Courtesy of Plenum Press and Dr. J.B. Park.)

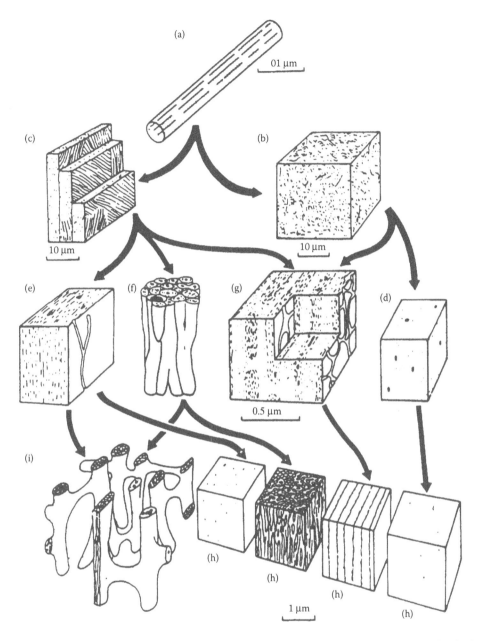

FIGURE 1.2 Diagram showing the structure of mammalian bone at different levels. Bone at the same level is drawn at the same magnification. The arrows show what types may contribute to structures at higher levels. (From Wainwright SA. et al. *Mechanical Design in Organisms*. Princeton, NJ: Princeton University Press, 1982. Courtesy Princeton University Press.) (a) Collagen fibril with associated mineral crystals. (b) Woven bone. The collagen fibrils are arranged more or less randomly. Osteocytes are not shown. (c) Lamellar bone. There are separate lamellae, and the collagen fibrils are arranged in "domains" of preferred fibrillar orientation in each lamella. Osteocytes are not shown. (d) Woven bone. Blood channels are shown as large black spots. At this level woven bone is indicated by light dotting. (e) Primary lamellar bone. At this level lamellar bone is indicated by fine dashes. (f) Haversian bone. A collection of Haversian systems, each with concentric lamellae round a central blood channel. The large black area represents the cavity formed as a cylinder of bone is eroded away. It will be filled in with concentric lamellae and form a new Haversian system. (g) Laminar bone. Two blood channel networks are exposed. Note how layers of woven and lamellar bone alternate. (h) Compact bone of the types shown at the lower levels. (i) Cancellous bone.

TABLE 1.1 Composition of Adult Human and Bovine Cortical Bone

Species	% H$_2$O	Ap	% Dry Weight Collagen	GAG[a]	Reference
Bovine	9.1	76.4	21.5	N.D[b]	Herring (1977)
Human	7.3	67.2	21.2	0.34	Pellegrino and Blitz (1965); Vejlens (1971)

[a] Glycosaminoglycan.
[b] Not determined.

1.3 Composition of Bone

The composition of bone depends on a large number of factors: the species, which bone, the location from which the sample is taken, and the age, sex, and type of bone tissue, for example, woven, cancellous, cortical. However, a rough estimate for overall composition by volume is one-third Ap, one-third collagen and other organic components, and one-third H$_2$O. Some data in the literature for the composition of adult human and bovine cortical bone are given in Table 1.1.

1.4 Elastic Properties

Although bone is a viscoelastic material, at the quasi-static strain rates in mechanical testing and even at the ultrasonic frequencies used experimentally, it is a reasonable first approximation to model cortical bone as an anisotropic, linear elastic solid with Hooke's law as the appropriate constitutive equation. Tensor notation for the equation is written as

$$\sigma_{ij} = C_{ijkl}\varepsilon_{kl} \tag{1.1}$$

where σ_{ij} and ε_{kl} are the second-rank stress and infinitesimal second rank strain tensors, respectively, and C_{ijkl} is the fourth-rank elasticity tensor. Using the reduced notation, we can rewrite Equation 1.1 as

$$\sigma_i = C_{ij}\epsilon_j \quad i,j = 1 \text{ to } 6 \tag{1.2}$$

where the C_{ij} are the stiffness coefficients (elastic constants). The inverse of the C_{ij}, the S_{ij}, are known as the compliance coefficients.

The anisotropy of cortical bone tissue has been described in two symmetry arrangements. Lang (1969), Katz and Ukraincik (1971), and Yoon and Katz (1976a,b) assumed bone to be transversely isotropic with the bone axis of symmetry (the 3 direction) as the unique axis of symmetry. Any small difference in elastic properties between the radial (1 direction) and transverse (2 direction) axes, due to the apparent gradient in porosity from the periosteal to the endosteal sides of bone, was deemed to be due essentially to the defect and did not alter the basic symmetry. For a transverse isotropic material, the stiffness matrix $[C_{ij}]$ is given by

$$[C_{ij}] = \begin{bmatrix} C_{11} & C_{12} & C_{13} & 0 & 0 & 0 \\ C_{12} & C_{11} & C_{13} & 0 & 0 & 0 \\ C_{13} & C_{13} & C_{33} & 0 & 0 & 0 \\ 0 & 0 & 0 & C_{44} & 0 & 0 \\ 0 & 0 & 0 & 0 & C_{44} & 0 \\ 0 & 0 & 0 & 0 & 0 & C_{66} \end{bmatrix} \tag{1.3}$$

where $C_{66} = 1/2 \ (C_{11}-C_{12})$. Of the 12 nonzero coefficients, only 5 are independent.

However, Van Buskirk and Ashman (1981) used the small differences in elastic properties between the radial and tangential directions to postulate that bone is an orthotropic material; this requires that 9 of the 12 nonzero elastic constants be independent, that is,

$$
[C_{ij}] = \begin{bmatrix}
C_{11} & C_{12} & C_{13} & 0 & 0 & 0 \\
C_{12} & C_{22} & C_{23} & 0 & 0 & 0 \\
C_{13} & C_{23} & C_{33} & 0 & 0 & 0 \\
0 & 0 & 0 & C_{44} & 0 & 0 \\
0 & 0 & 0 & 0 & C_{55} & 0 \\
0 & 0 & 0 & 0 & 0 & C_{66}
\end{bmatrix}
\tag{1.4}
$$

Corresponding matrices can be written for the compliance coefficients, the S_{ij}, based on the inverse equation to Equation 1.2:

$$
\varepsilon_i = S_{ij}\sigma_j \quad i,j = 1 \text{ to } 6
\tag{1.5}
$$

where the S_{ij}th compliance is obtained by dividing the $[C_{ij}]$ stiffness matrix, minus the ith row and jth column, by the full $[C_{ij}]$ matrix and vice versa to obtain the C_{ij} in terms of the S_{ij}. Thus, although $S_{33} = 1/E_3$, where E_3 is Young's modulus in the bone axis direction, $E_3 \neq C_{33}$, since C_{33} and S_{33}, are not reciprocals of one another even for an isotropic material, let alone for transverse isotropy or orthotropic symmetry.

The relationship between the compliance matrix and the technical constants such as Young's modulus (E_i) shear modulus (G_i), and Poisson's ratio (v_{ij}) measured in mechanical tests such as uniaxial or pure shear is expressed in Equation 1.6.

$$
[S_{ij}] = \begin{bmatrix}
\dfrac{1}{E_1} & \dfrac{-v_{21}}{E_2} & \dfrac{-v_{31}}{E_3} & 0 & 0 & 0 \\[2mm]
\dfrac{-v_{12}}{E_1} & \dfrac{1}{E_2} & \dfrac{-v_{32}}{E_3} & 0 & 0 & 0 \\[2mm]
\dfrac{-v_{13}}{E_1} & \dfrac{-v_{23}}{E_2} & \dfrac{1}{E_3} & 0 & 0 & 0 \\[2mm]
0 & 0 & 0 & \dfrac{1}{G_{23}} & 0 & 0 \\[2mm]
0 & 0 & 0 & 0 & \dfrac{1}{G_{31}} & 0 \\[2mm]
0 & 0 & 0 & 0 & 0 & \dfrac{1}{G_{12}}
\end{bmatrix}
\tag{1.6}
$$

Again, for an orthotropic material, only 9 of the above 12 nonzero terms are independent, due to the symmetry of the S_{ij} tensor:

$$
\frac{v_{12}}{E_1} = \frac{v_{21}}{E_2}, \quad \frac{v_{13}}{E_1} = \frac{v_{31}}{E_3}, \quad \frac{v_{23}}{E_2} = \frac{v_{32}}{E_3}
\tag{1.7}
$$

For the transverse isotropic case, Equation 1.5 reduces to only 5 independent coefficients, since

$$
E_1 = E_2, \quad v_{12} = v_{21}, \quad v_{31} = v_{32} = v_{13} = v_{23},
$$

$$
G_{23} = G_{31}, \quad G_{12} = \frac{E_1}{2(1 + v_{12})}
\tag{1.8}
$$

In addition to the mechanical tests cited above, ultrasonic wave propagation techniques have been used to measure the anisotropic elastic properties of bone (Lang, 1969; Yoon and Katz, 1976a,b; Van Buskirk and Ashman, 1981). This is possible, since combining Hooke's law with Newton's second law results in a wave equation which yields the following relationship involving the stiffness matrix:

$$\rho V^2 U_m = C_{mrns} N_r N_s U_n \tag{1.9}$$

where ρ is the density of the medium, V is the wave speed, and U and N are unit vectors along the particle displacement and wave propagation directions, respectively, so that U_m, N_r, and others are direction cosines.

Thus to find the five transverse isotropic elastic constants, at least five independent measurements are required, for example, a dilatational longitudinal wave in the 2 and 1(2) directions, a transverse wave in the 13(23) and 12 planes, and so on. The technical moduli must then be calculated from the full set of C_{ij}. For improved statistics, redundant measurements should be made. Correspondingly, for orthotropic symmetry, enough independent measurements must be made to obtain all nine C_{ij}; again, redundancy in measurements is a suggested approach.

One major advantage of the ultrasonic measurements over mechanical testing is that the former can be done with specimens too small for the latter technique. Second, the reproducibility of measurements using the former technique is greater than for the latter. Still a third advantage is that the full set of either five or nine coefficients can be measured on one specimen, a procedure not possible with the latter techniques. Thus, at present, most of the studies of elastic anisotropy in both human and other mammalian bone are done using ultrasonic techniques. In addition to the bulk wave-type measurements described above, it is possible to obtain Young's modulus directly. This is accomplished by using samples of small cross sections with transducers of low frequency so that the wavelength of the sound is much larger than the specimen size. In this case, an extensional longitudinal (bar) wave is propagated (which experimentally is analogous to a uniaxial mechanical test experiment), yielding

$$V^2 = \frac{E}{\rho} \tag{1.10}$$

This technique was used successfully to show that bovine plexiform bone was definitely orthotropic while the bovine Haversian bone could be treated as transversely isotropic (Lipson and Katz, 1984). The results were subsequently confirmed using bulk wave propagation techniques with considerable redundancy (Maharidge, 1984).

Table 1.2 lists the C_{ij} (in GPa) for human (Haversian) bone and bovine (both Haversian and plexiform) bone. With the exception of Knet's (1978) measurements, which were made using quasi-static mechanical testing, all the other measurements were made using bulk ultrasonic wave propagation.

TABLE 1.2 Elastic Stiffness Coefficients for Various Human and Bovine Bones; All Measurements Made with Ultrasound except for Knets (1978) Mechanical Tests

Experiments	C_{11}	C_{22}	C_{33}	C_{44}	C_{55}	C_{66}	C_{12}	C_{13}	C_{23}
(Bone Type)	(GPa)	(GPa)	(GPa)	(GPa)	(GPa)	(GPa)	(GPa)	(GPa)	(GPa)
Van Buskirk and Ashman (1981) (bovine femur)	14.1	18.4	25.0	7.00	6.30	5.28	6.34	4.84	6.94
Knets (1978) (human tibia)	11.6	14.4	22.5	4.91	3.56	2.41	7.95	6.10	6.92
Van Buskirk and Ashman (1981) (human femur)	20.0	21.7	30.0	6.56	5.85	4.74	10.9	11.5	11.5
Maharidge (1984) (bovine femur Haversian)	21.2	21.0	29.0	6.30	6.30	5.40	11.7	12.7	11.1
Maharidge (1984) (bovine femur plexiform)	22.4	25.0	35.0	8.20	7.10	6.10	14.0	15.8	13.6

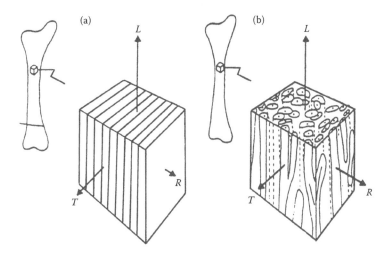

FIGURE 1.3 Diagram showing how laminar (plexiform) bone (a) differs more between radial and tangential directions (*R* and *T*) than does Haversian bone (b). The arrows are vectors representing the various directions. (From Wainwright SA et al. *Mechanical Design in Organisms*. Princeton, NJ: Princeton University Press, 1982. Courtesy Princeton University Press.)

In Maharidge's study (1984), both types of tissue specimens, the Haversian and plexiform, were obtained from different aspects of the same level of an adult bovine femur. Thus, the differences in C_{ij} reported between the two types of bone tissue are hypothesized to be due essentially to the differences in microstructural organization (Figure 1.3) (Wainwright et al., 1982). The textural symmetry at this level of structure has dimensions comparable to those of the ultrasound wavelengths used in the experiment, and the molecular and ultrastructural levels of organization in both types of tissues are essentially identical. Note that while C_{11}, almost equals C_{22} and that C_{44} and C_{55} are equal for bovine Haversian bone, C_{11} and C_{22} and C_{44} and C_{55} differ by 11.6% and 13.4%, respectively, for bovine plexiform bone. Similarly, although C_{66} and $\frac{1}{2}(C_{11}-C_{12})$ differ by 12.0% for the Haversian bone, they differ by 31.1% for plexiform bone. Only the differences between C_{13} and C_{23} are somewhat comparable: 12.6% for the Haversian bone and 13.9% for plexiform. These results reinforce the importance of modeling bone as a hierarchical ensemble in order to understand the basis for bone's elastic properties as a composite material–structure system in which the collagen–Ap components define the material composite property. When this material property is entered into calculations based on the microtextural arrangement, the overall anisotropic elastic anisotropy can be modeled.

The human femur data (Van Buskirk and Ashman, 1981) support this description of bone tissue. Although they measured all nine individual C_{ij}, treating the femur as an orthotropic material, their results are consistent with a near transverse isotropic symmetry. However, their nine C_{ij} for bovine femoral bone clearly shows the influence of the orthotropic microtextural symmetry of tissue's plexiform structure.

The data of Knets (1978) on the human tibia are difficult to analyze. This could be due to the possibility of significant systematic errors due to mechanical testing on a large number of small specimens from a multitude of different positions in the tibia.

The variations in bone's elastic properties cited earlier above due to location is appropriately illustrated in Table 1.3, where the mean values and standard deviations (all in GPa) for all *g* orthotropic C_{ij} are given for bovine cortical bone at each aspect over the entire length of bone.

Since the C_{ij} are simply related to the "technical" elastic moduli, such as Young's modulus (*E*), shear modulus (*G*), bulk modulus (*K*), and others, it is possible to describe the moduli along any given direction. The full equations for the most general anisotropy are too long to present here. However, they can

TABLE 1.3 Mean Values and Standard Deviations for the C_{ij} Measured by Van Buskirk and Ashman (1981) at Each Aspect over the Entire Length of Bone

	Anterior	Medial	Posterior	Lateral
C_{11}	18.7 ± 1.7	20.9 ± 0.8	20.1 ± 1.0	20.6 ± 1.6
C_{22}	20.4 ± 1.2	22.3 ± 1.0	22.2 ± 1.3	22.0 ± 1.0
C_{33}	28.6 ± 1.9	30.1 ± 2.3	30.8 ± 1.0	30.5 ± 1.1
C_{44}	6.73 ± 0.68	6.45 ± 0.35	6.78 ± 1.0	6.27 ± 0.28
C_{55}	5.55 ± 0.41	6.04 ± 0.51	5.93 ± 0.28	5.68 ± 0.29
C_{66}	4.34 ± 0.33	4.87 ± 0.35	5.10 ± 0.45	4.63 ± 0.36
C_{12}	11.2 ± 2.0	11.2 ± 1.1	10.4 ± 1.0	10.8 ± 1.7
C_{13}	11.2 ± 1.1	11.2 ± 2.4	11.6 ± 1.7	11.7 ± 1.8
C_{23}	10.4 ± 1.4	11.5 ± 1.0	12.5 ± 1.7	11.8 ± 1.1

Note: All values in GPa.

be found in Yoon and Katz (1976a). Presented below are the simplified equations for the case of transverse isotropy. Young's modulus is

$$\frac{1}{E(\gamma_3)} = S'_{33} = (1 - \gamma_3^2)2S_{11} + \gamma_3^4 S_{33} + \gamma_3^2(1 - \gamma_3^2)(2S_{13} + S_{44}) \tag{1.11}$$

where $\gamma_3 = \cos \phi$, and ϕ is the angle made with respect to the bone (3) axis.

The shear modulus (rigidity modulus or torsional modulus for a circular cylinder) is

$$\frac{1}{G(\gamma_3)} = \frac{1}{2}(S'_{44} + S'_{55}) = S_{44} + (S_{11} - S_{12}) - \frac{1}{2}S_{44}(1 - \gamma_3^2)$$
$$+ 2(S_{11} + S_{33} - 2S_{13} - S_{44})\gamma_3^2(1 - \gamma_3^2) \tag{1.12}$$

where, again $\gamma_3 = \cos \phi$.

The bulk modulus (reciprocal of the volume compressibility) is

$$\frac{1}{K} = S_{33} + 2(S_{11} + S_{12} + 2S_{13}) = \frac{C_{11} + C_{12} + 2C_{33} - 4C_{13}}{C_{33}(C_{11} + C_{12}) - 2C_{13}^2} \tag{1.13}$$

Conversion of Equations 1.11 and 1.12 from S_{ij} to C_{ij} can be done by using the following transformation equations:

$$S_{11} = \frac{C_{22}C_{33} - C_{23}^2}{\Delta}, \quad S_{22} = \frac{C_{33}C_{11} - C_{13}^2}{\Delta},$$
$$S_{33} = \frac{C_{11}C_{22} - C_{12}^2}{\Delta}, \quad S_{12} = \frac{C_{13}C_{23} - C_{12}C_{33}}{\Delta},$$
$$S_{13} = \frac{C_{12}C_{23} - C_{13}C_{22}}{\Delta}, \quad S_{23} = \frac{C_{12}C_{13} - C_{23}C_{11}}{\Delta}, \tag{1.14}$$
$$S_{44} = \frac{1}{C_{44}}, \quad S_{55} = \frac{1}{C_{55}}, \quad S_{66} = \frac{1}{C_{66}}$$

where

$$\Delta = \begin{bmatrix} C_{11} & C_{12} & C_{13} \\ C_{12} & C_{22} & C_{23} \\ C_{13} & C_{23} & C_{33} \end{bmatrix} = C_{11}C_{22}C_{33} + 2C_{12}C_{23}C_{13} - (C_{11}C_{23}^2 + C_{22}C_{13}^2 + C_{33}C_{12}^2) \tag{1.15}$$

In addition to data on the elastic properties of cortical bone presented above, there is also a considerable set of data available on the mechanical properties of cancellous (trabecullar) bone, including measurements of the elastic properties of single trabeculae. Indeed, as early as 1993, Keaveny and Hayes (1993) presented an analysis of 20 years of studies on the mechanical properties of trabecular bone. Most of the earlier studies used mechanical testing of bulk specimens of a size reflecting a cellular solid, that is, of the order of cubic millimeters or larger. These studies showed that both the modulus and strength of trabecular bone are strongly correlated to the apparent density, where apparent density, ρ_a, is defined as the product of individual trabeculae density, ρ_t, and the volume fraction of bone in the bulk specimen, V_f, and is given by $\rho_a = \rho_t V_f$.

Elastic moduli, E, from these measurements generally ranged from approximately 10 MPa to the order of 1 GPa depending on the apparent density and could be correlated to the apparent density in g/cm^3 by a power-law relationship, $E = 6.13 P_a^{144}$, calculated for 165 specimens with an $r^2 = 0.62$ (Keaveny and Hayes, 1993).

With the introduction of micromechanical modeling of bone, it became apparent that in addition to knowing the bulk properties of trabecular bone it was necessary to determine the elastic properties of the individual trabeculae. Several different experimental techniques have been used for these studies. Individual trabeculae have been machined and measured in buckling, yielding a modulus of 11.4 GPa (wet) and 14.1 GPa (dry) (Townsend et al., 1975), as well as by other mechanical testing methods providing average values of the elastic modulus ranging from less than 1 GPa to about 8 GPa (Table 1.4). Ultrasound measurements (Ashman and Rho, 1988; Rho et al., 1993) have yielded values commensurate with the measurements of Townsend et al. (1975) (Table 1.4). More recently, acoustic microscopy and nanoindentation have been used, yielding values significantly higher than those cited above. Rho et al. (1999) using nanoindentation obtained average values of modulus ranging from 15.0 to 19.4 GPa depending on orientation, as compared to 22.4 GPa for osteons and 25.7 GPa for the interstitial lamellae in cortical bone (Table 1.4). Turner et al. (1999) compared nanoindentation and acoustic microscopy at 50 MHz on the same specimens of trabecular and cortical bone from a common human donor. While the nanoindentation resulted in Young's moduli greater than those measured by acoustic microscopy by 4–14%, the anisotropy ratio of longitudinal modulus to transverse modulus for cortical bone was similar for both modes of measurement; the trabecular values are given in Table 1.4. Acoustic microscopy at 400 MHz has also been used to measure the moduli of both human trabecular and cortical bone (Bumrerraj and Katz, 2001), yielding results comparable with those of Turner et al. (1999) for both types of bone (Table 1.4).

These recent studies provide a framework for micromechanical analyses using material properties measured on the microstructural level. They also point to using nano-scale measurements, such as those

TABLE 1.4   Elastic Moduli of Trabecular Bone Material Measured by Different Experimental Methods

Study	Method	Average Modulus	(GPa)
Townsend et al. (1975)	Buckling	11.4	(Wet)
	Buckling	14.1	(Dry)
Ryan and Williams (1989)	Uniaxial tension	0.760	
Choi and Goldstein (1992)	4-point bending	5.72	
Ashman and Rho (1988)	Ultrasound	13.0	(Human)
	Ultrasound	10.9	(Bovine)
Rho et al. (1993)	Ultrasound	14.8	
	Tensile test	10.4	
Rho et al. (1999)	Nanoindentation	19.4	(Longitudinal)
	Nanoindentation	15.0	(Transverse)
Turner et al. (1999)	Acoustic microscopy	17.5	
	Nanoindentation	18.1	
Bumrerraj and Katz (2001)	Acoustic microscopy	17.4	

provided by atomic force microscopy (AFM), to analyze the mechanics of bone on the smallest unit of structure shown in Figure 1.1.

1.5 Characterizing Elastic Anisotropy

Having a full set of five or nine C_{ij} does permit describing the anisotropy of that particular specimen of bone, but there is no simple way of comparing the relative anisotropy between different specimens of the same bone or between different species or between experimenters' measurements by trying to relate individual C_{ij} between sets of measurements. Adapting a method from crystal physics (Chung and Buessem, 1968), Katz and Meunier (1987) presented a description for obtaining two scalar quantities defining the compressive and shear anisotropy for bone with transverse isotropic symmetry. Later, they developed a similar pair of scalar quantities for bone exhibiting orthotropic symmetry (Katz and Meunier, 1990). For both cases, the percentage compressive (Ac^*) and shear (As^*) elastic anisotropy are given, respectively, by

$$Ac^* (\%) = 100 \frac{K_V - K_R}{K_V + K_R}$$
$$As^* (\%) = 100 \frac{G_V - G_R}{G_V + G_R} \tag{1.16}$$

where K_V and K_R are the Voigt (uniform strain across an interface) and Reuss (uniform stress across an interface) bulk moduli, respectively, and G_V and G_R are the Voigt and Reuss shear moduli, respectively. The equations for K_V, K_R, G_V, and G_R are provided for both transverse isotropy and orthotropic symmetry in Appendix A.

Table 1.5 lists the values of $As^*(\%)$ and $Ac^*(\%)$ for various types of hard tissues and apatites. The graph of $As^*(\%)$ versus $Ac^*(\%)$ is given in Figure 1.4.

$As^*(\%)$ and $Ac^*(\%)$ have been calculated for a human femur, having both transverse isotropic and orthotropic symmetry, from the full set of Van Buskirk and Ashman (1981) C_{ij} data at each of the four aspects around the periphery, anterior, medial, posterior, lateral, as denoted in Table 1.3, at fractional proximal levels along the femur's length, $Z/L = 0.3–0.7$. The graph of $As^*(\%)$ versus Z/L, assuming transverse isotropy, is given in Figure 1.5. Note that the anterior aspect, that is in tension during loading, has values of $As^*(\%)$ in some positions considerably higher than those of the other aspects. Similarly, the graph of $Ac^*(\%)$ versus Z/L is given in Figure 1.6. Note here it is the posterior aspect, that is in compression during loading, that has values of $Ac^*(\%)$ in some positions considerably higher than those of the other aspects. Both graphs are based on the transverse isotropic symmetry calculations, however, the

TABLE 1.5 $As^*(\%)$ versus $Ac^*(\%)$ for Various Types of Hard Tissues and Apatites

Experiments (Specimen Type)	$Ac^*(\%)$	$As^*(\%)$
Van Buskirk et al. (1981) (bovine femur)	1.522	2.075
Katz and Ukraincik (1971) (OHAp)	0.995	0.686
Yoon (redone) in Katz (1984) (FAp)	0.867	0.630
Lang (1969, 1970) (bovine femur dried)	1.391	0.981
Reilly and Burstein (1975) (bovine femur)	2.627	5.554
Yoon and Katz (1976) (human femur dried)	1.036	1.055
Katz et al. (1983) (Haversian)	1.080	0.775
Van Buskirk and Ashman (1981) (human femur)	1.504	1.884
Kinney et al. (2004) (human dentin dry)	0.006	0.011
Kinney et al. (2004) (human dentin wet)	1.305	0.377

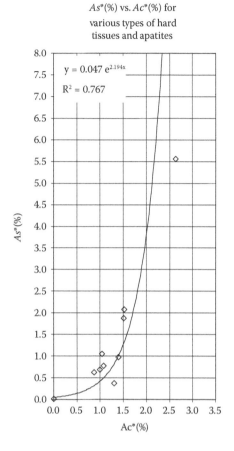

FIGURE 1.4 Values of As^*(%) versus Ac^*(%) from Table 1.5 are plotted for various types of hard tissues and apatites.

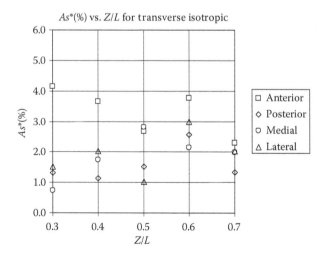

FIGURE 1.5 Values As^*(%) calculated from the data in Table 1.3 for human femoral bone, treated as having transverse isotropic symmetry, is plotted versus Z/L for all four aspects, anterior, medial, posterior, lateral around the bone's periphery; Z/L is the fractional proximal distance along the femur's length.

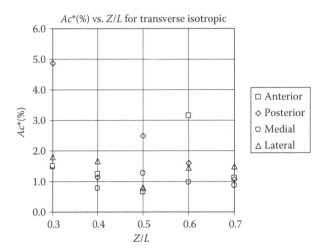

FIGURE 1.6   Values $Ac^*(\%)$ calculated from the data in Table 1.3 for human femoral bone, treated as having transverse isotropic symmetry, is plotted versus Z/L for all four aspects, anterior, medial, posterior, lateral around the bone's periphery; Z/L is the fractional proximal distance along the femur's length.

identical trends were obtained based on the orthotropic symmetry calculations. It is clear that in addition to the moduli varying along the length and over all four aspects of the femur, the anisotropy varies as well, reflecting the response of the femur to the manner of loading.

Recently, Kinney et al. (2004) used the technique of resonant ultrasound spectroscopy (RUS) to measure the elastic constants (C_{ij}) of human dentin from both wet and dry samples. $As^*(\%)$ and $Ac^*(\%)$ calculated from these data are included in both Table 1.5 and Figure 1.4. Their data showed that the samples exhibited transverse isotropic symmetry. However, the C_{ij} for dry dentin implied even higher symmetry. Indeed, the result of using the average value for C_{11} and $C_{12} = 36.6$ GPa and the value for $C_{44} = 14.7$ GP for dry dentin in the calculations suggests that dry human dentin is very nearly elastically isotropic. This isotropic-like behavior of the dry dentin may have clinical significance. There is independent experimental evidence to support this calculation of isotropy based on the ultrasonic data. Small-angle x-ray diffraction of human dentin yielded results implying isotropy near the pulp and mild anisotropy in mid-dentin (Kinney et al. 2001).

It is interesting to note that Haversian bones, whether human or bovine, have both their compressive and shear anisotropy factors considerably lower than the respective values for plexiform bone. Thus, not only is plexiform bone both stiffer and more rigid than the Haversian bone, it is also more anisotropic. These two scalar anisotropy quantities also provide a means of assessing whether there is the possibility either of systematic errors in the measurements and/or artifacts in the modeling of the elastic properties of hard tissues. This is determined when the values of $Ac^*(\%)$ and/or $As^*(\%)$ are much greater than the close range of lower values obtained by calculations on a variety of different ultrasonic measurements (Table 1.5). A possible example of this is the value of $As^*(\%) = 7.88$ calculated from the mechanical testing data of Knets (1978), Table 1.2.

1.6 Modeling Elastic Behavior

Currey (1964) first presented some preliminary ideas of modeling bone as a composite material composed of a simple linear superposition of collagen and Ap. He followed this later (1969) with an attempt to take into account the orientation of the Ap crystallites using a model proposed by Cox (1952) for fiber-reinforced composites. Katz (1971a) and Piekarski (1973) independently showed that the use of Voigt and Reuss or even Hashin and Shtrikman (1963) composite modeling showed the limitations of using linear combinations of either elastic moduli or elastic compliances. The failure of all these early models could be traced to the fact that they were based only on considerations of material properties. This is comparable to trying to determine the properties of an Eiffel Tower built using a composite material by simply modeling the composite material properties without considering void spaces and the interconnectivity of the structure (Lakes, 1993). In neither case is the complexity of the structural organization involved. This consideration of hierarchical organization clearly must be introduced into the modeling.

Katz in a number of papers (1971b, 1976) and meeting presentations put forth the hypothesis that the Haversian bone should be modeled as a hierarchical composite, eventually adapting a hollow fiber composite model by Hashin and Rosen (1964). Bonfield and Grynpas (1977) used extensional (longitudinal) ultrasonic wave propagation in both wet and dry bovine femoral cortical bone specimens oriented at angles of 5°, 10°, 20°, 40°, 50°, 70°, 80°, and 85° with respect to the long bone axis. They compared their experimental results for Young's moduli with the theoretical curve predicted by Currey's model (1969); this is shown in Figure 1.7. The lack of agreement led them to "conclude, therefore that an alternative model is required to account for the dependence of Young's modulus on orientation" (Bonfield and Grynpas, 1977, p. 454). Katz (1980, 1981), applying his hierarchical material–structure composite model, showed that the data in Figure 1.7 could be explained by considering different amounts of Ap crystallites aligned parallel to the long bone axis; this is shown in Figure 1.8. This early attempt at hierarchical micromechanical modeling is now being extended with more sophisticated modeling using either finite-element micromechanical computations (Hogan, 1992) or homogenization theory (Crolet et al., 1993). Further improvements will come by including more definitive information on the structural organization of collagen and Ap at the molecular–ultrastructural level (Wagner and Weiner, 1992; Weiner and Traub, 1989).

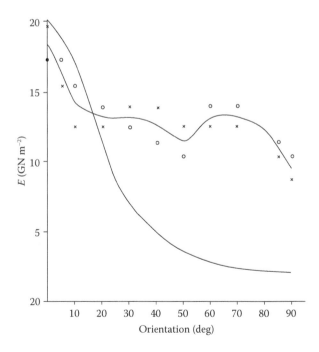

FIGURE 1.7 Variation in Young's modulus of bovine femur specimens (E) with the orientation of specimen axis to the long axis of the bone, for wet (o) and dry (x) conditions compared with the theoretical curve (———) predicted from a fiber-reinforced composite model. (Reprinted by permission from Macmillan Publishers Ltd. *Nature, London*, Bonfield W, Grynpas MD. Anisotropy of Young's modulus of bone. 270:453, Copyright 1977.)

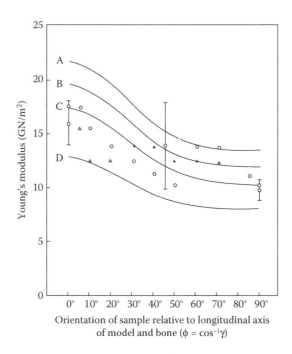

FIGURE 1.8 Comparison of predictions of Katz two-level composite model with the experimental data of Bonfield and Grynpas. Each curve represents a different lamellar configuration within a single osteon, with longitudinal fibers; A, 64%; B, 57%; C, 50%; D, 37%; and the rest of the fibers assumed horizontal. (From Katz JL, *Mechanical Properties of Bone*, AMD, Vol. 45, New York, American Society of Mechanical Engineers, 1981, with permission.)

1.7 Viscoelastic Properties

As stated earlier, bone (along with all other biologic tissues) is a viscoelastic material. Clearly, for such materials, Hooke's law for linear elastic materials must be replaced by a constitutive equation which includes the time dependency of the material properties. The behavior of an anisotropic linear viscoelastic material may be described by using the Boltzmann superposition integral as a constitutive equation:

$$\sigma_{ij}(t) = \int_{-\infty}^{t} C_{ijkl}(t - \tau)\frac{d\epsilon_{kl}(\tau)}{d\tau}d\tau \tag{1.17}$$

where $\sigma_{ij}(t)$ and $\varepsilon_{kl}(\tau)$ are the time-dependent second rank stress and strain tensors, respectively, and $C_{ijkl}(t-\tau)$ is the fourth-rank relaxation modulus tensor. This tensor has 36 independent elements for the lowest symmetry case and 12 nonzero independent elements for an orthotropic solid. Again, as for linear elasticity, a reduced notation is used, that is, $11 \rightarrow 1$, $22 \rightarrow 2$, $33 \rightarrow 3$, $23 \rightarrow 4$, $31 \rightarrow 5$, and $12 \rightarrow 6$. If we apply Equation 1.17 to the case of an orthotropic material, for example, plexiform bone, in uniaxial tension (compression) in the 1 direction (Lakes and Katz, 1974), in this case using the reduced notation, we obtain

$$\sigma_1(t) = \int_{-\infty}^{t}\left[C_{11}(t - \tau)\frac{d\epsilon_1(\tau)}{d\tau} + C_{12}(t - \tau)\frac{d\epsilon_2(\tau)}{d\tau} + C_{13}(t - \tau)\frac{d\epsilon_3(\tau)}{d\tau}\right]d\tau \tag{1.18}$$

$$\sigma_2(t) = \int_{-\infty}^{t}\left[C_{21}(t - \tau)\frac{d\epsilon_1(\tau)}{d\tau} + C_{22}(t - \tau)\frac{d\epsilon_2(\tau)}{d\tau} + C_{23}(t - \tau)\frac{d\epsilon_3(\tau)}{d\tau}\right] = 0 \tag{1.19}$$

for all t, and

$$\sigma_3(t) = \int_{-\infty}^{t}\left[C_{31}(t-\tau)\frac{d\epsilon_1(\tau)}{d\tau} + C_{32}(t-\tau)\frac{d\epsilon_2(\tau)}{d\tau} + C_{33}(t-\tau)\frac{d\epsilon_3(\tau)}{d\tau}\right]d\tau = 0 \qquad (1.20)$$

for all t.

Having the integrands vanish provides an obvious solution to Equations 1.19 and 1.20. Solving them simultaneously for $[d\epsilon_2^{(\tau)}]/d\tau$ and $[d\epsilon_3^{(\tau)}]/d\tau$ substituting these values into Equation 1.17 yields

$$\sigma_1(t) = \int_{-\infty}^{t} E_1(t-\tau)\frac{d\epsilon_1(\tau)}{d\tau}d\tau \qquad (1.21)$$

where, if for convenience we adopt the notation C_{ij}; $C_{ij}(t-\tau)$, then Young's modulus is given by

$$E_1(t-\tau) = C_{11} + C_{12}\frac{[C_{31} - (C_{21}C_{33}/C_{23})]}{[(C_{21}C_{33}/C_{23}) - C_{32}]} + C_{13}\frac{[C_{21} - (C_{31}C_{22}/C_{32})]}{[(C_{22}C_{33}/C_{32})/ - C_{23}]} \qquad (1.22)$$

In this case of uniaxial tension (compression), only nine independent orthotropic tensor components are involved, the three shear components being equal to zero. Still, this time-dependent Young's modulus is a rather complex function. As in the linear elastic case, the inverse form of the Boltzmann integral can be used; this would constitute the compliance formulation.

If we consider the bone being driven by a strain at a frequency ω, with a corresponding sinusoidal stress lagging by an angle δ, then the complex Young's modulus $E^*(\omega)$ may be expressed as

$$E^*(\omega) = E'(\omega) + iE''(\omega) \qquad (1.23)$$

where $E'(\omega)$, which represents the stress–strain ratio in phase with the strain, is known as the storage modulus, and $E''(\omega)$, which represents the stress–strain ratio 90° out of phase with the strain, is known as the loss modulus. The ratio of the loss modulus to the storage modulus is then equal to tan d. Usually, data are presented by a graph of the storage modulus along with a graph of tan d, both against frequency. For a more complete development of the values of $E'(\omega)$ and $E''(\omega)$, as well as for the derivation of other viscoelastic technical moduli, see Lakes and Katz (1974); for a similar development of the shear storage and loss moduli, see Cowin (1989).

Thus, for a more complete understanding of bone's response to applied loads, it is important to know its rheologic properties. There have been a number of early studies of the viscoelastic properties of various long bones (Sedlin, 1965; Smith and Keiper, 1965; Lugassy, 1968; Laird and Kingsbury, 1973; Black and Korostoff, 1973). However, none of these was performed over a wide enough range of frequency (or time) to completely define the viscoelastic properties measured, for example, creep or stress relaxation. Thus it is not possible to mathematically transform one property into any other to compare results of three different experiments on different bones (Lakes and Katz, 1974).

In the first experiments over an extended frequency range, the biaxial viscoelastic as well as uniaxial viscoelastic properties of wet cortical human and bovine femoral bone were measured using both dynamic and stress relaxation techniques over eight decades of frequency (time) (Lakes et al., 1979). The results of these experiments showed that bone was both nonlinear and thermorheologically complex, that is, time–temperature superposition could not be used to extend the range of viscoelastic measurements. A nonlinear constitutive equation was developed based on these measurements (Lakes and Katz, 1979a). In addition, relaxation spectrums for both human and bovine cortical bone were obtained; Figure 1.9 shows the former (Lakes and Katz, 1979b). The contributions of several mechanisms to the

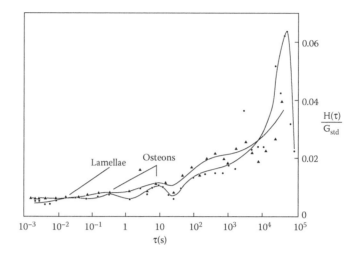

FIGURE 1.9 Comparison of relaxation spectra for wet human bone, specimens 5 and 6 (Lakes et al., 1979) in simple torsion; $T = 37°C$. First approximation from relaxation and dynamic data. • Human tibial bone, specimen 6. △ Human tibial bone, specimen 5, $G_{std} = G(10\ s)$. $G_{std}(5) = G(10\ s)$. $G_{std}(5) = 0.590 \times 10^6\ lb/in^2$. $G_{std}(6) \times 0.602 \times 10^6$ lb/in². (Courtesy *Journal of Biomechanics*, Pergamon Press.)

loss tangent of cortical bone are shown in Figure 1.10 (Lakes and Katz, 1979b). It is interesting to note that almost all the major loss mechanisms occur at frequencies (times) at or close to those in which there are "bumps," indicating possible strain energy dissipation, on the relaxation spectra shown in Figure 1.9. An extensive review of the viscoelastic properties of bone can be found in *Natural and Living Biomaterials*, CRC Press (Lakes and Katz, 1984).

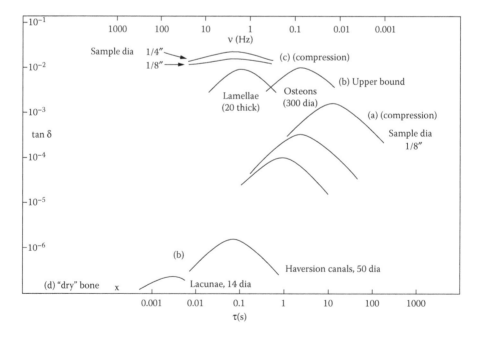

FIGURE 1.10 Contributions of several relaxation mechanisms to the loss tangent of cortical bone. (a) Homogeneous thermoelastic effect. (b) Inhomogeneous thermoelastic effect. (c) Fluid flow effect. (d) Piezoelectric effect. (From Lakes RS, Katz JL. *Natural and Living Tissues*. Boca Raton, FL: CRC Press; 1984. pp. 1–87. Courtesy CRC Press.)

Following on Katz's (1976, 1980) adaptation of the Hashin–Rosen hollow fiber composite model (1964), Gottesman and Hashin (1979) presented a viscoelastic calculation using the same major assumptions.

1.8 Related Research

As stated earlier, this chapter has concentrated on the elastic and viscoelastic properties of compact cortical bone and the elastic properties of trabecular bone. At present there is considerable research activity on the fracture properties of the bone. Professor William Bonfield and his associates at Queen Mary and Westfield College, University of London and Professor Dwight Davy and his colleagues at Case Western Reserve University are among those who publish regularly in this area. Review of the literature is necessary in order to become acquainted with the state of bone fracture mechanics.

An excellent introductory monograph which provides a fascinating insight into the structure–property relationships in bones including aspects of the two areas discussed immediately above is Professor John D. Currey's *Bones Structure and Mechanics* (2002), the 2nd edition of his book, *The Mechanical Adaptations of Bones,* Princeton University Press (1984).

1.9 Dentin Structure and Composition

Dentin is the hydrated composite structure that constitutes the body of each tooth, providing both a protective covering for the pulp and serving as a support for the overlying enamel. Dentin is composed of approximately 45–50% inorganic material, 30–35% organic material, and 20% fluid by volume. Dentin mineral is a carbonate rich, calcium-deficient apatite (Marshall et al. 1997). The organic component is predominantly type I collagen with minor contribution from other proteins (Gage et al. 1989; Linde 1989; Butler 1992). The apatite mineralites are of very small size and are deposited almost exclusively within the collagen fibril (see, e.g., Arsenault 1989). The interactions between collagen and nanocrystalline mineralite gives rise to the stiffness of the dentin structure. The consequent dentin elasticity is an important feature that determines the mechanical behavior of the tooth structure.

The structural characteristics of sound dentin are well known at the micro-scale (~100 μm). Dentin is described as a system of dentinal tubules surrounded by a collar of highly mineralized peritubular dentin (Wang and Weiner 1998). The tubules traverse the structure from the pulp cavity to the region just below the dentin–enamel junction (DEJ) or the dentin–cementum junction (CEJ). The tubules, which are described as narrow tunnels a few microns or less in diameter as shown in Figure 1.11, represent the tracks taken by the odontoblastic cells from the pulp chamber to the respective junctions. Tubule density, size, and orientation vary from location to location. The density and size are lowest close to the DEJ and highest at the predentin surface at the junction to the pulp chamber. Dentinal tubule diameter measures approximately 2.5 μm near the pulp and 0.9 μm near the DEJ (Ten Cate 1994). The porosity of dentin varies from 0 to 0.25 from the DEJ to the pulp (Manly and Deakins 1940; Koutsi et al. 1994; Sumikawa et al. 1999). The rate of change in porosity with depth depends on the tooth type. In primary tooth dentin, the dentinal tubule density and size is, in general, larger than in permanent dentin (Sumikawa et al. 1999).

The composition of the peritubular dentin is carbonated apatite with very small amounts of organic matrix whereas intertubular dentin, that is, the dentin separating the tubules, is type I collagen matrix reinforced with apatite. Based upon electron microscopic studies, peritubular dentin in primary teeth has been found to be 2–5 times thicker than that of permanent teeth (Hirayama et al. 1986). The composition of intertubular dentin is primarily mineralized collagen fibrils; the fibrils are described as a composite of a collagen framework and thin plate-shaped carbonate apatite crystals whose *c*-axes are aligned with the collagen fibril axis (Weiner et al. 1999). In sound dentin, the majority of the mineralized collagen fibrils are perpendicular to the tubules (Jones and Boyde 1984). The crystal organization in peritubular and intertubular dentin are similar, but the macromolecular constituents are not. The amino acid compositions of the principal proteins in peritubular dentin are high in

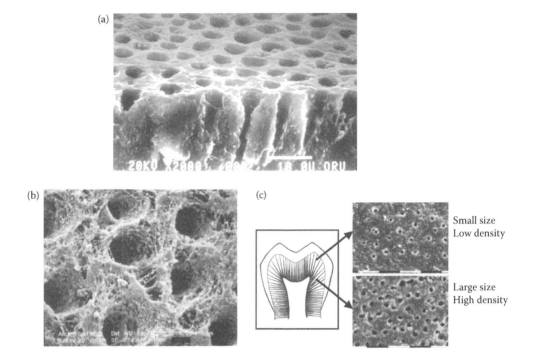

FIGURE 1.11 SEM micrograph showing (a) the spatial distribution of dentin tubules, (b) partially demineralized dentin indicating the orientations of inter-tubular collagen fibrils, and (c) that tubule opening is larger and spacing is denser for deep dentin as opposed to shallow dentin. As shown, the structure and properties of dentin substrate vary with location. (From Marshall GW et al. *J Dent* 1997; 25(6):441–458.)

serine and probably phosphoserine, but they are not similar to the phosphophoryns of intertubular dentin (Weiner et al. 1999). Water in dentin may be classified as either free or bound. Water is present within the dentinal tubules as pulpal fluid and within the interstitial spaces between collagen fibrils. Based upon experimental chemical microanalyses, bound water is likely present as hydroxyl groups bound to the mineral component (Gruner et al. 1937; LeFevre and Hodge 1937; Bird et al. 1940). Mass density measurements were completed more than a century ago. Mass densities of permanent and deciduous dentin were determined by direct measurement of mass and volume of moist dentin slabs (Boyd et al. 1938) and by considering dry powdered fractions of teeth (Manly et al. 1939; Berghash and Hodge 1940). More recently, mineral densities of dentin have been measured using x-ray tomographic microscopy (Kinney et al. 1994) and back scattered scanning electron microscopy (BSEM) (Angker et al. 2004b).

1.10 Dentin Elasticity

Beginning in the 1960s, macro-scale elastic moduli of dentin have been measured by a variety of methods as reviewed by Kinney et al. (2003). Using nanoindentation methods, Kinney et al. (1999), have measured the elastic modulus of peri-tubular dentin and inter-tubular dentin. At somewhat larger, unspecified scales, Katz et al. (2001) measured similar values of dentin elastic modulus using scanning acoustic microscopy (SAM). At even higher scales, Lees and Rollins (1972) used longitudinal and shear wave velocity measurements, Kinney et al. (2004) used resonant ultrasound spectroscopy to determine elastic moduli of millimeter scale samples, and John (2006) used longitudinal velocity measurements on approximately millimeter thick slices to find location-dependent elastic moduli. Primary tooth dentin

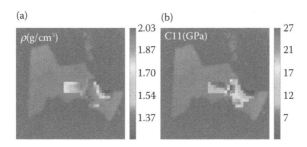

FIGURE 1.12 Micro-scale distribution of (a) density and (b) elastic modulus of carious, caries-affected and sound regions of primary dentin using homotopic measurements from SAM and BSEM. Background image is the SAM C-scan of the tooth sample. (From Marangos, O. et al. *Acta Biomaterial* 2009; 5:1338–1348.)

mechanical properties have been studied at nano-scales using nanoindentation (Hosoya and Marshall 2004; Hosoya and Marshall 2005; Hosoya and Tay 2007). Mechanical properties of primary dentin have also been studied at somewhat higher, unspecified scales (Angker et al. 2003, 2004a).

Recently, Marangos et al. (2009) have performed homotopic (same location) measurements with SAM and BSEM to obtain the micromechanical properties of carious, caries-affected, and sound primary tooth dentin. As a result, the relationships between micro-scale elastic moduli, density and composition of sound, carious, and caries-affected primary dentin were obtained. In Figure 1.12, we show the maps of mass density and the corresponding elastic moduli. In the sound dentin region, the mean and standard deviation of elastic modulus was found to be 10 ± 2 GPa. These values are somewhat lower than Young's moduli reported for inner primary tooth dentin at locations close to the pulp wall (ranging from 2.88 to 19.68 GPa in Angker et al. (2003), and 14.00–22.84 GPa in Hosoya and Marshall (2005)). The low values observed in our measurement were likely caused by resorption prior to natural exfoliation. We further observe that in caries-affected locations, the elastic modulus is higher than the carious or sound dentin regions. Previous studies have indicated the presence of hypermineralized dentin or sclerotic dentin in the vicinity of carious lesions (Driessens and Woltgens 1986; Ten Cate 1994; Nakajima et al. 1999; Marshall et al. 2001). The higher values of elastic modulus could be attributed to a higher level of mineralization in these locations. It is noteworthy however that sclerotic dentin is not always present below carious lesions (Hosoya and Marshall 2004). The conditions under which hypermineralization occurs in proximity of carious dentin remains unclear and needs further investigation. In region 2, that is locations in carious dentin, the elastic modulus varies over a large range. It is well known that carious locations are highly heterogeneous with widely varying degree and extent of demineralization.

Clearly, the mineral content has a significant effect on the elastic modulus. Previous investigators have attempted to correlate the mineral content to elastic modulus in dentin (Angker et al. 2004a; Bembey et al. 2005). Figure 1.13 shows the plot of elastic modulus versus the mineral volume fraction and total porosity for the 89 locations displayed in Figure 1.12. In general, the elastic modulus increases with the mineral content, and it decreases with the porosity. However, a single correlation cannot be used to describe the relationship between the elastic modulus and composition. At certain mineral volume fraction and porosity, the elastic modulus variation is found to be as large as five times. Thus, the mineral content or porosity alone cannot be used to uniquely determine the elastic modulus. Similar observations have been made regarding the elastic properties of bone (Oyen et al. 2008). At the fundamental level, the interactions between collagen and nanocrystalline mineralite gives rise to the stiffness of the dentin structure. Indeed, the various efforts (Hellmich et al. 2004; Nikolov and Raabe 2008) to calculate calcified tissue moduli based upon constituent phases suggest that the mechanical behavior of these tissues at various hierarchical scales may not be determined by simply considering the composition but rather additional interaction at the collagen/mineral interface must be considered.

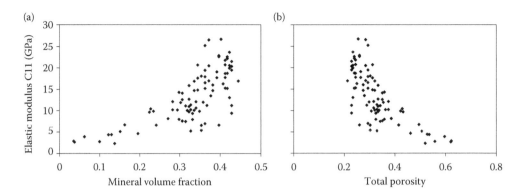

FIGURE 1.13 Elastic modulus plotted against (a) the mass density, and (b) mineral volume fraction. Using data from Figure 1.2. (From Marangos, O. et al. *Acta Biomaterial* 2009; 5:1338–1348.)

Defining Terms

Apatite: Calcium phosphate compound, stoichiometric chemical formula $Ca_5(PO_4)_3 \cdot X$, where X is OH– (hydroxyapatite), F– (fluorapatite), Cl– (chlorapatite), and so on. There are two molecules in the basic crystal unit cell.

Cancellous bone: Also known as porous, spongy, trabecular bone. Found in the regions of the articulating ends of tubular bones, in vertebrae, ribs, and so on.

Cortical bone: The dense compact bone found throughout the shafts of long bones such as the femur, tibia, and so on also found in the outer portions of other bones in the body.

Haversian bone: Also called osteonic. The form of bone found in adult humans and mature mammals, consisting mainly of concentric lamellar structures, surrounding a central canal called the Haversian canal, plus lamellar remnants of older Haversian systems (osteons) called interstitial lamellae.

Interstitial lamellae: See Haversian bone above.

Orthotropic: The symmetrical arrangement of structure in which there are three distinct orthogonal axes of symmetry. In crystals this symmetry is called orthothombic.

Osteons: See Haversian bone above.

Plexiform: Also called laminar. The form of parallel lamellar bone found in younger, immature nonhuman mammals.

Transverse isotropy: The symmetry arrangement of structure in which there is a unique axis perpendicular to a plane in which the other two axes are equivalent. The long bone direction is chosen as the unique axis. In crystals this symmetry is called hexagonal.

References

Angker L, Nijhof N, Swain MV, Kilpatrick NM. Influence of hydration and mechanical characterization of carious primary dentine using an ultra-micro indentation system (UMIS). *Eur J Oral Sci* 2004b; 112(3):231–6.

Angker L, Nockolds C, Swain MV, Kilpatrick N. Correlating the mechanical properties to the mineral content of carious dentine—A comparative study using an ultra-micro indentation system (UMIS) and SEM-BSE signals. *Arch Oral Biol* 2004a; 49(5):369–78.

Angker L, Swain MV, Kilpatrick N. Micro-mechanical characterisation of the properties of primary tooth dentine. *J Dent* 2003; 31(4):261–7.

Arsenault AL. A comparative electron microscopic study of apatite crystals in collagen fibrils of rat bone, dentin and calcified turkey leg tendons. *Bone Miner* 1989; 6(2):165–77.

Ashman RB, Rho JY. Elastic modulus of trabecular bone material. *J Biomech* 1988; 21:177.

Bembey AK, Oyen ML, Ko C-C, Bushby AJ, Boyde A. Elastic modulus and mineral density of dentine and enamel in natural caries lesions. In: Fratzl P, Landis WJ, Wang R, Silver FH (Eds). *Structure and Mechanical Behavior of Biological Materials*. Warrendale: MRS; 2005. pp. 125–130.

Berghash, SR, Hodge HC. Density and refractive index studies of dental hard tissues III: Density distribution of deciduous enamel and dentin. *J Dent Res* 1940; 19(5):487–95.

Bird MJ, French EL, Woodside MR, Morrison MI, Hodge HC. Chemical analyses of deciduous enamel and dentin. *J Dent Res* 1940; 19(4):413–23.

Black J, Korostoff E. Dynamic mechanical properties of viable human cortical bone. *J Biomech* 1973; 6:435.

Bonfield W, Grynpas MD. Anisotropy of Young's modulus of bone. *Nature, London* 1977; 270:453.

Boyd JD, Drain CL, Deakins ML. Method for determining the specific gravity of dentin and its application to permanent and deciduous teeth. *J Dent Res* 1938; 17(6):465–469.

Bumrerraj S, Katz JL. Scanning acoustic microscopy study of human cortical and trabecular bone. *Ann Biomed Eng* 2001; 29:1.

Butler WT. Dentin extracellular matrix and dentinogenesis. *Oper Dent* 1992; Suppl 5:18–23.

Choi K, Goldstein SA. A comparison of the fatigue behavior of human trabecular and cortical bone tissue. *J Biomech* 1992; 25:1371.

Chung DH, Buessem WR. In: Vahldiek FW and Mersol SA (eds), *Anisotropy in Single-Crystal Refractory Compounds*, Vol. 2, New York: Plenum Press; 1968. p. 217.

Cowin SC. *Bone Mechanics*. Boca Raton, FL: CRC Press; 1989

Cowin SC. *Bone Mechanics Handbook*. Boca Raton, FL: CRC Press; 2001.

Cox HL. The elasticity and strength of paper and other fibrous materials. *Br Appl Phys* 1952; 3:72.

Crolet JM, Aoubiza B, Meunier A. Compact bone: Numerical simulation of mechanical characteristics. *J Biomech* 1993; 26(6):677.

Currey JD. *Bone Structure and Mechanics*. New Jersey: Princeton University Press; 2002.

Currey JD. *The Mechanical Adaptations of Bones*. New Jersey: Princeton University Press; 1984.

Currey JD. The relationship between the stiffness and the mineral content of bone. *J Biomech* 1969; (2):477.

Currey JD. Three analogies to explain the mechanical properties of bone. *Biorheology* 1964; (2):1.

Driessens FCM, Woltgens JHM. *Tooth Development and Caries*. Boca Raton, FL: CRC Press; 1986. pp. 132–137.

Gage JP, Francis MJO, Triffitt JT. *Collagen and Dental Matrices*. Boston: Wright; 1989. pp. 21–24.

Gottesman T, Hashin Z. Analysis of viscoelastic behavior of bones on the basis of microstructure. *J Biomech* 1979; 13:89.

Gruner JW, McConnell D, Armstrong WD. The relationship between crystal structure and chemical composition of enamel and dentin. *J Biol Chem* 1937; 121(2):771–781.

Hashin Z, Rosen BW. The elastic moduli of fiber reinforced materials. *J Appl Mech* 1964; (31):223.

Hashin Z, Shtrikman S. A variational approach to the theory of elastic behavior of multiphase materials. *J Mech Phys Solids* 1963; (11):127.

Hastings GW, Ducheyne P (eds). *Natural and Living Biomaterials*, Boca Raton, FL: CRC Press; 1984.

Hellmich C, Ulm FJ, Dormieux L. Can the diverse elastic properties of trabecular and cortical bone be attributed to only a few tissue-independent phase properties and their interactions? *Biomech Model Mechanobiol* 2004; 2(4):219–38.

Herring GM. Methods for the study of the glycoproteins and proteoglycans of bone using bacterial collagenase. Determination of bone sialoprotein and chondroitin sulphate. *Calcif Tiss Res* 1977; (24):29.

Hirayama A, Yamada M, Miake K. An electron microscopic study on dentinal tubules of human deciduous teeth. *Shikwa Gakuho* 1986; 86(6):1021–31.

Hogan HA. Micromechanics modeling of haversian cortical bone properties. *J Biomech* 1992; 25(5):549.

Hosoya Y, Marshall GW. The nano-hardness and elastic modulus of carious and sound primary canine dentin. *Oper Dent* 2004; 29(2):142–9.

Hosoya Y, Marshall GW. The nano-hardness and elastic modulus of sound deciduous canine dentin and young premolar dentin—Preliminary study. *J Mater Sci Mater Med* 2005; 16(1):1–8.

Hosoya Y, Tay FR. Hardness, elasticity, and ultrastructure of bonded sound and caries-affected primary tooth dentin. *J Biomed Mater Res B Appl Biomater* 2007; 81B(1):135–141.

John C. Lateral distribution of ultrasound velocity in horizontal layers of human teeth. *J Acoust Soc Am* 2006; 119(2):1214–1226.

Jones SJ, Boyde A. Ultrastructure of dentine and dentinogenesis. In: Linde A. (ed), *Dentine and Dentinogenesis*. Boca Raton, FL: CRC Press; 1984. pp. 81–134.

Katz JL. Anisotropy of Young's modulus of bone. *Nature* 1980; 283:106.

Katz JL. Composite material models for cortical bone. In: Cowin SC (ed), *Mechanical Properties of Bone*, AMD, Vol. 45, New York: American Society of Mechanical Engineers; 1981. pp. 171–184.

Katz JL. Elastic properties of calcified tissues. *Isr J Med Sci* 1971b; 7:439.

Katz JL. Hard tissue as a composite material: I. Bounds on the elastic behavior. *J Biomech* 1971a; 4:455.

Katz JL. Hierarchical modeling of compact haversian bone as a fiber reinforced material. In: Mates, RE and Smith, CR (eds), *Advances in Bioengineering*. New York: American Society of Mechanical Engineers; 1976. pp. 17–18.

Katz JL, Bumrerraj S, Dreyfuss J, Wang Y, Spencer P. Micromechanics of the dentin/adhesive interface. *J Biomed Mater Res* 2001; 58(4):366.

Katz JL, Meunier A. The elastic anisotropy of bone. *J Biomech* 1987; 20:1063.

Katz JL, Meunier A. A generalized method for characterizing elastic anisotropy in solid living tissues. *J Mat Sci Mater Med* 1990; 1:1.

Katz JL, Ukraincik K. A fiber-reinforced model for compact haversian bone. *Program and Abstracts of the 16th Annual Meeting of the Biophysical Society*, 28a FPM-C15, Toronto, 1972.

Katz JL, Ukraincik K. On the anisotropic elastic properties of hydroxyapatite. *J Biomech* 1971; 4:221.

Keaveny TM, Hayes WC. A 20-year perspective on the mechanical properties of trabecular bone. *J Biomech Eng* 1993; 115:535.

Kinney JH, Balooch M, Marshall GW, Marshall SJ. A micromechanics model of the elastic properties of human dentine. *Arch Oral Biol* 1999; 44(10):813–22.

Kinney JH, Gladden JR, Marshall GW, Marshall SJ, So JH, Maynard JD. Resonant ultrasound spectroscopy measurements of the elastic constants in human dentin. *J Biomech* 2004; 37(4):437–41.

Kinney JH, Marshall GW Jr, Marshall SJ. Three-dimensional mapping of mineral densities in carious dentin: Theory and method. *Scanning Microsc* 1994; 8(2):197–205.

Kinney JH, Marshall SJ, Marshall GW. The mechanical properties of human dentin: A critical review and re-evaluation of the dental literature. *Crit Rev Oral Biol Med* 2003; 14(1):13–29.

Kinney JH, Pople JA, Marshall GW, Marshall SJ. Collagen orientation and crystallite size in human dentin: A small angle x-ray scattering study. *Calcif Tissue Inter* 2001; 69:31.

Knets IV. Mechanics of biological tissues. A review. *Mekhanika Polimerov* 1978; 13:434.

Koutsi V, Noonan RG, Horner JA, Simpson MD, Matthews WG, Pashley DH. The effect of dentin depth on the permeability and ultrastructure of primary molars. *Pediatr Dent* 1994; 16(1):29–35.

Laird GW, Kingsbury HB. Complex viscoelastic moduli of bovine bone. *J Biomech* 1973; 6:59.

Lakes RS. Materials with structural hierarchy. *Nature* 1993; 361:511.

Lakes RS, Katz JL. Interrelationships among the viscoelastic function for anisotropic solids: Application to calcified tissues and related systems. *J Biomech* 1974; 7:259.

Lakes RS, Katz JL. Viscoelastic properties and behavior of cortical bone. Part II. Relaxation mechanisms. *J Biomech* 1979a; 12:679.

Lakes RS, Katz JL. Viscoelastic properties of bone. In: GW Hastings and P Ducheyne (eds), *Natural and Living Tissues*. Boca Raton, FL: CRC Press; 1984. pp. 1–87.

Lakes RS, Katz JL. Viscoelastic properties of wet cortical bone: III. A nonlinear constitutive equation. *J Biomech* 1979b; 12:689.

Lakes RS, Katz JL, Sternstein SS. Viscoelastic properties of wet cortical bone: I. Torsional and biaxial studies. *J Biomech* 1979; 12:657.

Lang SB. Elastic coefficients of animal bone. *Science* 1969; 165:287.

Lees S, Rollins FR. Anisotropy in hard dental tissues. *J Biomech* 1972; 5(6):557–66.

LeFevre ML, Hodge HC. Chemical analysis of tooth samples composed of enamel, dentine and cementum. II. *J Dent Res* 1937; 16(4):279–87.

Linde A. Dentin matrix proteins: Composition and possible functions in calcification. *Anat Record* 1989; 224(2): 154–66.

Lipson SF, Katz JL. The relationship between elastic properties and microstructure of bovine cortical bone. *J Biomech* 1984; 4:231.

Lugassy AA. Mechanical and viscoelastic properties of bone and dentin in compression. Thesis, Metallurgy and Materials Science, University of Pennsylvania, 1968.

Maharidge R. Ultrasonic properties and microstructure of bovine bone and Haversian bovine bone modeling. Thesis, Rensselaer Polytechnic Institute, Troy, NY, 1984.

Manly RS, Deakins ML. Changes in the volume per cent of moisture, organic and inorganic material in dental caries. *J Dent Res* 1940; 19(2):165–70.

Manly RS, Hodge CH, Ange LE. Density and refractive index studies of dental hard tissues II: Density distribution curves. *J Dent Res* 1939; 18(3):203–11.

Marangos O, Misra A, Spencer P, Bohaty B, Katz JL. Physico-mechanical properties determination using microscale homotopic measurement: Application to sound and caries-affected primary tooth dentin. *Acta Biomaterial* 2009; 5:1338–1348.

Marshall GW, Habelitz S, Gallagher R, Balooch M, Balooch G, Marshall SJ. Nanomechanical properties of hydrated carious human dentin. *J Dent Res* 2001; 80(8):1768–1771.

Marshall GW, Marshall SJ, Kinney JH, Balooch M. The dentin substrate: Structure and properties related to bonding. *J Dent* 1997; 25(6):441–458.

Nakajima M, Ogata M, Okuda M, Tagami J, Sano H, Pashley DH. Bonding to caries-affected dentin using self-etching primers. *Am J Dent* 1999; 12(6):309–314.

Nikolov S, Raabe D. Hierarchical modeling of the elastic properties of bone at submicron scales: The role of extrafibrillar mineralization. *Biophys J* 2008; 94(11):4220–4232.

Oyen ML, Ferguson VL, Bembey AK, Bushby AJ, Boyde A. Composite bounds on the elastic modulus of bone. *J Biomech* 2008; 41(11):2585–2588.

Park JB. *Biomaterials: An Introduction*. New York: Plenum, 1979.

Pellegrino ED, Biltz RM. The composition of human bone in uremia. *Medicine* 1965; 44:397.

Piekarski K. Analysis of bone as a composite material. *Int J Eng Sci* 1973; 10:557.

Reuss A. Berechnung der fliessgrenze von mischkristallen auf grund der plastizitatsbedingung fur einkristalle, A. *Zeits Angew Math Mech* 1929; 9:49–58.

Rho JY, Ashman RB, Turner CH. Young's modulus of trabecular and cortical bone material; ultrasonic and microtensile measurements. *J Biomech* 1993; 26:111.

Rho JY, Roy ME, Tsui TY, Pharr GM. Elastic properties of microstructural components of human bone tissue as measured by indentation. *J Biomed Mat Res* 1999; 45:48.

Ryan SD, Williams JL. Tensile testing of rodlike trabeculae excised from bovine femoral bone. *J Biomech* 1989; 22:351.

Sedlin E. A rheological model for cortical bone. *Acta Orthop Scand* 1965; 36 (suppl 83).

Smith R, Keiper D. Dynamic measurement of viscoelastic properties of bone. *Am J Med Elec* 1965; 4:156.

Sumikawa DA, Marshall GW, Gee L, Marshall SJ. Microstructure of primary tooth dentin. *Pediatr Dent* 1999; 21(7): 439–44.

Ten Cate AR. Repair and regeneration of dental tissue. In: Ten Cate AR (ed), *Oral Histology. Development, Structure, and Function*. St. Louis: Mosby; 1994. pp. 456–468.

Townsend PR, Rose RM, Radin EL. Buckling studies of single human trabeculae. *J Biomech* 1975; 8:199.

Turner CH, Rho JY, Takano Y, Tsui TY, Pharr GM. The elastic properties of trabecular and cortical bone tissues are similar: Results from two microscopic measurement techniques. *J Biomech* 1999; 32:437.

Van Buskirk WC, Ashman RB. The elastic moduli of bone. In: Cowin SC (ed), *Mechanical Properties of Bone AMD*, Vol. 45, New York: American Society of Mechanical Engineers; 1981. pp. 131–143.

Vejlens L. Glycosaminoglycans of human bone tissue: I. Pattern of compact bone in relation to age. *Calcif Tiss Res* 1971; 7:175.

Voigt W. Lehrbuch der Kristallphysik Teubner, Leipzig 1910; *Reprinted (1928) with an additional appendix.* Leipzig, Teubner, New York: Johnson Reprint; 1966.

Wagner HD, Weiner S. On the relationship between the microstructure of bone and its mechanical stiffness. *J Biomech* 1992; 25:1311.

Wainwright SA, Briggs WD, Currey JD, Gosline JM. *Mechanical Design in Organisms.* Princeton, NJ: Princeton University Press, 1982.

Wang R, Weiner S. Human root dentin: Structure anisotropy and Vickers microhardness isotropy. *Connect Tissue Res* 1998;39(4):269–279.

Weiner S, Traub W. Crystal size and organization in bone. *Conn Tissue Res* 1989; 21:259.

Weiner S, Veis A, Beniash E, Arad T, Dillon JW, Sabsay B, Siddiqui F. Peritubular dentin formation: Crystal organization and the macromolecular constituents in human teeth. *J Struct Biol* 1999; 126(1):27–41.

Yoon HS, Katz JL. Ultrasonic wave propagation in human cortical bone: I. Theoretical considerations of hexagonal symmetry. *J Biomech* 1976a; 9:407.

Yoon HS, Katz JL. Ultrasonic wave propagation in human cortical bone: II. Measurements of elastic properties and microhardness. *J Biomech* 1976b; 9:459.

Zheng, L, Hilton JF, Habelitz S, Marshall SJ, Marshall GW. Dentin caries activity status related to hardness and elasticity. *Eur J Oral Sci* 2003; 111(3):243–252.

Further Information

Several societies both in the United States and abroad hold annual meetings during which many presentations, both oral and poster, deal with hard tissue biomechanics. In the United States these societies include the Orthopaedic Research Society, the American Society of Mechanical Engineers, the Biomaterials Society, the American Society of Biomechanics, the Biomedical Engineering Society, and the Society for Bone and Mineral Research. In Europe there are alternate year meetings of the European Society of Biomechanics and the European Society of Biomaterials. Every four years there is a World Congress of Biomechanics; every three years there is a World Congress of Biomaterials. All of these meetings result in documented proceedings; some with extended papers in book form.

The two principal journals in which bone mechanics papers appear frequently are the *Journal of Biomechanics* published by Elsevier and the *Journal of Biomechanical Engineering* published by the American Society of Mechanical Engineers. Other society journals which periodically publish papers in the field are the *Journal of Orthopaedic Research* published for the Orthopaedic Research Society, the *Annals of Biomedical Engineering* published for the Biomedical Engineering Society, and the *Journal of Bone and Joint Surgery* (both American and English issues) for the American Academy of Orthopaedic Surgeons and the British Organization, respectively. Additional papers in the field may be found in the journal *Bone and Calcified Tissue International.*

The 1984 CRC volume, *Natural and Living Biomaterials* (Hastings GW and Ducheyne P, Eds.) provides a good historical introduction to the field. A recent more advanced book is *Bone Mechanics Handbook* (Cowin SC, Ed. 2001) the 2nd edition of *Bone Mechanics* (Cowin SC, Ed. 1989).

Many of the biomaterials journals and society meetings will have occasional papers dealing with hard tissue mechanics, especially those dealing with implant–bone interactions.

Appendix A

The Voigt and Reuss moduli for both transverse isotropic and orthotropic symmetry are given below:

Voigt Transverse Isotropic

$$K^V = \frac{2(C_{11} + C_{12}) + 4(C_{13} + C_{33})}{9}$$

$$G^V = \frac{(C_{11} + C_{12}) - 4C_{13} + 2C_{33} + 12(C_{44} + C_{66})}{30}$$

(A.1)

Reuss Transverse Isotropic

$$K_R = \frac{C_{33}(C_{11} + C_{12}) - 2C_{13}^2}{(C_{11} + C_{12} - 4C_{13} + 2C_{33})}$$

$$G_R = \frac{5[C_{33}(C_{11} + C_{12}) - 2C_{13}^2]C_{44}C_{66}}{2\{[C_{33}(C_{11} + C_{12}) - 2C_{13}^2](C_{44} + C_{66}) + [C_{44}C_{66}(2C_{11} + C_{12}) + 4C_{13} + C_{33}]/3\}}$$

(A.2)

Voigt Orthotropic

$$K^V = C_{11} + C_{22} + C_{33} + 2(C_{12} + C_{13} + C_{23})$$

$$G^V = \frac{[C_{11} + C_{22} + C_{33} + 3(C_{44} + C_{55} + C_{66}) - (C_{12} + C_{13} + C_{23})]}{15}$$

(A.3)

Reuss Orthotropic

$$K_R = \frac{\Delta}{C_{11}C_{22} + C_{22}C_{33} + C_{33}C_{11}} - 2(C_{11}C_{23} + C_{22}C_{13} + C_{33}C_{12})$$
$$+ 2(C_{12}C_{23} + C_{23}C_{13} + C_{13}C_{12}) - (C_{12}^2 + C_{13}^2 + C_{23}^2)$$

$$G_R = 15/(4\{(C_{11}C_{22} + C_{22}C_{33} + C_{33}C_{11} + C_{11}C_{23} + C_{22}C_{13} + C_{33}C_{22})$$
$$- [C_{12}(C_{12} + C_{23}) + C_{23}(C_{23} + C_{13}) + C_{13}(C_{13} + C_{12})]\}/\Delta$$
$$+ 3(1/C_{44} + 1/C_{55} + 1/C_{66}))$$

(A.4)

where *D* is given in Equation 1.15.

2

Richard L. Lieber
*University of California,
San Diego*

*Veterans Administration
Medical Centers*

Samuel R. Ward
*University of California,
San Diego*

*Veterans Administration
Medical Centers*

Thomas J.
Burkholder
*Georgia Institute of
Technology*

Musculoskeletal Soft-Tissue Mechanics

2.1 Structure of Soft Tissues

2.1.1 Cartilage

Articular cartilage is found at the ends of bones, where it serves as a shock absorber and reduces friction between articulating bones. It is best described as a hydrated proteoglycan (PG) gel supported by a sparse population of chondrocytes, and its composition and properties vary dramatically over its 1–2 mm thickness. The bulk composition of articular cartilage consists of approximately 20% collagen, 5% PG, primarily aggrecan bound to hyaluronic acid, with most of the remaining 75% water (Ker, 1999). At the articular surface, collagen fibrils are most dense, and arranged primarily in parallel with the surface. PG content is very low and chondrocytes are rare in this region. At the bony interface, collagen fibrils are oriented perpendicular to the articular surface, chondrocytes are more abundant, but PG content is low. PGs are most abundant in the middle zone, where collagen fibrils lack obvious orientation in association with the transition from parallel to perpendicular alignment.

Collagen itself is a fibrous protein composed of tropocollagen molecules. Tropocollagen is a triple-helical protein, which self-assembles into the long collagen fibrils observable at the ultrastructural level. These fibrils, in turn, aggregate and intertwine to form the ground substance of articular cartilage. When crosslinked into a dense network, as in the superficial zone of articular cartilage, collagen has a low permeability to water and helps to maintain the water cushion of the middle and deep zones. Collagen fibrils arranged in a random network, as in the middle zone, structurally immobilize the large PG aggregates, creating the solid phase of the composite material.

PGs consist of a number of negatively charged glycosaminoglycan chains bound to an aggrecan protein core. Aggrecan molecules, in turn, bind to a hyaluronic acid backbone, forming a PG of 50–100 MDa which carries a dense negative charge. This negative charge attracts positively charged ions (Na^+) from the extracellular fluid, and the resulting Donnan equilibrium results in rich hydration of the tissue creating an osmotic pressure that enables the tissue to function well as a shock absorber.

The overall structure of articular cartilage is analogous to a jelly-filled balloon. The PG-rich middle zone is osmotically pressurized, with fluid restrained from exiting the tissue by the dense collagen network of the superficial zone and the calcified structure of the deep bone. The interaction between the mechanical loading forces and osmotic forces yields the complex material properties of articular cartilage.

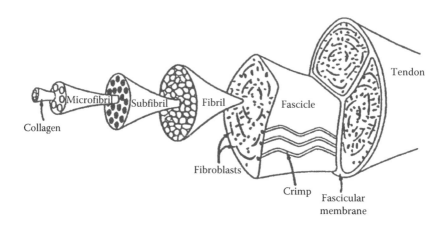

FIGURE 2.1 Tendons are organized in progressively larger filaments, beginning with molecular tropocollagen, and building to a complete tendon encased in a reticular sheath.

2.1.2 Tendon and Ligament

The passive tensile tissues, tendon and ligament, are also composed largely of water and collagen, but contain very little of the PGs that give cartilage its unique mechanical properties. In keeping with the functional role of these tissues, the collagen fibrils are organized primarily in long strands parallel to the axis of loading (Figure 2.1; Kastelic et al., 1978). The collagen fibrils, which may be hollow tubes (Gutsmann et al., 2003), combine in a hierarchical structure, with the 20–40 nm fibrils being bundled into 0.2–12 μm fibers. These fibers are birefringent under polarized light, reflecting an underlying wave or crimp structure with a periodicity between 20 and 100 μm. The fibers are bundled into fascicles, supported by fibroblasts or tenocytes, and surrounded by a fascicular membrane. Finally, multiple fascicles are bundled into a complete tendon or ligament encased in a reticular membrane.

As the tendon is loaded, the bending angle of the crimp structure of the collagen fibers can be seen to reversibly decrease, indicating that deformation of this structure is one source of elasticity. Individual collagen fibrils also display some inherent elasticity, and these two features are believed to determine the bulk properties of passive tensile tissues.

2.1.3 Muscle

2.1.3.1 Gross Morphology

Muscles are described as running from a proximal origin to a distal insertion. While these attachments are frequently discrete, distributed attachments, or even distinctly bifurcated attachments, are also common. The main mass of muscle fibers can be referred to as the belly. In a muscle with distinctly divided origins, the separate origins are often referred to as heads, and in a muscle with distinctly divided insertions, each mass of fibers terminating on distinct tendons is often referred to as a separate belly.

A muscle generally receives its blood supply from one main artery, which enters the muscle in a single, or sometimes two branches. Likewise, the major innervation is generally by a single nerve, which carries both motor efferents and sensory afferents.

Some muscles are functionally and structurally subdivided into compartments. A separate branch of the principle nerve generally innervates each compartment, and motor units of the compartments do not overlap. Generally, a dense connective tissue, or fascial, plane separates the compartments.

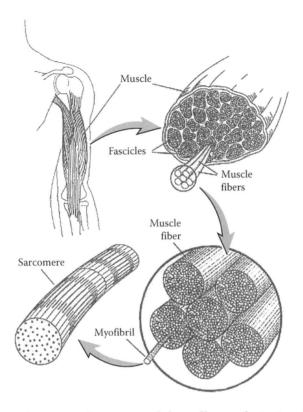

FIGURE 2.2 Skeletal muscle is organized in progressively larger filaments, beginning with molecular actin and myosin, arranged as myofibrils. Myofibrils assemble into sarcomeres and myofilaments. Myofilaments are assembled into myofibers, which are organized into the fascicles that form a whole muscle.

2.1.3.2 Fiber Architecture

Architecture, the arrangement of fibers within a muscle, determines the relationship between whole muscle length changes and force generation. The stereotypical muscle architecture is fusiform, with the muscle originating from a small tendonous attachment, inserting into a discrete tendon, and having fibers running generally parallel to the muscle axis (Figure 2.2). Fibers of unipennate muscles run parallel to each other but at an angle (pennation angle) to the muscle axis. Bipennate muscle fibers run in two distinct directions. Multipennate or fan-like muscles have one distinct attachment and one broad attachment, and pennation angle is different for every fiber. Strap-like muscles have parallel fibers that run from a broad bony origin to a broad insertion. As the length of each of these muscles is changed, the change in length of its fibers depends on fiber architecture. For example, fibers of a strap-like muscle undergo essentially the same length change as the muscle, where the length change of highly pennate fibers is reduced by their angle.

2.1.3.3 Sarcomere

Force generation in skeletal muscle results from the interaction between myosin and actin proteins. These molecules are arranged in antiparallel filaments, a 2–3 nm diameter thin filament composed mainly of actin, and a 20 nm diameter thick filament composed mainly of myosin. Myosin filaments are arranged in a hexagonal array, rigidly fixed at the M-line, and are the principal constituent of the A-band (anisotropic, light bending). Actin filaments are arranged in a complimentary hexagonal array and rigidly fixed at the Z-line, comprising the I-band (isotropic, light transmitting). The sarcomere is a nearly crystalline structure, composed of an A-band and two adjacent I-bands, and is the fundamental unit of muscle force generation. Sarcomeres are arranged into arrays of myofibrils, and one muscle cell or myofiber contains many myofibrils. Myofibers themselves are multinucleated syncitia, hundreds of microns in diameter and may be tens of millimeters in length that are derived during development by the fusion of myoblasts.

The myosin protein occurs in several different isoforms, each with different force generating characteristics, and each associated with expression of characteristic metabolic and calcium-handling proteins. Broadly, fibers can be characterized as either fast or slow, with slow fibers having a lower rate of actomyosin ATPase activity, slower velocity of shortening, slower calcium dynamics, and greater activity of oxidative metabolic enzymes. The lower ATPase activity makes these fibers more efficient for generating force, while the high oxidative capacity provides a plentiful energy source, making slow fibers ideal for extended periods of activity. Their relatively slow speed of shortening results in poor performance during fast or ballistic motions.

2.1.4 Material Properties

2.1.4.1 Cartilage

The behavior of cartilage is highly viscoelastic. A compressive load applied to articular cartilage drives the positively charged fluid phase through the densely intermeshed and negatively charged solid phase while deforming the elastic PG–collagen structure. The mobility of the fluid phase is relatively low, and, for rapid changes in load, cartilage responds nearly as a uniform linear elastic solid with a Young's modulus of approximately 6 MPa (Carter and Wong, 2003).

At lower loading rates, cartilage displays more nonlinear properties. Ker (1999) reports that human limb articular cartilage stiffness can be described as $E = E_0(1 + \sigma^{0.366})$, with $E_0 = 3.0$ MPa and σ expressed in MPa.

2.1.4.2 Tendon and Ligament

At rest, collagen fibrils are significantly crimped or wavy so that initial loading acts primarily to straighten these fibrils. At higher strains, the straightened collagen fibrils must be lengthened. Thus, tendons are more compliant at low loads and less compliant at high loads. The highly nonlinear low load region has been referred to as the "toe" region and occurs up to approximately 3% strain and 5 MPa (Butler et al. 1978; Zajac, 1989). Typically, tendons have nearly linear properties from about 3% strain until ultimate strain, which ranges from 9% to 10% (Table 2.1). The tangent modulus in this linear region is approximately 1.5 GPa. Ultimate tensile stress reported for tendons is approximately 100 MPa (McElhaney et al., 1976). However, under physiological conditions, tendons operate at stresses of only 5–10 MPa (Table 2.1) yielding a typical safety factor of 10.

2.1.4.3 Muscle

Tension generated by skeletal muscle depends on length, velocity, level of activation, and history. Performance characteristics of a muscle depend on both its intrinsic properties and the extrinsic organization of that tissue. Whole muscle maximum shortening velocity depends both upon the sliding velocity of its component sarcomeres and on the number of those sarcomeres arranged in series. Likewise, maximum isometric tension depends on both the intrinsic tension generating capacity of the actomyosin cross-bridges and on the number of sarcomeres arranged in parallel. The relationship between intrinsic properties and extrinsic function is further complicated by pennation of the fibers. Given the orthotropic nature of the muscle fiber, material properties should be considered relative to the fiber axis. That is, the relevant area for stress determination is not the geometric cross section, but the physiological cross section, perpendicular to the fiber axis. The common form for estimation of the physiological cross-sectional area (PCSA) is

$$\text{PCSA} = \frac{M \cos\theta}{\rho F L}$$

TABLE 2.1 Tendon Biomechanical Properties

Tendon	Ultimate Stress (MPa)	Ultimate Strain (%)	Stress under Normal Loads (MPa)	Strain under Normal Loads (%)	Tangent Modulus (GPa)	Reference
	40	9				Woo et al. (1980)
Wallaby			15–40		1.56	Bennett et al. (1986)
Porpoise					1.53	Bennett et al. (1986)
Dolphin					1.43	Bennett et al. (1986)
Deer			28–74		1.59	Bennett et al. (1986)
Sheep					1.65	Bennett et al. (1986)
Donkey			22–44		1.25	Bennett et al. (1986)
Human leg			53		1.0–1.2	Bennett et al. (1986)
Cat leg					1.21	Bennett et al. (1986)
Pig tail					0.9	Bennett et al. (1986)
Rat tail					0.8–1.5	Bennett et al. (1986)
Horse				4–10		Ker et al. (1988)
Dog leg			84			Ker et al. (1988)
Camel ankle			18			Ker et al. (1988)
Human limb (various)	60–120					McElhaney et al. (1976)
Human calcaneal	55	9.5				McElhaney et al. (1976)
Human wrist	52–74	11–17	3.2–3.3	1.5–3.5		Loren and Lieber (1994)

where M is muscle mass, θ is pennation angle, ρ is muscle density (1.06 g/cm³), and FL is fiber length. Likewise, the relevant gage length for strain determination is not muscle length, but fiber length, or fascicle length in muscles composed of serial fibers.

Maximum muscle stress: Maximum active stress, or specific tension, varies somewhat among fiber types and species (Table 2.2) around a generally accepted average of 250 kPa. This specific tension can be determined in any system in which it is possible to measure force and estimate the area of contractile material. Given muscle PCSA, maximum force produced by a muscle can be predicted by multiplying this PCSA by specific tension (Table 2.2). Specific tension can also be calculated for isolated muscle fibers or motor units in which estimates of cross-sectional area have been made.

Maximum muscle contraction velocity: Muscle maximum contraction velocity is primarily dependent on the type and number of sarcomeres in series along the muscle fiber length (Gans, 1982). The intrinsic velocity of shortening has been experimentally determined for a number of muscle types (Table 2.3). Maximum contraction velocity of a given muscle can thus be calculated based on knowledge of the number of serial sarcomeres within the muscle multiplied by the maximum contraction velocity of an individual sarcomere (Tables 2.4 through 2.6). Sarcomere shortening velocity varies widely among species and fiber types (Table 2.3).

Muscle force–length relationship: Under conditions of constant length, muscle force generated is proportional to the magnitude of the interaction between the actin and myosin contractile filaments. Myosin filament length in most species is approximately 1.6 μm, but actin filament length varies (Table 2.7). Optimal sarcomere length and maximum sarcomere length can be calculated using these filament lengths. For optimal force generation, each half myosin filament must completely overlap an actin filament, without opposing actin filaments overlapping, so peak force generation occurs at a sarcomere length of twice the thin filament length. No active force is produced at sarcomere spacings shorter than 1.3 μm or longer than the sum of the myosin and the pair of actin filament lengths. The range of operating sarcomere lengths varies among muscles, but generally covers a range of ±15% of optimal length (Burkholder and Lieber, 2003). At submaximal activation, the peak of the force–length relationship shifts to longer lengths (Rack and Westbury, 1969; Balnave and Allen, 1996).

TABLE 2.2   Skeletal Muscle-Specific Tension

Species	Muscle Type	Preparation	Specific Tension (kPa)	Reference
		Synthesis	300	Josephson (1989)
Rat	SO	Single fiber	134	Fitts et al. (1991)
Human	Slow	Single fiber	133	Fitts et al. (1991)
Rat	FOG	Single fiber	108	Fitts et al. (1991)
Rat	FG	Single fiber	108	Fitts et al. (1991)
Human	Fast	Single fiber	166	Fitts et al. (1991)
Cat	1	Motor unit	59	Dum et al, (1982)
Cat	S	Motor unit	172	Bodine et al. (1987)
Cat	2A	Motor unit	284	Dum et al, (1982)
Cat	FR	Motor unit	211	Bodine et al. (1987)
Cat	2B + 2AB	Motor unit	343	Dum et al, (1982)
Cat	FF/FI	Motor unit	249	Bodine et al. (1987)
Human	Elbow	Whole muscle	230–420	Edgerton et al. (1990)
Human	Ankle	Whole muscle	45–250	Fukunaga et al. (1996)
Rat	TA	Whole muscle	272	Wells (1965)
Rat	Soleus	Whole muscle	319	Wells (1965)
Guinea pig	Hindlimb	Whole muscle	225	Powell et al. (1984)
Guinea pig	Soleus	Whole muscle	154	Powell et al. (1984)

TABLE 2.3   Muscle Dynamic Properties

Species	Muscle Type	Preparation	V_{max}^a	a/P_o	b/V_{max}	Reference
Rat	SO	Single fiber	1.49 L/s			Fitts et al. (1991)
Human	Slow	Single fiber	0.86 L/s			Fitts et al. (1991)
Rat	FOG	Single fiber	4.91 L/s			Fitts et al. (1991)
Rat	FG	Single fiber	8.05 L/s			Fitts et al. (1991)
Human	Fast	Single fiber	4.85 L/s			Fitts et al. (1991)
Mouse	Soleus	Whole muscle	31.7 μm/s			Close (1972)
Rat	Soleus	Whole muscle	18.2 μm/s			Close (1972)
Rat	Soleus	Whole muscle	5.4 cm/s	0.214	0.23	Wells (1965)
Cat	Soleus	Whole muscle	13 μm/s			Close (1972)
Mouse	EDL	Whole muscle	60.5 μm/s			Close (1972)
Rat	EDL	Whole muscle	42.7 μm/s			Close (1972)
Cat	EDL	Whole muscle	31 μm/s			Close (1972)
Rat	TA	Whole muscle	14.4 cm/s	0.356	0.38	Wells (1965)

[a] L/s fiber or sarcomere lengths per second, μm/s sarcomere velocity; cm/s whole muscle velocity.

Muscle force–velocity relationship: Under conditions of constant load the relationship between force and velocity is nearly hyperbolic during shortening (Hill, 1938, Figure 2.5). The normalized shortening force–velocity relation can be described by

$$(F + a)v = b(1 - F)$$

TABLE 2.4 Architectural Properties of the Human Arm and Forearm[a]

Muscle	Muscle Mass (g)	Muscle Length (mm)	Fiber Length (mm)	Pennation Angle (deg.)	Cross-Sectional Area (cm²)	FL/ML Ratio
BR (*n* = 8)	16.6 ± 2.8	175 ± 8.3	121 ± 8.3	2.4 ± .6	1.33 ± .22	.69 ± .062
PT (*n* = 8)	15.9 ± 1.7	130 ± 4.7	36.4 ± 1.3	9.6 ± .8	4.13 ± .52	.28 ± .012
PQ (*n* = 8)	5.21 ± 1.0	39.3 ± 2.3	23.3 ± 2.0	9.9 ± .3	2.07 ± .33	.58 ± .021
EDC I (*n* = 8)	3.05 ± .45	114 ± 3.4	56.9 ± 3.6	3.1 ± .5	.52 ± .08	.49 ± .024
EDC M (*n* = 5)	6.13 ± 1.2	112 ± 4.7	58.8 ± 3.5	3.2 ± 1.0	1.02 ± .20	.50 ± .014
EDC R (*n* = 7)	4.70 ± .75	125 ± 10.7	51.2 ± 1.8	3.2 ± .54	.86 ± .13	.42 ± .023
EDC S (*n* = 6)	2.23 ± .32	121 ± 8.0	52.9 ± 5.2	2.4 ± .7	.40 ± .06	.43 ± .029
EDQ (*n* = 7)	3.81 ± .70	152 ± 9.2	55.3 ± 3.7	2.6 ± .6	.64 ± .10	.36 ± .012
FPLEIP (*n* = 6)	2.86 ± .61	105 ± 6.6	48.4 ± 2.3	6.3 ± .8	.56 ± .11	.46 ± .023
EPL (*n* = 7)	4.54 ± .68	138 ± 7.2	43.6 ± 2.6	5.6 ± 1.3	.98 ± .13	.31 ± .020
PL (*n* = 6)	3.78 ± .82	134 ± 11.5	52.3 ± 3.1	3.5 ± 1.2	.69 ± .17	.40 ± .032
FDS I(P) (*n* = 6)	6.0 ± 1.1	92.5 ± 8.4	31.6 ± 3.0	5.1 ± 0.2	1.81 ± .83	.34 ± .022
FDS I(D) (*n* = 9)	6.6 ± 0.8	119 ± 6.1	37.9 ± 3.0	6.7 ± 0.3	1.63 ± .22	.32 ± .013
FDS I(C) (*n* = 6)	12.4 ± 2.1	207 ± 10.7	67.6 ± 2.8	5.7 ± 0.2	1.71 ± .28	.33 ± .025
FDS M (*n* = 9)	16.3 ± 2.2	183 ± 11.5	60.8 ± 3.9	6.9 ± 0.7	2.53 ± .34	.34 ± .014
FDS R (*n* = 9)	10.2 ± 1.1	155 ± 7.7	60.1 ± 2.7	4.3 ± 0.6	1.61 ± .18	.39 ± .023
FDS S (*n* = 9)	1.8 ± 0.3	103 ± 6.3	42.4 ± 2.2	4.9 ± 0.7	0.40 ± .05	.42 ± .014
FDP I (*n* = 9)	11.7 ± 1.2	149 ± 3.8	61.4 ± 2.4	7.2 ± 0.7	1.77 ± .16	.41 ± .018
FDP M (*n* = 9)	16.3 ± 1.7	200 ± 8.2	68.4 ± 2.7	5.7 ± 0.3	2.23 ± .22	.34 ± .011
FDP R (*n* = 9)	11.9 ± 1.4	194 ± 7.0	64.6 ± 2.6	6.8 ± 0.5	1.72 ± .18	.33 ± .009
FDP S (*n* = 9)	13.7 ± 1.5	150 ± 4.7	60.7 ± 3.9	7.8 ± 0.9	2.20 ± .30	.40 ± .015
FPL (*n* = 9)	10.0 ± 1.1	168 ± 10.0	45.1 ± 2.1	6.9 ± 0.2	2.08 ± .22	.24 ± .010

Source: Data from Lieber, R.L. et al. 1990. *J. Hand Surg.* 15:244–250; Lieber, R.L. et al. 1992. *J. Hand Surg.* 17:787–798.

[a] BR, brachioradialis; EDC I, EDC M, EDC R, and EDC S, extensor digitorum communis to the index, middle, ring, and small fingers, respectively; EDQ, extensor digiti quinti; EIP, extensor indicis proprious; EPL, extensor pollicis longus; FDP I, FDP M, FDP R, and FDP S, flexor digitorum profundus muscles; FDS I, FDS M, FDS R, and FDS S, flexor digitorum superficialis muscles; FDS I (P) and FDS I (D), proximal and distal bellies of the FDS I; FDS I (C), the combined properties of the two bellies as if they were a single muscle; FPL, flexor pollicis longus; PQ, pronator quadratus; PS, palmaris longus; PT, pronator teres.

while the lengthening relation can be described by

$$F = 1.8 - 0.8 \, \frac{V_{max} + v}{V_{max} - 7.6 \, v}$$

The dynamic parameters (*a*, *b*, and V_{max}) vary across species and fiber types (Table 2.3).

2.1.5 Modeling

2.1.5.1 Cartilage

Although cartilage can be modeled as a simple elastic element, more accurate results are obtained using a biphasic model (Mow et al., 1980), which describes the motion of the hydrating fluid relative to the charged organic matrix. The total stress acting on the cartilage is separated into independent solid and fluid phases:

$$\sigma^T = \sigma^s + \sigma^f$$

TABLE 2.5 Architectural Properties of Human Lower Limb[a]

Muscle	Muscle Mass (g)	Muscle Length (cm)	Fiber Length (cm)	Pennation Angle (deg.)	Cross-Sectional Area (cm²)	FL/ML Ratio
Psoas	97.69 ± 33.58	24.25 ± 4.75	11.69 ± 1.66	10.66 ± 3.20	7.73 ± 2.31	0.50 ± 0.14
Iliacus	113.74 ± 37.01	20.61 ± 4.02	10.66 ± 1.86	14.29 ± 5.32	9.88 ± 3.40	0.56 ± 0.26
Gluteus maximus	547.24 ± 162.17	26.95 ± 6.42	15.69 ± 2.57	21.94 ± 26.24	28.17 ± 11.05	0.62 ± 0.22
Glut. medius	273.45 ± 76.86	19.99 ± 2.86	7.33 ± 1.57	20.47 ± 17.34	33.78 ± 14.39	0.37 ± 0.08
Sartorius	78.45 ± 31.13	44.81 ± 4.19	40.30 ± 4.63	1.33 ± 1.76	1.86 ± 0.74	0.90 ± 0.04
Rectus femoris	110.55 ± 43.33	36.28 ± 4.73	7.59 ± 1.28	13.93 ± 3.49	13.51 ± 4.97	0.21 ± 0.03
Vastus lateralis	375.85 ± 137.18	27.34 ± 4.62	9.94 ± 1.76	18.38 ± 6.78	35.09 ± 16.14	0.38 ± 0.11
Vastus intermedius	171.86 ± 72.89	41.20 ± 8.17	9.93 ± 2.03	4.54 ± 4.45	16.74 ± 6.91	0.24 ± 0.04
Vastus medialis	239.44 ± 94.83	43.90 ± 9.85	9.68 ± 2.30	29.61 ± 6.89	20.58 ± 7.17	0.22 ± 0.04
Gracilis	52.53 ± 16.72	28.69 ± 3.29	22.78 ± 4.38	8.16 ± 2.51	2.23 ± 0.81	0.79 ± 0.08
Adductor longus	74.67 ± 28.42	21.84 ± 4.46	10.82 ± 2.02	7.08 ± 3.43	6.50 ± 2.17	0.50 ± 0.07
Adductor brevis	54.56 ± 24.83	15.39 ± 2.46	10.31 ± 1.42	6.10 ± 3.14	4.95 ± 2.11	0.68 ± 0.06
Adductor magnus	324.72 ± 127.82	37.90 ± 7.36	14.44 ± 2.74	15.54 ± 7.27	20.48 ± 7.82	0.39 ± 0.07
Biceps femoris LH	113.37 ± 48.53	34.73 ± 3.65	9.76 ± 2.62	11.58 ± 5.50	11.33 ± 4.75	0.28 ± 0.08
Biceps femoris SH	59.79 ± 22.62	22.39 ± 2.50	11.03 ± 2.06	12.33 ± 3.61	5.06 ± 1.69	0.49 ± 0.07
Semitendinosus	99.74 ± 37.81	29.67 ± 3.86	19.30 ± 4.12	12.86 ± 4.94	4.82 ± 2.01	0.65 ± 0.11
Semimembranosus	134.31 ± 57.56	29.34 ± 3.42	6.90 ± 1.83	15.09 ± 3.43	18.40 ± 7.53	0.24 ± 0.06
Tibialis anterior	80.13 ± 26.63	25.98 ± 3.25	6.83 ± 0.79	9.56 ± 3.11	10.89 ± 3.01	0.27 ± 0.05
Extensor hallucis longus	20.93 ± 9.86	24.25 ± 3.27	7.48 ± 1.13	9.44 ± 2.15	2.67 ± 1.52	0.31 ± 0.06
Extensor digitorum longus	40.98 ± 12.62	29.00 ± 2.33	6.93 ± 1.14	10.83 ± 2.75	5.55 ± 1.68	0.24 ± 0.04
Peroneus longus	57.74 ± 22.64	27.08 ± 3.02	5.08 ± 0.63	14.08 ± 5.14	10.39 ± 3.75	0.19 ± 0.03
Peroneus brevis	24.15 ± 10.59	23.75 ± 3.11	4.54 ± 0.65	11.46 ± 2.96	4.91 ± 2.01	0.19 ± 0.03
GastrocnemiusMH	113.46 ± 31.97	26.94 ± 4.65	5.10 ± 0.98	9.88 ± 4.39	21.12 ± 5.66	0.19 ± 0.03
Gastrocnemius	62.24 ± 24.56	22.35 ± 3.70	5.88 ± 0.95	12.04 ± 3.11	9.72 ± 3.26	0.27 ± 0.03
Soleus	275.77 ± 98.50	40.54 ± 8.32	4.40 ± 0.99	28.25 ± 10.05	51.79 ± 14.91	0.11 ± 0.02
Flexor hallucis longus	38.89 ± 17.09	26.88 ± 3.55	5.27 ± 1.29	16.89 ± 4.62	6.85 ± 2.72	0.20 ± 0.05
Flexor digitorum longus	20.27 ± 10.75	27.33 ± 5.62	4.46 ± 1.06	13.64 ± 4.73	4.37 ± 2.02	0.16 ± 0.09
Tibialis posterior	58.44 ± 19.20	31.03 ± 4.68	3.78 ± 0.49	13.71 ± 4.11	14.42 ± 4.94	0.12 ± 0.02

[a] Data from Ward J.S. et al. 2009. *Clin Orthop Relat Res.* 467:1074–82.

where s denotes the solid phase and f the fluid phase. The relative motion of the phases defines the equilibrium equations

$$\nabla \cdot \sigma^s = \frac{(v^s - v^f)}{k(1 + \alpha)^2} = -\nabla \cdot \sigma^f$$

where α is tissue solid content and k the tissue permeability coefficient. In addition to the equilibrium equations, each phase is subject to separate constitutive relations:

$$\sigma^f = -p_a \underline{I} \quad \text{and} \quad \sigma^s = -\alpha p_a \underline{I} + \underline{D}\underline{e}$$

where p_a is the apparent tissue stress, $\underline{D}$ is the material property tensor and $\underline{e}$ is the strain tensor. For a hyperelastic solid phase

TABLE 2.6 Architectural Properties of Human Foot[a]

Muscle	Muscle Volume (cm³)	Muscle Length (mm)	Fiber Length (mm)	Cross-Sectional Area (cm²)
ABDH	15.2 ± 5.3	115.8 ± 4.9	23.0 ± 5.5	6.68 ± 2.07
ABDM	8.8 ± 4.7	112.8 ± 19.0	23.9 ± 7.4	3.79 ± 1.83
ADHT	1.1 ± 0.6	24.8 ± 4.2	18.7 ± 5.2	0.62 ± 0.26
ADHO	9.1 ± 3.1	67.4 ± 4.6	18.6 ± 5.3	4.94 ± 1.36
EDB2	2.1 ± 1.2	69.8 ± 16.8	28.0 ± 6.5	0.79 ± 0.43
EDB3	1.3 ± 0.7	82.2 ± 20.7	26.4 ± 5.1	0.51 ± 0.30
EDB4	1.0 ± 0.7	70.4 ± 21.1	23.1 ± 3.8	0.44 ± 0.29
EHB	3.6 ± 1.5	65.7 ± 8.5	27.9 ± 5.7	1.34 ± 0.66
FDB2	4.5 ± 2.3	92.9 ± 15.0	25.4 ± 4.5	1.78 ± 0.79
FDB3	3.2 ± 1.5	98.8 ± 18.1	22.8 ± 4.0	1.49 ± 0.71
FDB4	2.6 ± 1.0	103.0 ± 9.2	20.8 ± 4.5	1.26 ± 0.47
FDB5	0.7 ± 0.3	83.2 ± 3.0	18.2 ± 2.2	0.35 ± 0.16
FDMB	3.4 ± 1.7	51.0 ± 5.3	17.7 ± 3.8	2.00 ± 1.02
FHBM	3.1 ± 1.3	76.0 ± 19.8	17.5 ± 4.8	1.80 ± 0.75
FHBL	3.4 ± 1.4	65.3 ± 7.1	16.5 ± 3.4	2.12 ± 0.84
DI1	2.7 ± 1.4	51.0 ± 4.9	16.1 ± 4.4	1.70 ± 0.64
DI2	2.5 ± 1.4	49.9 ± 5.1	15.3 ± 4.0	1.68 ± 0.80
DI3	2.5 ± 1.2	44.3 ± 5.6	15.6 ± 5.4	1.64 ± 0.58
DI4	4.2 ± 2.0	61.4 ± 4.5	16.0 ± 4.8	2.72 ± 1.33
LB2	0.6 ± 0.4	53.9 ± 11.8	22.4 ± 6.5	0.28 ± 0.17
LB3	0.5 ± 0.4	45.2 ± 8.7	22.3 ± 6.7	0.28 ± 0.09
LB4	0.6 ± 0.4	37.3 ± 19.9	21.1 ± 9.3	0.30 ± 0.32
LB5	0.4 ± 0.4	41.0 ± 12.1	16.2 ± 7.0	0.18 ± 0.13
PI1	1.5 ± 0.5	46.2 ± 4.0	13.6 ± 3.7	1.23 ± 0.65
PI2	1.9 ± 0.7	56.6 ± 6.6	13.9 ± 3.5	1.41 ± 0.48
PI3	1.8 ± 0.6	48.8 ± 9.9	14.2 ± 5.9	1.38 ± 0.55
QPM	5.6 ± 3.4	81.3 ± 20.1	27.5 ± 7.0	1.96 ± 0.94
QPL	2.4 ± 1.2	55.3 ± 3.9	23.4 ± 7.1	1.00 ± 0.41

Source: Data from Kura, H. et al. 1997. *Anat. Rec.* 249:143–151.

[a] ABDH, abductor hallucis; FHBM flexor hallucis brevis medialis; FHBL, flexor hallucis brevis lateralis; ADHT, adductor hallucis transverse; ADHO, adductor hallucis oblique; ABDM, abductor digiti minimi; FDMB, flexor digiti minimi brevis; DI, dorsal interosseous; PI, plantar interosseous; FDB, flexor digitorum brevis; LB, lumbrical; QPM, quadratus plantaris medialis; QPL, quadratus plantaris lateralis; EHB, extensor hallucis brevis; EDB, extensor digitorum brevis.

$$\underline{D}\underline{e} = \lambda Tr(\underline{e})\underline{I} + 2\mu\underline{e}$$

where λ and μ are the Lamé constants.

These equations can be solved analytically for the special case of confined compression against a porous platen (Mow et al., 1980). The surface displacement during creep under an applied load f_0 is

$$\frac{u}{h} = \frac{f_0}{H_A}\left(1 - \frac{2}{\pi^2}\sum_{n=0}^{\infty}(n+12)^{-2}\exp\left\{-\pi^2(n+12)^2\frac{H_A k f}{(1+2a_0)h^2}\right\}\right)$$

where h is the tissue thickness, and H_A is the aggregate modulus ($\lambda + 2\mu$). Those authors estimate k as $7.6 \pm 3.0 \times 10^{-13}\,m^4/Ns$ and H_A as 0.70 ± 0.09 MPa for bovine articular cartilage. Chen et al. (2001) report

TABLE 2.7   Actin Filament Lengths

Species	Actin Filament Length (μm)	Optimal Length (μm)	Reference
Cat	1.12	2.24	Herzog et al. (1992)
Rat	1.09	2.18	Herzog et al. (1992)
Rabbit	1.09	2.18	Herzog et al. (1992)
Frog	0.98	1.96	Page and Huxley (1963)
Monkey	1.16	2.32	Walker and Schrodt (1973)
Human	1.27	2.54	Walker and Schrodt (1973)
Hummingbird	1.75	3.50	Mathieu-Costello et al. (1992)
Chicken	0.95	1.90	Page (1969)
Wild rabbit	1.12	2.24	Dimery (1985)
Carp	0.98	1.92	Sosnicki et al. (1991)

strongly depth-dependent values for H_A ranging between 1.16 ± 0.20 MPa in the superficial zone to 7.75 ± 1.45 MPa in the deep zone in human articular cartilage. The biphasic approach has been extended to finite element modeling, resulting in the u–p class of models (Wayne et al., 1991).

2.1.5.2 Tendon and Ligament

The composition and structure of the tensile soft tissues is quite similar to that of cartilage, and the biphasic theory can be applied to them as well (Yin and Elliott, 1983). Fluid pressure serves a smaller role in tissues loaded in tension, and the complication of the biphasic model is generally unnecessary. For modeling of segmental mechanics, it is frequently sufficient to treat these structures according to a one-dimensional approximation.

While considering tendons and ligaments as simple nonlinear elastic elements (Table 2.6) is often sufficient, additional accuracy can be obtained by incorporating viscous damping. The quasi-linear viscoelastic approach (Fung, 1967) introduces a stress relaxation function, $G(t)$, that depends only on time, is convoluted with the elastic response, $T^e(\lambda)$, that depends only on the stretch ratio, to yield the complete stress response, $K(\lambda,t)$. To obtain the stress at any point in time requires that the contribution of all preceding deformations be assessed:

$$T(t) = \int G(t - \tau) \frac{\partial T^e(\lambda)}{\partial \lambda} \frac{\partial \lambda}{\partial \tau} d\tau$$

Both the elastic response and the relaxation function are empirically determined. The common form for the relaxation function is a sum of exponentials

$$G(t) = A + \sum_i B_i e^{-t/\tau_i}$$

The form of the elastic response varies, but usually includes a power or exponential term to accommodate the toe region.

2.1.5.3 Muscle

2.1.5.3.1 Types of Muscle Models

There are three general classes of models for predicting muscle force: biochemical, or crossbridge, models, constitutive models, and phenomenological, or Hill, models. Cross-bridge models (Huxley, 1957;

Huxley and Simmons, 1971) attempt to determine force from the chemical reactions of the cross-bridge cycle. Though accurate at the cross-bridge level, it is generally computationally prohibitive to model a whole muscle in this manner. Constitutive models, such as that described by Zahalak and Ma (1990), generally attempt to determine muscle behavior by describing populations of cross-bridges. A potentially powerful approach, this technique has not yet been widely adopted. In the context of whole-body biomechanics, the primary modeling approach uses the phenomenological model first described by Hill (1939), which incorporates the steady-state force–length and force–velocity properties into a contractile element, which is dynamically isolated by a series elastic element (Figure 2.3). The parallel elastic element represents the passive properties of the muscle, which reflect the properties of titin and extracellular connective tissue. The series elastic element provides the dynamic response during time-varying force and velocity conditions. Some of this elasticity resides in extracellular connective tissue, including tendon and aponeurosis, but series elasticity of 5–10% Lo/Po is found even in muscles lacking any external tendon or in segments of single fibers. The contractile component is described by independent isometric force–length (Figure 2.4) and isotonic force–velocity relations (Figure 2.5) and an activation function (Zajac, 1989).

Force production by the contractile component can be calculated as the product of three independent functions, each bounded by 0 and 1, and the maximal isometric tension, F_0: $F = a * afl * afv * F_0$. The activation function (a) depends only on an input representing neural drive or a descending command if excitation–contraction coupling is intact. Often, it is a first-order transformation intended to represent calcium and troponin dynamics, but activation dynamics and series elasticity are both first-order processes, so the extent to which the activation function improves model results depends strongly on the extent to which modeled series elasticity accurately represents muscle mechanics. The active force–length function (afl) depends only on muscle fiber or sarcomere length. The active force–velocity function (afv) depends only on fiber velocity.

In forward simulation, initial conditions are known and an activation function is given or derived from a control model. The muscle model is coupled with a physical model, and the physical model provides a muscle–tendon unit (MTU) length. The muscle model must calculate force

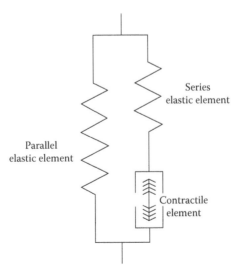

FIGURE 2.3 The Hill model of muscle separates the active properties of muscle into a contractile element, in series with a purely elastic element. The properties of the passive muscle are represented by the parallel elastic element.

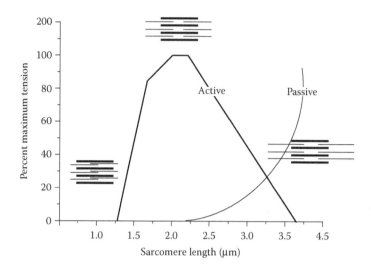

FIGURE 2.4 The force generating capacity of a sarcomere depends strongly on the degree of overlap of myosin and actin filaments.

production in order to update the physical model. Mathematically, this reduces to solving the following equations:

$$\frac{dx}{dt} = f(F)$$

$$\frac{dF}{dt} = k\left(\frac{dx}{dt} - \frac{dL}{dt}\right)$$

$$\frac{dL}{dt} = afv^{-1}\left(\frac{F}{F_0 a(t)afl(L)}\right)$$

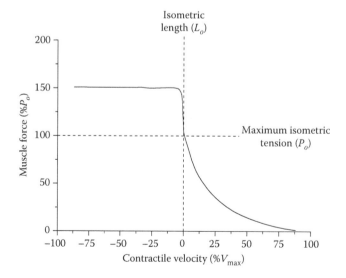

FIGURE 2.5 Active force generation depends strongly on shortening velocity.

where x is MTU length, calculated from the physical model; F is the force in the series elastic and contractile elements, calculated from the elasticity of the SEE; L is the length of the contractile element, calculated from the applied force and inversion of the force–velocity relationship.

It should be noted that this formulation omits several potentially important force-generating phenomena. Notable among these are the persistent extra tension obtained following stretch (Edman et al., 1982) and changes in the force–length relation associated with activation level (Rack and Westbury, 1969). Some of these features can be accommodated by considering series elasticity and sarcomere length inhomogeneity (Morgan, 1990), and each represents a nonlinearity that substantially complicates modeling and may not be necessary for first approximations of muscle function.

Common applications of muscle modeling include forward simulation to predict output forces or motions, as for control of functional electrical stimulation (Park and Durand 2008), and inverse analysis to estimate the muscle forces that produced an observed motion (Thelen and Anderson 2006). In neither of these cases is it necessarily practical to determine muscle contractile properties empirically, and it is frequently necessary to resort to estimation of the force–length and force–velocity relations from muscle structure. If a muscle is considered to be a composition of uniform sarcomeres in series and in parallel, then the deformation of single sarcomeres can be estimated from whole muscle length changes. A simplified view of a muscle is an array of identical fibers of uniform length arranged at a common pennation angle to the line of force. Peak isometric tension can be estimated from PCSA. Pennation angle determines the relationship between muscle and fiber length changes:

$$\frac{\Delta L_m}{L_m} = \frac{\Delta L_f}{L_f} \cos\theta$$

If sarcomere length is known at any muscle length, it is then possible to scale the sarcomere length-tension and velocity–tension relations to the whole muscle. When reporting architectural data (tables), muscle and fiber lengths should be normalized to optimal sarcomere length. Even with direct measurements of the steady-state afl and afv, errors in force estimates during dynamic, submaximal activations can be substantial (Perreault and Heckman, 2003).

References

Balnave, C.D. and Allen, D.G. 1996. The effect of muscle length on intracellular calcium and force in single fibres from mouse skeletal muscle. *J Physiol.* 492(Pt 3):705–713.

Bennett, M.B., Ker, R.F., Dimery, N.J., and Alexander, R. M. 1986. Mechanical properties of various mammalian tendons. *J Zoology* 209, 537–548.

Bodine, S.C., Roy, R.R., Eldred, E., and Edgerton, V.R. 1987. Maximal force as a function of anatomical features of motor units in the cat tibialis anterior. *J Neurophysiol.* 57, 1730–45.

Burkholder, T.J. and Lieber, R.L. Sarcomere length operating range of vertebrate muscles during movement. *J Exp Biol.* 204:1529–36.

Butler, D.L., Grood, E.S., Noyes, F.R., and Zernicke, R.F. 1978. Biomechanics of ligaments and tendons. *Exerc. Sport Sci. Rev.* Vol. 6: 125–181, Hutton, R.S. (Ed.). The Franklin Institute Press.

Carter, D.R. and Wong, M. 2003. Modeling Cartilage mechanobiology. *Philos Trans R Soc Lond B Biol Sci.* 29; 358(1437): 1461–1471.

Close, R.I. 1972. Dynamic properties of mammalian skeletal muscles. *Physiological Reviews* 52, 129–97.

Chen, A.C., Bae, W.C., Schinagl, R.M., and Sah, R.L. 2001. Depth- and strain-dependent mechanical and electromechanical properties of full-thickness bovine articular cartilage in confined compression. *J Biomech.* 34(1):1–12.

Dimery, N.J. 1985. Muscle and sarcomere lengths in the hind limb of the rabbit (Oryctolagus cuniculus) during a galloping stride. *J Zoology* 205, 373–383.

Dum, R.P., Burke, R.E., O'Donovan, M.J., Toop, J., and Hodgson, J.A. 1982. Motor-unit organization inflexor digitorum longus muscle of the cat. *J Neurophysiol.* 47(6):1108–25.

Edgerton, V.R., Apor, P., and Roy, R.R. 1990. Specific tension of human elbow flexor muscles. *Acta Physiologica Hungarica.* 75, 205–16.

Edman, K.A., Elzinga, G., and Noble, M.I. 1982. Residual force enhancement after stretch of contracting frog single muscle fibers. *J Gen Physiol.* 80(5):769–784.

Fitts, R.H., McDonald, K.S., and Schluter, J.M. 1991. The determinants of skeletal muscle force and power: their adaptability with changes in activity pattern. *J Biomech.* 24 Suppl 1, 111–22.

Fukunaga, T., Roy, R.R., Shellock, F.G., Hodgson, J.A., and Edgerton, V.R. 1996. Specific tension ofhuman plantar flexors and dorsiflexors. *J Appl Physiol.* 80(1):158–65.

Fung, Y.C. 1967. Elasticity of soft tissues in simple elongation. *Am. J. Physiol.* 213(6):1532–1544.

Gans, C. 1982. Fiber architecture and muscle function. *Exerc. Sport Sci. Rev.* 10:160–207.

Gordon, A.M., Huxley, A.F., and Julian, F.J. 1966. The variation in isometric tension with sarcomere length in vertebrate muscle fibres. *J. Physiol.* 184:170–192.

Gutsmann, T., Fantner, G.E., Venturoni, M., Ekani-Nkodo, A., Thompson, J.B., Kindt, J.H., Morse, D.E., Fygenson, D.K., and Hansma, P.K. 2003. Evidence that collagen fibrils in tendons are inhomogeneously structured in a tubelike manner. *Biophys. J.* 84(4):2593–2598.

Herzog, W., Leonard, T.R., Renaud, J.M., Wallace, J., Chaki, G., and Bornemisza, S. 1992. Force-length properties and functional demands of cat gastrocnemius, soleus andplantaris muscles. *J Biomech.* 25(11):1329–35.

Hill, A.V. 1938. The heat of shortening and the dynamic constants of muscle. *Proc. R. Soc. Lond. Series B: Biol. Sci.* 126:136–195.

Huxley, A.F. 1957. Muscle structure and theories of contraction. *Prog. Biophys. Mol. Biol.* 7:255–318.

Huxley, A.F. and Simmons, R.M. 1971. Proposed mechanism of force generation in striated muscle. *Nature* 233:533–538.

Josephson, R.K. 1989. Power output from skeletal muscle during linear and sinusoidal shortening. *J Exp Biol.* 147:533–37.

Kastelic, J., Galeski, A., and Baer, E. 1978. The multicomposite structure of tendon. *Connect. Tissue Res.* 6:11–23.

Ker, R.F. 1999. The design of soft collagenous load-bearing tissues. *J. Exp. Biol.* 202(Pt 23):3315–3324.

Ker, R.F., Alexander, R.M. and Bennett, M.B. 1988. Why are mammalian tendons so thick. *J Zoolog.* 216:309–24.

Kura, H., Luo, Z., Kitaoka, H.B., and An, K. 1997. Quantitative analysis of the intrinsic muscles of the foot. *Anat. Rec.* 249:143–151.

Lieber, R.L., Fazeli, B.M., and Botte, M.J. 1990. Architecture of selected wrist flexor and extensor muscles. *J. Hand Surg.* 15:244–250.

Lieber, R.L., Jacobson, M.D., Fazeli, B.M., Abrams, R.A., and Botte, M.J. 1992. Architecture of selected muscles of the arm and forearm: Anatomy and implications for tendon transfer. *J. Hand Surg.* 17:787–798.

Loren, G.J. and Lieber, R.L. 1995. Tendon biomechanical properties enhance human wrist muscle specialization. *J Biomech.* 28:791–9.

Mathieu-Costello, O., Suarez, R.K., and Hochachka, P.W. 1992. Capillary-to-fiber geometry andmitochondrial density in hummingbird flight muscle. *Respir Physiol.* 89(1):113–32.

McElhaney, J.H., Roberts, V.L., and Hilyard, J.F. 1976. *Handbook of Human Tolerance.* Japan Automobile Research Institute, Inc. (JARI), Tokyo, Japan.

Morgan, D.L. 1990. New insights into the behavior of muscle during active lengthening. *Biophys J.* 57(2):209–221.

Mow, V.C., Kuei, S.C., Lai, W.M., and Armstrong, C.G. 1980. Biphasic creep and stress relaxation of articular cartilage in compression: Theory and experiments. *J Biomech. Eng.* 102:73–84.

Page, S.G. 1969. Structure and some contractile properties of fast and slow muscles of the chicken. *J Physiol.* 205(1):131–45.

Page, S.G. and Huxley, H.E. 1996. Filament lengths in striated muscle. *J Cell Biol.* 19:369–90.

Park, H. and Durand, D.M. 2008. Motion control of musculoskeletal systems with redundancy. *Biol. Cybern.* 99(6):503–516.

Perreault, E.J., Heckman, C.J., and Sandercock, T.G. 2003. Hill muscle model errors during movement are greatest within the physiologically relevant range of motor unit firing rates. *J. Biomech.* 36(2):211–218.

Powell, P.L., Roy, R.R., Kanim, P., Bello, M.A., and Edgerton, V.R. 1984. Predictability of skeletal muscle tension from architectural determinations in guinea pig hindlimbs. *J. Appl. Physiol.* 57:1715–1721.

Rack, P.M. and Westbury, D.R. 1969. The effects of length and stimulus rate on tension on the isometric cat soleus muscle. *J. Physiol.* 204(2): 443–460.

Sosnicki, A.A., Loesser, K.E., and Rome, L.C. 1991. Myofilament overlap in swimming carp. I. Myofilament lengths of red and white muscle. *Am J Physiol.* 260(2 Pt1):C283–8.

Thelen, D.G. and Anderson, F.C. 2006. Using computed muscle control to generate forward dynamic simulations of human walking from experimental data. *J. Biomech.* 39(6):1107–1115.

Walker, S.M. and Schrodt, G.R. 1974. I segment lengths and thin filament periods in skeletal muscle fibers of the Rhesus monkey and the human. *Anatomical Record* 178, 63–81.

Ward, S.R., Eng, C.M., Smallwood, L.H. and Lieber, R.L. 2009. Are current measurements of lower extremity muscle architecture accurate? *Clin Orthop Relat Res.* 467:1074–82.

Wayne, J.S., Woo, S.L., and Kwan, M.K. 1991. Application of the u-p finite element method to the study of articular cartilage. *J. Biomech. Eng.* 113:397–403.

Weiss, J.A. and Gardiner, J.C. 2001. Computational modeling of ligament mechanics. *Crit. Rev. Biomed. Eng.* 29:303–371.

Wells, J.B. 1965. Comparison of Mechanical Properties between Slow and Fast Mammalian Muscles. *J Physiol.* 178, 252–69.

Wickiewicz, T.L., Roy, R.R., Powell, P.L., and Edgerton, V.R. 1983. Muscle architecture of the human lower limb. *Clin. Orthop. Rel. Res.* 179:275–283.

Woo, S.L., Ritter, M.A., Amiel, D., Sanders, T.M., Gomez, M.A., Kuei, S.C., Garfin, S.R., and Akeson, W.H. 1980. The biomechanical and biochemical properties of swine tendons—long term effects of exercise on the digital extensors. *Connect Tissue Res.* 7(3):177–183.

Yin, Y. and Elliott, D.M. 2003. A biphasic and transversely isotropic mechanical model for tendon: Application to mouse tail fascicles in uniaxial tension. *J. Biomech.* 37(6):907–914.

Zahalak, G.I. and Ma S.P. 1990. Muscle activation and contraction: Constitutive relations based directly on cross-bridge kinetics. *J. Biomech. Eng.* 112:52–62.

Zajac, F.E. 1989. Muscle, and tendon: Properties, models, scaling and application to biomechanics and motor control. *CRC Crit. Rev. Biomed. Eng.* CRC Press, Inc. 17:359–411.

3

Joint-Articulating Surface Motion

Kenton R. Kaufman
Mayo Clinic

Kai-Nan An
Mayo Clinic

3.1 Introduction

Knowledge of joint-articulating surface motion is essential for design of prosthetic devices to restore function; assessment of joint wear, stability, and degeneration; and determination of proper diagnosis and surgical treatment of joint disease. In general, kinematic analysis of human movement can be arranged into two separate categories, (1) gross movement of the limb segments interconnected by joints, or (2) detailed analysis of joint articulating surface motion which is described in this chapter. Gross movement is the relative three-dimensional joint rotation as described by adopting the Eulerian angle system. Movement of this type is described in Chapter 5: Analysis of Gait. In general, the three-dimensional unconstrained rotation and translation of an articulating joint can be described utilizing the concept of the screw displacement axis. The most commonly used analytic method for the description

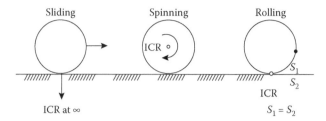

FIGURE 3.1   Three types of articulating surface motion in human joints.

of 6-degree-of-freedom displacement of a rigid body is the screw displacement axis (Kinzel et al., 1972; Spoor and Veldpaus, 1980; Woltring et al., 1985).

Various degrees of simplification have been used for kinematic modeling of joints. A hinged joint is the simplest and most common model used to simulate an anatomic joint in planar motion about a single axis embedded in the fixed segment. Experimental methods have been developed for determination of the instantaneous center of rotation for planar motion. The *instantaneous center of rotation* is defined as the point of zero velocity. For a true hinged motion, the instantaneous center of rotation will be a fixed point throughout the movement. Otherwise, loci of the instantaneous center of rotation or centrodes will exist. The center of curvature has also been used to define joint anatomy. The *center of curvature* is defined as the geometric center of coordinates of the articulating surface.

For more general planar motion of an articulating surface, the term *sliding, rolling,* and *spinning* are commonly used (Figure 3.1). Sliding (gliding) motion is defined as the pure translation of a moving segment against the surface of a fixed segment. The contact point of the moving segment does not change, while the contact point of the fixed segment has a constantly changing contact point. If the surface of the fixed segment is flat, the instantaneous center of rotation is located at infinity. Otherwise, it is located at the center of curvature of the fixed surface. Spinning motion (rotation) is the exact opposite of sliding motion. In this case, the moving segment rotates, and the contact points on the fixed surface does not change. The instantaneous center of rotation is located at the center of curvature of the spinning body that is undergoing pure rotation. Rolling motion occurs between moving and fixed segments where the contact points in each surface are constantly changing and the arc lengths of contact are equal on each segment. The instantaneous center of rolling motion is located at the contact point. Most planar motion of anatomic joints can be described by using any two of these three basic descriptions.

In this chapter, various aspects of joint-articulating motion are covered. Topics include the anatomical characteristics, joint contact, and axes of rotation. Joints of both the upper and lower extremity are discussed.

3.2 Ankle

The ankle joint is composed of two joints: the talocrural (ankle) joint and the talocalcaneal (subtalar joint). The talocrural joint is formed by the articulation of the distal tibia and fibula with the trochlea of the talus. The talocalcaneal joint is formed by the articulation of the talus with the calcaneus.

3.2.1 Geometry of the Articulating Surfaces

Morphological measurements of the ankle joint were collected in 36 normal subjects using a radiographic measurement method (Stagni et al., 2005). Three-dimensional characteristics of this articulation were collected (Figure 3.2, Table 3.1). A significant correlation was found among some of the measures but none of the measures correlated with malleolar width. Most measurements were larger in the male group than in the female group but these differences were not significantly different.

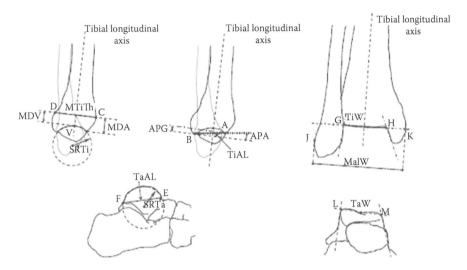

FIGURE 3.2 Sketch of the sagittal (a) and frontal (b) profiles of the tibio-fibular and talar segments. The relevant measurements taken in this work are schematically illustrated. (From Stagni R. et al., 2005. *Clin Biomech*, 20, 307–311. With permission.)

The upper articular surface of the talus is wedge-shaped, its width diminishing from front to back. The talus can be represented by a conical surface. The superior talar dome surface has an average anterior width of 29.9 ± 2.6 mm, a middle width of 27.9 ± 3.0 mm, and a posterior width of 25.2 ± 3.7 mm. Thus, the wedge shape of the talus is about 20% wider in front than behind. The talar dome radius is 20.7 ± 2.6 mm (Hayes et al., 2006). The wedge shape of the talus is about 25% wider in front than behind with an average difference of 2.4 ± 1.3 mm and a maximal difference of 6 mm (Inman, 1976).

3.2.2 Joint Contact

The talocrural joint contact area varies with flexion of the ankle (Table 3.2). During plantarflexion, such as would occur during the early stance phase of gait, the contact area is limited and the joint is incongruous. As the position of the joint progresses from neutral to dorsiflexion, as would occur during the midstance of gait, the contact area increases and the joint becomes more stable. The area of the subtalar articulation is smaller than that of the talocrural joint. The contact area of the subtalar joint is 0.89 ± 0.21 cm^2 for the posterior facet and 0.28 ± 15 cm^2 for the anterior and middle facets (Wang et al., 1994). The total contact area (1.18 ± 0.35 cm^2) is only 12.7% of the whole subtalar articulation area (9.31 ± 0.66 cm^2) (Wang et al., 1994). The contact area/joint area ratio increases with increases in applied load (Figure 3.3).

3.2.3 Axes of Rotation

Joint motion of the talocrural joint has been studied to define the axes of rotation and their location with respect to specific anatomic landmarks (Table 3.3). The axis of motion of the talocrural joint essentially passes through the inferior tibia at the fibular and tibial malleoli (Figure 3.4). Three types of motion have been used to describe the axes of rotation: fixed, quasi-instantaneous, and instantaneous axes. The motion that occurs in the ankle joints consists of dorsiflexion and plantarflexion. Minimal or no transverse rotation takes place within the talocrural joint. The motion in the talocrural joint is intimately related to the motion in the talocalcaneal joint which is described next.

The motion axes of the talocalcaneal joint have been described by several authors (Table 3.4). The axis of motion in the talocalcaneal joint passes from the anterior medial superior aspect of the navicular bone to the posterior lateral inferior aspect of the calcaneus (Figure 3.5). The motion that occurs in the talocalcaneal joint consists of inversion and eversion.

TABLE 3.1 Morphometry of the Ankle Joint

Measurement	Abbreviation Used in Figure 3.2	All (n = 36)					Male (n = 23)					Female (n = 13)					Male > Female
		Mean	SD	Max	Min	Median	Mean	SD	Max	Min	Median	Mean	SD	Max	Min	Median	P Value
Tibial arc length	TiAL	31.4	3.5	39.8	24.3	31.5	33.1	2.7	39.8	28.8	33.3	28.1	2.5	34.6	24.3	27.8	0.99
Sagittal radius of the tibial mortise	SRTi	27.8	4.4	34.9	21.2	26.8	29.3	4.2	41.5	23.1	27.9	24.7	4.4	32.4	21.2	24.1	0.97
Anteroposterior gap	APG	2.7	1.8	6.8	0.0	2.5	2.6	1.6	5.5	0.1	2.6	2.7	2.3	6.8	0.0	2.4	0.01
Anteroposterior inclination angle of the tibial mortise	APA	5.0	3.4	12.4	0.0	5.1	4.7	2.9	10.1	0.2	4.8	5.5	4.3	12.4	0.0	5.4	0.03
Tibial width	TiW	31.9	3.5	40.4	25.9	32.1	33.6	2.8	40.4	27.0	33.6	28.6	2.1	31.9	25.9	29.1	0.99
Malleolar width	MalW	69.0	7.6	79.6	54.0	69.9	71.0	7.4	79.6	54.0	71.9	63.5	5.1	70.3	55.1	63.4	0.91
Trochlea tali length	TaAL	41.7	4.4	49.6	34.2	41.5	43.6	3.9	49.6	35.1	44.2	37.9	2.4	41.6	34.2	37.6	0.99
Sagittal radius of the trochlea tali arc	SRTa	23.4	3.1	32.5	19.1	23.3	24.5	3.0	32.5	19.9	24.5	21.1	1.9	26.4	19.1	20.9	0.98
Tarsal width	TaW	30.4	3.3	40.2	24.2	30.1	31.5	3.5	40.2	24.2	31.9	28.3	1.4	31.0	26.2	28.1	0.97
Maximal tibial thickness	MTiTh	41.4	3.9	48.9	33.7	41.2	42.2	3.6	48.9	33.7	43.2	38.3	2.2	41.2	33.7	38.7	0.99
Distance of level of MTiTh from the vertex of the mortise	MDV	8.7	3.5	18.0	3.2	8.0	9.3	2.9	16.5	5.6	8.1	7.7	4.2	18.0	3.2	7.3	0.29
Distance of level of MTiTh from the anterior limit of the mortise	MDA	11.5	3.5	21.4	6.7	10.7	12.2	3.2	20.4	8.0	11.2	10.4	3.9	21.4	6.7	9.6	0.14

Source: Stagni R et al., 2005. *Clin. Biomech.*, 20: 307–311.
Note: All measurements in mm but APA in degrees.

TABLE 3.2 Talocalcaneal (Ankle) Joint Contact Area

Investigators	Plantarflexion	Neutral	Dorsiflexion
Ramsey and Hamilton (1976)		4.40 ± 1.21	
Kimizuka et al. (1980)		4.83	
Libotte et al. (1982)	5.01 (30°)	5.41	3.60 (30°)
Paar et al. (1983)	4.15 (10°)	4.15	3.63 (10°)
Macko et al. (1991)	3.81 ± 0.93 (15°)	5.2 ± 0.94	5.40 ± 0.74 (10°)
Driscoll et al. (1994)	2.70 ± 0.41 (20°)	3.27 ± 0.32	2.84 ± 0.43 (20°)
Hartford et al. (1995)		3.37 ± 0.52	
Pereira et al. (1996)	1.49 (20°)	1.67	1.47 (10°)
Rosenbaum et al. (2003)		2.11 ± 0.72	

Note: The contact area is expressed in square centimeters.

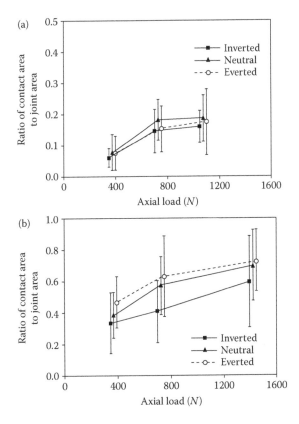

FIGURE 3.3 Ratio of total contact area to joint area in the (a) anterior/middle facet and (b) posterior facet of the subtalar joint as a function of applied axial load for three different positions of the foot. (From Wagner U.A. et al. 1992. *J. Orthop. Res.* 10: 535. With permission.)

3.3 Knee

The knee is the intermediate joint of the lower limb. It is composed of the distal femur and proximal tibia. It is the largest and most complex joint in the body. The knee joint is composed of the tibiofemoral articulation and the patellofemoral articulation.

TABLE 3.3 Axis of Rotation for the Ankle

Investigators	Axis[a]	Position
Elftman (1945)	Fix.	67.6 ± 7.4° with respect to sagittal plane
Isman and Inman (1969)	Fix.	8 mm anterior, 3 mm inferior to the distal tip of the lateral malleolus; 1 mm posterior, 5 mm inferior to the distal tip of the medial malleolus
Inman and Mann (1979)	Fix.	79° (68–88°) with respect to the sagittal plane
Allard et al. (1987)	Fix.	95.4 ± 6.6° with respect to the frontal plane, 77.7 ± 12.3° with respect to the sagittal plane, and 17.9 ± 4.5° with respect to the transverse plane
Singh et al. (1992)	Fix.	3.0 mm anterior, 2.5 mm inferior to distal tip of lateral malleolus; 2.2 mm posterior, 10 mm inferior to distal tip of medial malleolus
Sammarco et al. (1973)	Ins.	Inside and outside the body of the talus
D'Ambrosia et al. (1976)	Ins.	No consistent pattern
Parlasca et al. (1979)	Ins.	96% within 12 mm of a point 20 mm below the articular surface of the tibia along the long axis
Van Langelaan (1983)	Ins.	At an approximate right angle to the longitudinal direction of the foot, passing through the corpus tali, with a direction from anterolaterosuperior to posteromedioinferior
Barnett and Napier	Q-I	Dorsiflexion: down and lateral
		Plantarflexion: down and medial
Hicks (1953)	Q-I	Dorsiflexion: 5 mm inferior to tip of lateral malleolus to 15 mm anterior to tip of medial malleolus
		Plantarflexion: 5 mm superior to tip of lateral malleolus to 15 mm anterior, 10 mm inferior to tip of medial malleolus

[a] Fix. = fixed axis of rotation; Ins. = instantaneous axis of rotation; Q-I = quasi-instantaneous axis of rotation.

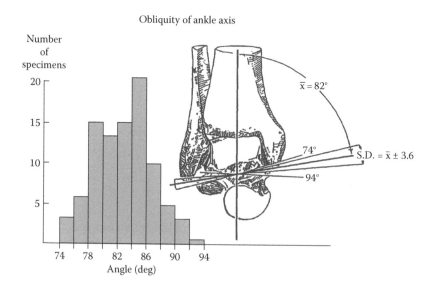

FIGURE 3.4 Variations in angle between middle of tibia and empirical axis of ankle. The histogram reveals a considerable spread of individual values. (From Inman V.T. 1976. *The Joints of the Ankle*, Baltimore, Williams and Wilkins. With permission.)

TABLE 3.4   Axis of Rotation for the Talocalcaneal (Subtalar) Joint

Investigators	Axis[a]	Position
Manter (1941)	Fix.	16° (8–24°) with respect to sagittal plane, and 42° (29–47°) with respect to transverse plane
Shephard (1951)	Fix.	Tuberosity of the calcaneus to the neck of the talus
Hicks (1953)	Fix.	Posterolateral corner of the heel to superomedial aspect of the neck of the talus
Root et al. (1966)	Fix.	17° (8–29°) with respect to sagittal plane, and 41° (22–55°) with respect to transverse plane
Isman and Inman (1969)	Fix.	23° ± 11° with respect to sagittal plane, and 41° ± 9° with respect to transverse plane
Kirby (1947)	Fix.	Extends from the posterolateral heel, posteriorly, to the first intermetatarsal space, anteriorly
Rastegar et al. (1980)	Ins.	Instant centers of rotation pathways in posterolateral quadrant of the distal articulating tibial surface, varying with applied load
Van Langelaan (1983)	Ins.	A bundle of axes that make an acute angle with the longitudinal direction of the foot passing through the tarsal canal having a direction from anteromediosuperior to posterolateroinferior
Engsberg (1987)	Ins.	A bundle of axes with a direction from anteromediosuperior to posterolateroinferior

[a] Fix. = fixed axis of rotation; Ins. = instantaneous axis of rotation.

3.3.1 Geometry of the Articulating Surfaces

The shape of the articular surfaces of the proximal tibia and distal femur must fulfill the requirement that they move in contact with one another. The profile of the femoral condyles varies with the condyle examined (Figure 3.6 and Table 3.5). The tibial plateau widths are greater than the corresponding widths of the femoral condyles (Figure 3.7 and Table 3.6). However, the tibial plateau depths are less than those of the femoral condyle distances. The medial and lateral tibial plateaus have a posterior slope in the sagittal plane (Table 3.7). The medial and lateral tibial slopes are greater in female subjects than in male subjects ($p < 0.05$) (Hashemi et al., 2008). There is also a slope in the coronal plane with the lateral point of the tibial plateau located proximal to the medial point (Table 3.7). The medial condyle of the tibia is concave superiorly (the center of curvature lies above the tibial surface) with a radius of curvature of 80 mm (Kapandji, 1987). The lateral condyle is convex superiorly (the center of curvature lies below the tibial surface) with a radius of curvature of 70 mm (Kapandji, 1987). The shape of the femoral surfaces is complementary to the shape of the tibial plateaus. The shape of the posterior femoral condyles may be approximated by spherical surfaces (Table 3.8).

The geometry of the patellofemoral articular surfaces remains relatively constant as the knee flexes. The knee sulcus angle changes only ±3.4° from 15° to 75° of knee flexion (Figure 3.8). The mean depth index varies by only ±4% over the same flexion range (Figure 3.8). Similarly, the medial and lateral patellar facet angles (Figure 3.9) change by less than a degree throughout the entire knee flexion range (Table 3.9). However, there is a significant difference between the magnitude of the medial and lateral patellar facet angles.

3.3.2 Joint Contact

The mechanism for movement between the femur and tibia is a combination of rolling and gliding. Backward movement of the femur on the tibia during flexion has long been observed in the human knee. The magnitude of the rolling and gliding changes through the range of flexion. The tibiofemoral contact area decreases as the knee flexion increases (Table 3.10). The tibial–femoral contact point has been shown to move posteriorly as the knee is flexed, reflecting the coupling of posterior motion with

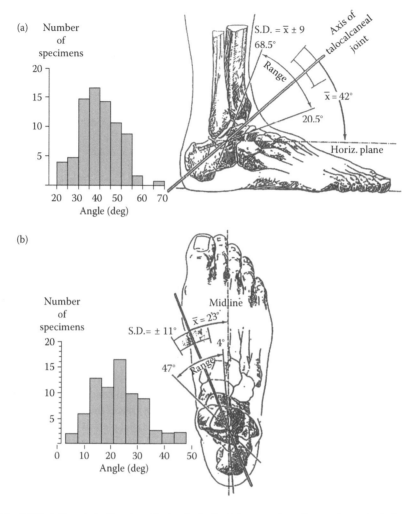

FIGURE 3.5   (a) Variations in inclination of axis of subtalar joint as projected upon the sagittal plane. The distribution of the measurements on the individual specimens is shown in the histogram. The single observation of an
angle of almost 70° was present in a markedly cavus foot. (b) Variations in position of subtalar axis as projected onto
the transverse plane. The angle was measured between the axis and the midline of the foot. The extent of individual
variation is shown on the sketch and revealed in the histogram. (From Inman V.T. 1976. *The Joints of the Ankle*,
Baltimore, Williams and Wilkins. With permission.)

flexion (Figure 3.10). In the intact knee at full extension, the center of pressure is approximately 25 mm
from the anterior edge of the tibial plateau (Andriacchi et al., 1986). The medial femoral condyle rests
further anteriorly on the tibial plateau than the lateral plateau. The medial femoral condyle is positioned
35 ± 4 mm from the posterior edge while the lateral femoral condyle is positioned 25 ± 4 mm from the
posterior edge (Figure 3.10). During knee flexion to 90°, the medial femoral condyle moves back by
15 ± 2 mm and the lateral femoral condyle moves back by 12 ± 2 mm. Thus, during flexion, the femur
moves posteriorly on the tibia (Table 3.11).

The patellofemoral contact area is smaller than the tibiofemoral contact area (Table 3.12). As the
knee joint moves from extension to flexion, a band of contact moves upward over the patellar surface
(Figure 3.11). As knee flexion increases, not only does the contact area move superiorly, but it also becomes
larger. At 90° of knee flexion, the contact area has reached the upper level of the patella. As the knee

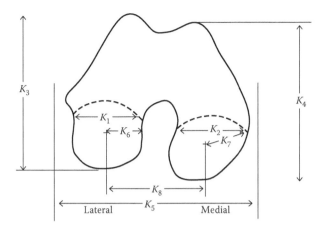

FIGURE 3.6 Geometry of the distal femur. The distances are defined in Table 3.5.

TABLE 3.5 Geometry of the Distal Femur

| Parameter | Condyle | | | | | | | |
| | Lateral | | Medial | | Overall | | | |
	Symbol	Distance (mm)	Symbol	Distance (mm)	Symbol	Distance (mm)
Medial/lateral distance	K_1	31 ± 2.3 (male)	K_2	32 ± 31 (male)		
		28 ± 1.8 (female)		27 ± 3.1 (female)		
Anterior/posterior distance	K_3	72 ± 4.0 (male)	K_4	70 ± 4.3 (male)		
		65 ± 3.7 (female)		63 ± 4.5 (female)		
Posterior femoral condyle spherical radii	K_6	19.2 ± 1.7	K_7	20.8 ± 2.4		
Epicondylar width					K_5	90 ± 6 (male)
						80 ± 6 (female)
Medial/lateral spacing of center of spherical surfaces					K_8	45.9 ± 3.4

Source: Yoshioka Y., Siu D., and Cooke T.D.V. 1987. *J. Bone Joint Surg.* 69A: 873–880; Kurosawa H. et al. 1985. *J. Biomech.* 18: 487.

Note: See Figure 3.6 for location of measurements.

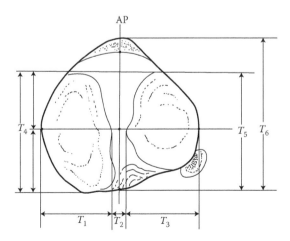

FIGURE 3.7 Contour of the tibial plateau (transverse plane). The distances are defined in Table 3.6.

TABLE 3.6   Geometry of the Proximal Tibia

Parameter	Symbols	All Limbs	Male	Female
Tibial plateau with widths (mm)				
Medial plateau	T_1	32 ± 3.8	34 ± 3.9	30 ± 22
Lateral plateau	T_3	33 ± 2.6	35 ± 1.9	31 ± 1.7
Overall width	$T_1 + T_2 + T_3$	76 ± 6.2	81 ± 4.5	73 ± 4.5
Tibial plateau depths (mm)				
AP depth, medial	T_4	48 ± 5.0	52 ± 3.4	45 ± 4.1
AP depth, lateral	T_5	42 ± 3.7	45 ± 3.1	40 ± 2.3
Interspinous width (mm)	T_2	12 ± 1.7	12 ± 0.9	12 ± 2.2
Intercondylar depth (mm)	T_6	48 ± 5.9	52 ± 5.7	45 ± 3.9

Source: Yoshioka Y. et al. 1989. *J. Orthop. Res.* 7: 132.

TABLE 3.7   Tibial Plateau Slope (deg)

Gender	Sagittal Plane		Coronal Plane
	Medial Plateau	Lateral Plateau	
Female ($n = 33$)	5.9 ± 3.0	7.0 ± 3.1	2.5 ± 1.9
Male ($n = 22$)	3.7 ± 3.1	5.4 ± 2.8	3.5 ± 1.9
P Value	0.01	0.02	0.03

Source: Hashemi J et al. 2008. *J. Bone Joint Surg.—Am.* Vol. 90: 2724–2734.

TABLE 3.8   Posterior Femoral Condyle Spherical Radius

	Normal Knee	Varus Knees	Valgus Knees
Medial condyle	20.3 ± 3.4 (16.1–28.0)	21.2 ± 2.1 (18.0–24.5)	21.1 ± 2.0 (17.84–24.1)
Lateral condyle	19.0 ± 3.0 (14.7–25.0)	20.8 ± 2.1 (17.5–30.0)	$21.1^a \pm 2.1$ (18.4–25.5)

Source: Matsuda S. et al. 2004. *J. Ortho. Res.* 22: 104–109.
[a] Significantly different from normal knees ($p < 0.05$).

continues to flex, the contact area is divided into separate medial and lateral zones. Under weight-bearing conditions, the contact area is increased by an average of 24% (Besier et al., 2005). When normalized by patellar dimensions (*Ht* × *Wt*), the contact areas are no different between genders (Besier et al., 2005).

3.3.3 Axes of Rotation

The tibiofemoral joint is mainly a joint with two degrees of freedom. The first degree of freedom allows movements of flexion and extension in the sagittal plane. The axis of rotation lies perpendicular to the sagittal plane and intersects the femoral condyles. Both fixed axes and screw axes have been calculated (Figure 3.12). In Figure 3.12, the optimal axes are fixed axes, whereas the screw axis is an instantaneous axis. The symmetric optimal axis is constrained such that the axis is the same for both the right and left knee. The screw axis may sometimes coincide with the optimal axis but not always, depending upon the motions of the knee joint. The second degree of freedom is the axial rotation around the long axis of the tibia. Rotation of the leg around its long axis can only be performed with the knee flexed. There is also an automatic axial rotation which is involuntarily linked to flexion and extension. When the knee is flexed, the tibia internally rotates. Conversely, when the knee is extended, the tibia externally rotates.

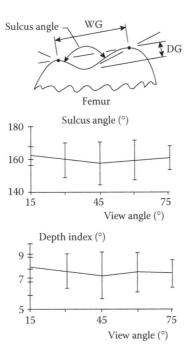

FIGURE 3.8 The trochlear geometry indices. The sulcus angle is the angle formed by the lines drawn from the top of the medial and lateral condyles to the deepest point of the sulcus. The depth index is the ratio of the width of the groove (WG) to the depth (DG). Mean and SD; $n = 12$. (From Farahmand et al. 1988. *J. Orthop. Res.* 16: 1, 136.)

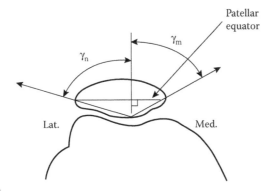

FIGURE 3.9 Medial (γ_m) and lateral (γ_n) patellar facet angles. (From Ahmed A.M., Burke D.L., and Hyder A. 1987. *J. Orthop. Res.* 5: 69–85.)

TABLE 3.9 Patellar Facet Angles

Facet angle (deg)	Knee Flexion Angle				
	0	30	60	90	120
γ_m (deg)	60.88	60.96	61.43	61.30	60.34
	3.89[a]	4.70	4.12	4.18	4.51
γ_n (deg)	67.76	68.05	68.36	68.39	68.20
	4.15	3.97	3.63	4.01	3.67

Source: Ahmed A.M., Burke D.L., and Hyder A. 1987. *J. Orthop. Res.* 5: 69–85.
[a] SD.

TABLE 3.10   Tibiofemoral Contact Area

Knee Flexion (deg)	Contact Area (cm²)
−5	20.2
5	19.8
15	19.2
25	18.2
35	14.0
45	13.4
55	11.8
65	13.6
75	11.4
85	12.1

Source: Maquet P.G., Vandberg A.J., and Simonet J.C. 1975. *J. Bone Joint Surg.* 57A: 766–771.

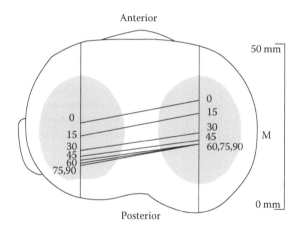

FIGURE 3.10   Diagram of the tibial plateau, showing the tibiofemoral contact pattern from 0° to 90° of knee flexion, in the loaded knee. In both medial and lateral compartments, the femoral condyle rolls back along the tibial plateau from 0° to 30°. Between 30° and 90° the lateral condyle continues to move posteriorly, while the medial condyle moves back little. (From Scarvell, J.M. et al. 2004. *J. Orthop. Res.* 22: 788–793.)

TABLE 3.11   Posterior Displacement of the Femur Relative to the Tibia

Authors	Condition	A/P Displacement (mm)
Kurosawa (1985)	*In vitro*	14.8
Andriacchi (1986)	*In vitro*	13.5
Draganich et al. (1987)	*In vitro*	13.5
Nahass et al. (1991)	*In vivo* (walking)	12.5
	In vivo (stairs)	13.9

During knee flexion, the patella makes a rolling/gliding motion along the femoral articulating surface. Throughout the entire flexion range, the gliding motion is clockwise (Figure 3.13). In contrast, the direction of the rolling motion is counter-clockwise between 0° and 90° and clockwise between 90° and 120° (Figure 3.13). The mean amount of patellar gliding for all knees is approximately 6.5 mm per 10° of flexion between 0° and 80° and 4.5 mm per 10° of flexion between 80° and 120°. The relationship

TABLE 3.12 Patellofemoral Contact Area

Knee Flexion (deg)	Contact Area (cm²)
20	2.6 ± 0.4
30	3.1 ± 0.3
60	3.9 ± 0.6
90	4.1 ± 1.2
120	4.6 ± 0.7

Source: Huberti H.H. and Hayes W.C. 1984. *J. Bone Joint Surg.* 66A: 715–725.

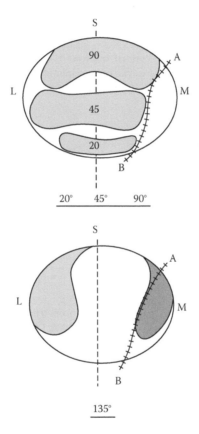

FIGURE 3.11 Diagrammatic representation of patella contact areas for varying degrees of knee flexion. (From Goodfellow J., Hungerford D.S., and Zindel M., 1976. *J. Bone Joint Surg.* 58-B: 3, 288. With permission.)

between the angle of flexion and the mean rolling/gliding ratio for all knees is shown in Figure 3.14. Between 80° and 90° of knee flexion, the rolling motion of the articulating surface comes to a standstill and then changes direction. The reversal in movement occurs at the flexion angle where the quadriceps tendon first contacts the femoral groove.

3.4 Hip

The hip joint is composed of the head of the femur and the acetabulum of the pelvis. The hip joint is one of the most stable joints in the body. The stability is provided by the rigid ball-and-socket configuration.

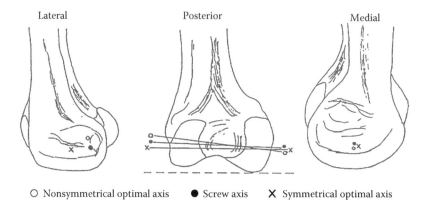

Lateral   Posterior   Medial

O Nonsymmetrical optimal axis   ● Screw axis   X Symmetrical optimal axis

FIGURE 3.12   Approximate location of the optimal axis (case 1—nonsymmetric, case 3—symmetric), and the screw axis (case 2) on the medial and lateral condyles of the femur of a human subject for the range of motion of 0–90° flexion (standing to sitting, respectively). (From Lewis J.L. and Lew W.D. 1978. *J. Biomech. Eng.* 100: 187. With permission.)

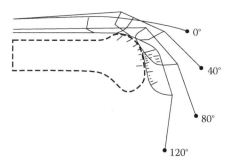

FIGURE 3.13   Position of patellar ligament, patella, and quadriceps tendon and location of the contact points as a function of the knee flexion angle. (From van Eijden T.M. et al. 1986. *J Biomech.* 19: 227. With permission.)

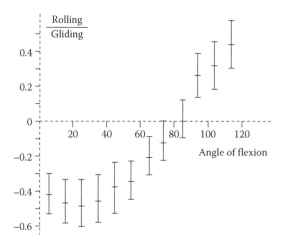

FIGURE 3.14   Calculated rolling/gliding ratio for the patellofemoral joint as a function of the knee flexion angle. (From van Eijden T.M. et al. 1986. *J Biomech.* 19: 226. With permission.)

3.4.1 Geometry of the Articulating Surfaces

The femoral head is spherical in its articular portion which forms two-thirds of a sphere. The diameter of the femoral head is smaller for female than for male individuals (Table 3.13). In the normal hip, the center of the femoral head coincides exactly with the center of the acetabulum. The rounded part of the femoral head is spheroidal rather than spherical because the uppermost part is flattened slightly. This causes the load to be distributed in a ringlike pattern around the superior pole. The geometrical center of the femoral head is traversed by the three axes of the joint, the horizontal axis, the vertical axis, and the anterior/posterior axis. The head is supported by the neck of the femur, which joins the shaft. The axis of the femoral neck is obliquely set and runs superiorly, medially, and anteriorly. The angle of inclination of the femoral neck to the shaft in the frontal plane is the neck–shaft angle (Figure 3.15). In most adults, this angle is about 130° (Table 3.13). An angle exceeding 130° is known as *coxa valga*; an angle less than 130° is known as *coxa vara*. The femoral neck forms an acute angle with the transverse axis of the femoral condyles. This angle faces medially and anteriorly and is called the *angle of anteversion* (Figure 3.16). In the adult, this angle averages about 7.5° (Table 3.13).

The acetabulum receives the femoral head and lies on the lateral aspect of the hip. The acetabulum of the adult is a hemispherical socket. Its cartilage area is approximately 16 cm² [(Von Lanz and Wauchsmuth, 1938). Together with the labrum, the acetabulum covers slightly more than 50% of the femoral head (Tönnis, 1987). Only the sides of the acetabulum are lined by articular cartilage, which is interrupted inferiorly by the deep acetabular notch. The central part of the cavity is deeper than the articular cartilage and is nonarticular. This part is called the *acetabular fossae* and is separated from the interface of the pelvic bone by a thin plate of bone.

TABLE 3.13   Geometry of the Proximal Femur

Parameter	Females	Males
Femoral head diameter (mm)	45.0 ± 3.0	52.0 ± 3.3
Neck shaft angle (deg)	133 ± 6.6	129 ± 7.3
Anteversion (deg)	8 ± 10	7.0 ± 6.8

Source: Yoshioka Y., Siu D., and Cooke T.D.V. 1987. *J. Bone Joint Surg.* 69A: 873.

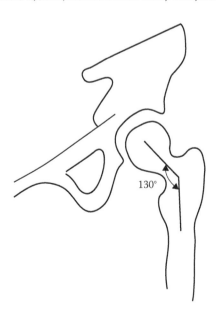

FIGURE 3.15   The neck–shaft angle.

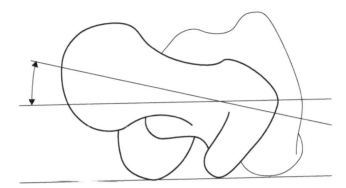

FIGURE 3.16 The normal anteversion angle formed by a line tangent to the femoral condyles and the femoral neck axis, as displayed in the superior view.

3.4.2 Joint Contact

Miyanaga et al. (1984) studied the deformation of the hip joint under loading, the contact area between the articular surfaces, and the contact pressures. They found that at loads up to 1000 N, pressure was distributed largely to the anterior and posterior parts of the lunate surface with very little pressure applied to the central portion of the roof itself. As the load increased, the contact area enlarged to include the outer and inner edges of the lunate surface (Figure 3.17). However, the highest pressures

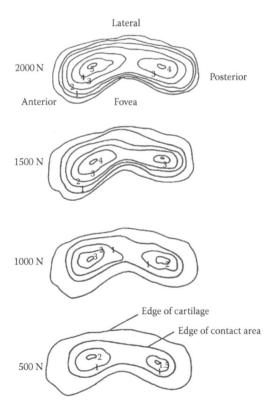

FIGURE 3.17 Pressure distribution and contact area of hip joint. The pressure is distributed largely to the anterior and posterior parts of the lunate surface. As the load increased, the contact area increased. (From Miyanaga Y., Fukubayashi T., and Kurosawa H. 1984. *Arch. Orth. Trauma Surg.* 103: 13–17. With permission.)

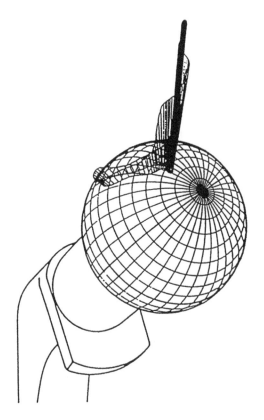

FIGURE 3.18 Scaled three-dimensional plot of resultant force during the gait cycle with crutches. The lengths of the lines indicate the magnitude of force. Radial line segments are drawn at equal increments of time, so the distance between the segments indicates the rate at which the orientation of the force was changing. For higher amplitudes of force during stance phase, line segments in close proximity indicate that the orientation of the force was changing relatively little with the cone angle between 30° and 40° and the polar angle between −25° and −15°. (From Davy D.T. et al. 1989. *J. Bone Joint Surg.* 70A: 45. With permission.)

were still measured anteriorly and posteriorly. Of five hip joints studied, only one had a pressure maximum at the zenith or central part of the acetabulum.

Davy et al. (1989) utilized a telemetered total hip prosthesis to measure forces across the hip after total hip arthroplasty. The orientation of the resultant joint contact force varies over a relatively limited range during the weight-load-bearing portions of gait. Generally, the joint contact force on the ball of the hip prosthesis is located in the anterior/superior region. A three-dimensional plot of the resultant joint force during the gait cycle, with crutches, is shown in Figure 3.18.

3.4.3 Axes of Rotation

The human hip is a modified spherical (ball-and-socket) joint. Thus, the hip possesses three degrees of freedom of motion with three correspondingly arranged, mutually perpendicular axes that intersect at the geometric center of rotation of the spherical head. The transverse axis lies in the frontal plane and controls movements of flexion and extension. An anterior/posterior axis lies in the sagittal plane and controls movements of adduction and abduction. A vertical axis which coincides with the long axis of the limb when the hip joint is in the neutral position controls movements of internal and external rotation. Surface motion in the hip joint can be considered as spinning of the femoral head on the acetabulum. The pivoting of the bone socket in three planes around the center of rotation in the femoral head produces the spinning of the joint surfaces.

3.5 Shoulder

The shoulder represents the group of structures connecting the arm to the thorax. The combined movements of four distinct articulations—glenohumeral, acromioclavicular, sternoclavicular, and scapulo-thoracic—allow the arm to be positioned in space.

3.5.1 Geometry of the Articulating Surfaces

The articular surface of the humerus is approximately one-third of a sphere (Figure 3.19). The articular surface is oriented with an upward tilt of approximately 45° and is retroverted approximately 30° with respect to the condylar line of the distal humerus (Morrey and An, 1990). The average radius of curvature of the humeral head in the coronal plane is 24.0 ± 2.1 mm (Iannotti et al., 1992). The radius of curvature in the anteroposterior and axillary-lateral view is similar, measuring 13.1 ± 1.3 and 22.9 ± 2.9 mm, respectively (McPherson et al., 1997). The humeral articulating surface is spherical in the center. However, the peripheral radius is 2 mm less in the axial plane than in the coronal plane. Thus, the peripheral contour of the articular surface is elliptical with a ratio of 0.92 (Iannotti et al., 1992). The major axis is superior to inferior and the minor axis is anterior to posterior (McPherson et al., 1997). More recently, the three-dimensional geometry of the proximal humerus has been studied extensively. The articular surface, which is part of a sphere, varies individually in its orientation with respect to inclination and retroversion, and it has variable medial and posterior offsets (Boileau and Walch, 1997). These findings have great impact in implant design and placement in order to restore soft-tissue function.

The glenoid fossa consists of a small, pear-shaped, cartilage-covered bony depression that measures 39.0 ± 3.5 mm in the superior/inferior direction and 29.0 ± 3.2 mm in the anterior/posterior direction (Iannotti et al., 1992). The anterior/posterior dimension of the glenoid is pear-shaped with the lower half being larger than the top half. The ratio of the lower half to the top half is 1:0.80 ± 0.01 (Iannotti et al., 1992). The glenoid radius of curvature is 32.2 ± 7.6 mm in the anteroposterior view and 40.6 ± 14.0 mm in the axillary–lateral view (McPherson et al., 1997). The glenoid is therefore more curved superior to inferior (coronal plane) and relatively flatter in an anterior to posterior direction (sagittal plane). Glenoid

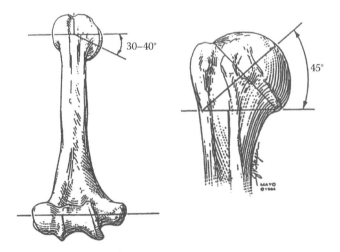

FIGURE 3.19 The two-dimensional orientation of the articular surface of the humerus with respect to the bicondylar axis. (With permission of the Mayo Foundation.)

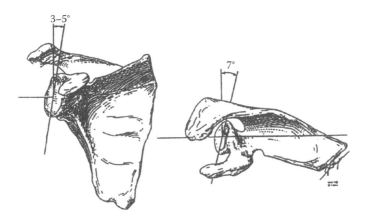

FIGURE 3.20 The glenoid faces slightly superior and posterior (retroverted) with respect to the body of the scapula. (With permission of the Mayo Foundation.)

depth is 5.0 ± 1.1 mm in the anteroposterior view and 2.9 ± 1.0 mm in the axillary–lateral (McPherson et al., 1997), again confirming that the glenoid is more curved superior to inferior. In the coronal plane the articular surface of the glenoid comprises an arc of approximately 75° and in the transverse plane the arc of curvature of the glenoid is about 50° (Morrey and An, 1990). The glenoid has a slight upward tilt of about 5° (Basmajian and Bazant, 1959) with respect to the medial border of the scapula (Figure 3.20) and is retroverted a mean of approximately 7° (Saha, 1971). The relationship of the dimension of the humeral head to the glenoid head is approximately 0.8 in the coronal plane and 0.6 in the horizontal or transverse plane (Saha, 1971). The surface area of the glenoid fossa is only one-third to one-fourth that of the humeral head (Kent, 1971). The arcs of articular cartilage on the humeral head and glenoid in the frontal and axial planes were measured (Jobe and Iannotti, 1995). In the coronal plane, the humeral heads had an arc of 159° covered by 96° of glenoid, leaving 63° of cartilage uncovered. In the transverse plane, the humeral arc of 160° is opposed by 74° of glenoid, leaving 86° uncovered.

3.5.2 Joint Contact

The degree of conformity and constraint between the humeral head and glenoid has been represented by conformity index (radius of head/radius of glenoid) and constraint index (arc of enclosure/360) (McPherson et al., 1997). Based on the study of 93 cadaveric specimens, the mean conformity index was 0.72 in the coronal and 0.63 in the sagittal plane. There was more constraint to the glenoid in the coronal versus sagittal plane (0.18 versus 0.13). These anatomic features help prevent superior–inferior translation of the humeral head but allow translation in the sagittal plane. Joint contact areas of the glenohumeral joint tend to be greater at mid-elevation positions than at either of the extremes of joint position (Table 3.14). These results suggest that the glenohumeral surface is maximum at these more functional positions, thus distributing joint load over a larger region in a more stable configuration. In general, the contact area between the glenohumeral joint over the glenolabral complex was between 49.0% and 61.5% of the calculated surface area for the intact specimens (Greis et al., 2002). The contact point moves forward and inferior during internal rotation (Figure 3.21). With external rotation, the contact is posterior/inferior. With elevation, the contact area moves superiorly. Lippitt and associates (1993) calculated the stability ratio, which is defined as a force necessary to translate the humeral head from the glenoid fossa divided by the compressive load times 100. The stability ratios were in the range of 50–60% in the superior–inferior direction and 30–40% in the anterior–posterior direction. After the labrum was removed, the ratio decreased by approximately 20%. Joint conformity was found to have significant influence on translations of humeral head during active positioning by muscles (Karduna et al., 1996).

TABLE 3.14   Glenohumeral Contact Areas

Elevation Angle (deg)	Contact Areas at SR (cm²)	Contact Areas at 20° Internal to SR (cm²)
0	0.87 ± 1.01	1.70 ± 1.68
30	2.09 ± 1.54	2.44 ± 2.15
60	3.48 ± 1.69	4.56 ± 1.84
90	4.95 ± 2.15	3.92 ± 2.10
120	5.07 ± 2.35	4.84 ± 1.84
150	3.52 ± 2.29	2.33 ± 1.47
180	2.59 ± 2.90	2.51 ± NA

Source: Soslowsky L.J. et al. 1992. *J. Orthop. Res.* 10: 524.

Note: SR, starting external rotation which allowed the shoulder to reach maximal elevation in the scapular plane (≈40° ± 8°); NA, not applicable.

The glenohumeral articular contact kinematics of normal healthy subjects and patients after total shoulder arthroplasty was assessed by using dual-plane fluoroscopic images and computer-aided design models (Boyer et al., 2008, Massimini et al., 2010). In all positions studied at 0°, 45°, and 90° of abduction, and maximal internal and external rotation, the centroid of contact on the glenoid surface for each individual, on average, was more than 5 mm away from the geometric center of the glenoid articular surface and on the humeral head surface, the centroids of contact were located at the superomedial quarter (Boyer et al., 2008). For patients with joint replacement, the superior–posterior quadrant seems to experience the most articular contact in all the shoulder positions tested. In a cadaveric experiment using Fiji film, the posterior edge loading was also consistently observed in the total shoulder specimens in positions of increased horizontal adduction and variably in positions of less adduction (Schamblin et al., 2009).

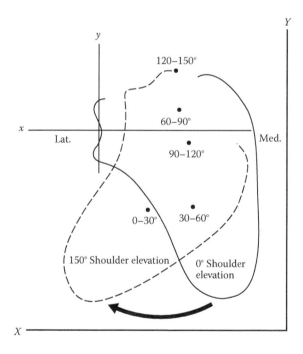

FIGURE 3.21   Humeral contact positions as a function of glenohumeral motion and positions. (From Morrey B.F. and An K.N. 1990. *The Shoulder*, pp. 208–245, Philadelphia, Saunders. With permission.)

TABLE 3.15   Arm Elevation: Glenohumeral–Scapulothoracic Rotation

Investigator	Glenohumeral/Scapulothoracic Motion Ratio
Inman et al. (1944)	2:1
Freedman and Munro (1966)	1.35:1
Doody et al. (1970)	1.74:1
Poppen and Walker (1976)	4.3:1 (<24° elevation)
	1.25:1 (>24° elevation)
Saha (1971)	2.3:1 (30–135° elevation)
Sugamoto (2002)	2.4 (Low speed)
	2.9 (High speed, 60° elevation)
	1.7 (High speed, 150° elevation)

3.5.3 Axes of Rotation

The shoulder complex consists of four distinct articulations: the glenohumeral joint, the acromioclavicular joint, the sternoclavicular joint, and the scapulothoracic articulation. The wide range of motion of the shoulder (exceeding a hemisphere) is the result of synchronous, simultaneous contributions from each joint. The most important function of the shoulder is arm elevation. Several investigators have attempted to relate glenohumeral and scapulothoracic motion during arm elevation in various planes (Table 3.15). About two-thirds of the motion takes place in the glenohumeral joint and about one-third in the scapulothoracic articulation, resulting in a 2:1 ratio. By using image intensifier combined with a video system, Sugamoto et al. (2002) found that the ratio can be influenced by the speed of rotation (Table 3.15).

Surface motion at the glenohumeral joint is primarily rotational. The center of rotation of the glenohumeral joint has been defined as a locus of points situated within 6.0 ± 1.8 mm of the geometric center of the humeral head (Poppen and Walker, 1976). However, the motion is not purely rotational. The humeral head displaces, with respect to the glenoid. From 0° to 30°, and often from 30° to 60°, the humeral head moves upward in the glenoid fossa by about 3 mm, indicating that rolling and/or gliding has taken place. Thereafter, the humeral head has only about 1 mm of additional excursion. During arm elevation in the scapular plane, the scapula moves in relation to the thorax (Poppen and Walker, 1976). From 0° to 30° the scapula rotates about its lower mid-portion, and then from 60° onward the center of rotation shifts toward the glenoid, resulting in a large lateral displacement of the inferior tip of the scapula (Figure 3.22). The center of rotation of the scapula for arm elevation is situated at the tip of the acromion as viewed from the edge on (Figure 3.23). The mean amount of scapular twisting at maximum arm elevation is 40°. The superior tip of the scapula moves away from the thorax, and the inferior tip moves toward it.

Recently, relative motion of the scapula with respect to the clavicle or the acromioclavicular joint motion was studied *in vivo* using 3D MR images obtained by a vertically open MRI (Sahara et al., 2006). They found that the scapula rotated about the clavicle at a specific screw axis passing through the insertions of both the acromioclavicular and the coracoclavicular ligaments on the coracoid process and the average rotation was 35° (Figure 3.24).

3.6 Elbow

The bony structures of the elbow are the distal end of the humerus and the proximal ends of the radius and ulna. The elbow joint complex allows two degrees of freedom in motion: flexion/extension and pronation/supination. The elbow joint complex is three separate synovial articulations. The humeral–ulnar joint is the articulation between the trochlea of the distal radius and the trochlear fossa of the proximal ulna. The humero–radial joint is formed by the articulation between the capitulum of the distal humerus and the head of the radius. The proximal radioulnar joint is formed by the head of the radius and the radial notch of the proximal ulna.

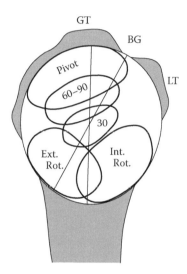

FIGURE 3.22 Rotation of the scapula on the thorax in the scapular plane. Instant centers of rotation (solid dots) are shown for each 30° interval of motion during shoulder elevation in the scapular plane from 0 to 150°. The *x* and *y* axes are fixed in the scapula, whereas the *X* and *Y* axes are fixed in the thorax. From 0 to 30° in the scapula rotated about its lower midportion; from 60° onward, rotation took place about the glenoid area, resulting in a medial and upward displacement of the glenoid face and a large lateral displacement of the inferior tip of the scapula. (From Poppen N.K. and Walker P.S. 1976. *J. Bone Joint Surg.* 58A: 195. With permission.)

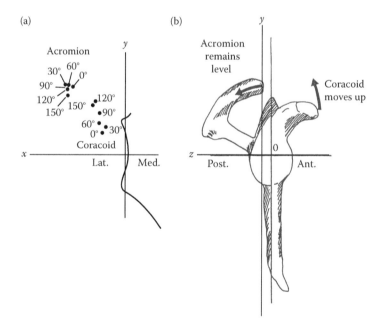

FIGURE 3.23 (a) A plot of the tips of the acromion and coracoid process on roentgenograms taken at successive intervals of arm elevation in the scapular plane shows upward movement of the coracoid and only a slight shift in the acromion relative to the glenoid face. This finding demonstrates twisting, or external rotation, of the scapula about the *x*-axis. (b) A lateral view of the scapula during this motion would show the coracoid process moving upward while the acromion remains on the same horizontal plane as the glenoid. (From Poppen N.K. and Walker P.S. 1976. *J. Bone Joint Surg.* 58A: 195. With permission.)

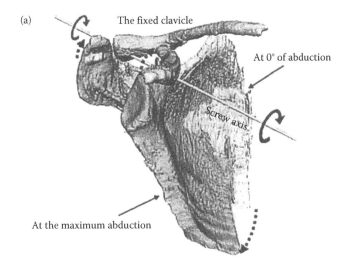

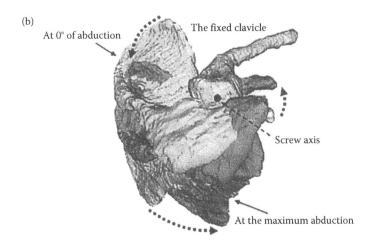

FIGURE 3.24 These figures show the motion of a representative case. The models of the scapula at both 0° (white) and the maximum abduction (gray) are shown when the clavicular motion is fixed. (a) Is in the anterior view. The white pole is the screw axis. (b) Is in the superolateral view of the acromion parallel to the screw axis. The black dot is the screw axis. The scapula relative to the clavicle was rotated counterclockwise on the screw axis in this view, and the average rotation around this axis was approximately 35°. (From Sahara W. et al. 2006. *J. Orthop. Res.*, 24, 1823–1831. With permission.)

3.6.1 Geometry of the Articulating Surfaces

The curved, articulating portions of the trochlea and capitulum are approximately circular in a cross-section. The radius of the capitulum is larger than the central trochlear groove (Table 3.16). The centers of curvature of the trochlea and capitulum lie in a straight line located on a plane that slopes at 45°–50° anterior and distal to the transepicondylar line and is inclined at 2.5° from the horizontal transverse plane (Shiba et al., 1988). The curves of the ulnar articulations form two surfaces (coronoid and olecranon) with centers on a line parallel to the transepicondylar line but are distinct from it (Shiba et al., 1988). The carrying angle is an angle made by the intersection of the longitudinal axis of the humerus and the forearm in the frontal plane with the elbow in an extended position. The carrying angle is contributed to, in part, by the oblique axis of the distal humerus and, in part, by the shape of the proximal ulna (Figure 3.25).

TABLE 3.16   Elbow Joint Geometry

Parameter	Size (mm)
Capitulum radius	10.6 ± 1.1
Lateral trochlear flange radius	10.8 ± 1.0
Central trochlear groove radius	8.8 ± 0.4
Medial trochlear groove radius	13.2 ± 1.4
Distal location of flexion/extension axis from transepicondylar line:	
Lateral	6.8 ± 0.2
Medial	8.7 ± 0.6

Source: Shiba R. et al. 1988. *J. Orthop. Res.* 6: 897.

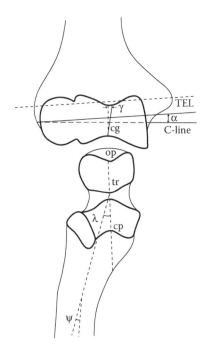

FIGURE 3.25   Components contributing to the carrying angles: $\alpha + \lambda + \psi$. α, angle between C-line and TEL; γ, inclination of central groove (cg); λ, angle between trochlear notch (tn); ψ, reverse angulation of shaft of ulna; TLE, transepicondylar line; C-line, line joining centers of curvature of the trochlea and capitellum; cg, central groove; op, olecranon process; tr, trochlear ridge; cp, coronoid process. $\alpha = 2.5 \pm 0.0$; $\lambda = 17.5 \pm 5.0$ (females) and 12.0 ± 7.0 (males); $\psi = -6.5 \pm 0.7$ (females) and -9.5 ± 3.5 (males). (From Shiba R. 1988. *J. Orthop. Res.* 6: 897. With permission.)

3.6.2 Joint Contact

The contact area on the articular surfaces of the elbow joint depends on the joint position and the loading conditions. Increasing the magnitude of the load not only increases the size of the contact area but shifts the locations as well (Figure 3.26). As the axial loading is increased, there is an increased lateralization of the articular contact (Stormont et al., 1985). The area of contact, expressed as a percentage of the total articulating surface area, is given in Table 3.17. Based on a finite element model of the humero–ulnar joint, Merz et al. (1997) demonstrated that the humero–ulnar joint incongruity brings about a bicentric distribution of contact pressure, a tensile stress exists in the notch that is the same order of magnitude as the compressive stress (Merz et al., 1997).

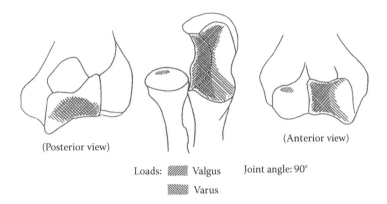

(Posterior view)   (Anterior view)

Loads: ▨ Valgus   Joint angle: 90°
       ▨ Varus

FIGURE 3.26 Contact of the ulnohumeral joint with varus and valgus loads and the elbow at 90°. Notice only minimal radiohumeral contact in this loading condition. (Reprinted from *J. Biomech.*, 18, Stormont T.J. et al. Elbow joint contact study: Comparison of technique, 329, Copyright 1985, with permission of Elsevier.)

TABLE 3.17 Elbow Joint Contact Area

Position	Total Articulating Surface Area of Ulna and Radial Head (mm²)	Contact Area (%)
Full extension	1598 ± 103	8.1 ± 2.7
90° flexion	1750 ± 123	10.8 ± 2.0
Full flexion	1594 ± 120	9.5 ± 2.1

Source: Goel V.K., Singh D., and Bijlani V. 1982. *J. Biomech. Eng.* 104: 169–175.

By using pressure-sensitive film, Ahmad et al. (2004) found that release of the medial ulnar collateral ligament condition and valgus load had significant effects on contact area and pressure. For a given load and flexion angle, in general, the contact area in the posteromedial olecranon decreased and the pressure increased with increasing medial ulnar collateral ligament insufficiency, especially when the elbow was at 30° of flexion.

Using magnetic resonance images and 3D registration, the *in vivo* three-dimensional kinematics of the elbow joint during elbow flexion was carried out by Goto et al. (2004). The inferred contact areas based on the proximity on the ulna against the trochlea tended to occur only on the medial facet of the trochlear notch in all of the elbow positions, and those on the radial head against the capitellum occurred on the central depression of the radial head (Goto et al., 2004).

3.6.3 Axes of Rotation

The axes of flexion and extension can be approximated by a line passing through the center of the trochlea, bisecting the angle formed by the longitudinal axes of the humerus and the ulna (Morrey and Chao, 1976). The instant centers of flexion and extension vary within 2–3 mm of this axis (Figures 3.27 through 3.29). With the elbow fully extended and the forearm fully supinated, the longitudinal axes of humerus and ulna normally intersect at a valgus angle referred to as the *carrying angle*. In adults, this angle is usually 10–15° and normally is greater on average in women (Zuckerman and Matsen, 1989). As the elbow flexes, the carrying angle varies as a function of flexion (Figures 3.30 through 3.32). In extension there is a valgus angulation of 10°; at full flexion there is a varus angulation of 8° (Morrey and Chao, 1976). More recently, the three-dimensional kinematics of the ulno–humeral joint under simulated active elbow joint flexion–extension was obtained by using an electromagnetic tracking device (Tanaka et al., 1998). The optimal axis to best represent flexion–extension motion was found to be close to the line joining the centers of the capitellum and the trochlear groove. Furthermore, the joint laxity

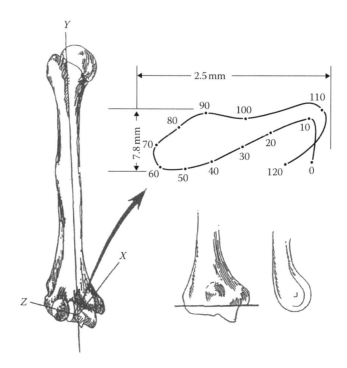

FIGURE 3.27 Very small locus of instant center of rotation for the elbow joint demonstrates that the axis may be replicated by a single line drawn from the inferior aspect of the medial epicondyle through the center of the lateral epicondyle, which is in the center of the lateral projected curvature of the trochlea and capitellum. (From Morrey B.F. and Chao E.Y.S. 1976. *J. Bone Joint Surg.* 58A: 501. With permission.)

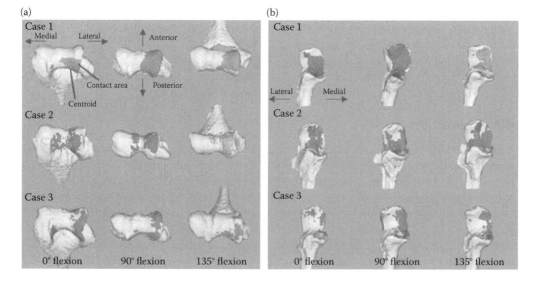

FIGURE 3.28 The inferred contact areas of articular surfaces and their centroids of the ulnohumeral joint in 0°, 90°, and 135° flexion. (a) Contact areas on the humerus. (b) Contact areas on the ulna. (From Goto A. et al. 2004. *J. Shoulder Elbow Surg.* 13, 441–447. With permission.)

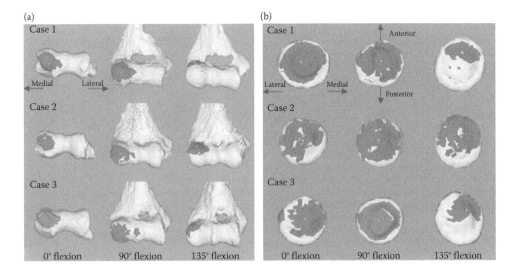

FIGURE 3.29 The inferred contact areas of articular surfaces and their centroids of the ulnohumeral joint in 0°, 90°, and 135° flexion. (a) Contact areas on the humerus. (b) Contact areas on the radius. (From Goto A. et al. 2004. *J. Shoulder Elbow Surg.* 13, 441–447. With permission.)

under valgus–varus stress was also examined. With the weight of the forearm as the stress, a maximum of 7.6° valgus–varus and 5.3° of axial rotation laxity were observed.

The screw axes of rotation of the elbow joint were evaluated *in vivo* using magnetic resonance images and 3D registration (Goto et al., 2004). They found that the pathway of the axis exhibits a roller configuration tracing the surface of a double conic shape, with the frustum waist being located in the medial portion of the trochlea (Figure 3.27). The locus of the axis of rotation traced on the surface of the condyles tended to be larger on the lateral side than on the medial side and that the locus of the averaged axis of rotation on the lateral condyle showed a counterclockwise circular pattern (Goto et al., 2004).

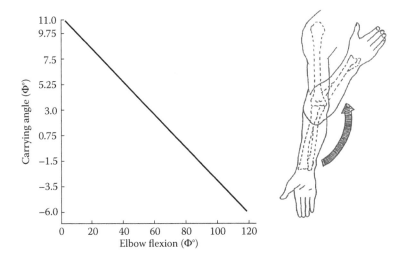

FIGURE 3.30 During elbow flexion and extension, a linear change in the carrying angle is demonstrated, typically going from the valgus in extension to the varus in flexion. (From Morrey B.F. and Chao E.Y.S. 1976. *J. Bone Joint Surg.* 58A: 501. With permission.)

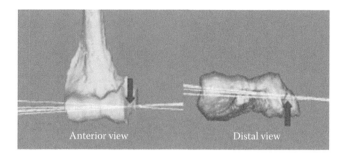

FIGURE 3.31 Superimposed images of the instantaneous axes of rotation of the ulnohumeral joint showing roller configuration tracing the surface of a double conic shape, with the frustum waist being located in the medial portion of the trochlea (arrows). (From Goto A. et al. 2004. *J. Shoulder Elbow Surg.* 13, 441–447. With permission.)

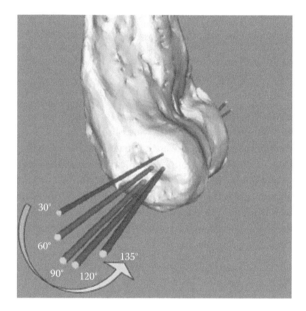

FIGURE 3.32 The locus of the averaged axis of rotation on the lateral condyle shows a counterclockwise circular pattern, where it initially moves anteriorly in the range from 0° to 60° flexion and then returns posteriorly. (From Goto A. et al. 2004. *J. Shoulder Elbow Surg.* 13, 441–447. With permission.)

3.7 Wrist

The wrist functions by allowing changes of orientation of the hand relative to the forearm. The wrist joint complex consists of multiple articulations of eight carpal bones with the distal radius, the structures of the ulnocarpal space, the metacarpals, and each other. This collection of bones and soft tissues is capable of a substantial arc of motion that augments hand and finger function.

3.7.1 Geometry of the Articulating Surfaces

The global geometry of the carpal bones has been quantified for grasp and active isometric contraction of the elbow flexors (Schuind et al., 1992). During grasping there is a significant proximal migration of the radius

TABLE 3.18   Changes of Wrist Geometry with Grasp

	Resting	Grasp	Analysis of Variance (p = Level)
Distal radioulnar joint space (mm)	1.6 ± 0.3	1.8 ± 0.6	0.06
Ulnar variance (mm)	−0.2 ± 1.6	0.7 ± 1.8	0.003
Lunate, uncovered length (mm)	6.0 ± 1.9	7.6 ± 2.6	0.0008
Capitate length (mm)	21.5 ± 2.2	20.8 ± 2.3	0.0002
Carpal height (mm)	33.4 ± 3.4	31.7 ± 3.4	0.0001
Carpal ulnar distance (mm)	15.8 ± 4.0	15.8 ± 3.0	NS
Carpal radial distance (mm)	19.4 ± 1.8	19.7 ± 1.8	NS
Third metacarpal length (mm)	63.8 ± 5.8	62.6 ± 5.5	NS
Carpal height ratio	52.4 ± 3.3	50.6 ± 4.1	0.02
Carpal ulnar ratio	24.9 ± 5.9	25.4 ± 5.3	NS
Lunate uncovering index	36.7 ± 12.1	45.3 ± 14.2	0.002
Carpal radial ratio	30.6 ± 2.4	31.6 ± 2.3	NS
Radius—third metacarpal angle (deg)	−0.3 ± 9.2	−3.1 ± 12.8	NS
Radius—capitate angle (deg)	0.4 ± 15.4	−3.8 ± 22.2	NS

Source: Schuind F.A. et al. 1992. *J. Hand Surg.* 17A: 698.
Note: 15 normal subjects with forearm in neutral position and elbow at 90° flexion.

of 0.9 mm, apparent shortening of the capitate, a decrease in the carpal height ratio, and an increase in the lunate uncovering index (Table 3.18). There is also a trend toward increase of the distal radioulnar joint with grasping. The addition of elbow flexion with concomitant grasping did not significantly change the global geometry, except for a significant decrease in the forearm interosseous space (Schuind et al., 1992).

3.7.2 Joint Contact

Studies of the normal biomechanics of the proximal wrist joint have determined that the scaphoid and lunate bones have separate, distinct areas of contact on the distal radius/triangular fibrocartilage complex surface (Viegas et al., 1987) so that the contact areas were localized and accounted for a relatively small fraction of the joint surface, regardless of wrist position (average of 20.6%). The contact areas shift from a more volar location to a more dorsal location as the wrist moves from flexion to extension. Overall, the scaphoid contact area is 1.47 times greater than that of the lunate. The scapho-lunate contact area ratio generally increases as the wrist position is changed from radial to ulnar deviation and/or from flexion to extension. Palmer and Werner (1984) also studied pressures in the proximal wrist joint and found that there are three distinct areas of contact: the ulno-lunate, radio-lunate, and radio-scaphoid. They determined that the peak articular pressure in the ulno-lunate fossa is 1.4 N/mm², in the radio-ulnate fossa is 3.0 N/mm², and in the radio-scaphoid fossa is 3.3 N/mm². Viegas et al. (1989) found a nonlinear relationship between increasing load and the joint contact area (Figure 3.33). In general, the distribution of load between the scaphoid and lunate was consistent with all loads tested, with 60% of the total contact area involving the scaphoid and 40% involving the lunate. Loads greater than 46 lbs were found to not significantly increase the overall contact area. The overall contact area, even at the highest loads tested, was not more than 40% of the available joint surface.

Horii et al. (1990) calculated the total amount of force borne by each joint with the intact wrist in the neutral position in the coronal plane and subjected to a total load of 143 N (Table 3.19). They found that 22% of the total force in the radio-ulno–carpal joint is dissipated through the ulna (14% through the ulno-lunate joint, and 18% through the ulno–triquetral joint) and 78% through the radius (46% through the scaphoid fossa and 32% through the lunate fossa). At the midcarpal joint, the scapho–trapezial joint transmits 31% of the total applied force, the scapho–capitate joint transmits 19%, the luno-capitate joint transmits 29%, and the triquetral-hamate joints transmits 21% of the load.

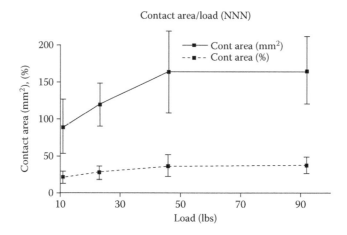

FIGURE 3.33 The nonlinear relation between the contact area and the load at the proximal wrist joint. The contact area was normalized as a percentage of the available joint surface. The load of 11, 23, 46, and 92 lbs was applied at the position of neutral pronation/supination, neutral radioulnar deviation, and neutral flexion/extension. (From Viegas S.F. et al. 1989. *J. Hand Surg.* 14A: 458. With permission.)

A limited amount of studies have been done to determine the contact areas in the midcarpal joint. Viegas et al. (1990) have found four general areas of contact: the scapho-trapezial-trapezoid (STT), the scapho-capitate (SC), the capito-lunate (CL), and the triquetral-hamate (TH). The high-pressure contact area accounted for only 8% of the available joint surface with a load of 32 lbs and increased to a maximum of only 15% with a load of 118 lbs. The total contact area, expressed as a percentage of the total available joint area for each fossa was: STT = 1.3%, SC = 1.8%, CL = 3.1%, and TH = 1.8%.

The correlation between the pressure loading in the wrist and the progress of degenerative osteoarthritis associated with pathological conditions of the forearm was studied in a cadaveric model (Sato, 1995). Malunion after distal radius fracture, tear of triangular fibrocartilage, and scapholunate dissociation were all responsible for the alteration of the articulating pressure across the wrist joint. Residual articular incongruity of the distal radius following intra-articular fracture has been correlated with early osteoarthritis. In an *in vitro* model, step-offs of the distal radius articular incongruity were created. Mean contact stress was significantly greater than the anatomically reduced case at only 3 mm of step-off (Anderson et al., 1996).

TABLE 3.19 Force Transmission at the Intercarpal Joints

Joint	Force (N)
Radio-ulno-carpal	
Ulno-triquetral	12 ± 3
Ulno-lunate	23 ± 8
Radio-lunate	52 ± 8
Radio-scaphoid	74 ± 13
Midcarpal	
Triquetral-hamate	36 ± 6
Luno-capitate	51 ± 6
Scapho-capitate	32 ± 4
Scapho-trapezial	51 ± 8

Source: Horii E. et al. 1990. *J. Bone Joint Surg.* 15A: 393.
Note: A total of 143 N axial force applied across the wrist.

3.7.3 Axes of Rotation

The complexity of joint motion at the wrist makes it difficult to calculate the instant center of motion. However, the trajectories of the hand during radioulnar deviation and flexion/extension, when they occur in a fixed plane, are circular, and the rotation in each plane takes place about a fixed axis. These axes are located within the head of the capitate and are not altered by the position of the hand in the plane of rotation (Youm et al., 1978). During radioulnar deviation, the instant center of rotation lies at a point in the capitate situated distal to the proximal end of this bone by a distance equivalent to approximately one-quarter of its total length (Figure 3.34). During flexion/extension, the instant center is close to the proximal cortex of the capitate, which is somewhat more proximal than the location for the instant center of radioulnar deviation.

Recently, an in vivo kinematic study of normal forearm rotation used computed tomographic (CT) images in five positions: neutral, 60° pronation, maximal pronation, 60° supination, and maximal supination. Surface registration of the image with the neutral position was performed, and the kinematics were expressed as motion of the radius relative to the ulna (Tay et al., 2008). The axes of the forearm rotation passed through the volar region of the radial head at the proximal radioulnar joint extending toward the dorsal region of the ulnar head at the distal radioulnar joint (Tay et al., 2008) (Figure 3.35).

Normal carpal kinematics was studied in 22 cadaver specimens using a biplanar radiography method. The kinematics of the trapezium, capitate, hamate, scaphoid, lunate, and triquetrum were determined during wrist rotation in the sagittal and coronal plane (Kobayashi et al., 1997). The results were expressed using the concept of the screw displacement axis and covered to describe the magnitude of rotation about and translation along three orthogonal axes. The orientation of these axes is expressed relative to the radius during sagittal plane motion of the wrist (Table 3.20). The scaphoid exhibited the greatest magnitude of rotation and the lunate displayed the least rotation. The proximal carpal bones exhibited some ulnar deviation in 60° of wrist flexion. During coronal plane motion (Table 3.21), the magnitude of radial–ulnar deviation of the distal carpal bones was mutually similar and generally of a greater magnitude than that of the proximal carpal bones. The proximal carpal bones experienced some flexion during radial deviation of the wrist and extension during ulnar deviation of the wrist.

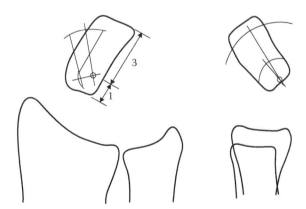

FIGURE 3.34 The location of the center of rotation during ulnar deviation (a) and extension (b), determined graphically using two metal markers embedded in the capitate. Note that during radial–ulnar deviation the center lies at a point in the capitate situated distal to the proximal end of this bone by a distance equivalent to approximately one-quarter of its total longitudinal length. During flexion–extension, the center of rotation is close to the proximal cortex of the capitate. (From Youm Y. et al. 1978. *J. Bone Joint Surg.* 60A: 423. With permission.)

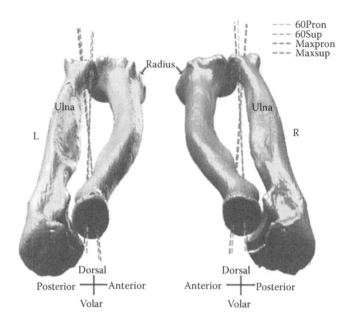

FIGURE 3.35 Distal view of three-dimensional reconstructions of the subject's left and right forearms in neutral rotation. The FHA of the four forearm positions (60° pronation, 60° supination, maximal pronation, and maximal supination), are distinctly shown. They all pass through the colar region of the proximal radial head and dorsal region of the distal ulnar head. The axis of forearm rotation appears to move largely in a linear manner during pronation and supination. (From Tay S.C. et al. 2008. *J. Biomech.* 41, 56–62. With permission.)

3.8 Hand

The hand is an extremely mobile organ that is capable of conforming to a large variety of object shapes and coordinating an infinite variety of movements in relation to each of its components. The mobility of this structure is possible through the unique arrangement of the bones in relation to one another, the articular contours, and the actions of an intricate system of muscles. Theoretical and empirical evidence suggest that limb joint surface morphology is mechanically related to joint mobility, stability, and strength (Hamrick, 1996).

3.8.1 Geometry of the Articulating Surfaces

Three-dimensional geometric models of the articular surfaces of the hand have been constructed. The sagittal contours of the metacarpal head and proximal phalanx grossly resemble the arc of a circle (Tamai et al., 1988). The radius of curvature of a circle fitted to the entire proximal phalanx surface ranges from 11 to 13 mm, almost twice as much as that of the metacarpal head, which ranges from 6 to 7 mm (Table 3.22). The local centers of curvature along the sagittal contour of the metacarpal heads are not fixed. The locus of the center of curvature for the subchondral bony contour approximates the locus of the center for the acute curve of an ellipse (Figure 3.36). However, the locus of center of curvature for the articular cartilage contour approximates the locus of the obtuse curve of an ellipse.

The surface geometry of the thumb carpometacarpal (CMC) joint has also been quantified (Athesian et al., 1992). The surface area of the CMC joint is significantly greater for male than for female individuals (Table 3.23). The minimum, maximum, and mean square curvature of these joints is reported in Table 3.23. The curvature of the surface is denoted by κ and the radius of curvature is $\rho = 1/\kappa$. The curvature is negative when the surface is concave and positive when the surface is convex.

TABLE 3.20 Individual Carpal Rotation Relative to the Radius (Deg) (Sagittal Plane Motion of the Wrist)

Wrist Motion[a] Carpal Bone	Axis of Rotation											
	X (+) Pronation; (−) Supination				Y (+) Flexion; (−) Extension				Z (+) Ulnar Deviation; (−) Radial Deviation			
	N-E60	N-E30	N-F30	N-F60	N-E60	N-E30	N-F30	N-F60	N-E60	N-E30	N-F30	N-F60
Trapezium (N = 13)	−0.9	−1.3	0.9	−1.4	−59.4	−29.3	28.7	54.2	1.2	0.3	−0.4	2.5
SD	2.8	2.2	2.6	2.7	2.3	1	1.8	3	4	2.7	1.3	2.8
Capitate (N = 22)	0.9	−1	1.3	−1.6	60.3	−30.2	21.5	63.5	0	0	0.6	3.2
SD	2.7	1.8	2.5	3.5	2.5	1.1	1.2	2.8	2	1.4	1.6	3.6
Hamate (N = 9)	0.4	−1	1.3	−0.3	−59.5	−29	28.8	62.6	2.1	0.7	0.1	1.8
SD	3.4	1.7	2.5	2.4	1.4	0.8	10.2	3.6	4.4	1.8	1.2	4.1
Scaphoid (N = 22)	−2.5	−0.7	1.6	2	−52.3	−26	20.6	39.7	4.5	0.8	2.1	7.8
SD	3.4	2.6	2.2	3.1	3	3.2	2.8	4.3	3.7	2.1	2.2	4.5
Lunate (N = 22)	1.2	0.5	0.3	−2.2	−29.7	−15.4	11.5	23	4.3	0.9	3.3	11.1
SD	2.8	1.8	1.7	2.8	6.6	3.9	3.9	5.9	2.6	1.5	1.9	3.4
Triquetrum (N = 22)	−3.5	−2.5	2.5	−0.7	−39.3	−20.1	15.5	30.6	0	−0.3	2.4	9.8
SD	3.5	2	2.2	3.7	4.8	2.7	3.8	5.1	2.8	1.4	2.6	4.3

Source: Kobayashi M. et al. 1997. J. Biomech. 30: 787.

Note: SD, standard deviation.

[a] N-E60: neutral to 60° of extension; N-E30: neutral to 30° of extension; N-F30: neutral to 30° of flexion; N-F60: neutral to 60° of flexion.

TABLE 3.21 Individual Carpal Rotation to the Radius (Deg) (Coronal Plane Motion of the Wrist)

| | Axis of Rotation | | | | | | | | |
| Wrist Motion[a] Carpal Bone | X (+) Pronation; (−) Supination | | | Y (+) Flexion; (−) Extension | | | Z (+) Ulnar Deviation; (−) Radial Deviation | | |
	N-RD15	N-UD15	N-UD30	N-RD15	N-UD15	N-UD30	N-RD15	N-UD15	N-UD30
Trapezium (N = 13)	−4.8	9.1	16.3	0	4.9	9.9	−14.3	16.4	32.5
SD	2.4	3.6	3.6	1.5	1.3	2.1	2.3	2.8	2.6
Capitate (N = 22)	−3.9	6.8	11.8	1.3	2.7	6.5	−14.6	15.9	30.7
SD	2.6	2.6	2.5	1.5	1.1	1.7	2.1	1.4	1.7
Hamate (N = 9)	−4.8	6.3	10.6	1.1	3.5	6.6	−15.5	15.4	30.2
SD	1.8	2.4	3.1	3	3.2	4.1	2.4	2.6	3.6
Scaphoid (N = 22)	0.8	2.2	6.6	8.5	−12.5	−17.1	−4.2	4.3	13.6
SD	1.8	2.4	3.1	3	3.2	4.1	2.4	2.6	3.6
Lunate (N = 22)	−1.2	1.4	3.9	7	−13.9	−22.5	−1.7	5.7	15
SD	1.6	0	3.3	3.1	4.3	6.9	1.7	2.8	4.3
Triquetrum (N = 22)	−1.1	−1	0.8	4.1	−10.5	−17.3	−5.1	7.7	18.4
SD	1.4	2.6	4	3	3.8	6	2.4	2.2	4

Source: Kobayashi M. et al. 1997. J. Biomech. 30: 787.

Note: SD, standard deviation.

[a] N-RD15: neutral to 15° of radial deviation; N-UD30: neutral to 30° of ulnar deviation; N-UD15: neutral to 15° of ulnar deviation.

TABLE 3.22 Radius of Curvature of the Middle Sections of the
Metacarpal Head and Proximal Phalanx Base

	Radius (mm)	
	Bony Contour	Cartilage Contour
MCH index	6.42 ± 1.23	6.91 ± 1.03
Long	6.44 ± 1.08	6.66 ± 1.18
PPB index	13.01 ± 4.09	12.07 ± 3.29
Long	11.46 ± 2.30	11.02 ± 2.48

Source: Tamai K. et al. 1988. *J. Hand Surg.* 13A: 521.

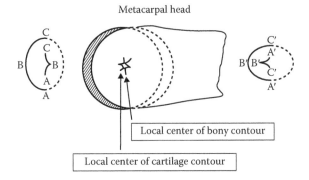

FIGURE 3.36 The loci of the local centers of curvature for subchondral bony contour of the metacarpal head approximates the loci of the center for the acute curve of an ellipse. The loci of the local center of curvature for articular cartilage contour of the metacarpal head approximates the loci of the bony center of the obtuse curve of an ellipse. (From Tamai K. et al. 1988. *J. Hand Surg.* 13A: 521. Reprinted with permission of Churchill Livingstone.)

TABLE 3.23 Curvature of Carpometacarpal Joint Articular Surfaces

	n	Area (cm²)	$\bar{\kappa}_{min}$ (m⁻¹)	$\bar{\kappa}_{max}$ (m⁻¹)	$\bar{\kappa}_{rms}$ (m⁻¹)
Trapezium					
Female	8	1.05 ± 0.21	−61 ± 22	190 ± 36	165 ± 32
Male	5	1.63 ± 0.18	−87 ± 17	114 ± 19	118 ± 6
Total	13	1.27 ± 0.35	−71 ± 24	161 ± 48	147 ± 34
Female versus male		$p \le 0.01$	$p \le 0.05$	$p \le 0.01$	$p \le 0.01$
Metacarpal					
Female	8	1.22 ± 0.36	−49 ± 10	175 ± 25	154 ± 20
Male	5	1.74 ± 0.21	−37 ± 11	131 ± 17	116 ± 8
Total	13	1.42 ± 0.40	−44 ± 12	158 ± 31	140 ± 25
Female versus male		$p \le 0.01$	$p \le 0.05$	$p \le 0.01$	$p \le 0.01$

Source: Athesian J.A., Rosenwasser M.P., and Mow V.C. 1992. *J. Biomech.* 25: 591.
Note: Radius of curvature: $\rho = 1/\kappa$.

3.8.2 Joint Contact

The size and location of joint contact areas of the metacarpophalangeal (MCP) joint changes as a function of the joint flexion angle (Figure 3.37). The radioulnar width of the contact area becomes narrow in the neutral position and expands in both the hyperextended and fully flexed positions (An and Cooney, 1991). In the neutral position, the contact area occurs in the center of the phalangeal base, this area being slightly larger on the ulnar than on the radial side.

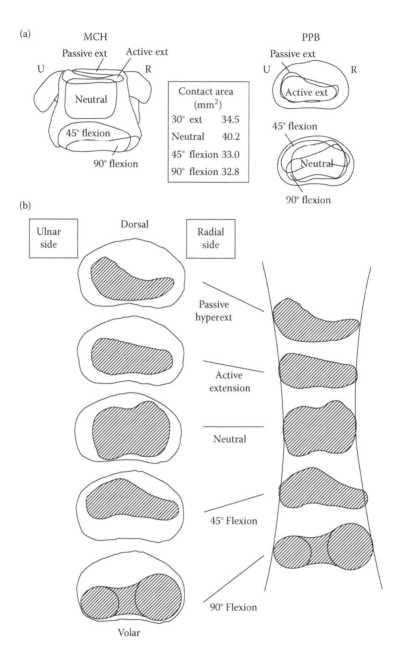

FIGURE 3.37 (a) Contact area of the MCP joint in five joint positions. (b) End on view of the contact area on each of the proximal phalanx bases. The radioulnar width of the contact area becomes narrow in the neutral position and expands in both the hyperextended and fully flexed positions. (From An K.N. and Cooney W.P. 1991. *Joint Replacement Arthroplasty*, pp. 137–146, New York, Churchill Livingstone. By permission of Mayo Foundation.)

The contact areas of the thumb carpometacarpal joint under the functional position of lateral key pinch and in the extremes of range of motion were studied using a stereophotogrammetric technique (Ateshian et al., 1995). The lateral pinch position produced contact predominately on the central, volar, and volar–ulnar regions of the trapezium and the metacarpals (Figure 3.38). Pellegrini et al. (1993) noted that the palmar compartment of the trapeziometacarpal joint was the primary contact area during

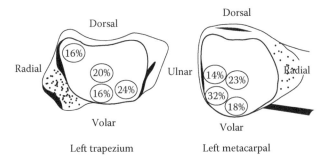

FIGURE 3.38 Summary of the contact areas for all specimens, in lateral pinch with a 25 N load. All results from the right hand are transposed onto the schema of a carpometacarpal joint from the left thumb. (From Ateshian G.A. et al. 1995. *J. Orthop. Res.* 13: 450.)

flexion adduction of the thumb in lateral pinch. Detachment of the palmar beak ligament resulted in dorsal translation of the contact area producing a pattern similar to that of cartilage degeneration seen in the osteoarthritic joint.

3.8.3 Axes of Rotation

Rolling and sliding actions of articulating surfaces exist during finger joint motion. The geometric shapes of the articular surfaces of the metacarpal head and proximal phalanx, as well as the insertion location of the collateral ligaments, significantly govern the articulating kinematics, and the center of rotation is not fixed but rather moves as a function of the angle of flexion (Pagowski and Piekarski, 1977). The instant centers of rotation are within 3 mm of the center of the metacarpal head (Walker and Erhman, 1975). Recently the axis of rotation of the MCP joint has been evaluated *in vivo* by Fioretti (1994). The instantaneous helical axis of the MCP joint tends to be more palmar and tends to be displaced distally as flexion increases (Figure 3.39).

The axes of rotation of the CMC joint have been described as being fixed (Hollister et al., 1992), but others believe that a polycentric center of rotation exists (Imaeda et al., 1994). Hollister et al. (1992) found

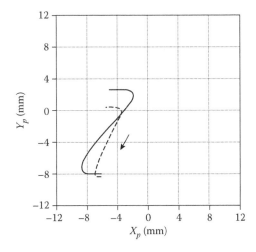

FIGURE 3.39 Intersections of the instantaneous helical angles with the metacarpal sagittal plane. They are relative to one subject tested twice in different days. The origin of the graph is coincident with the calibrated center of the metacarpal head. The arrow indicates the direction of flexion. (From Fioretti S. 1994. *Advances in the Biomechanics of the Hand and Wrist*, pp. 363–375, New York, Plenum Press. With permission.)

TABLE 3.24   Location of Center of Rotation of Trapeziometacarpal Joint

	Mean ± SD (mm)
Circumduction	
X	0.1 ± 1.3
Y	−0.6 ± 1.3
Z	−0.5 ± 1.4
Flexion/extension (in x–y plane)	
X	
Centroid	−4.2 ± 1.0
Radius	2.0 ± 0.5
Y	
Centroid	−0.4 ± 0.9
Radius	1.6 ± 0.5
Abduction/adduction (in x–z plane)	
X	
Centroid	6.7 ± 1.7
Radius	4.6 ± 3.1
Z	
Centroid	−0.2 ± 0.7
Radius	1.7 ± 0.5

Source: Imaeda T. et al. 1994. *J. Orthop. Res.* 12: 197.

Note: The coordinate system is defined with the x-axis corresponding to internal/external rotation, the y-axis corresponding to abduction/adduction, and the z-axis corresponding to flexion/extension. The x-axis is positive in the distal direction, the y-axis is positive in the dorsal direction for the left hand and in the palmar direction for the right hand, and the z-axis is positive in the radial direction. The origin of the coordinate system was at the intersection of a line connecting the radial and ulnar prominences and a line connecting the volar and dorsal tubercles.

that axes of the CMC joint are fixed and are not perpendicular to each other, or to the bones, and do not intersect. The flexion/extension axis is located in the trapezium, and the abduction/adduction axis is on the first metacarpal. In contrast, Imaeda et al. (1994) found that there was no single center of rotation, but rather the instantaneous motion occurred reciprocally between centers of rotations within the trapezium and the metacarpal base of the normal thumb. In flexion/extension, the axis of rotation was located within the trapezium, but for abduction/adduction the center of rotation was located distally to the trapezium and within the base of the first metacarpal. The average instantaneous center of circumduction was at approximately the center of the trapezial joint surface (Table 3.24).

The axes of rotation of the thumb interphalangeal and MCP joint were located using a mechanical device (Hollister et al., 1995). The physiological motion of the thumb joints occur about these axes (Figure 3.40 and Table 3.25). The interphalangeal joint axis is parallel to the flexion crease of the joint and is not perpendicular to the phalanx. The MCP joint has two fixed axes: a fixed flexion–extension axis just distal and volar to the epicondyles, and an abduction–adduction axis related to the proximal phalanx passing between the sesamoids. Neither axis is perpendicular to the phalanges.

3.9 Summary

It is important to understand the biomechanics of joint-articulating surface motion. The specific characteristics of the joint will determine the musculoskeletal function of that joint. The unique geometry of the joint surfaces and the surrounding capsule ligamentous constraints will guide the unique characteristics of the articulating surface motion. The range of joint motion, the stability of

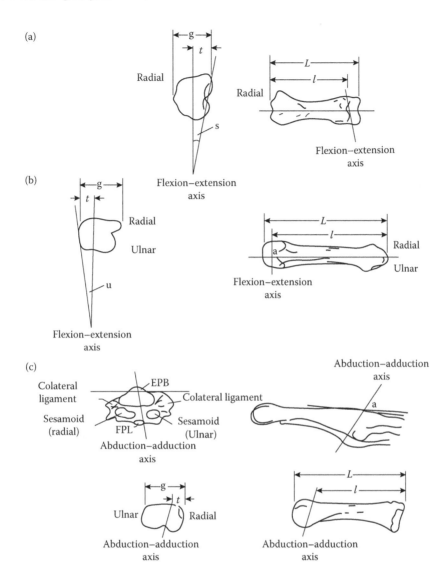

FIGURE 3.40 (a) The angles and length and breadth measurements defining the axis of rotation of the interphalangeal joint of the right thumb. (t/T = ratio of anatomic plane diameter; l/L = ratio of length). (b) The angles and length and breadth measurements of the MCP flexion–extension axis' position in the metacarpal. (c) The angles and length and breadth measurements that locate the MCP abduction–adduction axis. The measurements are made in the metacarpal when the metacarpophalangeal joint is at neutral flexion extension. The measurements are made relative to the metacarpal because the axis passes through this bone, not the proximal phalanx with which it moves. This method of recording the abduction–adduction measurements allows the measurements of the axes to each other at a neutral position to be made. The MCP abduction–adduction axis passes through the volar plate of the proximal phalanx. (From Hollister A. et al. 1995. *Clin. Orthop. Relat. Res.* 320: 188.)

TABLE 3.25   Measurement of Axis Location and Values for Axis Position in the Bone

Interphalangeal Joint Flexion–Extension Axis (Figure 3.40a)	
t/T	$44 \pm 17\%$
l/L	$90 \pm 5\%$
Θ	$5 \pm 2°$
β	$83 \pm 4°$
MCP Joint Flexion–Extension Axis (Figure 3.40b)	
t/T	$57 \pm 17\%$
l/L	$87 \pm 5\%$
α	$101 \pm 6°$
β	$5 \pm 2°$
MCP Joint Abduction–Adduction Axis (Figure 3.40c)	
t/T	$45 \pm 8\%$
l/L	$83 \pm 13\%$
α	$80 \pm 9°$
β	$74 \pm 8°$
M	

Source: Hollister A. et al. 1995. *Clin. Orthop. Relat. Res.* 320: 188.

Note: The angle of the abduction–adduction axis with respect to the flexion–extension axis is $84.8 \pm 12.2°$. The location and angulation of the K-wires of the axes with respect to the bones were measured (Θ, α, β) directly with a goniometer. The positions of the pins in the bones were measured (T, L) with a Vernier caliper.

the joint, and the ultimate functional strength of the joint will depend on these specific characteristics. A congruent joint usually has a relatively limited range of motion but a high degree of stability, whereas a less congruent joint will have a relatively larger range of motion but less degree of stability. The characteristics of the joint-articulating surface will determine the pattern of joint contact and the axes of rotation. These characteristics will regulate the stresses on the joint surface which will influence the degree of degeneration of articular cartilage in an anatomic joint and the amount of wear of an artificial joint.

Acknowledgment

The authors thank Barbara Iverson-Literski for her careful preparation of the manuscript.

References

Ahmad C.S., Park M.C., and Elattrache N.S. 2004. Elbow medial ulnar collateral ligament insufficiency alters posteromedial olecranon contact. *Am. J. Sports Med.,* 32: 1607–1612.

Ahmed A.M., Burke D.L., and Hyder A. 1987. Force analysis of the patellar mechanism. *J. Orthop. Res.* 5: 69–85.

Allard P., Duhaime M., Labelle H. et al. 1987. Spatial reconstruction technique and kinematic modeling of the ankle. *IEEE Eng. Med. Biol.* 6: 31.

An K.N. and Cooney W.P. 1991. Biomechanics, Section II. The hand and wrist. In B.F. Morrey (Ed.), *Joint Replacement Arthroplasty*, pp. 137–146, New York, Churchill Livingstone.

Anderson D.D., Bell A.L., Gaffney M.B. et al. 1996. Contact stress distributions in malreduced intraarticular distal radius fractures. *J. Orthop. Trauma* 10: 331.

Andriacchi T.P., Stanwyck T.S., and Galante J.O. 1986. Knee biomechanics in total knee replacement. *J. Arthroplasty* 1: 211.

Ateshian G.A., Ark J.W., Rosenwasser M.D. et al. 1995. Contact areas in the thumb carpometacarpal joint. *J. Orthop. Res.* 13: 450.

Athesian J.A., Rosenwasser M.P., and Mow V.C. 1992. Curvature characteristics and congruence of the thumb carpometacarpal joint: Differences between female and male joints. *J. Biomech.* 25: 591.

Barnett C.H. and Napier J.R. 1952. The axis of rotation at the ankle joint in man. Its influence upon the form of the talus and the mobility of the fibula. *J. Anat.* 86: 1.

Basmajian J.V. and Bazant F.J. 1959. Factors preventing downward dislocation of the adducted shoulder joint. An electromyographic and morphological study. *J. Bone Joint Surg.* 41A: 1182.

Besier T.F., Draper C.E., Gold G.E., Beaupre G.S., and Delp S.L. 2005. Patellofemoral joint contact area increases with knee flexion and weight-bearing. *J. Orthop. Res.* 23: 345–350.

Boileau P. and Walch G. 1997. The three-dimensional geometry of the proximal humerus. *J. Bone Joint Surg.* 79B: 857.

Boyer P.J., Massimini D.F., Gill T.J., Papannagari R., Stewart S.L., Warner J.P., and Li G. 2008. *In vivo* articular cartilage contact at the glenohumeral joint: Preliminary report. *J. Orthop. Sci.* 13: 359–365.

D'Ambrosia R.D., Shoji H., and Van Meter J. 1976. Rotational axis of the ankle joint: Comparison of normal and pathological states. *Surg. Forum* 27: 507.

Davy D.T., Kotzar D.M., Brown R.H. et al. 1989. Telemetric force measurements across the hip after total arthroplasty. *J. Bone Joint Surg.* 70A: 45.

Doody S.G., Freedman L., and Waterland J.C. 1970. Shoulder movements during abduction in the scapular plane. *Arch. Phys. Med. Rehabil.* 51: 595.

Draganich L.F., Andriacchi T.P., and Andersson G.B.J. 1987. Interaction between intrinsic knee mechanics and the knee extensor mechanism. *J. Orthop. Res.* 5: 539.

Driscoll H.L., Christensen J.C., and Tencer A.F. 1994. Contact characteristics of the ankle joint. *J. Am. Pediatr. Med. Assoc.* 84: 491.

Elftman H. 1945. The orientation of the joints of the lower extremity. *Bull. Hosp. Joint Dis.* 6: 139.

Engsberg J.R. 1987. A biomechanical analysis of the talocalcaneal joint *in vitro. J. Biomech.* 20: 429.

Farahmand F., Senavongse W., and Amis A.A. 1998. Quantitative study of the quadriceps muscles and trochlear groove geometry related to instability of the patellofemoral joint. *J. Orthop. Res.* 16: 136.

Fioretti S. 1994. Three-dimensional *in-vivo* kinematic analysis of finger movement. In F. Schuind et al. (Eds.), *Advances in the Biomechanics of the Hand and Wrist*, pp. 363–375, New York, Plenum.

Freedman L. and Munro R.R. 1966. Abduction of the arm in the scapular plane: Scapular and glenohumeral movements. A roentgenographic study. *J. Bone Joint Surg.* 48A: 1503.

Goel V.K., Singh D., and Bijlani V. 1982. Contact areas in human elbow joints. *J. Biomech. Eng.* 104: 169–175.

Goodfellow J., Hungerford D.S., and Zindel M. 1976. Patellofemoral joint mechanics and pathology. *J. Bone Joint Surg.* 58B: 287.

Goto A., Moritomo H., Murase T., Oka K., Sugamoto K., Arimura T., Nakajima Y. et al. 2004. *In vivo* elbow biomechanical analysis during flexion: Three-dimensional motion analysis using magnetic resonance imaging. *J. Shoulder Elbow Surg.* 13: 441–447.

Greis P.E., Scuderi M.G., Mohr A., Bachus K.N., and Burks R.T. 2002. Glenohumeral articular contact areas and pressures following labral and osseous injury to the anteroinferior quadrant of the glenoid. *J. Shoulder Elbow Surg.* 11: 442–451.

Hamrick M.W. 1996. Articular size and curvature as detriments of carpal joint mobility and stability in strepsirhine primates. *J. Morphol.* 230: 113.

Hartford J.M., Gorczyca J.T., McNamara J.L. et al. 1985. Tibiotalar contact area. *Clin. Orthop.* 320: 82.

Hashemi J., Chandrashekar N., Gill B., Beynnon B.D., Slauterbeck J.R., Schutt R.C., Jr., Mansouri H., and Dabezies E. 2008. The geometry of the tibial plateau and its influence on the biomechanics of the tibiofemoral joint. *J. Bone Joint Surg.—Am. Vol.* 90: 2724–2734.

Hayes A., Tochigi Y., and Saltzman C.L. 2006. Ankle morphometry on 3D-CT images. *Iowa Orthop. J.* 26: 1–4.

Hicks J.H. 1953. The mechanics of the foot. The joints. *J. Anat.* 87: 345–357.

Hollister A., Buford W.L., Myers L.M. et al. 1992. The axes of rotation of the thumb carpometacarpal joint. *J. Orthop. Res.* 10: 454.

Hollister A., Guirintano D.J., Bulford W.L. et al. 1995. The axes of rotation of the thumb interphalangeal and metacarpophalangeal joints. *Clin. Orthop. Relat. Res.* 320: 188.

Horii E., Garcia-Elias M., An K.N. et al. 1990. Effect of force transmission across the carpus in procedures used to treat Kienböck's disease. *J. Bone Joint Surg.* 15A: 393.

Huberti H.H. and Hayes W.C. 1984. Patellofemoral contact pressures: The influence of Q-angle and tendo-femoral contact. *J. Bone Joint Surg.* 66A: 715–725.

Iannotti J.P., Gabriel J.P., Schneck S.L. et al. 1992. The normal glenohumeral relationships: An anatomical study of 140 shoulders. *J. Bone Joint Surg.* 74A: 491.

Imaeda T., Niebur G., Cooney W.P. et al. 1994. Kinematics of the normal trapeziometacarpal joint. *J. Orthop. Res.* 12: 197.

Inman V.T. 1976. *The Joints of the Ankle*, Baltimore, MD. Williams and Wilkins.

Inman V.T. and Mann R.A. 1979. Biomechanics of the foot and ankle. In V.T. Inman (Ed.), *DuVrie's Surgery of the Foot*. St Louis, Mosby.

Inman V.T., Saunders J.B. deCM, and Abbott L.C. 1944. Observations on the function of the shoulder joint. *J. Bone Joint Surg.* 26A: 1.

Iseki F. and Tomatsu T. 1976. The biomechanics of the knee joint with special reference to the contact area. *Keio. J. Med.* 25: 37.

Isman R.E. and Inman V.T. 1969. Anthropometric studies of the human foot and ankle. *Pros. Res.* 10–11: 97.

Jobe C.M. and Iannotti J.P. 1995. Limits imposed on glenohumeral motion by joint geometry. *J. Shoulder Elbow Surg.* 4: 281.

Kapandji I.A. 1987. *The Physiology of the Joints*, Vol. 2, *Lower Limb*. Edinburgh, Churchill-Livingstone.

Karduna A.R., Williams G.R., Williams J.I. et al. 1996. Kinematics of the glenohumeral joint: Influences of muscle forces, ligamentous constraints, and articular geometry. *J. Orthop. Res.* 14: 986.

Kent B.E. 1971. Functional anatomy of the shoulder complex. A review. *Phys. Ther.* 51: 867.

Kimizuka M., Kurosawa H., and Fukubayashi T. 1980. Load-bearing pattern of the ankle joint. Contact area and pressure distribution. *Arch. Orthop. Trauma Surg.* 96: 45–49.

Kinzel G.L., Hall A.L., and Hillberry B.M. 1972. Measurement of the total motion between two body segments: Part I. Analytic development. *J. Biomech.* 5: 93.

Kirby K.A. 1947. Methods for determination of positional variations in the subtalar and transverse tarsal joints. *Anat. Rec.* 80: 397.

Kobayashi M., Berger R.A., Nagy L. et al. 1997. Normal kinematics of carpal bones: A three-dimensional analysis of carpal bone motion relative to the radius. *J. Biomech.* 30: 787.

Kurosawa H., Walker P.S., Abe S. et al. 1985. Geometry and motion of the knee for implant and orthotic design. *J. Biomech.* 18: 487.

Lewis J.L. and Lew W.D. 1978. A method for locating an optimal "fixed" axis of rotation for the human knee joint. *J. Biomech. Eng.* 100: 187.

Libotte M., Klein P., Colpaert H. et al. 1982. Contribution à l'étude biomécanique de la pince malléolaire. *Rev. Chir. Orthop.* 68: 299.

Lippitt B., Vanderhooft J.E., Harris S.L. et al. 1993. Glenohumeral stability from concavity-compression: A quantitative analysis. *J. Shoulder Elbow Surg.* 2: 27–35.

Macko V.W., Matthews L.S., Zwirkoski P. et al. 1991. The joint contract area of the ankle: The contribution of the posterior malleoli. *J. Bone Joint Surg.* 73A: 347.

Manter J.T. 1941. Movements of the subtalar and transverse tarsal joints. *Anat. Rec.* 80: 397–402.

Maquet P.G., Vandberg A.J., and Simonet J.C. 1975. Femorotibial weight bearing areas: Experimental determination. *J. Bone Joint Surg.* 57A: 766–771.

Massimini D.F., Li G., and Warner J.P. 2010. Glenohumeral contact kinematics in patients after total shoulder arthroplasty. *J. Bone Joint Surg.* 92: 916–926.

Matsuda S., Miura H., Nagamine R., Mawatari T., Tokunaga M., Nabeyama R., and Iwamoto Y. 2004. Anatomical analysis of the femoral condyle in normal and osteoarthritic knees. *J. Orthop. Res.* 22: 104–109.

McPherson E.J., Friedman R.J., An Y.H. et al. 1997. Anthropometric study of normal glenohumeral relationships. *J. Shoulder Elbow Surg.* 6: 105.

Merz B., Eckstein F., Hillebrand S. et al. 1997. Mechanical implication of humero-ulnar incongruity-finite element analysis and experiment. *J. Biomech.* 30: 713.

Miyanaga Y., Fukubayashi T., and Kurosawa H. 1984. Contact study of the hip joint: Load deformation pattern, contact area, and contact pressure. *Arch. Orth. Trauma Surg.* 103: 13–17.

Morrey B.F. and An K.N. 1990. Biomechanics of the shoulder. In C.A. Rockwood and F.A. Matsen (Eds.), *The Shoulder*, pp. 208–245, Philadelphia, Saunders.

Morrey B.F. and Chao E.Y.S. 1976. Passive motion of the elbow joint: A biomechanical analysis. *J. Bone Joint Surg.* 58A: 501.

Nahass B.E., Madson M.M., and Walker P.S. 1991. Motion of the knee after condylar resurfacing—An *in vivo* study. *J. Biomech.* 24: 1107.

Paar O., Rieck B., and Bernett P. 1983. Experimentelle untersuchungen über belastungsabhängige Drukund Kontaktflächenverläufe an den Fussgelenken. *Unfallheilkunde* 85: 531.

Pagowski S. and Piekarski K. 1977. Biomechanics of metacarpophalangeal joint. *J. Biomech.* 10: 205.

Palmer A.K. and Werner F.W. 1984. Biomechanics of the distal radio–ulnar joint. *Clin. Orthop.* 187: 26.

Parlasca R., Shoji H., and D'Ambrosia R.D. 1979. Effects of ligamentous injury on ankle and subtalar joints. A kinematic study. *Clin. Orthop.* 140: 266.

Pellegrini V.S., Olcott V.W., and Hollenberg C. 1993. Contact patterns in the trapeziometacarpal joint: The role of the palmar beak ligament. *J. Hand Surg.* 18A: 238.

Pereira D.S., Koval K.J., Resnick R.B. et al. 1996. Tibiotalar contact area and pressure distribution: The effect of mortise widening and syndesmosis fixation. *Foot Ankle* 17: 269.

Poppen N.K. and Walker P.S. 1976. Normal and abnormal motion of the shoulder. *J. Bone Joint Surg.* 58A: 195.

Ramsey P.L. and Hamilton W. 1976. Changes in tibiotalar area of contact caused by lateral talar shift. *J. Bone Joint Surg.* 58A: 356.

Rastegar J., Miller N., and Barmada R. 1980. An apparatus for measuring the load-displacement and load-dependent kinematic characteristics of articulating joints—Application to the human ankle. *J. Biomech. Eng.* 102: 208.

Root M.L., Weed J.H., Sgarlato T.E., and Bluth D.R. 1966. Axis of motion of the subtalar joint. *J. Am. Pediatry Assoc.* 56: 149.

Rosenbaum D., Eils E., and Hillmann A. 2003. Changes in talocrural joint contact stress characteristics after simulated rotationplasty. *J. Biomech.* 36: 81–86.

Saha A.K. 1971. Dynamic stability of the glenohumeral joint. *Acta Orthop. Scand.* 42: 491.

Sahara W., Sugamoto K., Murai M., Tanaka H., and Toshikawa H. 2006. 3D kinematic analysis of the acromioclavicular joint during arm abduction using vertically open MRI. *J. Orthop. Res.* 24: 1823–1831.

Sammarco G.J., Burstein A.J., and Frankel V.H. 1973. Biomechanics of the ankle: A kinematic study. *Orthop. Clin. North Am.* 4: 75–96.

Sato S. 1995. Load transmission through the wrist joint: A biomechanical study comparing the normal and pathological wrist. *Nippon Seikeigeka Gakkai Zasshi-Journal of the Japanese Orthopaedic Association* 69: 470–483.

Scarvell J.M., Smith P.N., Refshauge K.M., Galloway H.R., and Woods K.R. 2004. Evaluation of a method to map tibiofemoral contact points in the normal knee using MRI. *J. Orthop. Res.* 22: 788–793.

Schamblin M., Gupta R., Yang B.Y., Mcgarry M.H., Mcmaster W.C., and Lee T.Q. 2009. *In vitro* quantitative assessment of total and bipolar shoulder arthroplasties: A biomechanical study using human cadaver shoulders. *Clin Biomech (Bristol, Avon)*, 24: 626–631.

Schuind F.A., Linscheid R.L., An K.N. et al. 1992. Changes in wrist and forearm configuration with grasp and isometric contraction of elbow flexors. *J. Hand Surg.* 17A: 698.

Shephard E. 1951. Tarsal movements. *J. Bone Joint Surg.* 33B: 258.

Shiba R., Sorbie C., Siu D.W. et al. 1988. Geometry of the humeral–ulnar joint. *J. Orthop. Res.* 6: 897.

Singh A.K., Starkweather K.D., Hollister A.M. et al. 1992. Kinematics of the ankle: A hinge axis model. *Foot Ankle* 13: 439.

Soslowsky L.J., Flatow E.L., Bigliani L.U. et al. 1992. Quantitation of *in situ* contact areas at the glenohumeral joint: A biomechanical study. *J. Orthop. Res.* 10: 524.

Spoor C.W. and Veldpaus F.E. 1980. Rigid body motion calculated from spatial coordinates of markers. *J. Biomech.* 13: 391.

Stagni R., Leardini A., Ensini A., and Cappello A. 2005. Ankle morphometry evaluated using a new semi-automated technique based on X-ray pictures. *Clin. Biomech.,* 20: 307–311.

Stormont T.J., An K.A., Morrey B.F. et al. 1985. Elbow joint contact study: Comparison of techniques. *J. Biomech.* 18: 329.

Sugamoto K., Harada T., Machida A., Inui H., Miyamoto T., Takeuchi E., Yoshikawa H., and Ochi T. 2002. Scapulohumeral rhythm: Relationship between motion velocity and rhythm. *Clin. Orthop. Relat. Res.* 401: 119–124.

Tamai K., Ryu J., An K.N. et al. 1988. Three-dimensional geometric analysis of the metacarpophalangeal joint. *J. Hand Surg.* 13A: 521.

Tanaka S., An K.N., and Morrey B.F. 1998. Kinematics and laxity of ulnohumeral joint under valgus–varus stress. *J. Musculoskeletal Res.* 2: 45.

Tay S.C., Van Riet R., Kazunari T., Koff M.F., Amrami K.K., An K.N., and Berger R.A. 2008. A method for in-vivo kinematic analysis of the forearm. *J. Biomech.* 41: 56–62.

Tönnis D. 1987. *Congenital Dysplasia and Dislocation of the Hip and Shoulder in Adults*, pp. 1–12. Berlin, Springer-Verlag.

Van Eijden T.M.G.J., Kouwenhoven E., Verburg J. et al. 1986. A mathematical model of the patellofemoral joint. *J. Biomech.* 19: 219.

Van Langelaan E.J. 1983. A kinematical analysis of the tarsal joints. An x-ray photogrammetric study. *Acta Orthop. Scand.* 204: 211.

Viegas S.F., Patterson R.M., Peterson P.D. et al. 1989. The effects of various load paths and different loads on the load transfer characteristics of the wrist. *J. Hand Surg.* 14A: 458.

Viegas S.F., Patterson R.M., Todd P. et al. 1990. Load transfer characteristics of the midcarpal joint. *Wrist Biomechanics Symposium, Wrist Biomechanics Workshop*, Mayo Clinic, Rochester, MN.

Viegas S.F., Tencer A.F., Cantrell J. et al. 1987. Load transfer characteristics of the wrist: Part I. The normal joint. *J. Hand Surg.* 12A: 971.

Von Lanz D. and Wauchsmuth W. 1938. *Das Hüftgelenk, Praktische Anatomie* I Bd, pp. 138–175, Teil 4: *Bein und Statik*, Berlin, Springer-Verlag.

Wagner U.A., Sangeorzan B.J., Harrington R.M. et al. 1992. Contact characteristics of the subtalar joint: Load distribution between the anterior and posterior facets. *J. Orthop. Res.* 10: 535.

Walker P.S. and Erhman M.J. 1975. Laboratory evaluation of a metaplastic type of metacarpophalangeal joint prosthesis. *Clin. Orthop.* 112: 349.

Wang C.-L., Cheng C.-K., Chen C.-W. et al. 1994. Contact areas and pressure distributions in the subtalar joint. *J. Biomech.* 28: 269.

Woltring H.J., Huiskes R., deLange A., and Veldpaus F.E. 1985. Finite centroid and helical axis estimation from noisy landmark measurements in the study of human joint kinematics. *J. Biomech.* 18: 379.

Yoshioka Y., Siu D., and Cooke T.D.V. 1987. The anatomy and functional axes of the femur. *J. Bone Joint Surg.* 69A: 873.

Yoshioka Y., Siu D., Scudamore R.A. et al. 1989. Tibial anatomy in functional axes. *J. Orthop. Res.* 7: 132.

Youm Y., McMurty R.Y., Flatt A.E. et al. 1978. Kinematics of the wrist: An experimental study of radioulnar deviation and flexion/extension. *J. Bone Joint Surg.* 60A: 423.

Zuckerman J.D. and Matsen F.A. 1989. Biomechanics of the elbow. In M. Nordine and V.H. Frankel (Eds.), *Basic Biomechanics of the Musculoskeletal System*, pp. 249–260. Philadelphia, Lea & Febiger.

4

Joint Lubrication

Michael J. Furey
*Virginia Polytechnic
Institute and State
University*

The Fabric of the Joints in the Human Body is a subject so much the more entertaining, as it must strike every one that considers it attentively with an Idea of fine Mechanical Composition. Wherever the Motion of one Bone upon another is requisite, there we find an excellent Apparatus for rendering that Motion safe and free: We see, for Instance, the Extremity of one Bone molded into an orbicular Cavity, to receive the Head of another, in order to afford it an extensive Play. Both are covered with a smooth elastic Crust, to prevent mutual Abrasion; connected with strong Ligaments, to prevent Dislocation; and inclosed in a Bag that contains a proper Fluid Deposited there, for lubricating the Two contiguous Surfaces. So much in general.

The above is the opening paragraph of the classic paragraph of the classic paper by the surgeon, Sir William Hunter, "Of the Structure and Diseases of Articulating Cartilages" which he read at a meeting of the Royal Society, June 2, 1743 [1]. Since then, a great deal of research has been carried out on the subject of synovial joint lubrication. However, the mechanisms involved are still unknown.

4.1 Introduction

The purpose of this chapter is twofold: (1) to introduce the reader to the subject of tribology—the study of friction, wear, and lubrication; and (2) to extend this to the topic of *biotribology*, which includes the lubrication of natural synovial joints. It is not meant to be an exhaustive review of joint lubrication theories; space does not permit this. Instead, major concepts or principles will be discussed not only in the light of what is known about synovial joint lubrication but perhaps more importantly what is not known. Several references are given for those who wish to learn more about the topic. It is clear that synovial joints are by far the most complex and sophisticated tribological systems that exist. We shall see that although numerous theories have been put forth to attempt to explain joint lubrication, the mechanisms involved are still far from being understood. And when one begins to examine possible connections between tribology and degenerative joint disease or osteoarthritis (OA), the picture is even more complex and controversial. Finally, this chapter does not treat (1) the tribological behavior of artificial joints or partial joint replacements, (2) the possible use of elastic or poroplastic materials as artificial cartilage, and (3) new developments in cartilage repair using transplanted chondrocytes. These are separate topics, which would require detailed discussion and additional space.

4.2 Tribology

The word tribology, derived from the Greek "to rub," covers all frictional processes between solid bodies moving relative to one another that are in contact [2]. Thus, tribology may be defined as the study of friction, wear, and lubrication.

Tribological processes are involved whenever one solid slides or rolls against another, as in bearings, cams, gears, piston rings and cylinders, machining and metalworking, grinding, rock drilling, sliding electrical contacts, frictional welding, brakes, the striking of a match, music from a cello, articulation of human synovial joints (e.g., hip joints), machinery, and in numerous less obvious processes (e.g., walking, holding, stopping, writing, and the use of fasteners such as nails, screws, and bolts).

Tribology is a multidisciplinary subject involving at least the areas of materials science, solid and surface mechanics, surface science and chemistry, rheology, engineering, mathematics, and even biology and biochemistry. Although tribology is still an emerging science, interest in the phenomena of friction, wear, and lubrication is an ancient one. Unlike thermodynamics, there are no generally accepted laws in tribology. But there are some important basic principles that are needed to understand any study of lubrication and wear and even more so in a study of biotribology or biological lubrication phenomena. These basic principles follow.

4.2.1 Friction

Much of the early work in tribology was in the area of friction—possibly because frictional effects are more readily demonstrated and measured. Generally, early theories of friction dealt with dry or unlubricated systems. The problem was often treated strictly from a mechanical viewpoint, with little or no regard for the environment, surface films, or chemistry.

In the first place, *friction may be defined as the tangential resistance that is offered to the sliding of one solid body over another.* Friction is the result of many factors and cannot be treated as something as singular as density or even viscosity. Postulated sources of friction have included (1) the lifting of one asperity over another (increase in potential energy), (2) the interlocking of asperities followed by shear, (3) interlocking followed by plastic deformation or plowing, (4) adhesion followed by shear, (5) elastic hysteresis and waves of deformation, (6) adhesion or interlocking followed by tensile failure, (7) intermolecular attraction, (8) electrostatic effects, and (9) viscous drag. The coefficient of friction, indicated in the literature by μ or f, is defined as the ratio F/W where F = friction force and W = the normal load. It is emphasized that friction is a force and not a property of a solid material or lubricant.

4.2.2 Wear and Surface Damage

One definition of wear in a tribological sense is that it is the *progressive loss of substance from the operating surface of a body as a result of relative motion at the surface.* In comparison with friction, very little theoretical work has been done on the extremely important area of wear and surface damage. This is not too surprising in view of the complexity of wear and how little is known of the mechanisms by which it can occur. Variations in wear can be, and often are, enormous compared with variations in friction. For example, practically all the coefficients of sliding friction for diverse dry or lubricated systems fall within a relatively narrow range of 0.1–1. In some cases (e.g., certain regimes of hydrodynamic or "boundary" lubrication), the coefficient of friction may be <0.1 and as low as 0.001. In other cases (e.g., very clean unlubricated metals in vacuum), friction coefficients may exceed 1. Reduction of friction by a factor of 2 through changes in design, materials, or lubricant would be a reasonable, although not always attainable, goal. On the other hand, it is not uncommon for wear rates to vary by a factor of 100, 1000, or even more.

For systems consisting of common materials (e.g., metals, polymers, ceramics), there are at least four main mechanisms by which wear and surface damage can occur between solids in relative motion: (1) abrasive wear, (2) adhesive wear, (3) fatigue wear, and (4) chemical or corrosive wear. A fifth, fretting wear and fretting corrosion, combines elements of more than one mechanism. For complex biological materials such as articular cartilage, most likely other mechanisms are involved.

Again, wear is the removal of material. The idea that friction causes wear and therefore, low friction means low wear, is a common mistake. Brief descriptions of five types of wear; abrasive, adhesive, fatigue, chemical or corrosive, and fretting—may be found in Reference 2 as well as in other references in this chapter. Next, it may be useful to consider some of the major concepts of lubrication.

4.3 Lubrication

Lubrication is a process of reducing friction *and/or* wear (or other forms of surface damage) between relatively moving surfaces by the application of a solid, liquid, or gaseous substance (i.e., a lubricant). Since friction and wear do not necessarily correlate with each other, the use of the word *and* in place of *and/or* in the above definition is a common mistake to be avoided. The primary function of a lubricant is to reduce friction or wear or both between moving surfaces in contact with each other.

Examples of lubricants are wide and varied. They include automotive engine oils, wheel bearing greases, transmission fluids, electrical contact lubricants, rolling oils, cutting fluids, preservative oils, gear oils, jet fuels, instrument oils, turbine oils, textile lubricants, machine oils, jet engine lubricants, air, water, molten glass, liquid metals, oxide films, talcum powder, graphite, molybdenum disulfide, waxes, soaps, polymers, and the synovial fluid in human joints.

A few general principles of lubrication may be mentioned here:

1. The lubricant must be present at the place where it can function.
2. Almost any substance under carefully selected or special conditions can be shown to reduce friction or wear in a particular test, but that does not mean these substances are lubricants.
3. Friction and wear do not necessarily go together. This is an extremely important principle which applies to nonlubricated (dry) as well as lubricated systems. It is particularly true under conditions of "boundary lubrication," to be discussed later. An additive may reduce friction and increase wear, reduce wear and increase friction, reduce both or increase both. Although the reasons are not fully understood, this is an experimental observation. Thus, friction and wear should be thought of as separate phenomena—an important point when we discuss theories of synovial joint lubrication.
4. The effective or active lubricating film in a particular system may or may not consist of the original or bulk lubricant phase.

In a broad sense, it may be considered that the main function of a lubricant is to keep the surfaces apart so that interaction (e.g., adhesion, plowing, and shear) between the solids cannot occur; thus friction and wear can be reduced or controlled.

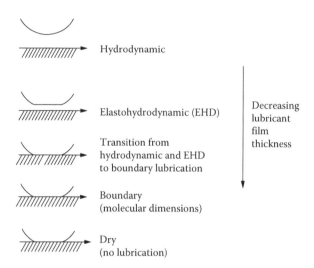

FIGURE 4.1   Regimes of lubrication.

The following regimes or types of lubrication may be considered in the order of increasing severity or decreasing lubricant film thickness (Figure 4.1):

1. Hydrodynamic lubrication
2. Elastohydrodynamic lubrication (EHL)
3. Transition from hydrodynamic and EHL to boundary lubrication
4. Boundary lubrication

A fifth regime, sometimes referred to as *dry* or *unlubricated*, may also be considered as an extreme or limit. In addition, there is another form of lubrication that does not require relative movement of the bodies either parallel or perpendicular to the surface, that is, as in externally pressurized hydrostatic or aerostatic bearings.

4.3.1 Hydrodynamic Lubrication Theories

In hydrodynamic lubrication, the load is supported by the pressure developed due to relative motion and the geometry of the system. In the regime of hydrodynamic or fluid film lubrication, there is no contact between the solids. The film thickness is governed by the bulk physical properties of the lubricants, the most important being viscosity; friction arises purely from shearing of viscous lubricant.

Contributions to our knowledge of hydrodynamic lubrication, with special focus on journal bearings, have been made by numerous investigators including Reynolds. The classic Reynolds treatment considered the equilibrium of a fluid element and the pressure and shear forces on this element. In this treatment, eight assumptions were made (e.g., surface curvature is large compared to lubricant film thickness, fluid is Newtonian, flow is laminar, viscosity is constant through film thickness). Velocity distributions due to relative motion and pressure buildup were developed and added together. The solution of the basic Reynolds equation for a particular bearing configuration results in a pressure distribution throughout the film as a function of viscosity, film shape, and velocity.

The total load W and frictional (viscous) drag F can be calculated from this information. For rotating disks with parallel axes, the "simple" Reynolds equation yields

$$\frac{h_o}{R} = 4.9 \left(\frac{\eta U}{W} \right) \tag{4.1}$$

where h_o is the minimum lubricant film thickness, η is the absolute viscosity, U is the average velocity $(U_1 + U_2)/2$, W is the applied normal load per unit width of disk, and R is the reduced radius of curvature $(1/R = 1/R_1 + 1/R_2)$.

The dimensionless term $(\eta U/W)$ is sometimes referred to as the hydrodynamic factor. It can be seen that doubling either the viscosity or velocity doubles the film thickness, and that doubling the applied load halves the film thickness. This regime of lubrication is sometimes referred to as the *rigid isoviscous or classical Martin condition*, since the solid bodies are assumed to be perfectly rigid (nondeformable), and the fluid is assumed to have a constant viscosity.

At high loads with systems such as gears, ball bearings, and other high-contact-stress geometries, two additional factors have been considered in further developments of the hydrodynamic theory of lubrication. One of these is that the surfaces deform elastically; this leads to a localized change in geometry more favorable to lubrication. The second is that the lubricant becomes more viscous under the high pressure existing in the contact zone, according to relationships such as

$$\eta/\eta_o = \exp\alpha(p - p_o) \tag{4.2}$$

where η is the viscosity at pressure p, η_o is the viscosity at atmospheric pressure p_o, and α is the pressure–viscosity coefficient (e.g., in Pa^{-1}). In this concept, the lubricant pressures existing in the contact zone approximate those of dry contact Hertzian stress. This is the regime of elastohydrodynamic lubrication, sometimes abbreviated as EHL or EHD. It may also be described as the elastic–viscous type or mode of lubrication, since elastic deformation exists and the fluid viscosity is considerably greater due to the pressure effect.

The comparable Dowson–Higginson expression for minimum film thickness between cylinders or disks in contact with parallel axes is

$$\frac{h_o}{R} = 2.6\left(\frac{\eta U}{W}\right)^{0.7}\left(\frac{\alpha W}{R}\right)^{0.54}\left(\frac{W}{RE'}\right)^{0.03} \tag{4.3}$$

The term E' represents the reduced modulus of elasticity:

$$\frac{1}{E'} = \frac{(1 - v_1^2)}{E_1} + \frac{(1 - v_2^2)}{E_2} \tag{4.4}$$

where E is the modulus, v is Poisson's ratio, and the subscripts 1 and 2 refer to the two solids in contact. All the other terms are the same as previously stated. In addition to the hydrodynamic factor $(\eta U/W)$, a pressure–viscosity factor $(\alpha W/R)$, and an elastic deformation factor (W/RE') can be considered. Thus, properties of both the lubricant and the solids as materials are included. In examining the elastohydrodynamic film thickness equations, it can be seen that the velocity U is an important factor $(h_o \propto U^{0.7})$ but the load W is rather unimportant $(h_o \propto W^{-0.13})$.

Experimental confirmation of the EHL theory has been obtained in certain selected systems using electrical capacitance, x-ray transmission, and optical interference techniques to determine film thickness and shape under dynamic conditions. Research is continuing in this area, including studies on micro-EHL or asperity lubrication mechanisms, since surfaces are never perfectly smooth. These studies may lead to a better understanding of not only lubricant film formation in high-contact-stress systems but lubricant film failure as well.

Two other possible types of hydrodynamic lubrication, rigid–viscous and elastic–isoviscous, complete the matrix of four, considering the two factors of elastic deformation and pressure–viscosity effects. In addition, *squeeze film* lubrication can occur when surfaces approach one another. For more information on hydrodynamic and EHL, see Cameron [3] and Dowson and Higginson [4].

4.3.2 Transition from Hydrodynamic to Boundary Lubrication

Although prevention of contact is probably the most important function of a lubricant, there is still much to be learned about the transition from hydrodynamic and EHL to boundary lubrication. This is the region in which lubrication goes from the desirable hydrodynamic condition of no contact to the less acceptable "boundary" condition, where increased contact usually leads to higher friction and wear. This regime is sometimes referred to as a condition of *mixed lubrication*.

Several examples of experimental approaches to thin-film lubrication have been reported [3]. It is important in examining these techniques to make the distinction between methods that are used to determine lubricant film thickness under hydrodynamic or elastohydrodynamic conditions (e.g., optical interference, electrical capacitance, or x-ray transmission), and methods that are used to determine the occurrence or frequency of contact. As we will see later, most experimental studies of synovial joint lubrication have focused on friction measurements, using the information to determine the lubrication regime involved; this approach can be misleading.

4.3.2.1 Boundary Lubrication

Although there is no generally accepted definition of boundary lubrication, it is often described as a condition of lubrication in which the friction and wear between two surfaces in relative motion are determined by the surface properties of the solids and the chemical nature of the lubricant rather than its viscosity. An example of the difficulty in defining boundary lubrication can be seen if the term *bulk viscosity* is used in place of viscosity in the preceding sentence—another frequent form. This opens the door to the inclusion of elastohydrodynamic effects which depend in part on the influence of pressure on viscosity. Increased friction under these circumstances could be attributed to increased viscous drag rather than solid–solid contact. According to another common definition, boundary lubrication occurs or exists when the surfaces of the bearing solids are separated by films of molecular thickness. That may be true, but it ignores the possibility that "boundary" layer surface films may indeed be very thick (i.e., 10, 20, or 100 molecular layers). The difficulty is that boundary lubrication is complex.

Although a considerable amount of research has been done on this topic, an understanding of the basic mechanisms and processes involved is by no means complete. Therefore, definitions of boundary lubrication tend to be nonoperational. This is an extremely important regime of lubrication because it involves more extensive solid–solid contact and interaction as well as generally greater friction, wear, and surface damage. In many practical systems, the occurrence of the boundary lubrication regime is unavoidable or at least quite common. The condition can be brought about by high loads, low relative sliding speeds (including zero for stop-and-go, motion reversal, or reciprocating elements) and low lubricant viscosity—factors that are important in the transition from hydrodynamic to boundary lubrication.

The most important factor in boundary lubrication is the chemistry of the tribological system—the contacting solids and total environment including lubricants. More particularly, the surface chemistry and interactions occurring with and on the solid surfaces are important. This includes factors such as physisorption, chemisorption, intermolecular forces, surface chemical reactions, and the nature, structure, and properties of thin films on solid surfaces. It also includes many other effects brought on by the process of moving one solid over another, such as (1) changes in topography and the area of contact, (2) high surface temperatures, (3) the generation of fresh reactive metal surfaces by the removal of oxide and other layers, (4) catalysis, (5) the generation of electrical charges, and (6) the emission of charged particles such as electrons.

In examining the action of boundary lubricant compounds in reducing friction or wear or both between solids in sliding contact, it may be helpful to consider at least the following five modes of film formation on or protection of surfaces: (1) physisorption, (2) chemisorption, (3) chemical reactions with the solid surface, (4) chemical reactions on the solid surface, and (5) mere interposition of a solid or other material. These modes of surface protection are discussed in more detail in Reference 2.

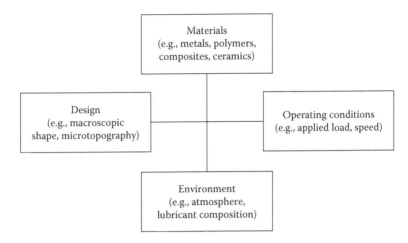

FIGURE 4.2 In any tribological system, friction, wear, and surface damage depend on four interrelated factors.

The beneficial and harmful effects of minor changes in chemistry of the environment (e.g., the lubricant) are often enormous in comparison with hydrodynamic and elastohydrodynamic effects. Thus, the surface and chemical properties of the solid materials used in tribological applications become especially important. One might expect that this would also be the case in biological (e.g., human joint) lubrication where biochemistry is very likely an important factor.

4.3.2.2 General Comments on Tribological Processes

It is important to recognize that friction and wear depend upon four major factors, that is, materials, design, operating conditions, and total environment (Figure 4.2). This four-block figure may be useful as a guide in thinking about synovial joint lubrication either from a theoretical or experimental viewpoint—the topic discussed in the next section.

Readers are cautioned against the use of various terms in tribology which are either vaguely defined or not defined at all. These would include such terms as "lubricating ability," "lubricity," and even "boundary lubrication." For example, do "boundary lubricating properties" refer to effects on friction or effects on wear and damage? It makes a difference. It is emphasized once again that friction and wear are different phenomena. Low friction does not necessarily mean low wear. We will see several examples of this common error in the discussion of joint lubrication research.

4.4 Synovial Joints

Examples of natural synovial or movable joints include the human hip, knee, elbow, ankle, finger, and shoulder. A simplified representation of a synovial joint is shown in Figure 4.3. The bones are covered by a thin layer of articular cartilage bathed in synovial fluid confined by synovial membrane. Synovial joints are truly remarkable systems—providing the basis of movement by allowing bones to articulate on one another with minimal friction and wear. Unfortunately, various joint diseases occur even among the young—causing pain, loss of freedom of movement, or instability.

Synovial joints are complex, sophisticated systems not yet fully understood. The loads are surprisingly high and the relative motion is complex. Articular cartilage has the deceptive appearance of simplicity and uniformity. But it is an extremely complex material with unusual properties. Basically, it consists of water (~75%) enmeshed in a network of collagen fibers and proteoglycans with high molecular weight. In a way, cartilage could be considered as one of nature's composite materials. Articular cartilage also has no blood supply, no nerves, and very few cells (chondrocytes).

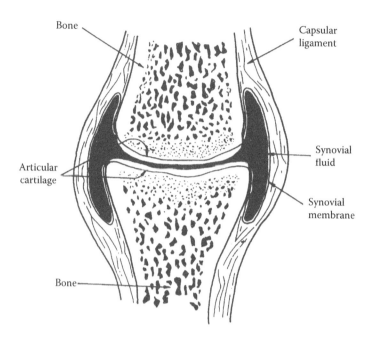

FIGURE 4.3   Representation of a synovial joint.

The other major component of an articular joint is *synovial fluid*, named by Paracelsus after "synovia" (egg-white). It is essentially a dialysate of blood plasma with added hyaluronic acid. Synovial fluid contains complex proteins, polysaccharides, and other compounds. Its chief constituent is water (~85%). Synovial fluid functions as a joint lubricant, nutrient for cartilage, and carrier for waste products.

For more information on the biochemistry, structure, and properties of articular cartilage, Freeman [5], Sokoloff [6], Stockwell [7], and articles referenced in these works are suggested.

4.5 Theories on the Lubrication of Natural and Normal Synovial Joints

As stated, the word *tribology* means the study of friction, wear, and lubrication. Therefore, *biotribology* may be thought of as the study of biological lubrication processes, for example, as in synovial joints. A surprisingly large number of concepts and theories of synovial joint lubrication have been proposed [8–10] (as shown in Table 4.1). And even if similar ideas are grouped together, there are still well over a dozen fundamentally different theories. These have included a wide range of lubrication concepts, for example, hydrodynamic, hydrostatic, elasto-hydrodynamic, squeeze-film, "boundary," mixed-regime, "weeping," osmotic, synovial mucin gel, "boosted," lipid, electrostatic, porous layers, and special forms of boundary lubrication (e.g., "lubricating glycoproteins," structuring of boundary water "surface-active" phospholipids). This chapter will not review these numerous theories, but excellent reviews on the lubrication of synovial joints have been written by McCutchen [11], Swanson [12], and Higginsworth and Unsworth [13]. The book edited by Dumbleton is also recommended [14]. In addition, theses by Droogendijk [15] and Burkhardt [16] contain extensive and detailed reviews of theories of joint lubrication.

McCutchen was the first to propose an entirely new concept of lubrication, "weeping lubrication," applied to synovial joint action [17,18]. He considered unique and special properties of cartilage and how this could affect flow and lubrication. The work of Mow et al. continued along a more complex and sophisticated approach in which a biomechanical model is proposed for the study of the dynamic

TABLE 4.1 Examples of Proposed Mechanisms and Studies of Synovial Joint Lubrication

Mechanism	Authors	Date
1. Hydrodynamic	MacConnail	1932
2. Boundary	Jones	1934
3. Hydrodynamic	Jones	1936
4. Boundary	Charnley	1959
5. Weeping	McCutchen	1959
6. Floating	Barnett and Cobbold	1962
7. Elastohydrodynamic	Tanner	1966
	Dowson	1967
8. Thixotropic/elastic fluid	Dintenfass	1963
9. Osmotic (boundary)	McCutchen	1966
10. Squeeze-film	Fein	1966
	Higginson et al.	1974
11. Synovial gel	Maroudas	1967
12. Thin-film	Faber et al.	1967
13. Combinations of hydrostatic, boundary, and EHL	Linn	1968
14. Boosted	Walker et al.	1968
15. Lipid	Little et al.	1969
16. Weeping + boundary	McCutchen and Wilkins	1969
	McCutchen	1969
17. Boundary	Caygill and West	1969
18. Fat (or mucin)	Freeman et al.	1970
19. Electrostatic	Roberts	1971
20. Boundary + fluid squeeze-film	Radin and Paul	1972
21. Mixed	Unsworth et al.	1974
22. Imbibe/exudate composite model	Ling	1974
23. Complex biomechanical model	Mow et al.	1974
	Mansour and Mow	1977
24. Two porous layer model	Dinnar	1974
25. Boundary	Reimann et al.	1975
26. Squeeze-film + fluid film + boundary	Unsworth, Dowson et al.	1975
27. Compliant bearing model	Rybicki	1977
28. Lubricating glycoproteins	Swann et al.	1977
29. Structuring of boundary water	Sokoloff et al.	1979
30. Surface flow	Kenyon	1980
31. Lubricin	Swann et al.	1985
32. Micro-EHL	Dowson and Jin	1986
33. Lubricating factor	Jay	1992
34. Lipidic component	LaBerge et al.	1993
35. Constitutive modeling of cartilage	Lai et al.	1993
36. Asperity model	Yao et al.	1993
37. Bingham fluid	Tandon et al.	1994
38. Filtration/gel/squeeze film	Hlavacek et al.	1995
39. Surface-active phospholipid	Schwarz and Hills	1998
40. Interstitial fluid pressurization	Ateshian et al.	1998

interaction between synovial fluid and articular cartilage [19,20]. These ideas are combined in the more recent work of Ateshian [21] which uses a framework of the biphasic theory of articular cartilage to model interstitial fluid pressurization. Several additional studies have also been made of effects of porosity and compliance, including the behavior of elastic layers, in producing hydrodynamic and squeeze-film lubrication. A good review in this area was given by Unsworth who discussed both human and artificial joints [22].

The following general observations are offered on the theories of synovial joint lubrication that have been proposed:

1. Most of the theories are strictly mechanical or rheological—involving such factors as deformation, pressure, and fluid flow.
2. There is a preoccupation with *friction*, which of course is very low for articular cartilage systems.
3. None of the theories consider *wear*—which is neither the same as friction nor related to it.
4. The detailed structure, biochemistry, complexity, and living nature of the total articular cartilage–synovial fluid system are generally ignored.

These are only general impressions. And although mechanical/rheological concepts seem dominant (with a focus on friction), wear and biochemistry are not completely ignored. For example, Simon [23] abraded articular cartilage from human patellae and canine femoral heads with a stainless-steel rotary file, measuring the depth of penetration with time and the amount of wear debris generated. Cartilage wear was also studied experimentally by Bloebaum and Wilson [24], Radin and Paul [25], and Lipshitz et al. [26–28]. The latter researchers carried out several *in vitro* studies of wear of articular cartilage using bovine cartilage plugs or specimens in sliding contact against stainless-steel plates. They developed a means of measuring cartilage wear by determining the hydroxyproline content of both the lubricant and solid wear debris. Using this system and technique, effects of variables such as time, applied load, and chemical modification of articular cartilage on wear and profile changes were determined. This work is of particular importance in that they addressed the question of *cartilage wear and damage* rather than friction, recognizing that wear and friction are different phenomena.

Special note is also made of two researchers, Swann and Sokoloff, who considered biochemistry as an important factor in synovial joint lubrication. Swann et al. very carefully isolated fractions of bovine synovial fluid using sequential sedimentation techniques and gel permeation chromatography. They found a high molecular weight glycoprotein to be the major constituent in the articular lubrication fraction from bovine synovial fluid and called this LGP-I (from lubricating glycoprotein). This was based on friction measurements using cartilage in sliding contact against a glass disc. An excellent summary of this work with additional references is presented in a chapter by Swann in *The Joints and Synovial Fluid: I* [6].

Sokoloff et al. [29] examined the "boundary lubricating ability" of several synovial fluids using a latex-glass test system and cartilage specimens obtained at necropsy from knees. Measurements were made of friction. The research was extended to other *in vitro* friction tests using cartilage obtained from the nasal septum of cows and widely differing artificial surfaces [30]. As a result of this work, a new model of boundary lubrication by synovial fluid was proposed—the structuring of boundary water. The postulate involves adsorption of one part of a glycoprotein on a surface followed by the formation of hydration shells around the polar portions of the adsorbed glycoprotein; the net result is a thin layer of viscous "structured" water at the surface. This work is of particular interest in that it involves not only a specific and more detailed mechanism of boundary lubrication in synovial joints but also takes into account the possible importance of water in this system.

In more recent research by Jay, an interaction between hyaluronic acid and a "purified synovial lubricating factor" (PSLF) was observed, suggesting a possible synergistic action in the boundary lubrication of synovial joints [31]. The definition of "lubricating ability" was based on friction measurements made with a latex-covered stainless-steel stud in oscillating contact against polished glass.

The above summary of major synovial joint lubrication theories is taken from References 10 and 31 as well as the thesis by Burkhardt [32].

Two more recent studies are of interest since cartilage wear was considered although not as a part of a theory of joint lubrication. Stachowiak et al. [33] investigated the friction and wear characteristics of adult rat femur cartilage against a stainless-steel plate using an environmental scanning microscope (ESM) to examine damaged cartilage. One finding was evidence of a load limit to lubrication of cartilage, beyond which high friction and damage occurred. Another study, by Hayes et al. [34] on the influence of crystals on cartilage wear, is particularly interesting not only in the findings reported (e.g., certain crystals can increase cartilage wear), but also in the full description of the biochemical techniques used.

A special note should be made concerning the doctoral thesis by Lawrence Malcom in 1976 [35]. This is an excellent study of cartilage friction and deformation, in which a device resembling a rotary plate rheometer was used to investigate the effects of static and dynamic loading on the frictional behavior of bovine cartilage. The contact geometry consisted of a circular cylindrical annulus in contact with a concave hemispherical section. It was found that dynamically loaded specimens in bovine synovial fluid yielded the more efficient lubrication based on friction measurements. The Malcom study is thorough and excellent in its attention to detail (e.g., specimen preparation) in examining the influence of type of loading and time effects on cartilage friction. It does not, however, consider cartilage wear and damage except in a very preliminary way. And it does not consider the influence of fluid biochemistry on cartilage friction, wear, and damage. In short, the Malcom work represents a superb piece of systematic research along the lines of mechanical, dynamic, rheological, and viscoelastic behavior—one important dimension of synovial joint lubrication.

4.6 *In Vitro* Cartilage Wear Studies

Over the last 15 years, studies aimed at exploring possible connections between tribology and mechanisms of synovial joint lubrication and degeneration (e.g., OA) have been conducted by the author and his graduate and undergraduate students in the Department of Mechanical Engineering at Virginia Polytechnic Institute and State University. The basic approach used involved *in vitro* tribological experiments using bovine articular cartilage, with an emphasis on the effects of fluid composition and biochemistry on cartilage wear and damage. This research is an outgrowth of earlier work carried out during a sabbatical study in the Laboratory for the Study of Skeletal Disorders, The Children's Hospital Medical Center, Harvard Medical School in Boston. In that study, bovine cartilage test specimens were loaded against a polished steel plate and subjected to reciprocating sliding for several hours in the presence of a fluid (e.g., bovine synovial fluid or a buffered saline reference fluid containing biochemical constituents kindly provided by Dr. David Swann). Cartilage wear was determined by sampling the test fluid and determining the concentration of 4-hydroxyproline—a constituent of collagen. The results of that earlier study have been reported and summarized elsewhere [36–39]. Figure 4.4 shows the average hydroxyproline contents of wear debris obtained from these *in vitro* experiments. These numbers are related to the cartilage wear which occurred. However, since the total quantities of collected fluids varied somewhat, the values shown in the bar graph should not be taken as exact or precise measures of fluid effects on cartilage wear.

The main conclusions of that study were as follows:

1. Normal bovine synovial fluid is very effective in reducing cartilage wear under these *in vitro* conditions as compared to the buffered saline reference fluid.
2. There is no significant difference in wear between the saline reference and distilled water.
3. The addition of hyaluronic acid to the reference fluid significantly reduces wear; but its effect depends on the source.
4. Under these test conditions, Swann's LGP-I, known to be extremely effective in reducing friction in cartilage-on-glass tests, does not reduce cartilage wear.
5. However, a protein complex isolated by Swann is extremely effective in reducing wear—producing results similar to those obtained with synovial fluid. The detailed structure of this constituent is complex and has not yet been fully determined.

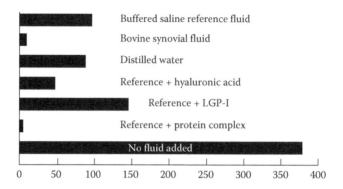

FIGURE 4.4   Relative cartilage wear based on hydroxyproline content of debris (*in vitro* tests with cartilage on stainless steel).

6. Last, the lack of an added fluid in these experiments leads to extremely high wear and damage of the articular cartilage.

In discussing the possible significance of these findings from a tribological point of view, it may be helpful first of all to emphasize once again that friction and wear are different phenomena. Furthermore, as suggested by Figure 4.5, certain constituents of synovial fluid (e.g., Swann's LGP) may act to reduce friction in synovial joints while other constituents (e.g., Swann's protein complex or hyaluronic acid) may act to reduce cartilage *wear*. Therefore, it is necessary to distinguish between biochemical antifriction and antiwear compounds present in synovial fluid.

In more recent years, this study has been greatly enhanced by the participation of interested faculty and students from the Virginia-Maryland College of Veterinary Medicine and Department of Biochemistry and Animal Science at Virginia Tech. One major hypothesis tested is a continuation of previous work showing that the detailed biochemistry of the fluid–cartilage system has a pronounced and possibly controlling influence on cartilage wear. A consequence of the above hypothesis is that a lack or deficiency of certain biochemical constituents in the synovial joint may be one factor contributing to the initiation and progression of cartilage damage, wear, and possibly OA. A related but somewhat different hypothesis concerns synovial fluid constituents which may act to increase the wear and further damage of articular cartilage under tribological contact.

To carry out continued research on biotribology, a new device for studies of cartilage deformation, wear, damage, and friction under conditions of tribological contact was designed by Burkhardt [32] and later modified, constructed, and instrumented. A simplified sketch is shown in Figure 4.6. The key features of this test device are shown in Table 4.2. The apparatus is designed to accommodate cartilage-on-cartilage specimens. Motion of the lower specimen is controlled by a computer-driven *x*–*y* table, allowing simple oscillating motion or complex motion patterns. An octagonal strain ring with two full semi-conductor bridges is used to measure the normal load as well as the tangential load (friction). An

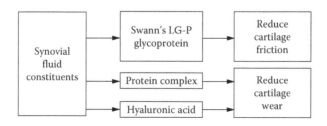

FIGURE 4.5   Friction and wear are different phenomena.

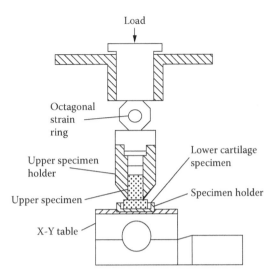

FIGURE 4.6 Device for *in vitro* cartilage-on-cartilage wear studies.

LVDT, not shown in the figure, is used to measure cartilage deformation and linear wear during a test. However, hydroxyproline analysis of the wear debris and washings is used for the actual determination of total cartilage wear on a mass basis.

In one study by Schroeder [40], two types of experiments were carried out, that is, cartilage-on-stainless steel and cartilage-on-cartilage at applied loads up to 70 N—yielding an average pressure of 2.2 MPa in the contact area. Reciprocating motion (40 cps) was used. The fluids tested included (1) a buffered saline solution, (2) saline plus hyaluronic acid, and (3) bovine synovial fluid. In cartilage-on-stainless-steel tests, scanning electron microscopy, and histological staining showed distinct effects of the lubricants on surface and subsurface damage. Tests with the buffered saline fluid resulted in the most damage, with large wear tracks visible on the surface of the cartilage plug, as well as subsurface voids and cracks. When hyaluronic acid, a constituent of the natural synovial joint lubricant, was added

TABLE 4.2 Key Features of Test Device Designed for Cartilage Wear Studies

Contact System	Cartilage-on-Cartilage
Contact geometry	Flat-on-flat, convex-on-flat, irregular-on-irregular
Cartilage type	Articular, any source (e.g., bovine)
Specimen size	Upper specimen, 4–6 mm diam., lower specimen, ca. 15–25 mm diam.
Applied load	50–660 N
Average pressure	0.44–4.4 MPa
Type of motion	Linear, oscillating; circular, constant velocity; more complex patterns
Sliding velocity	0–20 mm/s
Fluid temperature	Ambient (20°C); or controlled humidity
Environment	Ambient or controlled humidity
Measurements	Normal load, cartilage deformation, friction; cartilage wear and damage, biochemical analysis of cartilage specimens, synovial fluid, and wear debris; sub-surface changes

Source: Burkhardt, B.M. Development and design of a test device for cartilage wear studies, MS thesis, Mechanical Engineering, Virginia Polytechnic Institute and State University, Blacksburg, VA, December 1988.

to the saline reference fluid, less severe damage was observed. Little or no cartilage damage was evident in tests in which the natural synovial joint fluid was used as the lubricant.

These results were confirmed in a later study by Owellen [41] in which hydroxyproline analysis was used to determine cartilage wear. It was found that increasing the applied load from 20 to 65 N increased cartilage wear by eightfold for the saline solution and approximately threefold for synovial fluid. Furthermore, the coefficient of friction increased from an initial low value of 0.01–0.02 to a much higher value, for example, 0.20–0.30 and higher, during a normal test which lasted 3 h; the greatest change occurred during the first 20 min. Another interesting result was that a thin film of transferred or altered material was observed on the stainless-steel disks—being most pronounced with the buffered saline lubricant and not observed with synovial fluid. Examination of the film with Fourier transfer infrared microspectrometry shows distinctive bio-organic spectra which differs from that of the original bovine cartilage. We believe this to be an important finding since it suggests a possible bio-tribo-chemical effect [42].

In another phase of this research, the emphasis is on the cartilage-on-cartilage system and the influence of potentially beneficial as well as harmful constituents of synovial fluid on wear and damage. In cartilage-on-cartilage tests, the most severe wear and damage occurred during tests with buffered saline as the lubricant. The damage was less severe than in the stainless-steel tests, but some visible wear tracks were detectable with scanning electron microscopy. Histological sectioning and staining of both the upper and lower cartilage samples show evidence of elongated lacunae and coalesced voids that could lead to wear by delamination. An example is shown in Figure 4.7 (original magnification of 500 × on 35 mm slide). The proteoglycan content of the subsurface cartilage under the region of contact was also reduced. When synovial fluid was used as the lubricant, no visible wear or damage was detected [43]. These results demonstrate that even in *in vitro* tests with bovine articular cartilage, the nature of the fluid environment can have a dramatic effect on the severity of wear and subsurface damage.

In a more recent study carried out by Berrien in the biotribology program at Virginia Tech, a different approach was taken to examine the role of joint lubrication in joint disease, particularly OA. A degradative biological enzyme, collagenase-3, suspected of playing a role in a cartilage degeneration was used to create a physiologically adverse biochemical fluid environment. Tribological tests were performed with the same device and procedures described previously. The stainless-steel disk was replaced with a 1 in. diameter plug of bovine cartilage to create a cartilage sliding on cartilage configuration more closely related to the *in vivo* condition. Normal load was increased to 78.6 N and synovial fluid and buffered saline were used as lubricants. Prior to testing, cartilage plugs were exposed to a fluid medium containing three concentrations of collagenase-3 for 24 h. The major discovery of this work was that exposure to the collagenase-3 enzyme had a substantial adverse effect on cartilage wear *in vitro*, increasing average wear

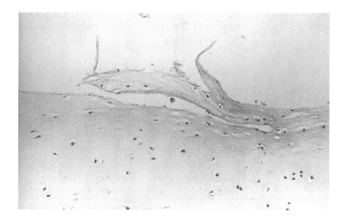

FIGURE 4.7 Cartilage damage produced by sliding contact.

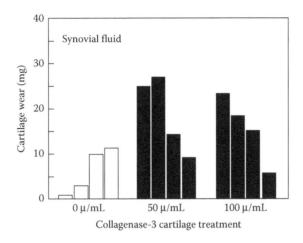

FIGURE 4.8   Effect of collagenase-3 on cartilage wear.

values by three and one-half times those of the unexposed cases. Figure 4.8 shows an example of the effect of enzyme treatment when bovine synovial fluid was used as the lubricant. Scanning electron microscopy showed disruption of the superficial layer and collagen matrix with exposure to collagenase-3, where unexposed cartilage showed none. Histological sections showed a substantial loss of the superficial layer of cartilage and a distinct and abnormal loss of proteoglycans in the middle layer of collagenase-treated cartilage. Unexposed cartilage showed only minor disruption of the superficial layer [44].

This study indicates that some of the biochemical constituents that gain access to the joint space, during normal and pathological functions, can have a significant adverse effect on the wear and damage of the articular cartilage. Future studies will include determination of additional constituents that have harmful effects on cartilage wear and damage. This research, using bovine articular cartilage in *in vitro* sliding contact tests, raises a number of interesting questions:

1. Has "Nature" designed a special biochemical compound which has as its function the protection of articular cartilage?
2. What is the mechanism (or mechanisms) by which biochemical constituents of synovial fluid can act to reduce wear of articular cartilage?
3. Could a lack of this biochemical constituent lead to increased cartilage wear and damage?
4. Does articular cartilage from osteoarthritic patients have reduced wear resistance?
5. Do any of the findings on the importance of synovial fluid biochemistry on cartilage wear in our *in vitro* studies apply to living or *in vitro* systems as well?
6. How does collagenase-3 treatment of cartilage lead to increased wear and does this finding have any significance in the *in vivo* situation? This question is addressed in the next section.

4.7 Biotribology and Arthritis: Are There Connections?

Arthritis is an umbrella term for more than 100 rheumatic diseases affecting joints and connective tissue. The two most common forms are OA and rheumatoid arthritis (RA). Osteoarthritis—also referred to as *osteoarthrosis or degenerative joint disease*—is the most common form of arthritis. It is sometimes simplistically described as the "wear and tear" form of arthritis. The causes and progression of degenerative joint disease are still not understood. RA is a chronic and often progressive disease of the synovial membrane leading to release of enzymes which attack, erode, and destroy articular cartilage. It is an inflammatory response involving the immune system and is more prevalent in female individuals. RA is extremely complex. Its causes are still unknown.

Sokoloff defines degenerative joint disease as "an extremely common, noninflammatory, progressive disorder of movable joints, particularly weight-bearing joints, characterized pathologically by deterioration of articular cartilage and by formation of new bone in the sub-chondral areas and at the margins of the 'joint'" [45]. As mentioned, osteoarthritis or osteoarthrosis is sometimes referred to as the "wear and tear" form of arthritis; but, wear itself is rarely a simple process even in well-defined systems.

It has been noted by the author that tribological terms occasionally appear in hypotheses which describe the etiology of OA (e.g., "reduced wear resistance of cartilage" or "poor lubricity of synovial fluid"). It has also been noted that there is a general absence of hypotheses connecting normal synovial joint *lubrication* (or lack thereof) and synovial joint *degeneration*. Perhaps it is natural (and unhelpful) for a tribologist to imagine such a connection and that, for example, cartilage wear under certain circumstances might be due to or influenced by a lack of proper "boundary lubrication" by the synovial fluid. In this regard, it may be of interest to quote Swanson [12] who said in 1979 that "there exists at present no experimental evidence which certainly shows that a failure of lubrication is or is not a causative factor in the first stages of cartilage degeneration." A statement made by Professor Glimcher (discussions with M.J. Glimcher, The Children's Hospital Medical Center) may also be appropriate here. Glimcher fully recognized the fundamental difference between friction and wear as well as the difference between joint lubrication (one area of study) and joint degeneration (another area of study). Glimcher said that wearing or abrading cartilage with a steel file is not OA; and neither is digesting cartilage in a test tube with an enzyme. But both forms of cartilage deterioration can occur in a living joint and in a way which is still not understood. It is interesting that essentially none of the many synovial joint lubrication theories consider enzymatic degradation of cartilage as a factor whereas practically all the models of the etiology of degenerative joint disease include this as an important factor.

It was stated earlier that there are at least two main areas to consider, that is, (1) mechanisms of synovial joint lubrication and (2) the etiology of synovial joint degeneration (e.g., as in osteoarthrosis). Both areas are extremely complex. And the key questions as to what actually happens in each have yet to be answered (and perhaps asked). It may therefore be presumptuous of the present author to suggest possible connections between two areas which in themselves are still not fully understood.

Tribological processes in a movable joint involve not only the contacting surfaces (articular cartilage), but the surrounding medium (synovial fluid) as well. Each of these depends on the synthesis and transport of necessary biochemical constituents to the contact region or interface. As a result of relative motion (sliding, rubbing, rolling, and impact) between the joint elements, friction and wear can occur.

It has already been shown and discussed—at least in *in vitro* tests with articular cartilage—that compounds which reduce friction do not necessarily reduce wear; the latter was suggested as being more important [10]. It may be helpful first of all to emphasize once again that friction and wear are different phenomena. Furthermore, certain constituents of synovial fluid (e.g., Swann's LGP) may act to reduce *friction* in synovial joints while other constituents (e.g., Swann's protein complex or hyaluronic acid) may act to reduce cartilage *wear*.

A significant increase in joint friction could lead to a slight increase in local temperatures or possibly to reduce mobility. But the effects of cartilage wear would be expected to be more serious. When cartilage wear occurs, a very special material is lost and the body is neither capable of regenerating cartilage of the same quality nor at the desired rate. Thus, there are at least two major tribological dimensions involved—one concerning the nature of the synovial fluid and the other having to do with the properties of articular cartilage itself. Changes in *either* the synovial fluid or cartilage could conceivably lead to increased wear or damage (or friction) as shown in Figure 4.9.

A simplified model or illustration of possible connections between OA and tribology is offered in Figure 4.10 taken from Furey [46]. Its purpose is to stimulate discussion. There are other pathways to the disease, pathways which may include genetic factors.

In some cases, the body makes an unsuccessful attempt at repair, and bone growth may occur at the periphery of contact. As suggested by Figure 4.10, this process and the generation of wear particles could lead to joint inflammation and the release of enzymes which further soften and degrade the articular cartilage.

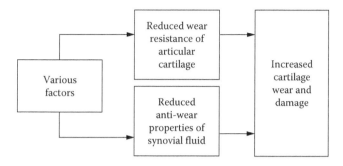

FIGURE 4.9 Two tribological aspects of synovial joint lubrication.

This softer, degraded cartilage does not possess the wear-resistance of the original. It has been shown previously that treatment of cartilage with collagenase-3 increases wear significantly, thus supporting the idea of enzyme release as a factor in OA. Thus, there exists a feedback process in which the occurrence of cartilage wear can lead to even more damage. Degradative enzymes can also be released by trauma, shock, or injury to the joint. Ultimately, as the cartilage is progressively thinned and bony growth occurs, a condition of OA or degenerative joint disease may exist. There are other pathways to the disease, pathways which may include genetic factors. It is not argued that arthritis is a tribological problem. However, the inclusion of tribological processes in one set of pathways to osteoarthrosis would not seem strange or unusual.

A specific example of a different tribological dimension to the problem of synovial joint lubrication (i.e., third-body abrasion), was shown by the work of Hayes et al. [47]. In an excellent study of the effect of crystals on the wear of articular cartilage, they carried out *in vitro* tests using cylindrical cartilage sub-chondral bone plugs obtained from equine fetlock joints in sliding contact against a stainless-steel plate. They examined the effects of three types of crystals (orthorhombic calcium pyrophosphate tetrahydrate, monoclinic calcium pyrophosphate dehydrate, and calcium hydroxyapatite) on wear using a Ringer's solution as the carrier fluid. Concentration of cartilage wear debris in the fluid was determined

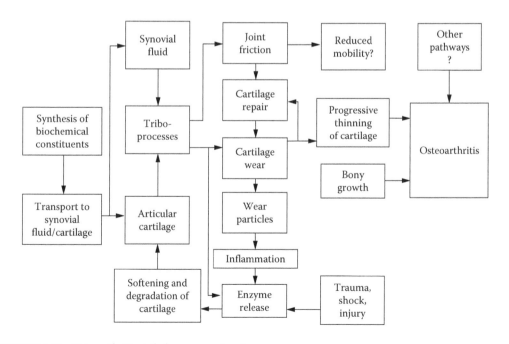

FIGURE 4.10 Osteoarthritis–tribology connections?

by analyzing for inorganic sulfate derived from the proteoglycans present. Several interesting findings were made, one of them being that the presence of the crystals roughly doubled cartilage wear. This is an important contribution which should be read by anyone seriously contemplating research on the tribology of articular cartilage. The careful attention to detail and potential problems, as well as the precise description of the biochemical procedures and diverse experimental techniques used, set a high standard.

4.8 Recapitulation and Final Comments

It is obvious from the unusually large number of theories of synovial joint lubrication proposed, that very little is known about the subject. Synovial joints are undoubtedly the most sophisticated and complex tribological systems that exist or will ever exist. It will require a great deal more research—possibly very different approaches—before we even begin to understand the processes involved.

Some general comments and specific suggestions are offered—not for the purpose of criticizing any particular study but hopefully to provide ideas which may be helpful in further research as well as in the re-interpretation of some past research.

4.8.1 Terms and Definitions

First of all, as mentioned earlier in this chapter, part of the problem has to do with the use and misuse of various terms in tribology—the study of friction, wear, and lubrication. A glance at any number of the published papers on synovial joint lubrication will reveal such terms and phrases as "lubricating ability," "lubricity," "lubricating properties," "lubricating component," and many others, all undefined. We also see terms such as "boundary lubricant," "lubricating glycoprotein," or "lubricin." There is nothing inherently wrong with this but one should remember that lubrication is a process of reducing friction and/or wear between rubbing surfaces. Saying that a fluid is a "good" lubricant does not distinguish between friction and wear. And assuming that friction and wear are correlated and go together is the first pitfall in any tribological study. It cannot be overemphasized that friction and wear are different, though sometimes related, phenomena. Low friction does not mean low wear. The terms and phrases used are therefore extremely important. For example, in a brief and early review article by Wright and Dowson [48], it was stated that "Digestion of hyaluronate does not alter the boundary lubrication," referring to the work of Radin et al. [49]. In another article, McCutchen re-states this conclusion in another way, saying "… the lubricating ability did not reside in the hyaluronic acid" and later asks the question "Why do the glycoprotein molecules (of Swann) lubricate?" [50] These statements are based on effects of various constituents on friction, not wear. The work of the present author showed that in tests with bovine articular cartilage, Swann's LGP-I which was effective in reducing friction did not reduce cartilage wear. However, hyaluronic acid—shown earlier not to be responsible for friction-reduction—did reduce cartilage wear. Thus, it is important to make the distinction between friction-reduction and wear-reduction. It is suggested that operational definitions be used in place of vague "lubricating ability," and other terms in future papers on the subject.

4.8.2 Experimental Contact Systems

Second, some comments are made on the experimental approaches that have been reported in the literature on synovial joint lubrication mechanisms. Sliding contact combinations in *in vitro* studies have consisted of (1) cartilage-on-cartilage, (2) cartilage-on-some other surface (e.g., stainless steel, glass), and (3) solids other than cartilage sliding against each other in X-on-X or X-on-Y combinations.

The cartilage-on-cartilage combination is of course the most realistic and yet most complex contact system. But variations in shape or macroscopic geometry, microtopography, and the nature of contact present problems in carrying out well-controlled experiments. There is also the added problem of acquiring suitable specimens which are large enough and reasonably uniform.

The next combination—cartilage-on-another material—allows for better control of contact, with the more elastic, deformable cartilage loaded against a well-defined hard surface (e.g., a polished, flat solid made of glass or stainless steel). This contact configuration can provide useful tribological information on effects of changes in biochemical environment (e.g., fluids), on friction, wear, and sub-surface damage. It also could parallel the situation in a partial joint replacement in which healthy cartilage is in contact with a metal alloy.

The third combination, which appears in some of the literature on synovial joint lubrication, does not involve any articular cartilage at all. For example, Jay made friction measurements using a latex-covered stainless-steel stud in oscillating contact against polished glass [31]. Williams et al., in a study of a lipid component of synovial fluid, used reciprocating contact of borosilicate glass-on-glass [51]. And in a recent paper on the action of a surface-active phospholipid as the "lubricating component of lubricin," Schwarz and Hills carried out friction measurements using two optically flat quartz plates in sliding contact [52]. In another study, a standard four-ball machine using alloy steel balls was used to examine the "lubricating ability" of synovial fluid constituents. Such tests, in the absence of cartilage, are easiest to control and carry out. However, they are not relevant to the study of synovial joint lubrication. With a glass sphere sliding against a glass flat, almost anything will reduce friction—including a wide variety of chemicals, biochemicals, semi-solids, and fluids. This has little if anything to do with the lubrication of synovial joints.

4.8.3 Fluids and Materials Used as Lubricants in *In Vitro* Biotribology Studies

Fluids used as lubricants in synovial joint lubrication studies have consisted of (1) "normal" synovial fluid (e.g., bovine), (2) buffered saline solution containing synovial fluid constituents (e.g., hyaluronic acid), and (3) various aqueous solutions of surface-active compounds neither derived from nor present in synovial fluid. In addition, a few studies used synovial fluids from patients suffering from either OA or RA.

The general comment made here is that the use of synovial fluids—whether derived from human or animal sources and whether "healthy" or "abnormal"—is important in *in vitro* studies of synovial joint lubrication. The documented behavior of synovial fluid in producing low friction and wear with articular cartilage sets a reference standard and demonstrates that useful information can indeed come from *in vitro* tests.

Studies that are based on adding synovial fluid constituents to a reference fluid (e.g., a buffered saline solution) can also be useful in attempting to identify which biochemical compound or compounds are responsible for reductions in frictions or wear. But if significant interactions between compounds exist, then such an approach may require an extensive program of tests. It should also be mentioned that in the view of the present author, the use of a pure undissolved constituent of synovial fluid, either derived or synthetic, in a sliding contact test is not only irrelevant but may be misleading. An example would be the use of a pure lipid (e.g., phospholipid) at the interface rather than in the concentration and solution form in which this compound would normally exist in synovial fluid. This is basic in any study of lubrication and particularly in the case of boundary lubrication where major effects on wear or friction can be brought on by minor, seemingly trivial, changes in chemistry.

4.8.4 The Preoccupation with Rheology and Friction

The synovial joint as a system—the articular cartilage and underlying bone structure as well as the synovial fluid as important elements—is extremely complex and far from being understood. It is noted that there is a proliferation of mathematical modeling papers stressing rheology and the mechanics of deformation, flow, and fluid pressures developed in the cartilage model. One recent example is the paper "The Role of Interstitial Fluid Pressurization and Surface Properties on the Boundary Friction of Articular Cartilage" by Ateshian et al. [21]. This study, a genuine contribution, grew out of the early work by Mow and connects also with the "weeping lubrication" model of McCutchen. Both McCutchen and

Mow have made significant contributions to our understanding of synovial joint lubrication, although each approach is predominantly rheological and friction-oriented with little regard for biochemistry and wear. This is not to say that rheology is unimportant. It could well be that, as suggested by Ateshian, the mechanism of interstitial fluid pressurization that leads to low friction in cartilage could also lead to low wear rates (private communication, letter to Michael J. Furey from Gerard A. Ateshian, July 1998).

4.8.5 The Probable Existence of Various Lubrication Regimes

In an article by Wright and Dowson, it is suggested that a variety of types of lubrication operate in human synovial joints at different parts of a walking cycle stating that, "At heel-strike a squeeze-film situation may develop, leading to elastohydrodynamic lubrication and possibly both squeeze-film and boundary lubrication, while hydrodynamic lubrication may operate during the free-swing phase of walking" [48].

In a simplified approach to examining the various regimes of lubrication that could exist in a human joint, it may be useful to look at Figure 4.11a which shows the variation in force (load) and velocity for a human hip joint at different parts of the walking cycle (taken from Graham and Walker [53]). As discussed earlier in this chapter, theories of hydrodynamic and EHL all include the hydrodynamic factor ($\eta U/W$) as the key variable, where η = fluid viscosity, U = the relative sliding velocity, and W = the normal load. High values of ($\eta U/W$) lead to thicker hydrodynamic films—a more desirable condition

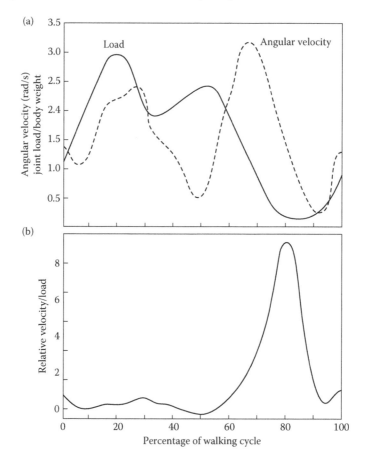

FIGURE 4.11 (a) Hip joint forces and angular velocities at different parts of the walking cycle. (After Graham, J.D. and Walker, T.W. *Perspectives in Biomedical Engineering*, University Park Press, Baltimore, MD, pp. 161–164, 1973.) (b) Calculated ratio of velocity to force for the hip joint (from (a)).

if one wants to keep surfaces apart. It can be seen from Figure 4.11a that there is considerable variation in load and velocity, with peaks and valleys occurring at different parts of the cycle. Note also that in this example, the loads can be quite high (e.g., up to three times body weight). The maximum load occurs at 20% of the walking cycle illustrated in Figure 4.11a, with a secondary maximum occurring at a little over the 50% point. The maximum angular velocity occurs at approximately 67% of the cycle. If one now creates a new curve of relative velocity/load or (U/W) from Figure 4.11a, the result obtained is shown in Figure 4.11b. We now see a very different and somewhat simplified picture. There is a clear and distinct maximum in the ratio of velocity to load (U/W) at 80% of walking cycle, favoring the formation of a hydrodynamic film of maximum thickness. However, for most of the cycle (e.g., from 0 to 60%), the velocity/load ratio is significantly lower, thus favoring a condition of minimum film thickness and "boundary lubrication." However, we also know that synovial fluid is non-Newtonian; at higher rates of shear, its viscosity decreases sharply, approaching that of water. The shear rate is equal to the relative velocity divided by fluid film thickness (U/h) and is expressed in per second. This means that at the regions of low (U/W) ratios or thinner hydrodynamic films, the viscosity term in ($\eta U/W$) is even lower, thus pushing the minima to lower values favoring a condition of boundary lubrication. This is only a simplified view and does not consider those periods in which the relative sliding velocity is zero at motion reversal and where squeeze-film lubrication may come into play. A good example of the complexity of load and velocity variation in a human knee joint—including several zero-velocity periods—may be found in the chapter by Higginson and Unsworth [54] citing the work of Seedhom et al., which deals with biomechanics in the design of a total knee replacement [55].

The major point made here is that (1) there are parts of a walking cycle that would be expected to approach a condition of minimum fluid film thickness and boundary lubrication and (2) it is during these parts of the cycle that cartilage wear and damage resulting from contact is more likely to occur. Thus, approaches to reducing cartilage wear in a synovial joint could be broken down into two categories (i.e., promoting thicker hydrodynamic films and providing special forms of "boundary lubrication").

4.8.6 Recent Developments

Recent developments in addressing some of the problems that involve cartilage damage and existing joint replacements include (1) progress in promoting cartilage repair [56], (2) possible use of artificial cartilage materials (e.g., synthetic hydrogels) [57,58], and (3) the development and application of more compliant joint replacement materials to promote a more favorable formation of an elastohydrodynamic film [59]. Although these are not strictly "lubricant-oriented" developments, they do and will involve important tribological aspects discussed in this chapter. For example, if new cartilage growth can be promoted by transplanting healthy chondrocytes to a platform in a damaged region of a synovial joint, how long will this cartilage last? If a hydrogel is used as an artificial cartilage, how long will it last? And if softer, elastomeric materials are used as partial joint replacements or coatings, how long will they last? These are questions of wear, not friction. And although the early fundamental studies of hydrogels as artificial cartilage measured only friction, and often only after a few moments of sliding, we know from recent work that even for hydrogels, low friction does not mean low wear [60].

4.9 Conclusions

The following main conclusions relating to the tribological behavior of natural, "normal" synovial joints are presented:

1. An unusually large number of theories and studies of joint lubrication have been proposed over the years. All of the theories focus on friction, none address wear, many do not involve experimental studies with cartilage, and very few consider the complexity and detailed biochemistry of the synovial-fluid articular-cartilage system.

2. It was shown by *in vitro* tests with bovine articular cartilage that the detailed biochemistry of synovial fluid has a significant effect on cartilage wear and damage. "Normal" bovine synovial fluid was found to provide excellent protection against wear. Various biochemical constituents isolated from bovine synovial fluid by Dr. David Swann, of the Shriners Burns Institute in Boston, showed varying effects on cartilage wear when added back to a buffered saline reference fluid. This research demonstrates once again the importance of distinguishing between friction and wear.

3. In a collaborative study of biotribology involving researchers and students in Mechanical Engineering, the Virginia-Maryland College of Veterinary Medicine, and Biochemistry, *in vitro* tribological tests using bovine articular cartilage demonstrated among other things that (1) normal synovial fluid provides better protection than a buffered saline solution in a cartilage-on-cartilage system, (2) tribological contact in cartilage systems can cause subsurface damage, delamination, changes in proteoglycan content, and in chemistry via a "biotribochemical" process not understood, and (3) pretreatment of articular cartilage with the enzyme collagenase-3—suspected as a factor in OA—significantly increases cartilage wear.

4. It is suggested that these results could change significantly the way mechanisms of synovial joint lubrication are examined. Effects of biochemistry of the system on wear of articular cartilage are likely to be important; such effects may not be related to physical/rheological models of joint lubrication.

5. It is also suggested that connections between tribology/normal synovial joint lubrication and degenerative joint disease are not only possible but likely; however, such connections are undoubtedly complex. It is *not* argued that OA is a tribological problem or that it is necessarily the result of a tribological deficiency. Ultimately, a better understanding of how normal synovial joints function from a tribological point of view could conceivably lead to advances in the prevention and treatment of OA.

6. Several problems exist that make it difficult to understand and interpret many of the published works on synovial joint lubrication. One example is the widespread use of nonoperational and vague terms such as "lubricating activity," "lubricating factor," "boundary lubricating ability," and similar undefined terms which not only fail to distinguish between friction (which is usually measured) and cartilage wear (which is rarely measured), but tend to lump these phenomena together—a common error. Another problem is that a significant number of the published experimental studies of biotribology do not involve cartilage at all—relying on the use of glass-on-glass, rubber-on-glass, and even steel-on-steel. Such approaches may be a reflection of the incorrect view that "lubricating activity" is a property of a fluid and can be measured independently. Some suggestions are offered.

7. Last, the topic of synovial joint lubrication is far from being understood. It is a complex subject involving at least biophysics, biomechanics, biochemistry, and tribology. For a physical scientist or engineer, carrying out research in this area is a humbling experience.

Acknowledgments

The author acknowledge the support of the Edward H. Lane, G. Harold, and Leila Y. Mathers Foundations for their support during the sabbatical study at The Children's Hospital Medical Center. He also thank Dr. David Swann for his invaluable help in providing the test fluids and carrying out the biochemical analyses as well as Ms Karen Hodgens for conducting the early scanning electron microscopy studies of worn cartilage specimens.

The author is also indebted to the following researchers for their encouraging and stimulating discussions of this topic over the years and for teaching a tribologist something of the complexity of synovial joints, articular cartilage, and arthritis: Drs. Leon Sokoloff, Charles McCutchen, Melvin Glimcher, David Swann, Henry Mankin, Clement Sledge, Helen Muir, Paul Dieppe, Heikki Helminen, as well as his colleagues at Virginia Tech—Hugo Veit, E. T. Kornegay, and E. M. Gregory.

Last, the author expresses his appreciation for and recognition of the valuable contributions made by students interested in biotribology over the years. These include graduate students Bettina Burkhardt, Michael Owellen, Matt Schroeder, Mark Freeman, and especially La Shaun Berrien, who contributed to this chapter, as well as the following summer undergraduate research students: Jean Yates, Elaine Ashby, Anne Newell, T. J. Hayes, Bethany Revak, Carolina Reyes, Amy Diegelman, and Heather Hughes.

Further Information

For more information on synovial joints and arthritis, the following books are suggested: *The Biology of Degenerative Joint Disease* [45], *Adult Articular Cartilage* [5], *The Joints and Synovial Fluid: I* [6], *Textbook of Rheumatology* [61], *Osteoarthritis: Diagnosis and Management* [62], Degenerative joints: Test tubes, tissues, models, and man [63], Biology of the articular cartilage in health and disease [64], and *Crystals and Joint Disease* [65].

References

1. Hunter, W. Of the structure and diseases of articulating cartilages, *Philos. Trans.*, 42, 514–521, 1742–1743.
2. Furey, M.J. Tribology, In: *Encyclopedia of Materials Science and Engineering*, Pergamon Press, Oxford, 1986, pp. 5145–5158.
3. Cameron, A. *The Principles of Lubrication*, Longmans Green & Co. Ltd, London, 1966.
4. Dowson, D. and Higginson, G.R. *Elastohydrodynamic Lubrication*, SI Edition, Pergamon Press, Oxford, 1977.
5. Freeman, M.A.R. *Adult Articular Cartilage*, 2nd ed., Pitman Medical Publishing Co., Ltd., Tunbridge Wells, Kent, England, 1979.
6. Sokoloff, L., Ed. *The Joints and Synovial Fluid*, Vol. I, Academic Press, New York, 1978.
7. Stockwell, R.A. *Biology of Cartilage Cells*, Cambridge University Press, Cambridge, 1979.
8. Furey, M.J. Biochemical aspects of synovial joint lubrication and cartilage wear, European Society of Osteoarthrology. *Symposium on Joint Destruction in Arthritis and Osteoarthritis*, Noordwijkerhout, the Netherlands, May 24–27, 1992.
9. Furey, M.J. Biotribology: Cartilage lubrication and wear, *6th International Congress on Tribology, EUROTRIB '93*, Budapest, Hungary, August 30–September 2, 1993.
10. Furey, M.J. and Burkhardt, B.M. Biotribology: Friction, wear, and lubrication of natural synovial joints, *Lubrication Sci.*, 255–271, 3–9, 1997.
11. McCutchen, C.W. Lubrication of joints. In: *The Joints and Synovial Fluid*, Vol. I, Academic Press, New York, 1978, pp. 437–483.
12. Swanson, S.A.V. Friction, wear and lubrication. In *Adult Articular Cartilage*, M.A.R. Freeman, Ed., Pitman Medical Publishing Co., Ltd., Tunbridge Wells, Kent, England, 2nd ed., 1979, pp. 415–460.
13. Higginson, G.R. and Unsworth, T. The lubrication of natural joints. In *Tribology of Natural and Artificial Joints*, J. H. Dumbleton, Ed. Elsevier Scientific Publishing Co., Amsterdam, 1981, pp. 47–73.
14. Dumbleton, J.H. *Tribology of Natural and Artificial Joints*, Elsevier Scientific Publishing Co., Amsterdam, the Netherlands, 1981.
15. Droogendijk, L. *On the Lubrication of Synovial Joints*, PhD Thesis, Twente University of Technology, the Netherlands, 1984.
16. Burkhardt, B.M. *Development and Design of a Test Device for Cartilage Wear Studies*, MS thesis, Mechanical Engineering, Virginia Polytechnic Institute & State University, Blacksburg, VA, December 1988.
17. McCutchen, C.W. Mechanisms of animal joints: Sponge-hydrostatic and weeping bearings, *Nature (Lond.)*, 184, 1284–1285, 1959.

18. McCutchen, C.W. The frictional properties of animal joints, *Wear*, 5, 1–17, 1962.
19. Torzilli, P.A. and Mow, V.C. On the fundamental fluid transport mechanisms through normal and pathological articular cartilage during friction-1. The formulation. *J. Biomech.*, 9, 541–552, 1976.
20. Mansour, J.M. and Mow, V.C. On the natural lubrication of synovial joints: Normal and degenerated. *J. Lubrication Technol.*, 163–173, 1977.
21. Ateshian, G. A., Wang, H., and Lai, W. M. The role of interstitial fluid pressurization and surface porosities on the boundary friction of articular cartilage, *ASMS J. Biomed. Eng.*, 120, 241–251, 1998.
22. Unsworth, A. Tribology of human and artificial joints. *Proc. I. Mech. E., Part II: J. Eng. Med.*, 205, 1991.
23. Simon, W.H. Wear properties of articular cartilage. *In vitro*, Section on Rheumatic Diseases, Laboratory of Experimental Pathology, National Institute of Arthritis and Metabolic Diseases, National Institutes of Health, February 1971.
24. Bloebaum, R.D. and Wilson, A.S. The morphology of the surface of articular cartilage in adult rats, *J. Anatomy*, 131, 333–346, 1980.
25. Radin, E.L. and Paul, I.L. Response of joints to impact loading I. *In vitro* wear tests, *Arthritis Rheumatism*, 14, 1971.
26. Lipshitz, H. and Glimcher, M.J. A technique for the preparation of plugs of articular cartilage and subchondral bone, *J. Biomech.*, 7, 293–298.
27. Lipshitz, H. and Etheredge, III, R. *In vitro* wear of articular cartilage. *J. Bone Joint Surg.*, 57-A, 527–534, 1975.
28. Lipshitz, H. and Glimcher, M.J. *In vitro* studies of wear of articular cartilage, II. Characteristics of the wear of articular cartilage when worn against stainless steel plates having characterized surfaces. *Wear*, 52, 297–337, 1979.
29. Sokoloff, L., Davis, W.H., and Lee, S.L. Boundary lubricating ability of synovial fluid in degenerative joint disease, *Arthritis Rheum.*, 21, 754–760, 1978.
30. Sokoloff, L., Davis, W.H., and Lee, S.L. A proposed model of boundary lubrication by synovial fluid: Structuring of boundary water, *J. Biomech. Eng.*, 101, 185–192, 1979.
31. Jay, D.J. Characterization of bovine synovial fluid lubricating factor, I. Chemical surface activity and lubrication properties, *Connective Tissue Res.*, 28, 71–88, 1992.
32. Burkhardt, B.M. *Development and Design of a Test Device for Cartilage Wear Studies*, MS thesis, Mechanical Engineering, Virginia Polytechnic Institute and State University, Blacksburg, VA, December 1988.
33. Stachowiak, G.W., Batchelor, A.W., and Griffiths, L.J. Friction and wear changes in synovial joints, *Wear*, 171, 135–142, 1994.
34. Hayes, A., Harris, B., Dieppe, P.A., and Clift, S.E. Wear of articular cartilage: The effect of crystals, *IMechE*, 41–58, 1993.
35. Malcolm, L.L. *An Experimental Investigation of the Frictional and Deformational Responses of Articular Cartilage Interfaces to Static and Dynamic Loading*, PhD thesis, University of California, San Diego, 1976.
36. Furey, M.J. Biotribology: An *in vitro* study of the effects of synovial fluid constituents on cartilage wear. *Proc., XVth Symposium of the European Society of Osteoarthrology*, Kuopio, Finland, June 25–27, 1986, abstract in *Scandanavian Journal of Rheumatology*, Supplement.
37. Furey, M.J. The influence of synovial fluid constituents on cartilage wear: A scanning electron microscope study. *Conference on Joint Destruction, XVth Symposium on the European Society of Osteoarthrology*, Sochi, USSR, September 28–October 3, 1987.
39. Furey, M.J. Biotribology: Cartilage lubrication and wear. *Proceedings of the 6th International Congress on Tribology EUROTRIB;* '93, Vol. 2, pp. 464–470, Budapest, Hungary, August 30–September 2, 1993.
40. Schroeder, M.O. *Biotribology: Articular Cartilage Friction, Wear, and Lubrication*, MS thesis, Mechanical Engineering, Virginia Polytechnic Institute and State University, Blacksburg, VA, July 1995.

41. Owellen, M.C. *Biotribology: The Effect of Lubricant and Load on Articular Cartilage Wear and Friction*, MS thesis, Mechanical Engineering, Virginia Polytechnic Institute and State University, Blacksburg, VA, July 1997.

42. Furey, M.J., Schroeder, M.O., Hughes, H.L., Owellen, M.C., Berrien, L.S., Veit, H., Gregory, E.M., and Kornegay, E.T. Observations of subsurface damage and cartilage degradation in *in vitro* tribological tests using bovine articular cartilage, *21st Symposium of the European Society for Osteoarthrology*, Vol. 15, Gent, Belgium, September 1996, 5, 3.2.

43. Furey, M.J., Schroeder, M.O., Hughes, H.L., Owellen, M.C., Berrien, L.S., Veit, H., Gregory, E.M., and Kornegay, E.T. *Biotribology, Synovial Joint Lubrication and Osteoarthritis*, Paper in Session W5 on Biotribology, *World Tribology Congress*, London, September 8–12, 1997.

44. Berrien, L.S., Furey, M.J., Veit, H.P., and Gregory, E.M. The Effect of collagenase-3 on the *in vitro* wear of bovine articular cartilage, paper, Biotribology Session, *Fifth International Tribology Conference*, Brisbane, Australia, December 6–9, 1998.

45. Sokoloff, L. *The Biology of Degenerative Joint Disease*, University of Chicago Press, Chicago, IL, 1969. Boston, MA, Fall 1983.

46. Furey, M.J. Exploring possible connections between tribology and osteoarthritis, *Lubricat. Sci.*, 273, May 1997.

47. Hayes, A., Harris, B., Dieppe, P.A., and Clift, S.E. Wear of articular cartilage: The effect of crystals, *Proc. I.Mech.E.*, 207, 41–58, 1993.

48. Wright, V. and Dowson, D. Lubrication and cartilage, *J. Anat.*, 121, 107–118, 1976.

49. Radin, E.L., Swann, D.A., and Weisser, P.A. Separation of a hyaluronate-free lubricating fraction from synovial fluid, *Nature*, 228, 377–378, 1970.

50. McCutchen, C.W. Joint lubrication, *Bull. Hosp. Joint Dis. Orthop. Inst.* XLIII, 118–129, 1983.

51. Williams, III, P.F., Powell, G.L., and LaBerge, M. Sliding friction analysis of phosphatidylcholine as a boundary lubricant for articular cartilage, *Proc. I. Mech. E.*, 207, 41–166, 1993.

52. Schwarz, I. M. and Hills, B. A. Surface-active phospholipid as the lubricating component of lubrician, *Br. J. Rheumatol.*, 37, 21–26, 1998.

53. Graham, J.D. and Walker, T.W. Motion in the hip: The relationship of split line patterns to surface velocities, a paper in *Perspectives in Biomedical Engineering*, R.M. Kenedi, Ed., University Park Press, Baltimore, MD, pp. 161–164, 1973.

54. Higginson, G.R. and Unsworth, T. The lubrication of natural joints. In *Tribology by Natural and Artificial Joints*, J.H. Dumbleton, Ed., Elsevier Scientific Publishing Co., Amsterdam, pp. 47–73, 1981.

55. Seedhom, B.B., Longton, E.B., Dowson, D., and Wright, V. Biomechanics background in the design of total replacement knee prosthesis. *Acta Orthop. Belgica*, 39(1), 164–180, 1973.

56. Brittberg, M. Cartilage repair, *A Collection of Five Articles on Cartilaginous Tissue Engineering with an Emphasis on Chondrocyte Transplantation*, 2nd ed., Institute of Surgical Sciences and Department of Clinical Chemistry and Institute of Laboratory Medicine, Goteborg University, Sweden, 1996.

57. Corkhill, P.H., Trevett, A.S., and Tighe, B.J. The potential of hydrogels as synthetic articular cartilage. *Proc. Inst. Mech. Eng.*, 204, 147–155, 1990.

58. Caravia, L., Dowson, D., Fisher, J., Corkhill, P.H., and Tighe, B.J.A comparison of friction in hydrogel and polyurethane materials for cushion form joints. *J. Mater. Sci.: Mater. Med.*, 4, 515–520, 1993.

59. Caravia, L., Dowson, D., Fisher, J., Corkhill, P.H., and Tighe, B.J. Friction of hydrogel and polyurethane elastic layers when sliding against each other under a mixed lubrication regime. *Wear*, 181–183, 236–240, 1995.

60. Freeman, M.E., Furey, M.J., Love, B.J., and Hampton, J.M. Friction, wear, and lubrication of hydrogels as synthetic articular cartilage, paper, Biotribology Session, *Fifth International Tribology Conference*, AUSTRIB '98, Brisbane, Australia, December 6–9, 1998.

61. Kelley, W.N., Harris, Jr., E.D., Ruddy, S., and Sledge, C.B. *Textbook of Rheumatology*, W.B. Saunders Co., Philadelphia, 1981.

62. Moskowitz, R.W., Howell, D.S., Goldberg, V.M., and Mankin, H.J. *Osteoarthritis: Diagnosis and Management*, W.B. Saunders Co., Philadelphia, 1984.

63. Verbruggen, G. and Veyes, E.M. Degenerative joints: Test tubes, tissues, models, and man. *Proceedings of the First Conference on Degenerative Joint Diseases*, Excerpta Medica, Amsterdam, 1982.

64. Gastpar, H. Biology of the articular cartilage in health and disease. *Proceedings of the Second Munich Symposium on Biology of Connective Tissue*, Munich, July 23–24, 1979; F.K. Schattauer Verlag, Stuttgart, 1980.

65. Dieppe, P. and Calvert, P. *Crystals and Joint Disease*, Chapman & Hall, London, 1983.

5

Analysis of Gait

Roy B. Davis III
Shriners Hospitals for Children

Sylvia Õunpuu
Connecticut Children's Medical Center

Peter A. DeLuca
Connecticut Orthopaedic Specialists

The analysis of gait is the quantitative measurement and assessment of human locomotion which may include walking, running, and stair assent and descent. A number of different disciplines use gait or movement analysis techniques. Basic scientists seek a better understanding of how typically developing ambulators use muscle contractions about articulating joints to accomplish functional tasks, such as level walking [1] and stair climbing [2]. Physicians seek a better understanding of atypical movement patterns to assist in treatment decision making. Sports biomechanists, athletes, and their coaches use movement analysis techniques to investigate performance improvement [3–5] and injury mechanisms [6]. Sports equipment manufacturers seek to quantify the perceived advantages of their products relative to a competitor's offering.

With respect to the analysis of gait in the clinical setting, medical professionals measure and analyze the walking patterns of patients with locomotor impairment in the planning of treatment protocols, for example, orthotic prescription and surgical intervention. Clinical gait analysis is an evaluation tool that may determine the extent to which an individual's gait has been affected by an already diagnosed disorder [7] or provide a baseline for gait disorders that are progressive. Examples of clinical pathologies currently served by gait analysis include

- Amputation [8]
- Cerebral palsy [9,10]
- Degenerative joint disease [11,12]
- Joint pain [13]
- Joint replacement [14]
- Poliomyelitis [15]
- Multiple sclerosis [16]
- Muscular dystrophy [17]
- Myelodysplasia [18,19]

- Rheumatoid arthritis [20]
- Spinal cord injury [21]
- Stroke [22]
- Traumatic brain injury [23]

Generally, gait analysis data collection protocols and data reduction models have been developed to meet the requirements specific to the research, sport or clinical setting. For example, gait measurement protocols in a research setting might include an extensive physical examination to detail the anthropometrics of each subject. This time expenditure may not be possible in a clinical setting. This chapter focuses on the methods to assess the walking patterns of persons with locomotor impairment, that is, clinical gait analysis. The discussion will include a description of the available measurement technology, the components of data collection and reduction, the type of gait information produced for clinical interpretation, and the strengths and limitations of clinical gait analysis.

5.1 Fundamental Concepts

5.1.1 Clinical Gait Analysis Components

A comprehensive clinical gait analysis consists of a variety of components, the final combination of which is predicated on the individual patient's movement-related pathology and ability. Data that are currently provided for the assessment of gait in a clinical setting may include

- A video recording of the individual's gait (before instrumentation) for qualitative review and quality control purposes.
- Static physical examination measures, such as passive joint range of motion, muscle strength, ability to isolate movement, muscle tone, and the presence and degree of bony deformity.
- Segment and joint angular positions associated with standing posture.
- Stride and temporal parameters, such as step length and walking velocity.
- Segment and joint angular displacements during gait (level walking), commonly referred to as *kinematics*.
- The forces and torque applied to the patient's foot by the ground, or ground reaction loads during gait.
- The reactive intersegmental moments produced about the lower extremity joints by active and passive soft-tissue forces as well as the associated mechanical power of the intersegmental moment during gait, collectively referred to as *kinetics*.
- Indications of muscle activity, that is, voltage potentials produced by contracting muscles, during gait, relaxed standing and muscle tone assessment, known as dynamic *electromyography* (EMG).
- The dynamic pressure distributions on the plantar surface of the foot during standing and gait, referred to as *pedobarography*.
- A measure of metabolic energy expenditure during rest (sitting) and gait, for example, oxygen consumption, energy cost.
- The time to complete these steps can range from 1 to 3 h (Table 5.1).

5.1.2 Gait Data Reference System

Gait is a cyclic activity for which certain discrete events have been defined as significant. Typically, the *gait cycle* is defined as a period of time from the point of *initial contact* (also referred to as *foot contact*) of the patient's foot with the ground to the next point of initial contact for that same limb. Dividing the gait cycle into stance and swing phases is the point in the cycle where the stance limb leaves the ground, called *toe off* or *foot off*. Gait variables that change over time such as the patient's joint angular displacements are normally presented for clinical analysis as a function of the individual's gait cycle. This is

TABLE 5.1 A Typical Gait Data Collection Protocol

Test Component	Approximate Time (min)
Pretest tasks: test explanation to the adult patient or the pediatric patient and parent, system calibration	10
Video taping: brace, barefoot, close-up, standing	5–10
Clinical examination: range of motion, muscle strength, etc.	15–30
Motion marker placement	15–20
Motion data collection: subject calibration and multiple walks, per test condition (barefoot and orthosis)	10–60
EMG (surface electrodes and fine wire electrodes)	20–60
Data reduction of all trials	15–90
Data interpretation	20–30
Report dictation, generation, and distribution	120–180

done to facilitate the comparison of different walking trials and the use of a reference database from a matched, typical population [24].

5.1.3 Motion Data Collection Protocol

Motion data collection is typically the longest component of a comprehensive clinical gait assessment. After anatomical measures are acquired from the patient, such as leg length and joint widths, the patient is equipped with external markers (see Section 5.2.2.3). A static calibration of the "instrumented" patient is then completed followed by multiple walks along a pathway that is commonly both level and smooth. While the baseline for analysis is typically barefoot gait, patients are tested in other conditions as well, for example, while using lower extremity orthoses and walking aids such as crutches or a walker. Requirements and constraints associated with clinical gait data collection include the following:

- The patient should not be intimidated or distracted by the testing environment.
- The measurement equipment and protocols should not alter the patient's gait.
- Patient preparation and testing time must be minimized, and rest (or play) intervals must be included in the process as needed.
- Data collection techniques must be repeatable.
- Methodology must be sufficiently robust and flexible to allow the evaluation of a variety of gait abnormalities where the patient's dynamic range of motion and anatomy may be significantly different from typically developing persons of a similar age.
- The quality of the collected data must be assured before the patient leaves the facility.

5.2 Measurement Approaches and Systems

The purpose of this section is to provide an overview of the several technologies that are available to measure the dynamic gait variables listed earlier, including stride and temporal parameters, kinematics, kinetics, and dynamic EMG. Methods of data reduction will be described in a following section.

5.2.1 Stride and Temporal Parameters

The gait cycle events of first and second initial contact and toe off must be identified for the computation of the stride and temporal parameters. These measures may be obtained through a wide variety of approaches ranging from the use of simple tools such as a stopwatch and tape measure to sophisticated arrays of photoelectric monitors. Foot switches may be applied to the plantar surface of the patient's foot, for example, under the heel, first and fifth metatarsal heads and great toe. In clinical populations, foot switch placement is challenging because of the variability of foot deformities and the associated foot-ground contact patterns. This foot switch placement difficulty is avoided through the use of either shoe insoles instrumented with one or two large foot switches or entire contact-sensitive walkways. These gait events may also be quantified using simultaneous synchronized video recordings, the camera-based motion measurement or the force platform technology described below.

5.2.2 Motion Measurement

A number of alternative technologies are available for the measurement of body segment spatial position and orientation. These include the use of electrogoniometry, accelerometry, and video-based digitizers. These approaches are described below.

5.2.2.1 Electrogoniometry

A simple electrogoniometer consists of a rotary potentiometer with arms fixed to the shaft and base for attachment to the body segments juxtaposed to the joint of interest. Multi-axial goniometers extend this capability by providing additional, simultaneous, orthogonal measures of rotational displacement, more appropriate for human joint motion measurement. Electrogoniometers offer the advantages of real-time display and the rapid collection of single joint information. These devices are, however, limited to the measurement of relative angles and may be cumbersome in typical clinical applications such as the simultaneous, bilateral assessment of hip, knee, and ankle motion during gait.

5.2.2.2 Accelerometry

Multi-axis accelerometers can be employed to measure both linear and angular accelerations (if multiple transducers are properly configured). Velocity and position data may then be derived through numerical integration although care must be taken with respect to the selection of initial conditions and the handling of gravitational effects.

5.2.2.3 Video Camera–Based Systems

This approach to human motion measurement involves the use of external markers that are placed on the patient's body segments and aligned with specific anatomical landmarks. Marker trajectories are then monitored by a system of motion capture cameras (generally from 6 to 12) placed around a measurement volume (Figure 5.1). In a frame-by-frame analysis, stereophotogrammetric techniques are then used to produce the instantaneous three-dimensional (3-D) coordinates of each marker (relative to a fixed laboratory coordinate system) from the set of two-dimensional camera images. The processing of the 3-D marker coordinate data is described in a later section.

The video camera-based systems employ either passive (retroreflective) or active (light-emitting diodes [LEDs]) markers. Passive marker camera systems incorporate strobe light sources (LED rings around the camera lens). The cameras then capture the light returned from the highly reflective markers (usually small spheres). Active marker camera systems record the light that is produced by small LED markers that are placed directly on the patient. Advantages and disadvantages are associated with each approach. For example, the anatomical location (or identity) of each marker used in an active marker system is immediately known because the markers are sequentially pulsed by a controlling computer. Active markers and the associated electronics worn by the patients are heavier and more cumbersome than comparable passive markers. Passive marker systems require user interaction for marker identification although algorithms have been developed to expedite this process through semi-automated tracking.

5.2.3 Ground Reaction Measurement

5.2.3.1 Force Platforms

The 3-D ground reaction force vector, the vertical ground reaction torque and the point of application of the ground reaction force vector (referred to as the center of pressure) are measured with force platforms

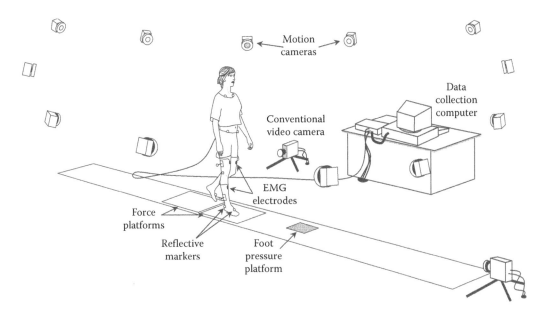

FIGURE 5.1 An "instrumented" patient with reflective spheres or markers and EMG electrodes. She walks along a level pathway while being monitored by 6–12 motion cameras (that monitor the displacement of the reflective markers) and 2–4 force platforms (that measure ground reaction loads). She might also walk over a foot pressure platform that measures the plantar pressure distribution. Her walk is also videotaped with 1 or 2 conventional video cameras. All of these signals (from the motion cameras, force platforms, EMG electrodes, foot pressure platform) are sent to the central data collection computer in the lab. These signals are then processed by the operator to produce the information used, along with the video recordings and other clinical examination data, to identify gait abnormalities and guide treatment planning.

embedded in the walkway. Force platforms with typical measurement surface dimensions of 0.5 × 0.5 m are comprised of several strain gauge or piezoelectric sensor arrays rigidly mounted together.

5.2.3.2 Pedobarography

The dynamic distributed load that corresponds to the vertical ground reaction force can be evaluated with the use of a flat, two-dimensional array of small piezoresistive force sensors. Overall resolution of the pedobarograph is dictated by the size of the individual sensor "cell." Sensor arrays configured as shoe insole inserts or flat plates offer the clinical user two measurement alternatives. Although this technology does afford the clinical practitioner better insight into the interaction between the plantar surface of the patient's foot and the ground, careful data interpretation is essential in patients with both foot deformity and altered gait patterns.

5.2.4 Dynamic EMG

Electrodes placed on the skin's surface and fine wires inserted into muscle are used to measure the voltage potentials produced by contracting muscles. The activity of the lower limb musculature is evaluated in this way with respect to the timing and the intensity of the contraction. Data collection variables that affect the quality of the EMG signal include the placement and distance between recording electrodes, skin surface conditions, distance between electrode and target muscle, signal amplification and filtering, and the rate of data acquisition. The quality of the EMG signal needs to be evaluated in all EMG data collection using the raw (unprocessed) signal. The phasic characteristics of the muscle activity may then be estimated from the raw EMG signal when referenced to the phases of the gait cycle. The EMG data may also be presented as a rectified and/or integrated waveform. To evaluate the intensity of the contraction, the dynamic EMG amplitudes are typically normalized by a reference value, for example, the EMG amplitude during a maximum voluntary contraction. This latter requirement is difficult to achieve consistently for patients who have limited isolated control of individual muscles, such as patients with cerebral palsy.

5.3 Gait Data Reduction: Kinematics and Kinetics

The predominant approach for the collection of clinical gait data involves the placement of external markers on the surface of body segments that are aligned with particular anatomical landmarks. These markers are commonly attached to the patient as either discrete units or in rigidly connected clusters. As described briefly above, the products of the data-acquisition process are the 3-D coordinates (relative to an inertially fixed laboratory coordinate system) of each marker trajectory over a gait cycle. If at least three markers or reference points are identified for each body segment, then the six degrees-of-freedom associated with the translation and attitude of the segment may be determined. The following example illustrates this relatively straightforward process.

Assume that a cluster of three markers has been attached to the thigh and shank of the patient as shown in Figure 5.2a. A body-fixed coordinate system may be computed for each marker cluster. For example, for the thigh, the cross product of the vectors from markers B to A and B to C produces a vector that is perpendicular to the cluster plane. From these vectors, the unit vectors T_{TX} and T_{TY} may be determined and used to compute the third orthogonal coordinate direction T_{TZ}. In a similar manner, the marker-based, or technical, coordinate system may be calculated for the shank, that is, S_{TX}, S_{TY}, and S_{TZ}. At this point, one might use these two technical coordinate systems to provide an estimate of

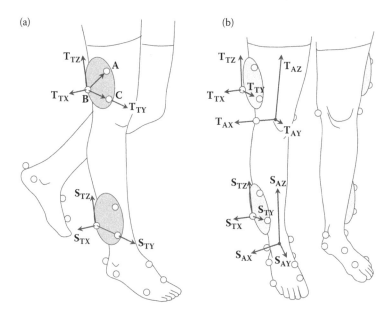

FIGURE 5.2 (a) Technical or marker-based coordinate systems "fixed" to the thigh and shank. A body fixed coordinate system may be computed for each cluster of three or more markers. On the thigh, for example, the vector cross product of the vectors from markers B to A and B to C produces a vector that is perpendicular to the cluster plane. From these vectors, the unit vectors T_{TX} and T_{TY} may be determined and used to compute the third orthogonal coordinate direction T_{TZ}. (b) A subject calibration relates technical coordinate systems with anatomical coordinate systems, for example, $\{T_T\}$ with $\{T_A\}$, through the identification of anatomical landmarks, for example, the medial and lateral femoral condyles and medial and lateral malleoli.

the absolute orientation of the thigh or shank or the relative angles between the thigh and shank. This assumes that the technical coordinate systems reasonably approximate the anatomical axes of the body segments, for example, that T_{TZ} approximates the long axis of the thigh. A more rigorous approach incorporates the use of a subject calibration procedure to relate technical coordinate systems with relevant anatomical axes [25].

In a subject calibration, usually performed with the patient in a relaxed standing position, additional data are collected by the motion measurement system that relates the technical coordinate systems to the underlying anatomical structure. For example, as shown in Figure 5.2b, the medial and lateral femoral condyles and the medial and lateral malleoli may be used as anatomical references with the application of additional markers. With the hip center location estimated from markers placed on the pelvis [26,27] and knee and ankle center locations based on the additional markers, anatomical coordinate systems may be computed, for example, $\{T_A\}$ and $\{S_A\}$. The relationship between the respective anatomical and technical coordinate system pairs as well as the location of the joint centers in terms of the appropriate technical coordinate system may be stored, to be recalled in the reduction of each frame of the walking data. In this way, the technical coordinate systems (shown in Figure 5.2b) are transformed into alignment with the anatomical coordinate systems.

Once anatomically aligned coordinate systems have been computed for each body segment under investigation, one may compute relative joint angles and absolute segment attitudes in a number of ways. The classical approach of Euler, or more specifically, Cardan angles is commonly used in clinical gait analysis to describe the motion of the thigh relative to the pelvis (or hip angles), the motion of the shank relative to the thigh (or knee angles), the motion of the foot relative to the shank (or ankle angles), as well as the absolute attitudes of the pelvis and foot in space. The joint rotation sequence commonly used for the Cardan angle computation is flexion–extension, adduction–abduction, and transverse plane rotation [28]. Alternatively, joint motion has been described through the use of helical axes [29].

The intersegmental moments that soft tissue (e.g., muscle, ligaments, joint capsule) forces produce about approximate joint centers may be computed using Newtonian mechanics. For example, the free body diagram of the foot shown in Figure 5.3 depicts the various external loads to the foot as well as the intersegmental reactions produced at the ankle. The mass, mass moments of inertia, and location of the center of mass may be estimated from regression-based anthropometric relationships [30–32], and linear and angular velocity and acceleration may be determined by numerical differentiation. If the ground reaction loads, F_G and T, are measured by a force platform, then the unknown ankle intersegmental force, F_A, may be solved for with Newton's translational equation of motion. Note that intersegmental force values underestimate the magnitude of the actual joint contact forces. Newton's rotational equation of motion may then be applied to compute the net ankle intersegmental moment, M_A. This process

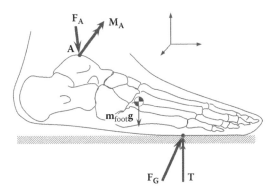

FIGURE 5.3   A free body diagram of the foot that illustrates the external loads to the foot, for example, the ground reaction loads, F_G and T, and the weight of the foot, $m_{foot}g$, as well as the unknown intersegmental reactions produced at the ankle, F_A and M_A, which may be solved for through the application of Newtonian mechanics.

may then be repeated for the shank and thigh by using computed (distal) intersegmental force and moment values to solve for the unknown (proximal) intersegmental reactions. The mechanical power associated with an intersegmental moment and the corresponding joint angular velocity may be computed from the vector dot product of the two vectors, for example, ankle intersegmental power is computed through $\mathbf{M}_A \cdot \omega_A$ where ω_A is the angular velocity of the foot relative to the shank. Readers are referred to descriptions by Õunpuu et al. [33] and Palladino and Davis [34] for more details associated with this process.

Although sometimes referred to as "muscle moments," these net intersegmental moments reflect the moments produced by several mechanisms, for example, bony restrictions to motion, ligamentous forces, passive muscle and tendon force, and active muscle contractile force, in response to external loads. Currently, the evaluation of individual muscle forces in a patient population is not feasible because optimization strategies that may be successful for typically developing ambulation [35,36] may not be appropriate for pathological muscle behavior, for example, spasticity, overactivity, hyper- or hypotonicity [37].

With respect to assumptions associated with these gait models, the body segments are assumed to be rigid, for example, soft-tissue movement relative to underlying bone is small. The external markers are assumed to move with the underlying anatomical references. In this way, estimated joint center locations are assumed to remain fixed relative to the respective segmental coordinate systems, for example, the knee center is fixed relative to the thigh coordinate system. Moreover, the mass distribution changes during motion are assumed to be negligible. Consequently, the marker or instrumentation attachment sites must be selected carefully, for example, over tendinous structures of the distal shank as opposed to the more proximal muscle masses of the gastrocnemius and soleus.

5.4 Illustrative Clinical Example

As indicated above, the information available for clinical gait interpretation may include static physical examination measures, stride and temporal data, segment and joint kinematics, joint kinetics, electromyograms, and a video record. With this information, the clinical team can assess the patient's gait deviations, attempt to identify the etiology of the abnormalities and recommend treatment alternatives. In this way, clinicians are able to isolate the biomechanical insufficiency that may produce a locomotor impairment and require a compensatory response from the patient. For example, a patient may excessively elevate a pelvis (compensatory) in order to gain additional foot clearance in swing which may be inadequate due to a weak ankle dorsiflexor muscle (primary problem).

The following example illustrates how gait analysis data are used in the treatment decision-making process for a six-year-old child with cerebral palsy, left spastic hemiplegia. All gait video records, clinical examination data, and quantitative gait data are reviewed and a list of primary problems and possible causes is generated. The reviewed gait data would include 3-D kinematic data (Figure 5.4) and kinetic data (Figure 5.5) and dynamic EMG data (Figure 5.6).

In the sagittal plane, increased left plantar flexion in stance and swing (Figure 5.4, Point **A**) is secondary to spasticity of the ankle plantar flexor muscles as the patient has a passive range of motion of the ankle that is within normal limits and can stand plantigrade. Premature plantar flexion of the right ankle in mid stance (Figure 5.4, Point **B**) is a vault compensation as the patient can isolate motion about the right ankle on clinical examination and produce an internal dorsiflexor moment following initial contact (Figure 5.5, Point **A**). Increased left knee flexion at initial contact (Figure 5.4, Point **C**) is secondary to hamstring muscle spasticity/tightness (appreciated during the clinical examination and evidenced by hamstring over-activity during gait, seen in the EMG data, Figure 5.6, Point **A**). Reduced left knee flexion in swing (Figure 5.4, Point **D**) is secondary to rectus femoris muscle over-activity in mid swing (Figure 5.6, Point **B**), an absence of ankle power generation in terminal stance (Figure 5.5, Point **B**), reduced hip power generation in pre-swing (Figure 5.5, Point **C**), and out-of-plane positioning of the lower extremity due to internal hip rotation (Figure 5.4, Point **E**). Increasing anterior pelvic

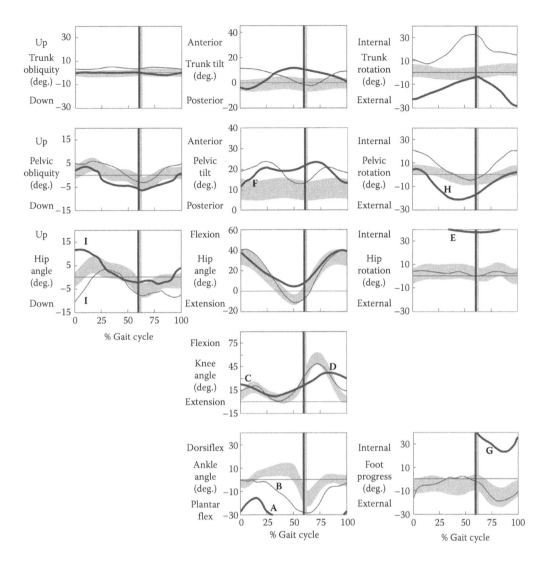

FIGURE 5.4 The left (thick lines) and right (thin lines) trunk, pelvic, and lower extremity kinematics for a six-year-old child with cerebral palsy, left spastic hemiplegia. Also shown are shaded bands that indicate one standard deviation about mean values associated with the reference (typically developing children) database used in the Motion Analysis Laboratory at Shriners Hospitals for Children, Greenville, South Carolina.

tilt during left-side stance (Figure 5.4, Point **F**) is related to the patient's limited ability to isolate movement between the pelvis and femur on the left side (determined from the clinical examination). In the transverse plane, increased left internal hip rotation (Figure 5.4, Point **E**), increased left internal foot progression (Figure 5.4, Point **G**), and asymmetric pelvic rotation with the left side externally rotated (Figure 5.4, Point **H**) are all secondary to increased internal femoral torsion (noted during the clinical examination). In the coronal plane, asymmetrical hip rotations (Figure 5.4, Point **I**) are secondary to pelvic transverse plane asymmetry.

After all of the primary gait issues are identified and possible causes are determined, treatment options for each primary issue are proposed. For the child presented above, treatment options include a left femoral derotation osteotomy to correct for internal femoral torsion and associated internal hip rotation (primary problem). Expected secondary outcomes of this intervention include improved foot

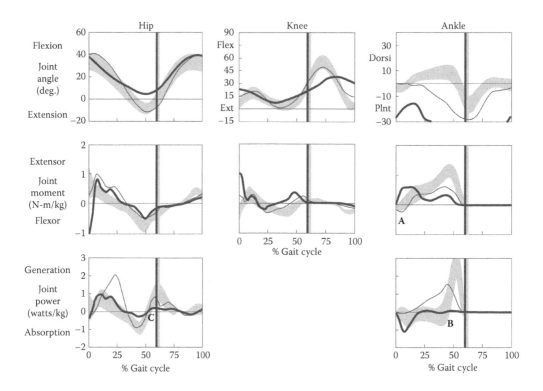

FIGURE 5.5   The left (thick lines) and right (thin lines) sagittal lower extremity kinetics for a six-year-old child with cerebral palsy, left spastic hemiplegia. Also shown are shaded bands that indicate one standard deviation about mean values associated with the reference (typically developing children) database used in the Motion Analysis Laboratory at Shriners Hospitals for Children, Greenville, South Carolina.

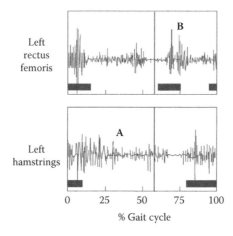

FIGURE 5.6   EMG tracing for the left rectus femoris and hamstring muscles for a six-year-old child with cerebral palsy, left spastic hemiplegia. The horizontal bars on the graphs indicate the approximate typical activity of these muscles during walking associated with the reference database used in the Motion Analysis Laboratory at Shriners Hospitals for Children, Greenville, South Carolina.

progression and symmetrical pelvic position in the transverse plane. A left intramuscular plantar flexor muscle lengthening is recommended to provide more length to the ankle plantar flexor muscles and reduce the impact of muscle stretch on the spastic plantar flexor muscles, thereby reducing (or resolving) the excessive ankle equinus and provide improved stability in stance and foot clearance in swing. A left hamstring muscle lengthening is also recommended to reduce the impact of muscle stretch on hamstring muscle spasticity, thereby improving knee extension at initial contact and overall knee motion in stance. A rectus femoris muscle transfer is recommended to reduce the impact of inappropriate activity of the rectus femoris muscle in mid swing and therefore improve peak knee flexion in swing and the associated clearance in swing. The premature plantar flexion of the right ankle in stance is secondary to a vault compensation and therefore, is predicted to resolve secondary to the surgery on the left side, that is, does not require any treatment. A standard protocol in most clinical gait laboratories is to repeat the gait analysis at about one year post surgery. At this time, surgical hypotheses and progress with respect to resolution of pretreatment gait abnormalities can be evaluated objectively.

5.5 Gait Analysis: Current Status

Comprehensive gait analysis techniques as described above have had a profound impact on the understanding of gait pathology, defining indications for specific treatments and ultimately, improving treatment outcomes. As with any kind of measurement, the utility of gait analysis information may be limited by sources of error, for example, soft-tissue displacement relative to the underlying bone. However, gains continue to be made with respect to analytical techniques to address this potential artifact [38–41]. The estimation of the location of the hip joint center is required in the determination of both hip kinematics and kinetics. Recent improvements in technology and computational techniques [42–44] have made the dynamic estimation of the instantaneous joint center locations, suggested by Cappozzo [25] in 1984, more viable clinically. Functional joint centering of the hip and all motion measurement using external markers, however, is challenged by excessive pelvic adipose tissue in patients who are overweight or obese. The evaluation of small patients weakens the quality of the data because inter-marker distances are reduced, thereby reducing the precision of angular computations, although recent improvements in camera resolution and camera image processing have addressed this limitation to a degree. Other errors associated with data collection alter the results as well, such as, a marker improperly placed or a force platform inadvertently contacted by the swing limb. To minimize the impact of these issues on motion data and its utility, it is essential that the potential adverse effects of these errors on the gait information be understood and appreciated by the clinical team in the interpretation process.

In addition to the kinematic (segment and joint angles), kinetic, and dynamic EMG data, estimations of musculo-tendon length are coming into use in clinical assessment and research [45,46]. This alternative expression of gait kinematics is also subject to the measurement and modeling issues associated with soft-tissue artifact and joint center determination with the additional challenge of approximating muscle origin and insertion anatomical locations. However, the assessment of musculo-tendon lengths in combination with other motion measurement and clinical data may assist in our understanding of the complex relationships between adjacent joints during gait. Gait forward simulation models are proving increasingly useful as exploratory tools in the investigation of the mechanisms associated with pathological gait [47,48]. These simulations will be strengthened when more is understood about the pathomechanics of impaired muscle and tendon and when they can be applied on an individual patient basis in the clinical setting.

Carefully performed gait analysis facilitates the systematic, quantitative documentation of walking patterns in comparison to qualitative observational techniques which represent the standard of care for the assessment of complex gait disorders in many medical facilities. With the various gait data, the clinician has the opportunity to separate the primary causes of a gait abnormality from the secondary deviations and compensatory gait mechanisms. Apparent contradictions between the different types of gait information, specifically visual impression versus joint angles (kinematics), can result in a more carefully developed understanding of the gait deviations and an appreciation for the additional knowledge and understanding gained through gait analysis data interpretation. Gait analysis provides the clinical user the ability to more precisely (than observational gait analysis alone) understand the gait pathomechanics; therefore, plan complex multi-level surgeries and ultimately objectively evaluate the efficacy of different interventions, for example, surgical approaches and orthotic designs. Through gait analysis, movement in planes of motion not easily observed, such as about the long axes of the lower limb segments, may be quantified. Finally, quantities that cannot be observed may be assessed, for example, muscular activity and joint kinetics. In the future, it is anticipated that our understanding of gait will be enhanced through the application of pattern recognition strategies, and coupled dynamics. The systematic and objective evaluation of gait both before and after intervention will continue to lead to improved treatment outcomes.

For Additional Information on Gait Analysis Techniques

Allard, P., Stokes, I.A.F., and Blanchi, J.P. (Eds.), *Three-Dimensional Analysis of Human Movement*, Human Kinetics, Champaign, Illinois, 1995.

Berme, N. and Cappozzo, A. (Eds.), *Biomechanics of Human Movement: Applications in Rehabilitation, Sports and Ergonomics*, Bertec Corporation, Worthington, Ohio, 1990.

Harris, G.F. and Smith, P.A., (Eds.), *Human Motion Analysis*, IEEE Press, Piscataway, New Jersey, 1996.

Rose, J. and Gamble, J.G. (Eds), *Human Walking*, 3rd Edition, Lippincott Williams & Wilkins, Philadelphia, 2006.

Winter, D.A., *Biomechanics and Motor Control of Human Movement*, John Wiley and Sons, New Jersey, 2009.

For Additional Information on Typically Developing and Pathological Gait

Gage, J.R., Koop, S.E., Schwartz, M.H., Novacheck, T.F. (Eds.), *The Treatment of Gait Problems in Cerebral Palsy*, 2nd Edition, Mac Keith Press, London, 2009.

Perry, J. and Burnfield, J.M., *Gait Analysis: Normal and Pathological Function*, 2nd Edition, Slack, New Jersey, 2010.

Rose, J. and Gamble, J.G. (Eds.), *Human Walking*, 3rd Edition, Lippincott Williams & Wilkins, Philadelphia, 2006.

Sutherland, D.H. et al., *The Development of Mature Walking*, Mac Keith Press, London, 1988.

References

1. Neptune, R.R., Zajac, F.E., and Kautz, S.A., Muscle force redistributes segmental power for body progression during walking, *Gait Posture*, 19, 194, 2004.

2. Heller, M.O. et al., Musculo-skeletal loading conditions at the hip during walking and stair climbing, *J. Biomech.*, 34, 883, 2001.

3. Ferber, R., Davis, I.M., and Williams, D.S. 3rd, Gender differences in lower extremity mechanics during running, *Clin. Biomech.*, 18, 350, 2003.

4. Kerrigan D.C. et al., The effect of running shoes on lower extremity joint torques, *Arch. Phys. Med. Rehabil.*, 1, 1058, 2009.

5. Kautz, S.A. and Hull, M.L., Dynamic optimization analysis for equipment setup problems in endurance cycling, *J. Biomech.*, 28, 1391, 1995.

6. Tashman, S. et al., Abnormal rotational knee motion during running after anterior cruciate ligament reconstruction, *Am. J. Sports Med.*, 32, 975, 2004.

7. Brand, R.A. and Crowninshield, R.D., Comment on criteria for patient evaluation tools, *J. Biomech.*, 14, 655, 1981.

8. Mâaref, K. et al., Kinematics in the terminal swing phase of unilateral transfemoral amputees: Microprocessor-controlled versus swing-phase control prosthetic knees, *Arch. Phys. Med. Rehabil.*, 91, 919, 2010.

9. Stebbins, J. et al., Gait compensations caused by foot deformity in cerebral palsy, *Gait Posture*, 32, 226, 2010.

10. Adolfsen, S.E. et al., Kinematic and kinetic outcomes after identical multilevel soft tissue surgery in children with cerebral palsy, *J. Pediatr. Orthop.*, 27, 658, 2007.

11. Kaufman, K.R. et al., Gait characteristics of patients with knee osteoarthritis, *J. Biomech.*, 34, 907, 2001.

12. Vanwanseele, B. et al., The relationship between knee adduction moment and cartilage and meniscus morphology in women with osteoarthritis, *Osteoarthritis Cartilage*, 18, 894, 2010.

13. Koutakis, P. et al., Abnormal joint powers before and after the onset of claudication symptoms, *J. Vasc. Surg.*, 52, 340, 2010.

14. Pospischill, M. et al., Minimally invasive compared with traditional transgluteal approach for total hip arthroplasty: A comparative gait analysis, *J. Bone Joint Surg. Am.*, 92, 328, 2010.

15. Perry, J., Mulroy, S.J., and Renwick, S.E., The relationship of lower extremity strength and gait parameters in patients with post-polio syndrome, *Arch. Phys. Med. Rehabil.*, 74, 165, 1993.

16. Kelleher, K.J. et al., The characterisation of gait patterns of people with multiple sclerosis, *Disabil. Rehabil.*, 32, 1242, 2010.

17. D'Angelo, M.G. et al., Gait pattern in Duchenne muscular dystrophy, *Gait Posture*, 29, 36, 2009.

18. Õunpuu, S. et al., An examination of knee function during gait in children with myelomeningocele, *J. Pediatr. Orthop.*, 20, 629, 2000.

19. Bartonek, A., Eriksson, M., and Gutierrez-Farewik, E.M., Effects of carbon fibre spring orthoses on gait in ambulatory children with motor disorders and plantarflexor weakness, *Dev. Med. Child. Neurol.*, 49, 615, 2007.

20. Weiss, R.J. et al., Gait pattern in rheumatoid arthritis, *Gait Posture*, 28, 229, 2008.

21. Gordon, K.E. et al., Ankle load modulates hip kinetics and EMG during human locomotion, *J. Neurophysiol.*, 101, 2062, 2009.

22. Mulroy, S. et al., Use of cluster analysis for gait pattern classification of patients in the early and late recovery phases following stroke, *Gait Posture*, 18, 114, 2003.

23. Perry, J., The use of gait analysis for surgical recommendations in traumatic brain injury, *J. Head Trauma Rehabil.*, 14, 116, 1999.

24. Õunpuu, S., Gage, J.R., and Davis, R.B., Three-dimensional lower extremity joint kinetics in normal pediatric gait, *J. Pediatr. Orthop.*, 11, 341, 1991.

25. Cappozzo, A., Gait analysis methodology, *Hum. Move. Sci.*, 3, 27, 1984.

26. Davis, R.B. et al., A gait analysis data collection and reduction technique, *Hum. Move. Sci.*, 10, 575, 1991.

27. Bell, A.L., Pederson, D.R., and Brand, R.A., Prediction of hip joint center location from external landmarks, *Hum. Move. Sci.*, 8, 3, 1989.

28. Grood, E.S. and Suntay, W.J., A joint coordinate system for the clinical description of three-dimensional motions: Application to the knee, *J. Biomech. Eng.*, 105, 136, 1983.

29. Woltring, H.J., Huskies, R., and DeLange, A., Finite centroid and helical axis estimation from noisy landmark measurement in the study of human joint kinematics, *J. Biomech.*, 18, 379, 1985.

30. Dempster, W.T., Space requirements of the seated operator: Geometrical, kinematic, and mechanical aspects of the body with special reference to the limbs, WADC-55-159, AD-087-892, Wright Air Development Center, Wright-Patterson Air Force Base, Ohio, 1955.

31. McConville, J.T. et al., Anthropometric relationships of body and body segment moments of inertia, Technical report AFAMRL-TR-80-119, Air Force Aerospace Medical Research Laboratory,

Aerospace Medical Division, Air Force Systems Command, Wright-Patterson Air Force Base, Ohio, 1980.

32. Jenson, R.K., Body segment mass, radius and radius of gyration proportions of children, *J. Biomech.*, 19, 359, 1986.

33. Õunpuu, S., Davis, R.B., and DeLuca, P.A., Joint kinetics: Methods, interpretation and treatment decision-making in children with cerebral palsy and myelomeningocele, *Gait Posture*, 4, 62, 1996.

34. Palladino, J. and Davis, R.B., Biomechanics, in *Introduction to Biomedical Engineering*, Enderle, J., Blanchard, S., and Bronzino, J., Eds., Elsevier Academic Press, Amsterdam, 133, 2012.

35. Chao, E.Y. and Rim, K., Application of optimization principles in determining the applied moments in human leg joints during gait, *J. Biomech.*, 6, 497, 1973.

36. Anderson, F.C. and Pandy, M.G., Static and dynamic optimization solutions for gait are practically equivalent, *J. Biomech.*, 34, 153, 2001.

37. Bleck, E.E., *Orthopaedic Management in Cerebral Palsy*, Mac Keith Press, Philadelphia, 1987, 87.

38. Stagni R., Fantozzi S., and Cappello A., Double calibration vs. global optimization: Performance and effectiveness for clinical application, *Gait Posture*, 1, 119, 2009.

39. Peters A. et al., Determination of the optimal locations of surface-mounted markers on the tibial segment, *Gait Posture*, 1, 42, 2009.

40. De Groote F. et al., Kalman smoothing improves the estimation of joint kinematics and kinetics in marker-based human gait analysis, *J. Biomech.*, 41, 3390, 2008.

41. Cappello A. et al., Soft tissue artifact compensation in knee kinematics by double anatomical landmark calibration: Performance of a novel method during selected motor tasks, *IEEE Trans Biomed Eng.*, 52, 992, 2005.

42. Leardini, A. et al., Validation of a functional method for the estimation of hip joint centre location, *J. Biomech.*, 32, 99, 1999.

43. Piazza, S.J. et al., Assessment of the functional method of hip joint center location subject to reduced range of hip motion, *J. Biomech.*, 37, 349, 2004.

44. Schwartz, M.H. and Rozumalskia, A., A new method for estimating joint parameters from motion data, *J. Biomech.*, 38, 107, 2005.

45. Jahn, J., Vasavada, A.N., and McMulkin, M.L., Calf muscle-tendon lengths before and after tendo-Achilles lengthenings and gastrocnemius lengthenings for equinus in cerebral palsy and idiopathic toe walking, *Gait Posture*, 29, 612, 2009.

46. van der Krogt, M.M. et al., Walking speed modifies spasticity effects in gastrocnemius and soleus in cerebral palsy gait, *Clin. Biomech.*, 24, 422, 2009.

47. Damiano, D.L. et al., Can strength training predictably improve gait kinematics? A pilot study on the effects of hip and knee extensor strengthening on lower-extremity alignment in cerebral palsy, *Phys. Ther.*, 90, 269, 2010.

48. Fox, M.D. et al., Mechanisms of improved knee flexion after rectus femoris transfer surgery, *J. Biomech.*, 42, 614, 2009.

6

Mechanics of Head/Neck

Albert I. King
Wayne State University

David C. Viano
Wayne State University

Injury is a major societal problem in the United States. Approximately 140,000 fatalities occur each year due to both intentional and unintentional injuries. Two-thirds of these are unintentional, and of these, about one-half are attributable to automotive-related injuries. In 1993, the estimated number of automotive-related fatalities dipped under 40,000 for the first time in the last three decades due to a continuing effort by both the industry and the government to render vehicles safer in crash situations. However, for people under 40 years of age, automotive crashes, falls, and other unintentional injuries are the highest risks of fatality in the United States in comparison with all other causes.

The principal aim of impact biomechanics is the prevention of injury through environmental modification, such as the provision of an airbag for automotive occupants to protect them during a frontal crash. To achieve this aim effectively, it is necessary that workers in the field have a clear understanding of the *mechanisms of injury*, be able to describe the *mechanical response* of the tissues involved, have some basic information on *human tolerance* to impact, and be in possession of tools that can be used as *human surrogates* to assess a particular injury (Viano et al., 1989). This chapter deals with the biomechanics of blunt impact injury to the head and neck.

6.1 Mechanisms of Injury

6.1.1 Head Injury Mechanisms

Among the more popular theories of brain injury due to blunt impact are changes in intracranial pressure and the development of shear strains in the brain. Positive pressure increases are found in the brain behind the site of impact on the skull. Rapid acceleration of the head, in-bending of the skull, and the propagation of a compressive pressure wave are proposed as mechanisms for the generation of intracranial compression that causes local contusion of brain tissue. At the contrecoup site, there is an opposite response in the form of a negative-pressure pulse that also causes bruising. It is not clear as to whether the injury is due to the negative pressure itself (tensile loading) or to a cavitation phenomenon similar to that seen on the surfaces of propellers of ships (compression loading). The pressure differential across the brain necessarily results in a pressure gradient that can give rise to shear strains developing within the deep structures of the brain. Furthermore, when the head is impacted, it not only translates but also rotates about the neck, causing relative motion of the brain with respect to the skull. Gennarelli (1983) has found that rotational acceleration of the head can cause a diffuse injury to the white matter of the brain in animal models, as evidenced by retraction balls developing along the axons of injured nerves. This injury was described by Strich (1961) as diffuse axonal injury (DAI) that she found in the white matter of autopsied human brains. Other researchers, including Lighthall et al. (1990), have been able to cause the development of DAI in the brain of an animal model (ferrets) by the application of direct impact to the brain without the associated head angular acceleration. Adams ct al. (1986) indicated that DAI is the most important factor in severe head injury because it is irreversible and leads to incapacitation and dementia. It is postulated that DAI occurs as a result of the mechanical insult but cannot be detected by staining techniques at autopsy unless the patient survives the injury for at least several hours.

6.1.2 Neck Injury Mechanisms

The neck or the cervical spine is subjected to several forms of unique injuries that are not seen in the thoracolumbar spine. Injuries to the upper cervical spine, particularly at the atlanto-occipital joint, are considered to be more serious and life threatening than those at the lower level. The atlanto-occipital joint can be dislocated either by an axial torsional load or a shear force applied in the anteroposterior direction, or vice versa. A large compression force can cause the arches of Cl to fracture, breaking it up into two or four sections. The odontoid process of C2 is also a vulnerable area. Extreme flexion of the neck is a common cause of odontoid fractures, and a large percentage of these injuries are related to automotive accidents (Pierce and Barr, 1983). Fractures through the pars interarticularis of C2, commonly known as "hangman's fractures" in automotive collisions, are the result of a combined axial compression and extension (rearward bending) of the cervical spine. Impact of the forehead and face of unrestrained occupants with the windshield can result in this injury. Garfin and Rothman (1983) discussed this injury in relation to hanging and traced the history of this mode of execution. It was estimated by a British judiciary committee that the energy required to cause a hangman's fracture was 1708 N m (1260 ft lb).

In automotive-type accidents, the loading on the neck due to head contact forces is usually a combination of an axial or shear load with bending. Bending loads are almost always present, and the degree of axial or shear force depends on the location and direction of the contact force. For impacts near the crown of the head, compressive forces predominate. If the impact is principally in the transverse plane, there is less compression and more shear. Bending modes are infinite in number because the impact can come from any angle around the head. To limit the scope of the discussion, the following injury modes are considered: tension–flexion, tension–extension, compression–flexion, and compression–extension in the midsagittal plane and lateral bending.

6.1.2.1 Tension–Flexion Injuries

Forces resulting from inertial loading of the head–neck system can result in flexion of the cervical spine while it is being subjected to a tensile force. In experimental impacts of restrained subjects undergoing forward deceleration, Thomas and Jessop (1983) reported atlanto-occipital separation and C1–C2 separation occurring in subhuman primates at 120 g. Similar injuries in human cadavers were found at 34–38 g by Cheng et al. (1982), who used a preinflated driver airbag system that restrained the thorax but allowed the head and neck to rotate over the bag.

6.1.2.2 Tension–Extension Injuries

The most common type of injury due to combined tension and extension of the cervical spine is the "whiplash" syndrome. However, a large majority of such injuries involve the soft tissues of the neck, and the pain is believed to reside in the joint capsules of the articular facets of the cervical vertebrae (Wallis et al., 1997).

In severe cases, teardrop fractures of the anterosuperior aspect of the vertebral body can occur. Alternately, separation of the anterior aspect of the disk from the vertebral endplate is known to occur. More severe injuries occur when the chin impacts the instrument panel or when the forehead impacts the windshield. In both cases, the head rotates rearward and applies a tensile and bending load on the neck. In the case of windshield impact by the forehead, hangman's fracture of C2 can occur. Garfin and Rothman (1983) suggested that it is caused by spinal extension combined with compression on the lamina of C2, causing the pars to fracture.

6.1.2.3 Compression–Flexion Injuries

When a force is applied to the posterosuperior quadrant of the head or when a crown impact is administered while the head is in flexion, the neck is subjected to a combined load of axial compression and forward bending. Anterior wedge fractures of vertebral bodies are commonly seen, but with increased load, burst fractures, and fracture-dislocations of the facets can result. The latter two conditions are unstable and tend to disrupt or injure the spinal cord, and the extent of the injury depends on the penetration of the vertebral body or its fragments into the spinal canal. Recent experiments by Pintar et al. (1989, 1990) indicate that burst fractures of lower cervical vertebrae can be reproduced in cadaveric specimens by a crown impact to a flexed cervical spine. A study by Nightingale et al. (1993) showed that fracture dislocations of the cervical spine occur very early in the impact event (within the first 10 ms) and that the subsequent motion of the head or bending of the cervical spine cannot be used as a reliable indicator of the mechanism of injury.

6.1.2.4 Compression–Extension Injuries

Frontal impacts to the head with the neck in extension will cause compression–extension injuries. These involve the fracture of one or more spinous processes and, possibly, symmetrical lesions of the pedicles, facets, and laminae. If there is a fracture dislocation, the inferior facet of the upper vertebra is displaced posteriorly and upward and appears to be more horizontal than normal on x-ray.

6.1.2.5 Injuries Involving Lateral Bending

If the applied force or inertial load on the head has a significant component out of the midsagittal plane, the neck will be subjected to lateral or oblique along with axial and shear loading. The injuries characteristic of lateral bending are lateral wedge fractures of the vertebral body and fractures to the posterior elements on one side of the vertebral column.

Whenever there is lateral or oblique bending, there is the possibility of twisting the neck. The associated torsional loads may be responsible for unilateral facet dislocations or unilateral locked facets (Moffat et al., 1978). However, the authors postulated that pure torsional loads on the neck are rarely encountered in automotive accidents.

6.2 Mechanical Response

6.2.1 Mechanical Response of the Brain

Skull impact response was presented in the previous edition in which remarks were made regarding the unavailability of data on the response of the brain during an injury-producing impact. Such data are now available. For intact heads, the motion of the brain inside the skull has been recently studied by Hardy et al. (2001). Isolated cadaveric heads were subjected to a combined linear and angular acceleration and exposed to a biplanar high-speed x-ray system. Neutral density targets made of tin or tungsten were preinserted into the brain. Video data collected from such impacts showed that most of the motion was in the center of the brain and that target motion was in the form of a figure 8, as shown in Figure 6.1. This motion was limited to ±5 mm regardless of the severity of the impact. Angular acceleration levels in excess of 10,000 rad/s^2 were reached.

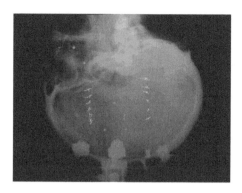

FIGURE 6.1 Brain response to blunt impact.

In another experiment, a Hybrid III dummy head and neck system was accelerated into a variety of plastic foams to assess head response with and without the use of a helmet used in American football. It was found that the helmet reduced the linear acceleration of the head substantially but did not change its angular acceleration significantly. However, it is believed by many that angular acceleration is the cause of brain injury. So if angular acceleration is the culprit, then how does the helmet protect the brain? In an attempt to answer this question, video data from NFL helmet impacts were analyzed and the helmet velocities were computed using stereophotogrammetric methods. The helmet impacts were reproduced in the laboratory by Newman et al. (1999) to yield head angular and linear accelerations, using helmeted Hybrid III dummies. These head accelerations were fed into a brain injury computer model developed by Zhang et al. (2001) to compute brain responses, such as strain (ε), strain rate ($d\varepsilon/dt$), and pressure. A total of 58 cases were studied, involving 25 cases of concussion or mild traumatic brain injury (MTBI), as reported by Pellman et al. (2003). The results of the model were analyzed statistically to determine the best predictors of MTBI, using the logist analysis. It was found brain response parameters such as the product of strain and strain rate, were good predictors whereas angular acceleration was a poor predictor, as shown in Table 6.1. The chi square value is a measure of the ability of the parameter to predict injury and in this analysis, its ability to predict injury is high if the chi square value is high. These results are consistent with the findings of Viano and Lövsund (1999) who used animal data to determine the parameter most likely to cause DAI in a living brain. It was the product of the velocity (V) of the impactor and depth of penetration of the impactor as percentage of the brain depth (C). For the brain, the product, $V \cdot C$, is analogous to $\varepsilon \cdot d\varepsilon/dt$. Note that head injury criterion (HIC) is the current criterion used in Federal Motor Vehicle Safety Standard (FMVSS) 208 to assess head injury and GSI (Gadd Severity Index) is the previous head injury criterion, now referred to as the Gadd Severity Index. The cumulative strain

TABLE 6.1 List of Best Predictors of MTBI

Rank Order	Predictor Variable	Chi Square	p-value
1	$\varepsilon \cdot d\varepsilon/dt$	41.0	0.0000
2	$d\varepsilon/dt$	33.1	0.0000
3	HIC	31.5	0.0000
4	SI	31.2	0.0000
5	Linear acceleration	28.3	0.0000
6	ε_{max}	28.0	0.0000
7	Max. principal stress	27.3	0.0000
8	Cumulative strain at 15%	26.0	0.0000
9	Angular acceleration	24.9	0.0000

at 15% is a measure of the volume of brain that experienced a strain of 15% or higher throughout the impact. It is concluded that response variable of the brain are better predictors of injury than input variables.

6.2.2 Mechanical Response of the Neck

The mechanical response of the cervical spine was studied by Mertz and Patrick (1967, 1971), Patrick and Chou (1976), Schneider et al. (1975), and Ewing et al. (1978). Mertz et al. (1973) quantified the response in terms of rotation of the head relative to the torso as a function of bending moment at the occipital condyles. Loading corridors were obtained for flexion and extension, as shown in Figures 6.2 and 6.3. An exacting definition of the impact environments to be used in evaluating dummy necks relative to the loading corridors illustrated in these figures is included in SAE J1460 (1985). It should be noted that the primary basis for these curves is volunteer data and that the extension of these corridors to dummy tests in the injury-producing range is somewhat surprising.

The issue of whiplash is a controversial one principally because researchers in the field cannot agree on an injury mechanism. Currently, five such mechanisms have been proposed. It began with the hyperextension theory, which was discarded when the automotive headrest did not reduce the incidence of injury. The flexion theory is also considered untenable because head and neck flexion after the rear end collision is much less severe than that resulting from a frontal impact and the whiplash syndrome is not frequently seen in frontal impacts. The theory that a momentary increase in pressure in the cerebrospinal fluid during whiplash could induce neck pain was also considered invalid because injury to the nerve roots require prolonged pressure and root compression leads to radiculopathy and not direct neck pain. The fourth theory of impingement of the facet joint surfaces was proposed but has not been demonstrated. It claims that the synovial lining can be trapped between the facets resulting in pain. Finally, the shear theory appears to be the most promising. A shear force is developed at every level of the cervical spine before the head and can be brought forward along with the torso, which is pushed forward by the seat back. This shear force causes relative motion between adjacent cervical vertebrae in the form of relative translation and rotation. Deng et al. (2000) performed a series of cadaveric tests and measured this relative displacement and also estimated the amount of stretch the facet capsules would undergo. Wallis et al. (1997) have shown that removal of nerve endings in the cervical facet capsules can relieve neck pain for an average of about nine

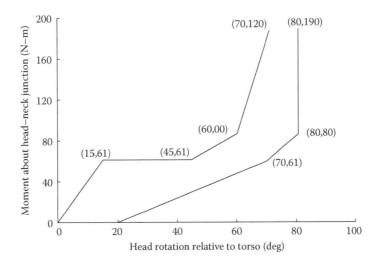

FIGURE 6.2 Loading corridor for neck flexion.

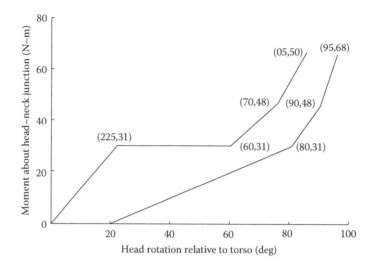

FIGURE 6.3   Loading corridor for neck extension.

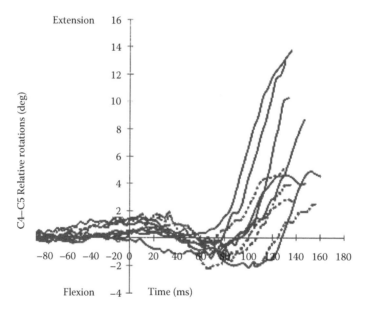

FIGURE 6.4   Relative displacement of C4 on C5 for 20° seat back angle tests (solid lines) and 0° seat back angle tests (dotted lines) simulating low-speed rear-end collisions, using a cadaver. (Reproduced from Deng, B. et al. 2000. *Stapp Car Crash J.* 44: 171–188. With permission.)

months. Figure 6.4 shows the amount of forward motion of C5 relative to C4 and Figure 6.5 shows the estimated stretch of the C4–5 and C5–6 facet capsule. Of interest is the time of occurrence of these events. They occur before the head hits the headrest. It not only explains why the present headrest is ineffective but also indicates to the safety engineer that the headrest needs to be much closer to the head if it is to be effective.

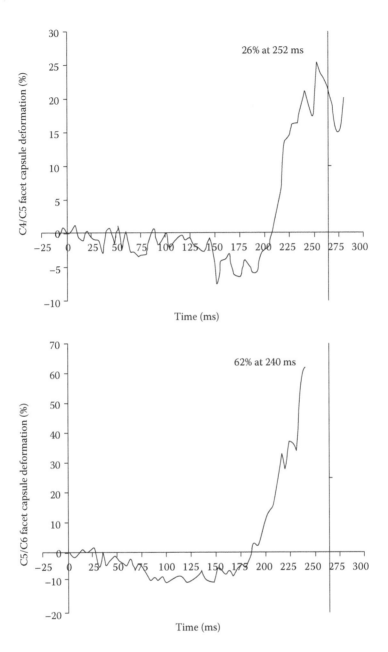

FIGURE 6.5 Estimated cervical facet capsule stretch during the simulated test described in Figure 6.4. (Reproduced from Deng, B. et al. 2000. *Stapp Car Crash J.* 44: 171–188. With permission.)

6.3 Regional Tolerance of the Head and Neck to Blunt Impact

6.3.1 Regional Tolerance of the Head

The most commonly measured parameter for head injury is acceleration. It is therefore natural to express human tolerance to injury in terms of head acceleration. The first known tolerance criterion is the Wayne State Tolerance Curve, proposed by Lissner et al. (1960) and subsequently modified by

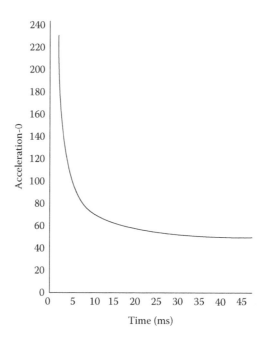

FIGURE 6.6   The Wayne State Tolerance Curve for head injury.

Patrick et al. (1965) by the addition of animal and volunteer data to the original cadaveric data. The modified curve is shown in Figure 6.6. The head can withstand higher accelerations for shorter durations and any exposure above the curve is injurious. When this curve is plotted on logarithmic paper, it becomes a straight line with a slope of −2.5. This slope was used as an exponent by Gadd (1961) in his proposed severity index, now known as the *Gadd Severity Index* (GSI):

$$\text{GSI} = \int_{0}^{T} a^{2.5}\,dt \tag{6.1}$$

where a is the instantaneous acceleration of the head, and T is the duration of the pulse.

If the integrated value exceeds 1000, a severe injury will result. A modified form of the GSI, now known as the *Head Injury Criterion* (HIC), was proposed by Versace (1970) to identify the most damaging part of the acceleration pulse by finding the maximum value of the following integral:

$$\text{HIC} = (t_2 - t_1)\left[(t_2 - t_1)^{-1}\int_{t_1}^{t_2} a(t)\,dt\right]^{2.5}\Bigg|_{\text{max}} \tag{6.2}$$

where $a(t)$ is the resultant instantaneous acceleration of the head, and $t_2 - t_1$ is the time interval over which HIC is a maximum.

A severe but not life-threatening injury would have occurred if the HIC reached or exceeded 1000. Subsequently, Prasad and Mertz (1985) proposed a probabilistic method of assessing head injury and developed the curve shown in Figure 6.7. At an HIC of 1000, approximately 16% of the population would sustain a severe-to-fatal injury. It is apparent that this criterion is useful in automotive safety design and in the design of protective equipment for the head, such as football and bicycle helmets. However, there is another school of thought that believes in the injurious potential of angular acceleration in its ability to cause DAI and rupture of the parasagittal bridging veins between the brain and

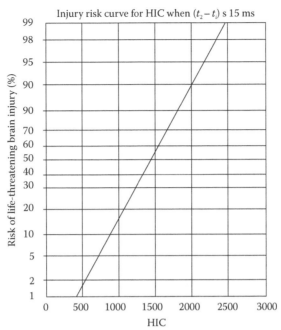

FIGURE 6.7   Head injury risk curve based on HIC.

TABLE 6.2   Tolerance Estimates for MTBI

	Tolerance Estimate (Probability of Injury)		
Variable	25%	50%	75%
HIC	136	235	333
Linear acceleration (m/s²)	559	778	965
Angular acceleration (rad/s²)	4384	5757	7130
Max. principal strain, ε (%)	25	37	49
Max. principal strain rate, $d\varepsilon/dt$ (s^{-1})	46	60	79
$\varepsilon \cdot d\varepsilon/dt$ (s^{-1})	14	20	25

Source: King, A.I. et al. 2003. *Bertil Aldman Lecture, Proceedings of the 2003 International IRCOBI Conference on the Biomechanics of Impact*, pp. 1–12.

dura mater. The MTBI data referred to above show that this may not be case and that a strain-related parameter should be designated as a brain injury criterion, regardless of the input. However, for the moment, HIC remains as the head injury criterion in FMVSS 208 and attempts to replace it have so far been unsuccessful.

As a matter of interest, tolerance data for MTBI, data obtained from the National Football League (NFL) data are presented in Table 6.2, taken from King et al. (2003).

6.3.2 Regional Tolerance of the Neck

Currently there are no universally accepted tolerance values for the neck for the various injury modes. This is not due to a lack of data but rather to the many injury mechanisms and several levels of injury severity, ranging from life-threatening injuries to the spinal cord to minor soft-tissue injuries that cannot be identified on radiographic or magnetic scans. It is likely that a combined criterion of axial load and bending moment about one or more axes will be adopted as a future FMVSS.

6.4 Human Surrogates of the Head and Neck

6.4.1 The Experimental Surrogate

The most effective experimental surrogate for impact biomechanics research is the unembalmed cadaver. This is also true for the head and neck, despite the fact that the cadaver is devoid of muscle tone because the duration of impact is usually too short for the muscles to respond adequately. It is true, however, that muscle pretensioning in the neck may have to be added under certain circumstances. Similarly, for the brain, the cadaveric brain cannot develop DAI, and the mechanical properties of the brain change rapidly after death. If the pathophysiology of the central nervous system is to be studied, the ideal surrogate is an animal brain. Currently, the rat is frequently used as the animal of choice and there is some work in progress using the mini-pig.

6.4.2 The Injury-Assessment Tool

The response and tolerance data acquired from cadaveric studies are used to design human-like surrogates, known as *anthropomorphic test devices* (ATD). These surrogates are required not only to have biofidelity and the ability to simulate human response but also need to provide physical measurements that are representative of human injury. In addition, they are designed to be repeatable and reproducible. The current frontal impact dummy is the Hybrid III family of dummies ranging from the 95th percentile male to the 3-year-old infant. The 50th percentile male dummy is human like in many of its responses, including that of the head and neck. The head consists of an aluminum headform covered by an appropriately designed vinyl "skin" to yield human-like acceleration responses for frontal and lateral impacts against a flat, rigid surface. Two-dimensional physical models of the brain were proposed by Margulies et al. (1990) using a silicone gel in which preinscribed grid lines would deform under angular acceleration. No injury criterion is associated with this gel model.

The dummy neck was designed to yield responses in flexion and extension that would fit within the corridors shown in Figures 6.2 and 6.3. The principal function of the dummy neck is to place the head in the approximate position of a human head in the same impact involving a human occupant.

6.4.3 Computer Models

Models of head impact first appeared over 50 years ago (Holbourn, 1943). Extensive reviews of such models were made by King and Chou (1977) and Hardy et al. (1994). The use of the finite-element method (FEM) to simulate the various components of the head appears to be the most effective and popular means of modeling brain response. A recent model by Zhang et al. (2001) is extremely detailed, with over 300,000 elements. It simulates the brain, the meninges, the cerebrospinal fluid and ventricles, the skull, scalp, and most of the facial bones and soft tissues. Validation was attempted against all available experimental data. It has been used in many applications, including the prediction of MTBI for helmeted football players described earlier. Other less detailed models include those by Kleiven and Hardy (2002), Willinger et al. (1999), and Takhounts et al. (2003).

A large number of neck and spinal models also have been developed over the past four decades. A paper by Kleinberger (1993) provides a brief and incomplete review of these models. However, the method of choice for modeling the response of the neck is the finite-element method, principally because of the complex geometry of the vertebral components and the interaction of several different materials.

A partially validated model for impact response was developed by Yang et al. (1998) to simulate both crown impact as well as the whiplash phenomenon due to a rear-end impact.

References

Adams, J.H., Doyle, D., Graham, D.I. et al. 1986. Gliding contusions in nonmissile head injury in humans. *Arch. Pathol. Lab. Med.* 110: 485.

Cheng, R., Yang, K.H., Levine, R.S. et al. 1982. Injuries to the cervical spine caused by a distributed frontal load to the chest. In *Proceedings of the 26th Stapp Car Crash Conference*, pp. 1–40.

Deng, B., Begeman, P.C., Yang, K.H. et al. 2000. Kinematics of human cadaver cervical spine during low speed rear-end impacts. *Stapp Car Crash J.* 44: 171–188.

Ewing, C.L., Thomas, D.J., Lustick, L. et al. 1978. Effect of initial position on the human head and neck response to + Y impact acceleration. In *Proceedings of the 22nd Stapp Car Crash Conference*, pp. 101–138.

Gadd, C.W. 1961. Criteria for injury potential. In *Impact Acceleration Stress Symposium, National Research Council Publication No. 977*, pp. 141–144. Washington, National Academy of Sciences.

Garfin, S.R. and Rothman, R.H. 1983. Traumatic spondylolisthesis of the axis (Hangman's fracture). In R.W. Baily (Ed.), *The Cervical Spine*, pp. 223–232. Philadelphia, PA, Lippincott.

Gennarelli, T.A. 1983. Head injuries in man and experimental animals: Clinical aspects. *Acta Neurochir. Suppl.* 32: 1.

Hardy, W.N., Foster, C.D., Mason, M.J. et al. 2001. Investigation of head injury mechanisms using neutral density technology and high-speed biplanar x-ray. *Stapp Car Crash J.* 45: 337–368.

Hardy, W.N., Khalil, T.B., and King, A.I. 1994. Literature review of head injury biomechanics. *Int. J. Impact Eng.* 15: 561–586.

Holbourn, A.H.S. 1943. Mechanics of head injury. *Lancet* 2: 438.

King, A.I. and Chou, C. 1977. Mathematical modelling, simulation and experimental testing of biomechanical system crash response. *J. Biomech.* 9: 3–10.

King, A.I., Yang, K.H., Zhang, L. et al. 2003. Is head injury caused by linear or angular acceleration? In *Bertil Aldman Lecture, Proceedings of the 2003 International IRCOBI Conference on the Biomechanics of Impact*, pp. 1–12.

Kleinberger, M. 1993. Application of finite element techniques to the study of cervical spine mechanics. In *Proceedings of the 37th Stapp Car Crash Conference*, pp. 261–272.

Kleiven, S. and Hardy, W.N. 2002. Correlation of an FE model of the human head with experiments on localized motion of the brain—Consequences for injury prediction. *Stapp Car Crash J.* 46: 123–144.

Lighthall, J.W., Goshgarian, H.G., and Pinderski, C.R. 1990. Characterization of axonal injury produced by controlled cortical impact. *J. Neurotrauma* 7(2): 65.

Lissner, H.R., Lebow, M., and Evans F.G. 1960. Experimental studies on the relation between acceleration and intracranial pressure changes in man. *Surg. Gynecol. Obstet.* 111: 329.

Margulies, S.S., Thibault, L.E., and Gennarelli, T.A. 1990. Physical model simulation of brain injury in the primate. *J. Biomech.* 23: 823.

Mertz, H.J., Neathery, R.F., and Culver, C.C. 1973. Performance requirements and characteristics of mechanical necks. In W.F. King and H.I. Mertz (Eds.), *Human Impact Response: Measurement and Simulations*, pp. 263–288. New York, Plenum Press.

Mertz, H.J. and Patrick, L.M. 1967. Investigation of the kinematics and kinetics of whiplash. In *Proceedings of the 11th Stapp Car Crash Conference*, pp. 267–317.

Mertz, H.J. and Patrick, L.M. 1971. Strength and response of the human neck. In *Proceedings of the 15th Stapp Car Crash Conference*, pp. 207–255.

Moffat, E.A., Siegel, A.W., and Huelke, D.F. 1978. The biomechanics of automotive cervical fractures. In *Proceedings of the 22nd Conference of American Association for Automotive Medicine*, pp. 151–168.

Newman, J., Beusenberg, M., Fournier, E. et al. 1999. A new biomechanical assessment of mild traumatic brain injury—Part I: methodology. In *Proceedings of the 1999 International IRCOBI Conference on the Biomechanics of Impact*, pp. 17–36.

Nightingale, R.W., McElhaney, J.H., Best, T.M. et al. 1993. The relationship between observed head motion and cervical spine injury mechanism. In *Proceedings of the 39th Meeting of the Orthopedic Research Society*, p. 233.

Patrick, L.M. and Chou, C. 1976. Response of the human neck in flexion, extension, and lateral flexion, Vehicle Research Institute Report No. VRI-7-3. Warrendale, PA, Society of Automotive Engineers.

Patrick, L.M., Lissner, H.R., and Gurdjian, E.S. 1965. Survival by design: Head protection. In *Proceedings of the 7th Stapp Car Crash Conference*, pp. 483–499.

Pellman, E.J., Viano D.C., Tucker, A.M. et al. 2003. Concussion in professional football: Reconstruction of game impacts and injuries. *Neurosurgery*, 53: 799–814.

Pierce, D.A. and Barr, J.S. 1983. Fractures and dislocations at the base of the skull and upper spine. In R.W. Baily (Ed.), *The Cervical Spine*, pp. 196–206. Philadelphia, PA, Lippincott.

Pintar, F.A., Sances, A. Jr, Yoganandan, N. et al. 1990. Biodynamics of the total human cadaveric spine. In *Proceedings of the 34th Stapp Car Crash Conference*, pp. 55–72.

Pintar, F.A., Yoganandan, N., Sances, A. Jr et al. 1989. Kinematic and anatomical analysis of the human cervical spinal column under axial loading. In *Proceedings of the 33rd Stapp Car Crash Conference*, pp. 191–214.

Prasad, P. and Mertz, H.J. 1985. The Position of the United States Delegation to the ISO Working Group 6 on the Use of HIC in the Automotive Environment, SAE Paper No. 851246. Warrendale, PA, Society of Automotive Engineers.

Schneider, L.W., Foust, D.R., Bowman, B.M. et al. 1975. Biomechanical properties of the human neck in lateral flexion. In *Proceedings of the 19th Stapp Car Crash Conference*, pp. 455–486.

Society of Automotive Engineers, Human Mechanical Response Task Force. 1985. *Human Mechanical Response Characteristics, SAE J1460*. Warrendale, PA, Society of Automotive Engineers.

Strich, S.J. 1961. Shearing of nerve fibres as a cause of brain damage due to head injury. *Lancet* 2: 443.

Takhounts, E.G., Eppinger, R.H., Campbell, J.Q. et al. 2003. On the development of the SIMon finite element head model. *Stapp Car Crash J.* 47: 107–134.

Thomas, D.J. and Jessop, M.E. 1983. Experimental head and neck injury. In C.L. Ewing et al. (Eds.), *Impact Injury of the Head and Spine*, pp. 177–217. Springfield, IL, Charles C. Thomas.

Versace, J. 1970. A review of the severity index. In *Proceedings of the 15th Stapp Car Crash Conference*, pp. 771–796.

Viano, D.C., King, A.I., Melvin, J.W., and Weber, K. 1989. Injury biomechanics research: An essential element in the prevention of trauma. *J. Biomech.* 21: 403.

Viano, D.C. and Lövsund, P. 1999. Biomechanics of brain and spinal cord injury: Analysis of neurophysiological experiments. *Crash Prevention and Injury Control* 1: 35–43.

Wallis, B.J., Lord, S.M., and Bogduk, N. 1997. Resolution of psychological distress of whiplash patients following treatment by radiofrequency neurotomy: A randomized, double-blind, placebo controlled trial. *Pain* 73: 15–22.

Willinger, R., Kang, H.S., and Diaw, B. 1999. Three-dimensional human head finite-element model validation against two experimental impacts. *Ann. Biomed. Eng.* 27(3): 403–410.

Yang, K.H., Zhu, F., Luan, F. et al. 1998. Development of a finite element model of the human neck. In *Proceedings of the 42nd Stapp Car Crash Conference*, pp. 195–205.

Zhang, L., Yang, K.H., Dwarampudi, R. et al. 2001. Recent advances in brain injury research: A new human head model, development and validation. *Stapp Car Crash J.* 45: 369–394.

7

Biomechanics of Chest and Abdomen Impact

David C. Viano
Wayne State University

Albert I. King
Wayne State University

7.1 Introduction

Injury is caused by energy transfer to the body by an impacting object. It occurs when sufficient force is concentrated on the chest or abdomen by striking a blunt object, such as a vehicle instrument panel or side interior, or being struck by a baseball or blunt ballistic mass. The risk of injury is influenced by the object's shape, stiffness, point of contact, and orientation. It can be reduced by energy-absorbing padding or crushable materials, which allow the surfaces in contact to deform, extend the duration of impact, and reduce loads. The torso is viscoelastic, so reaction force increases with the speed of body deformation.

The biomechanical response of the body has three components, (1) inertial resistance by acceleration of body masses, (2) elastic resistance by compression of stiff structures and tissues, and (3) viscous resistance by rate-dependent properties of tissue. For low-impact speeds, the elastic stiffness protects from crush injuries; whereas, for high rates of body deformation, the inertial and viscous properties determine the force developed and limit deformation. The risk of skeletal and internal organ injury relates to energy stored or absorbed by the elastic and viscous properties. The reaction load is related to these responses and inertial resistance of body masses, which combine to resist deformation and prevent injury. When tissues are deformed beyond their recoverable limit, injuries occur.

7.2 Chest and Abdomen Injury Mechanisms

The primary mechanism of chest and abdomen injury is compression of the body at high rates of loading. This causes deformation and stretching of internal organs and vessels. When torso compression exceeds the rib-cage tolerance, fractures occur and internal organs and vessels can be contused or ruptured. In some chest impacts, internal injury occurs without skeletal damage. This can happen during high-speed loading, such as with a baseball impact causing ventricular fibrillation in a child without rib fractures. Injury is due to the viscous or rate-sensitive nature of human tissue as biomechanical responses differ for low- and high-speed impact.

When organs or vessels are loaded slowly, the input energy is absorbed gradually through deformation, which is resisted by elastic properties and pressure buildup in tissue. This is the situation when the shoulder belt loads the upper body in a frontal crash. When loaded rapidly, reaction force is proportional to the speed of tissue deformation as the viscous properties of the body resist deformation and provide a natural protection from impact. However, there is also a considerable inertial component to the reaction force. In this case, the body develops high internal pressure and injuries can occur before the ribs deflect much. The ability of an organ or other biological system to absorb impact energy without failure is called tolerance.

If an artery is stretched beyond its tensile strength, the tissue will tear. Organs and vessels can be stretched in different ways, which result in different types of injury. Motion of the heart during chest compression stretches the aorta along its axis from points of tethering in the body. This elongation generally leads to a transverse laceration when the strain limit is exceeded. In contrast, an increase in vascular pressure dilates the vessel and produces biaxial strain, which is larger in the transverse than axial direction. If pressure rises beyond the vessel's limit, it will burst. For severe impacts, intra-aortic pressure exceeds 500–1000 mm Hg, which is a significant, nonphysiological level, but is tolerable for short durations. When laceration occurs, the predominant mode of aortic failure is axial so the combined effects of stretch and internal pressure contribute to injury. Chest impact also compresses the rib cage causing tensile strain on the outer surface of the ribs. As compression increases, the risk of rib fracture increases. In both cases, the mechanism of injury is tissue deformation. Shah et al. (2001) found right-side impacts caused a higher risk of aortic injury than other impact directions.

The abdomen is more vulnerable to injury than the chest, because there is little bony structure below the ribcage to protect internal organs in front and lateral impact. Blunt impact of the upper abdomen can compress and injure the liver and spleen, before significant whole-body motion occurs. In the liver, compression increases intrahepatic pressure and generates tensile or shear strains. If the tissue is sufficiently deformed, laceration of the major hepatic vessels can result in hemoperitoneum. The injury tolerance of the solid organs in the abdomen is rate sensitive. Abdominal deformation also causes lobes of the liver to move relative to each other, stretching and shearing the vascular attachment at the hilar region.

Effective occupant restraints, safety systems, and protective equipment not only spread impact energy over the strongest body structures but also reduce contact velocity between the body and the impacted surface or striking object. The design of protective systems is aided by an understanding of injury mechanisms, quantification of human tolerance levels and development of numerical relationships between measurable engineering parameter, such as force, acceleration or deformation, and human injury. These relationships are called injury criteria.

7.3 Injury Criteria and Tolerances

7.3.1 Acceleration Injury

Stapp (1970) conducted rocket-sled experiments in the 1940s on belt-restraint systems and achieved a substantial human tolerance to long-duration, whole-body acceleration. Safety belts protected military personnel exposed to rapid but sustained acceleration. The experiments enabled Eiband (1959) to show in Figure 7.1 that the tolerance to whole-body acceleration increased as the exposure duration decreased. This linked human tolerance and acceleration for exposures of 2–1000 ms duration. The tolerance data are based on average sled acceleration rather than the acceleration of the volunteer subject, which would be higher due to compliance of the restraint system. Even with this limitation, the data provide useful early guidelines for the development of military and civilian restraint systems.

More recent side impact tests have led to other tolerance formulas for chest injury. Morgan et al. (1986) evaluated rigid, side-wall cadaver tests and developed TTI, a thoracic trauma index, which is the average rib and spine acceleration. TTI limits human tolerance to 85–90 g in vehicle crash tests. Better

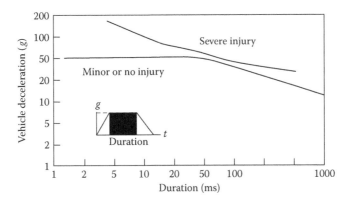

FIGURE 7.1 Whole-body human tolerance to vehicle acceleration based on impact duration. (Redrawn from Eiband A.M. Human tolerance to rapidly applied acceleration. A survey of the literature. National Aeronautics and Space Administration, Washington, DC, NASA Memo No. 5-19-59E, 1959; Viano D.C., *Bull. NY Acad. Med.*, 2nd Series, 64: 376–421, 1988. With permission.)

injury assessment was achieved by Cavanaugh et al. (1993) using average spinal acceleration (ASA), which is the average slope of the integral of spinal acceleration. ASA is the rate of momentum transfer during side impact, and a value of 30 g is proposed. In most cases, the torso can withstand 60–80 g peak, whole-body acceleration by a well-distributed load.

7.3.2 Force Injury

Whole-body tolerance is related to Newton's second law of motion, where acceleration of a rigid mass is proportional to the force acting on it, or $F = ma$. While the human body is not a rigid mass, a well-distributed restraint system allows the torso to respond as though it were fairly rigid when load is applied through the shoulder and pelvis. The greater the acceleration, the greater the force and risk of injury. For a high-speed frontal crash, a restrained occupant can experience 60 g acceleration. For a body mass of 76 kg, the inertial load is 44.7 kN (10,000 lb) and is tolerable if distributed over strong skeletal elements for a short period of time.

The ability to withstand high acceleration for short durations implies that tolerance is related to momentum transfer, because an equivalent change in velocity can be achieved by increasing the acceleration and decreasing its duration, as $\Delta V = a \Delta t$. The implication for occupant-protection systems is that the risk of injury can be decreased if the crash deceleration is extended over a greater period of time. For occupant restraint in 25 ms, a velocity change of 14.7 m/s (32.7 mph) occurs with 60 g whole-body acceleration. This duration can be achieved by crushable vehicle structures and occupant restraints (Mertz and Gadd, 1971).

Prior to the widespread use of safety belts, safety engineers needed information on the tolerance of the chest to design energy-absorbing instrument panels and steering systems. The concept was to limit impact force below human tolerance by crushable materials and structures. Using the highest practical crush force, safety was extended to the greatest severity of vehicle crashes. GM Research and Wayne State University collaborated on the development of the first crash sled, which was used to simulate progressively more severe frontal impacts. Embalmed human cadavers were exposed to head, chest, and knee impact on 15 cm (6″) diameter load cells until bone fracture was observed on x-ray. Patrick et al. (1965, 1967) demonstrated that blunt chest loading of 3.3 kN (740 lb) could be tolerated with minimal risk of serious injury. This is a pressure of 187 kPa. Gadd and Patrick (1968) later found a tolerance of 8.0 kN (1800 lb) if the load was distributed over the shoulders and chest by a properly designed steering wheel and column. Cavanaugh et al. (1993) found that side-impact tolerance is similar to frontal tolerance, and that shoulder contact is also an important load path. However, for the abdomen, side padding needs to crush at lower force than the abdominal tolerance to protect the liver and spleen (Viano and Andrzejak, 1993).

7.3.3 Compression Injury

High-speed films of cadaver impacts show that whole-body acceleration does not describe torso impact biomechanics. Tolerance of the chest and abdomen must consider body deformation. Force acting on the body causes two simultaneous responses, (1) compression of the compliant structures of the torso, and (2) acceleration of body masses. The neglected mechanism of injury was compression, which causes the sternum to displace toward the spine as ribs bend and possibly fracture. Acceleration and force, *per se*, are not sufficient indicators of impact tolerance because they cannot discriminate between the two responses. Numerous studies have shown that acceleration is less related to injury than compression.

The importance of chest deformation was confirmed by Kroell et al. (1971, 1974) in blunt thoracic impacts of unembalmed cadavers. Peak spinal acceleration and impact force were poorer injury predictors than the maximum compression of the chest, as measured by the percent change in the anteroposterior thickness of the body. A relationship was found between injury risk and compression and that it involves energy stored by elastic deformation of the body for moderate rates of chest compression. The stored energy (E_s) by a spring representing the ribcage and soft tissues is related to the displacement integral of force: $E_s = \int F dx$. Force in a spring is proportional to deformation: $F = kx$, where k is a spring constant representing the stiffness of the chest and is in the range of 26 kN/m. Stored energy is $E_s = k \int x dx = 0.5 kx^2$. Over a compression range of 20–40%, stored energy is proportional to deformation or compression, so $E_s \approx C$.

Tests with human volunteers showed that compression up to 20% during moderate-duration loading was fully reversible. Cadaver impacts with compression greater than 20% showed (Figure 7.2a) an increase in rib fractures and internal organ injury as the compression increased to 40%. The deflection tolerance was originally set at 8.8 cm (3.5″) for moderate but recoverable injury. This represents 39% compression. However, at this level of compression, multiple rib fractures and serious injury can occur, so a more conservative tolerance of 32% has been used to avert the possibility of flail chest (Figure 7.2b).

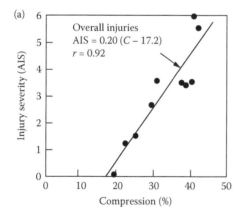 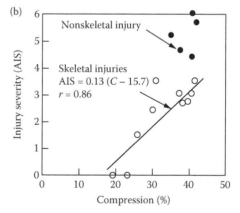

FIGURE 7.2   (a) Injury severity from blunt impact of human cadavers as a function of the maximum chest compression. (From Viano, D.C., *Bull. NY Acad. Med.*, 2nd Series, 64: 376–421, 1988. With permission.) (b) Severity of skeletal injury and incidence of internal organ injury as a function of maximum chest compression for blunt impacts of human cadavers. (From Viano D.C., *Bull. NY Acad. Med.*, 2nd Series, 64: 376–421, 1988. With permission.)

This reduces the risk of direct loading on the heart, lungs, and internal organs by a loss of the protective function of the ribcage.

7.3.4 Viscous Injury

The velocity of body deformation is an important factor in impact injury. For example, when a fluid-filled organ is compressed slowly, energy can be absorbed by tissue deformation without damage. When loaded rapidly, the organ cannot deform fast enough and rupture may occur without significant change in shape, even though the load is substantially higher than for the slow-loading condition. This situation depends on the viscous and inertial characteristics of the tissues.

The viscoelastic behavior of soft tissues becomes progressively more important as the velocity of body deformation exceeds 3 m/s. For lower speeds, such as in slow-crushing loads or for a belt-restrained occupant in a frontal crash, tissue compression is limited by elastic properties resisting skeletal and internal organ injury. For higher speeds of deformation, such as occupant loading by the door in a side impact, an unrestrained occupant or pedestrian impact, or chest impact by a nonpenetrating bullet, maximum compression does not adequately address the viscous and inertial properties of the torso, nor the time of greatest injury risk. In these conditions, the tolerance to compression is progressively lower as the speed of deformation increases, and the velocity of deformation becomes a dominant factor in injury.

Insight on a rate-dependent injury mechanism came from over 20 years of research by Jonsson et al. (1979) on high-speed impact and blast-wave exposures. The studies confirmed that tolerable compression inversely varied with the velocity of impact. The concept was further studied in relation to the abdomen by Lau and Viano (1981) for frontal impacts in the range of 5–20 m/s (10–45 mph). The liver was the target organ. Using a maximum compression of 16%, the severity of injury increased with the speed of loading, including serious mutilation of the lobes and major vessels in the highest-speed impacts. While the compression was within limits of volunteer loading at low speeds, the exposure produced critical injury at higher speeds. Subsequent tests on other animals and target organs verified an interrelationship between body compression, deformation velocity, and injury.

The previous observations led Viano and Lau (1988) to propose a viscous injury mechanism for soft biological tissues. The viscous response (VC) is defined as the product of velocity of deformation (V) and compression (C), which is a time-varying function in an impact. The parameter has physical meaning to absorbed energy (E_a) by a viscous dashpot under impact loading. Absorbed energy is related to the displacement integral of force: $E_a = \int F dx$, and force in a dashpot representing the viscous characteristics of the body is proportional to the velocity of deformation: $F = cV$, where c is a dashpot parameter in the range of 0.5 kN/m/s for the chest. Absorbed energy is $E_a = c \int V dx$, or a time integral by substitution: $E_a = c \int V^2 dt$. The integrand is composed of two responses, so: $E_a = c(\int d(Vx) - \int ax \, dt)$, where a is acceleration across the dashpot. The first term is the viscous response and the second an inertial term related to the deceleration of fluid set in motion. Absorbed energy is given by: $E_a = c(Vx - \int ax \, dt)$. The viscous response is proportional to absorbed energy, or $E_a \approx VC$, during the rapid phase of impact loading prior to peak compression.

Subsequent tests by Lau and Viano (1986, 1988) verified that serious injury occurred at the time of peak VC, much earlier than peak compression. For blunt chest impact, peak VC occurs in about half the time for maximum compression. Rib fractures also occur progressively with chest compression, as early as 9–14 ms—at peak VC—in a cadaver impact requiring 30 ms to reach peak compression. Upper-abdominal injury by steering wheel contact also relates to viscous loading. Lau et al. (1987) showed that limiting the viscous response by a self-aligning steering wheel reduced the risk of liver injury, as does force limiting an armrest in side impacts. Animal tests have also shown that VC is a good predictor of functional injury to heart and respiratory systems. In these experiments, Stein et al. (1982) found that the severity of cardiac arrhythmia and traumatic apnea was related to VC. This situation is important to baseball impact protection of children, Viano et al. (1992), and in the definition of human biomechanical responses used in the assessment of bullet-proof protective vests and blunt ballistics (Bir et al., 2004).

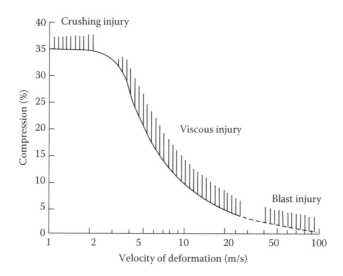

FIGURE 7.3 Biomechanics of chest injury by a crushing injury mechanism limited by tolerable compression at $C_{max} = 35\%$, a viscous injury mechanism limited by the product of velocity and extent of deformation at $VC_{max} = 1.0$ m/s, and a blast injury mechanism for shock wave loading.

With the increasing use of bullet-proof vests and nonpenetrating munitions by the police and military, blunt, high-velocity impacts are occurring to the chest. Although rarely lethal, there has been a concern for improving the understanding of injury mechanisms and means to establish standards for the technology. Behind-body-armor standards use the depth of the cavity created in clay after a bullet is stopped by the vest. The roots of this approach involve military research. However, the clay may not adequately simulate the human viscoelastic properties and biomechanical responses. Recent research has defined the blunt ballistic characteristics of the chest and the mechanisms for ventricular fibrillation (Bir and Viano, 1999; Bir et al., 2004).

Sturdivan et al. (2004) developed the blunt criterion (BC) in the 1970s. It is energy based and assesses vulnerability to blunt weapons, projectile impacts, and behind-body-armor exposures. $BC = \ln[E/(W^{0.33}TD)]$, where $E = 1\ 2\ MV^2$ is the kinetic energy of the projectile at impact in Joules, M is the projectile mass in kg, V is projectile velocity in m/s, D is the projectile diameter in cm, W is the mass of the individual in kg, and T is body-wall thickness in cm. BC is an energy ratio. The numerator is the striking kinetic energy of the blunt projectile, the energy available to cause injury. The denominator is a semiempirical expression of the capacity of the body to absorb the impact energy without lethal damage to the vulnerable organs, scaled by the mass of the individual. The viscous and blunt criteria are both energy-based and have been correlated for chest and abdominal impacts.

Figure 7.3 summarizes injury mechanisms associated with torso impact deformation. For low speeds of deformation, the limiting factor is crush injury from compression of the body (C). This occurs at $C = 35–40\%$ depending on the contact area and orientation of loading. For deformation speeds above 3 m/s, injury is related to a peak viscous response of $VC = 1.0$ m/s. In a particular situation, injury can occur by a compression or viscous responses, or both, as these responses occur at different times in an impact. At extreme rates of loading, such as in a blast-wave exposure, injury occurs with less than 10–15% compression by high-energy transfer to viscous elements of the body.

7.4 Biomechanical Responses during Impact

The reaction force developed by the chest varies with the velocity of deformation, and biomechanics is best characterized by a family of force–deflection responses. Figure 7.4 summarizes frontal and lateral

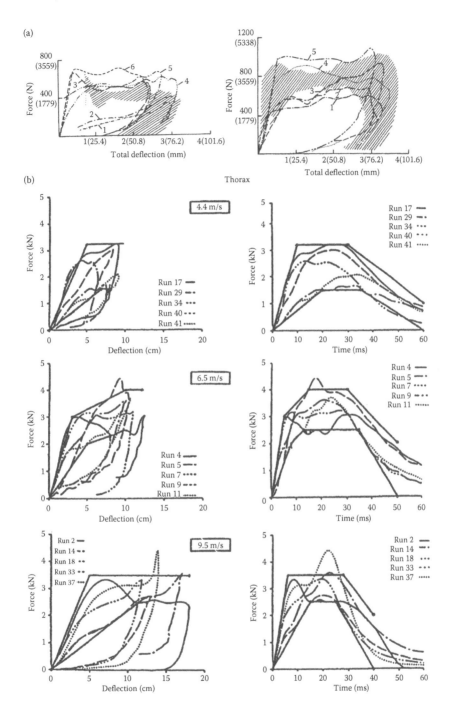

FIGURE 7.4 Frontal (a) and lateral (b) force–deflection response of the human cadaver chest at various speeds of blunt pendulum impact. The initial stiffness is followed by a plateau force until unloading. (From Kroell et al., *Proceedings of the 18th Stapp Car Crash Conference*, pp. 383–457, SAE Paper No. 741187, Society of Automotive Engineers, Warrendale, PA, 1974; Viano, D.C., *Proceedings of the 33rd Stapp Car Crash Conference*, pp. 113–142, SAE Paper No. 892432, Society of Automotive Engineers, Warrendale, PA, 1989; with kind permission from Springer Science+Business Media: *Accidental Injury: Biomechanics and Prevention*, The biomechanics of thoracic trauma, 1993, pp. 362–391, Cavanaugh, J.M.)

chest biomechanics for various impact speeds. The dynamic compliance is related to viscous, inertial, and elastic properties of the body. The initial rise in force is due to inertia as the sternal mass, which is rapidly accelerated to the impact speed as the chest begins to deform. The plateau force is related to the viscous component, which is rate-dependent, and a superimposed elastic stiffness, which increases force with chest compression. Unloading provides a hysteresis loop representing the energy absorbed by body deformation.

Melvin et al. (1988) analyzed frontal biomechanics of the chest. The dynamic compliance is related to viscous, inertial, and elastic properties of the body. There is an initial rise in force, which is related to the inertia of the sternal mass, which is rapidly accelerated to the impact speed. This is followed by a plateau in force, which is related to the viscous properties and is rate dependent. There is also an elastic stiffness component from chest compression that adds to the force. The force–deflection response can be modeled as an initial stiffness $k = 0.26 + 0.60(V - 1.3)$ and a plateau force $F = 1.0 + 0.75(V - 3.7)$, where k is in kN/cm, F is in kN, and the velocity of impact V is in m/s. The force F reasonably approximates the plateau level for lateral chest and abdominal impact, but the initial stiffness is lower at $F = 0.12(V - 1.2)$ for side loading (Melvin and Weber, 1988).

The reaction force developed by the chest varies with the velocity of impact, so biomechanics is best characterized by the force–deflection response of the torso (25.6). The dynamic compliance is related to viscous, inertial, and elastic properties of the body. There is an initial rise in force, which is related to inertial responses as the sternal mass is rapidly accelerated to the impact speed. This is followed by a plateau in force, which is related to the viscous response and is rate dependent, and a superimposed stiffness component related to chest compression. By analyzing frontal biomechanics, the chest response can be modeled as an initial stiffness $k = 0.26 + 0.60(V - 1.3)$ and a plateau force $F = 1.0 + 0.75(V - 3.7)$, where k is in kN/cm, F is in kN, and the velocity of impact V is in m/s. The force F reasonably approximates the plateau level for lateral chest and abdominal impact, but the initial stiffness is lower at $F = 0.12(V - 1.2)$ for side loading.

A simple, but relevant, lumped-mass model of the chest was developed by Lobdell et al. (1973) and is shown in Figure 7.5. The impacting mass is m_1 and skin compliance is represented by k_{12}. An energy-absorbing interface was added by Viano (1987) to evaluate protective padding. Chest structure is represented by a parallel Voigt and Maxwell spring–dashpot system, which couples the sternal m_2 and spinal m_3 masses. When subjected to a blunt sternal impact, the model follows established force–deflection corridors. The biomechanical model is effective in studying compression and viscous responses. It also simulates military exposures to high-speed, nonpenetrating projectiles (Figure 7.6), even though the loading conditions are quite different from the cadaver database used to develop the model. This mechanical system characterizes the elastic, viscous, and inertial components of the torso.

The Hybrid III dummy was the first to demonstrate humanlike chest responses typical of the biomechanical data for frontal impacts (Foster et al., 1977). Rouhana (1989) developed a frangible abdomen, useful in predicting injury for lap-belt submarining. More recent work by Schneider et al. (1992) led to a new prototype frontal dummy. Lateral impact tests of cadavers against a rigid wall and blunt pendulum led to side-impact dummies, such as the Eurosid and Biosid (Mertz, 1993). Even more recently, a small female-sized side-impact dummy has been developed (Scherer et al., 1998).

7.5 Injury Risk Assessment

Over years of study, tolerances have been established for most responses of the chest and abdomen. Table 7.1 provides tolerance levels from reviews by Cavanaugh (1993), Rouhana (1993), and Viano et al. (1989). While these are single thresholds, they are commonly used to evaluate safety systems. The implication is that for biomechanical responses below tolerance, there is no injury, and for responses above tolerance, there is injury. An additional factor is biomechanical response scaling for individuals of different size and weight. The commonly accepted procedure involves equal stress and velocity, which enabled Mertz et al. (1989) to predict injury tolerances and biomechanical responses for different size adult dummies.

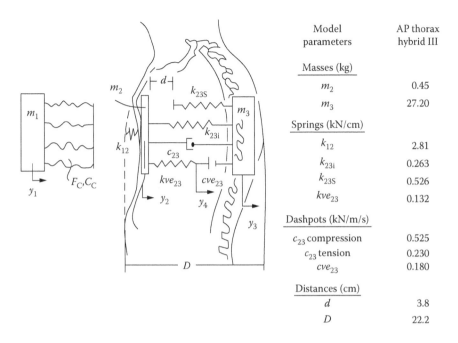

Model parameters	AP thorax hybrid III
Masses (kg)	
m_2	0.45
m_3	27.20
Springs (kN/cm)	
k_{12}	2.81
k_{23i}	0.263
k_{23S}	0.526
kve_{23}	0.132
Dashpots (kN/m/s)	
c_{23} compression	0.525
c_{23} tension	0.230
cve_{23}	0.180
Distances (cm)	
d	3.8
D	22.2

FIGURE 7.5 Lumped-mass model of the human thorax with impacting mass and energy-absorbing material interface. The biomechanical parameters are given for mass, spring, and damping characteristics of the chest in blunt frontal impact. (Modified from Lobdell T.E. et al., In *Human Impact Response Measurement and Simulation*, Plenum Press, New York, pp. 201–245, 1973; Viano, D.C., *Proceedings of the 31st Stapp Car Crash Conference*, pp. 185–224, SAE Paper No. 872213, Society of Automotive Engineers, Warrendale, PA, 1987. With permission.)

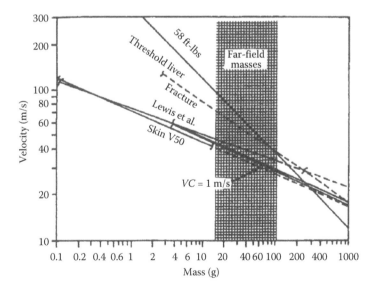

FIGURE 7.6 Tolerance levels for blunt loading as a function of impact mass and velocity. The plot includes information from automotive impact situations and from high-speed military projectile impacts. The Lobdell model is effective over the entire range of impact conditions. (Modified from Quatros J.H., *Proceedings of the 14th International Symposium on Ballistics*, Quebec, Canada, September 26–29, 1993. With permission.)

TABLE 7.1   Human Tolerance for Chest and Abdomen Impact

Criteria	Chest		Abdomen		Criteria
	Frontal	Lateral	Frontal	Lateral	
Acceleration					*Acceleration*
3 ms limit	60 g				
TTI		85–90 g			
ASA		30 g			
AIS 4+		45 g		39 g	AIS 4+
Force					*Force*
Sternum	3.3 kN				
Chest + shoulder	8.8 kN	10.2 kN			
AIS 3+			2.9 kN	3.1 kN	AIS 3+
AIS 4+		5.5 kN	3.8 kN	6.7 kN	AIS 4+
Pressure					*Pressure*
	187 kPa		166 kPa		AIS 3+
			216 kPa		AIS 4+
Compression					*Compression*
Rib fracture	20%				
Stable ribcage	32%		38%		AIS 3+
Flail chest	40%	38%	48%	44%	AIS 4+
Viscous					*Viscous*
AIS 3+	1.0 m/s				AIS 3+
AIS 4+	1.3 m/s	1.47 m/s	1.4 m/s	1.98 m/s	AIS 4+

Source: With kind permission from Springer Science+Business Media: *Accidental Injury: Biomechanics and Prevention*, The biomechanics of thoracic trauma, 1993, pp. 362–391, Cavanaugh, J.M.; *Accidental Injury: Biomechanics and Prevention*, Biomechanics of abdominal trauma, 1993, pp. 391–428, Rouhana, S.W.

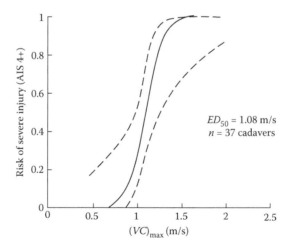

FIGURE 7.7   Typical logist injury probability function relating the risk of serious injury to the viscous response of the chest. (From Viano D.C., *Bull. NY Acad. Med.*, 2nd Series, 64: 376–421, 1988. With permission.)

TABLE 7.2 Injury Probability Functions for Blunt Impact

Body Region	$ED_{25\%}$	α	β	X^2	p	R
		Frontal Impact				
Chest (AIS 4+)						
VC	1.0 m/s	11.42	11.56	25.6	0.000	0.68
C	34%	10.49	0.277	15.9	0.000	0.52
		Lateral Impact				
Chest (AIS 4+)						
VC	1.5 m/s	10.02	6.08	13.7	0.000	0.77
C	38%	31.22	0.79	13.5	0.000	0.76
Abdomen (AIS 4+)						
VC	2.0 m/s	8.64	3.81	6.1	0.013	0.60
C	47%	16.29	0.35	4.6	0.032	0.48
Pelvis (pubic ramus facture)						
C	27%	84.02	3.07	11.5	0.001	0.91

Source: Modified from Viano, D.C. et al., *J. Biomech.*, 22: 403–417, 1989.

Injury risk assessment is frequently used. It evaluates the probability of injury as a continuous function of a biomechanical response. A logist function relates injury probability p to a biomechanical response x by $p(x) = [1 + \exp(\alpha - \beta x)]^{-1}$ where α and β are parameters derived from statistical analysis of biomechanical data. This function provides a sigmoidal relationship with three distinct regions in Figure 7.7. For low biomechanical response levels, there is a low probability of injury. Similarly, for very high levels, the risk asymptotes to 100%. The transition region between the two extremes involves risk, which is proportional to the biomechanical response. A sigmoidal function is typical of human tolerance because it represents the distribution in weak through strong subjects in a population exposed to impact. Table 7.2 summarizes available parameters for chest and abdominal injury risk assessment.

References

Bir, C. and Viano, D.C., Biomechanics of commotio cordis. *J. Trauma*, 47(3): 468–473, 1999.

Bir, C., Viano, D.C., and King, A.I., Human response of the thorax to blunt ballistic impacts. *J. Biomech.*, 37(1): 73–79, 2004.

Cavanaugh, J.M., The biomechanics of thoracic trauma, In *Accidental Injury: Biomechanics and Prevention*, Nahum A.M. and Melvin J.W. (Eds.), pp. 362–391, Springer-Verlag, New York, 1993.

Cavanaugh, J.M. et al., Injury and response of the thorax in side impact cadaveric tests, *Proceedings of the 37th Stapp Car Crash Conference*, pp. 199–222, SAE Paper No. 933127, Society of Automotive Engineers, Warrendale, PA, 1993.

Eiband, A.M., Human Tolerance to Rapidly Applied Acceleration. A Survey of the Literature. National Aeronautics and Space Administration, Washington DC, NASA Memo No. 5-19-59E, 1959.

Foster, J.K., Kortge, J.O., and Wolanin, M.J., Hybrid III—A biomechanically-based crash test dummy, *Stapp Car Crash Conference*, pp. 975–1014, SAE Paper No. 770938, Society of Automotive Engineers, Warrendale, PA, 1977.

Gadd, C.W. and Patrick, L.M., Systems versus laboratory impact tests for estimating injury hazards, SAE Paper No. 680053, Society of Automotive Engineers, Warrendale, PA, 1968.

Jonsson, A., Clemedson, C.J. et al., Dynamic factors influencing the production of lung injury in rabbits subjected to blunt chest wall impact, *Aviation, Space Environ. Med.*, 50: 325–337, 1979.

King, A.I., Regional tolerance to impact acceleration, In SP-622, SAE 850852, Society of Automotive Engineers, Warrendale, PA, 1985.

Kroell, C.K., Schneider, D.C., and Nahum, A.M., Impact tolerance and response to the human thorax, *Proceedings of the 15th Stapp Car Crash Conference*, pp. 84–134, SAE Paper No. 710851, Society of Automotive Engineers, Warrendale, PA, 1971.

Kroell, C.K., Schneider, D.C., and Nahum, A.M., Impact tolerance and response to the human thorax II, *Proceedings of the 18th Stapp Car Crash Conference*, pp. 383–457, SAE Paper No. 741187, Society of Automotive Engineers, Warrendale, PA, 1974.

Lau, I.V., Horsch, J.D. et al., Biomechanics of liver injury by steering wheel loading, *J. Trauma*, 27: 225–237, 1987.

Lau, I.V. and Viano, D.C., How and when blunt injury occurs: Implications to frontal and side impact protection. *Proceedings of the 32nd Stapp Car Crash Conference*, pp. 81–100, SAE Paper No. 881714, Society of Automotive Engineers, Warrendale, PA, 1988.

Lau, I.V. and Viano, D.C., Influence of impact velocity on the severity of nonpenetrating hepatic injury, *J. Trauma*, 21(2): 115–123, 1981.

Lau, I.V. and Viano, D.C., The viscous criterion—Bases and application of an injury severity index for soft tissue, *Proceedings of the 30th Stapp Car Crash Conference*, pp. 123–142, SAE Paper No. 861882, Society of Automotive Engineers, Warrendale, PA, 1986.

Lobdell, T.E., Kroell, C.K., Schneider, D.C., Hering, W.E., and Nahum, A.M., Impact response of the human thorax, In *Human Impact Response Measurement and Simulation*, King W.F. and Mertz H.J. (Eds.), Plenum Press, New York, pp. 201–245, 1973.

Melvin, J.W., King, A.I., and Alem, N.M., AATD system technical characteristics, design concepts, and trauma assessment criteria, AATD task E-F Final Report, DOT-HS-807-224, US Department of Transportation, National Highway Traffic Safety Administration, Washington, DC, 1988.

Melvin, J.W. and Weber, K. (Eds.), Review of biomechanical response and injury in the automotive environment, AATD Task B Final Report, DOT-HS-807-224, US Department of Transportation, National Highway Traffic Safety Administration, Washington, DC, 1988.

Mertz, H.J., Anthropomorphic test devices, In *Accidental Injury: Biomechanics and Prevention*, Nahum, A.M. and Melvin, J.W. (Eds.), pp. 66–84, Springer-Verlag, New York, 1993.

Mertz, H.J. and Gadd, C.W., Thoracic tolerance to whole-body deceleration, *Proceedings of the 15th Stapp Car Crash Conference*, pp. 135–157, SAE Paper No. 710852, Society of Automotive Engineers, Warrendale, PA, 1971.

Mertz, H.J., Irwin, A. et al., Size, weight and biomechanical impact response requirements for adult size small female and large male dummies, SAE Paper No. 890756, Society of Automotive Engineers, Warrendale, PA, 1989.

Morgan, R.M., Marcus, J.H., and Eppinger, R.H., Side impact—The biofidelity of NHTSA's proposed ATD and efficacy of TTI, *Proceedings of the 30th Stapp Car Crash Conference*, pp. 27–40, SAE Paper No. 861877, Society of Automotive Engineers, Warrendale, PA, 1986.

Patrick, L.M., Kroell, C.K., and Mertz, H.J., Forces on the human body in simulated crashes, *Proceedings of the 9th Stapp Car Crash Conference*, SAE, pp. 237–260, Society of Automotive Engineers, Warrendale, PA, 1965.

Patrick, L.M., Mertz, H.J., and Kroell, C.K., Cadaver knee, chest, and head impact loads, *Proceedings of the 11th Stapp Car Crash Conference*, pp. 168–182, SAE Paper No. 670913, Society of Automotive Engineers, Warrendale, PA, 1967.

Quatros, J.H., Terminal ballistics of non-lethal projectiles, *Proceedings of the 14th International Symposium on Ballistics*, Quebec, Canada, September 26–29, 1993.

Rouhana, S.W., Biomechanics of abdominal trauma, In *Accidental Injury: Biomechanics and Prevention*, Nahum A.M. and Melvin J.W. (Eds.), pp. 391–428, Springer-Verlag, New York, 1993.

Rouhana, S.W. et al., Assessing submarining and abdominal injury risk in the Hybrid III family of dummies, *Proceedings of the 33rd Stapp Car Crash Conference*, pp. 257–279, SAE Paper No. 892440, Society of Automotive Engineers, Warrendale, PA, 1989.

Scherer, R.D., Kirkish, S.L., McCleary, J.P., Rouhana, S.W. et al., SIDS-IIs Beta\u+– prototype dummy biomechanical responses. SAE 983151, *Proceedings of the 42nd Stapp Car Crash Conference*, Society of Automotive Engineers, Warrendale, PA, 1998.

Schneider, L.W., Haffner, M.P. et al., Development of an advanced ATD thorax for improved injury assessment in frontal crash environments, *Proceedings of the 36th Stapp Car Crash Conference*, pp. 129–156, SAE Paper No. 922520, Society of Automotive Engineers, Warrendale, PA, 1992.

Shah, C.S., Yang, K.H., Hardy, W.N., Wang, H.K., and King, A.I., Development of a computer model to predict aortic rupture due to impact loading. SAE 2001-22-0007, Society of Automotive Engineers, Warrendale, PA, *Stapp Car Crash J.*, 45: 161–182, 2001.

Society of Automotive Engineers, *Human Tolerance to Impact Conditions as Related to Motor Vehicle Design*, SAE J885, Society of Automotive Engineers, Warrendale, PA, 1986.

Stapp, J.P., Voluntary human tolerance levels, In *Impact Injury and Crash Protection*, Gurdjian, E.S., Lange, W.A., Patrick, L.M., and Thomas, L.M. (Eds.), pp. 308–349, Charles C. Thomas, Springfield, IL, 1970.

Stein, P.D., Sabbah, H.N. et al., Response of the heart to nonpenetrating cardiac trauma. *J. Trauma*, 22(5): 364–373, 1982.

Sturdivan, L.M., Viano, D.C., and Champion, H., Analysis of injury criteria to assess chest and abdominal injury risks in blunt and ballistic impacts. *J. Trauma*, 56: 651–663, 2004.

Viano, D.C., Biomechanical responses and injuries in blunt lateral impact, *Proceedings of the 33rd Stapp Car Crash Conference*, pp. 113–142, SAE Paper No. 892432, Society of Automotive Engineers, Warrendale, PA, 1989.

Viano, D.C., Cause and control of automotive trauma, *Bull. NY Acad. Med.*, 2nd Series, 64: 376–421, 1988.

Viano, D.C., Evaluation of the benefit of energy-absorbing materials for side impact protection, *Proceedings of the 31st Stapp Car Crash Conference*, pp. 185–224, SAE Paper No. 872213, Society of Automotive Engineers, Warrendale, PA, 1987.

Viano, D.C. and Andrzejak, D.V., Biomechanics of abdominal injury by armrest loading. *J. Trauma*, 34(1): 105–115, 1993.

Viano, D.C., Andrzejak, D.V., Polley, T.Z., and King, A.I., Mechanism of fatal chest injury by baseball impact: Development of an experimental model, *Clin. J. Sport Med.*, 2: 166–171, 1992.

Viano, D.C., King, A.I. et al., Injury biomechanics research: An essential element in the prevention of trauma, *J. Biomech.*, 22: 403–417, 1989.

Viano, D.C. and Lau, I.V., A viscous tolerance criterion for soft tissue injury assessment, *J. Biomech.*, 21: 387–399, 1988.

8

Cardiac Biomechanics

Andrew D.
McCulloch
*University of California,
San Diego*

Roy C. P. Kerckhoffs
*University of California,
San Diego*

8.1 Introduction

The primary function of the heart, to pump blood through the circulatory system, is fundamentally mechanical. In this chapter, cardiac function is discussed in the context of the mechanics of the ventricular walls from the perspective of the determinants of myocardial stresses and strains (Table 8.1). Many physiological, pathophysiological, and clinical factors are directly or indirectly affected by myocardial stress and strain (Table 8.2). Of course, the factors in Tables 8.1 and 8.2 are closely interrelated—most of the factors affected by myocardial stress and strain in turn affect the stress and strain in the ventricular wall. For example, changes in wall stress due to altered hemodynamic load may cause ventricular remodeling, which in turn alters the geometry, structure, and material properties. This chapter is organized around the governing determinants in Table 8.1, but mention is made where appropriate of some of the factors in Table 8.2.

8.2 Cardiac Geometry and Structure

The mammalian heart consists of four pumping chambers, the left and right atria and ventricles communicating through the atrioventricular (mitral and tricuspid) valves, which are structurally connected by chordae tendineae to papillary muscles that extend from the anterior and posterior aspects of the right and left ventricular lumens. The muscular cardiac wall is perfused via the coronary vessels that originate at the left and right coronary ostia located in the sinuses of Valsalva immediately distal to the aortic valve leaflets. Surrounding the whole heart is the collagenous parietal pericardium that fuses with the diaphragm and great vessels. These are the anatomical structures that are most commonly studied in the field of cardiac mechanics. Particular emphasis is given in this chapter to the ventricular walls, which are the most important for the pumping function of the heart. Most studies of cardiac mechanics have focused on the left ventricle, but many of the important conclusions apply equally to the right ventricle.

TABLE 8.1   Basic Determinants of Myocardial Stress and Strain

Geometry and Structure	
3D shape	Wall thickness
	Curvature
	Stress-free and unloaded reference configurations
Tissue structure	Muscle fiber architecture
	Connective tissue organization
	Pericardium, epicardium, and endocardium
	Coronary vascular anatomy
Boundary/Initial Conditions	
Pressure	Filling pressure (preload)
	Arterial pressure (afterload)
	Direct and indirect ventricular interactions
	Thoracic and pericardial pressure
Constraints	Effects of inspiration and expiration
	Constraints due to the pericardium and its attachments
	Valves and fibrous valve annuli, chordae tendineae
	Great vessels, lungs
Material Properties	
Resting or passive	Nonlinear finite elasticity
	Quasilinear viscoelasticity
	Anisotropy
	Biphasic poroelasticity
Active dynamic	Activation sequence
	Myofiber isometric and isotonic contractile dynamics
	Sarcomere length and length history
	Cellular calcium kinetics and metabolic energy supply

8.2.1 Ventricular Geometry

From the perspective of engineering mechanics, the ventricles are three-dimensional thick-walled pressure vessels with substantial variations in wall thickness and principal curvatures both regionally and temporally through the cardiac cycle. The ventricular walls in the normal heart are thickest at the equator and base of the left ventricle and thinnest at the left ventricular apex and right ventricular free wall. There are also variations in the principal dimensions of the left ventricle with species, age, phase of the cardiac cycle, and disease (Table 8.3). But, in general, the ratio of wall thickness to radius is too high to be treated accurately by all but the most sophisticated thick-wall shell theories [1].

Ventricular geometry has been studied in most quantitative detail in the dog heart [2,3]. Geometric models have been very useful in the analysis, especially the use of confocal and nonconfocal ellipses of revolution to describe the epicardial and endocardial surfaces of the left and right ventricular walls (Figure 8.1). The canine left ventricle is reasonably modeled by a thick ellipsoid of revolution truncated at the base. The crescentic right ventricle wraps about 180° around the heart wall circumferentially and extends longitudinally about two-thirds of the distance from the base to the apex. Using a truncated ellipsoidal model, the left ventricular geometry in the dog can be defined by the major and minor radii of two surfaces, the left ventricular endocardium, and a surface defining the free wall epicardium and the septal endocardium of the right ventricle. Streeter and Hanna [2] described the position of the basal plane using a truncation factor f_b defined as the ratio between the longitudinal distances from equator-to-base and equator-to-apex. Hence, the overall longitudinal distance from base to apex is $(1 + f_b)$ times

TABLE 8.2   Factors Affected by Myocardial Stress and Strain

Direct factors	Regional muscle work
	Myocardial oxygen demand and energetics
	Coronary blood flow
Electrophysiological responses	Action potential duration (QT interval)
	Repolarization (T wave morphology)
	Excitability
	Risk of arrhythmia
Development and morphogenesis	Growth rate
	Cardiac looping and septation
	Valve formation
Vulnerability to injury	Ischemia
	Arrhythmia
	Cell dropout
	Aneurysm rupture
Remodeling, repair, and adaptation	Eccentric and concentric hypertrophy
	Fibrosis
	Scar formation
Progression of disease	Transition from hypertrophy to failure
	Ventricular dilation
	Infarct expansion
	Response to reperfusion
	Aneurysm formation

TABLE 8.3   Representative Left Ventricular Minor-Axis Dimensions

Species	Comments	Inner Radius (mm)	Outer Radius (mm)	Wall Thickness: Inner Radius
Dog (21 kg)	Unloaded diastole (0 mm Hg)	16	26	0.62
Dog	Normal diastole (2–12 mm Hg)	19	28	0.47
Dog	Dilated diastole (24–40 mm Hg)	22	30	0.36
Dog	Normal systole (1–9 mm Hg EDP)	14	26	0.86
Dog	Long axis, apex-equator (normal diastole)	42	47	0.12
Young rats	Unloaded diastole (0 mm Hg)	1.4	3.5	1.50
Mature rats	Unloaded diastole (0 mm Hg)	3.2	5.8	0.81
Human	Normal	24	32	0.34
Human	Compensated pressure overload	27	42	0.56
Human	Compensated volume overload	32	42	0.33

Note: Dog data from Ross et al. [177] and Streeter and Hanna [2]. Human data from Grossman et al. [178,179]. Rat data are from unpublished observations in the author's laboratory.

the major radius of the ellipse. Since variations in f_b between diastole and systole are relatively small (0.45–0.51), they suggested a constant value of 0.5.

The focal length d of an ellipsoid is defined from the major and minor radii (a and b) by $d^2 = a^2 - b^2$, and varies only slightly in the dog from endocardium to epicardium between end-diastole (37.3–37.9 mm) and end-systole (37.7–37.1 mm) [2]. Hence, within the accuracy that the boundaries of the left ventricular wall can be treated as ellipsoids of revolution, the assumption that the ellipsoids are confocal appears to be a good one. This has motivated the choice of prolate spheroidal (elliptic–hyperbolic–polar) coordinates (λ, μ, θ) as a system for economically representing ventricular geometries obtained post mortem or by noninvasive tomography [3,4]. The Cartesian coordinates of a point are given in terms of its prolate spheroidal coordinates by

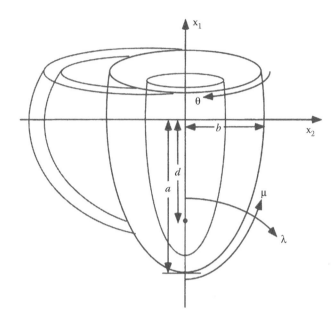

FIGURE 8.1 Truncated ellipsoid representation of ventricular geometry, showing major left ventricular radius (a), minor radius (b), focal length (d), and prolate spheroidal coordinates (λ, μ, θ).

$$x_1 = d \cosh \lambda \cos \mu,$$

$$x_2 = d \sinh \lambda \sin \mu \cos \theta, \tag{8.1}$$

$$x_3 = d \sinh \lambda \sin \mu \sin \theta.$$

Here, the focal length d defines a family of coordinate systems that vary from spherical polar when $d = 0$ to cylindrical polar in the limit when $d \to \infty$. A surface of constant transmural coordinate λ (Figure 8.1) is an ellipse of revolution with major radius $a = d \cosh \lambda$ and minor radius $b = d \sinh \lambda$. In an ellipsoidal model with a truncation factor of 0.5, the longitudinal coordinate μ varies from zero at the apex to 120° at the base. Integrating the Jacobian in prolate spheroidal coordinates gives the volume of the wall or cavity:

$$d^3 \int_0^{2\pi} \int_0^{\mu_2} \int_{\lambda_1}^{\lambda_2} ((\sinh^2 \lambda + \sin^2 \mu)\sinh \lambda \sin \mu) d\lambda \, d\mu \, d\theta = \frac{2\pi d^3}{3} \left| (1 - \cos \mu_2)\cosh^3 \lambda - (1 - \cos^3 \mu_2)\cosh \lambda \right|_{\lambda_1}^{\lambda_2}$$

$$\tag{8.2}$$

The scaling between heart mass M_H and body mass M within or between species is commonly described by the allometric formula

$$M_H = kM^\alpha. \tag{8.3}$$

Using combined measurements from a variety of mammalian species with M expressed in kilograms, the coefficient k is 5.8 g and the power α is close to unity (0.98) [5]. Within individual species, the ratio of heart weight to body weight is somewhat lower in mature rabbits and rats (about 2 g kg^{-1}) than in humans (5 g kg^{-1}), and higher in horses and dogs (8 g kg^{-1}) [6]. The rate α of heart growth with body weight decreases with age in most species but not humans. At birth, left and right ventricular weights are similar, but the left ventricle is substantially more massive than the right by adulthood.

8.2.2 Myofiber Architecture

The cardiac ventricles have a complex three-dimensional muscle fiber architecture (for a comprehensive review, see Reference 7). Although the myocytes are relatively short, they are connected such that at any point in the normal heart wall there is a clear predominant fiber axis that is approximately tangent to the wall (within 3–5° in most regions, except near the apex and papillary muscle insertions). Each ventricular myocyte is connected via gap junctions at intercalated disks to an average of 11.3 neighbors, 5.3 on the sides and 6.0 at the ends [8]. The classical anatomists dissected discrete bundles of fibrous swirls, though later investigations showed that the ventricular myocardium could be unwrapped by blunt dissection into a single continuous muscle "band" [9]. However, more modern histological techniques have shown that in the plane of the wall, the mean muscle fiber angle makes a smooth transmural transition from epicardium to endocardium (Figure 8.2). About the mean, myofiber angle dispersion is typically 10–15° [10] except in certain pathologies. Similar patterns have been described for humans, dogs, baboons, macaques, pigs, guinea pigs, and rats. In the human or dog left ventricle, the muscle fiber angle typically varies continuously from about −60° (i.e., 60° clockwise from the circumferential axis) at the epicardium to about +70° at the endocardium. The rate of change of fiber angle is usually greatest at the epicardium, so that circumferential (0°) fibers are found in the outer half of the wall, and begins to slow down on approaching the inner third near the trabeculata–compacta interface. There are also small increases in fiber orientation from end-diastole to systole (7–19°), with greatest changes at the epicardium and apex [11].

Regional variations in ventricular myofiber orientations are generally smooth except at the junction between the right ventricular free wall and septum. A detailed study in the dog that mapped fiber angles throughout the entire right and left ventricles described the same general transmural pattern in all regions, including the septum and right ventricular free wall, but with definite regional variations [3]. Transmural differences in the fiber angle were about 120–140° in the left ventricular free wall, larger in the septum (160–180°), and smaller in the right ventricular free wall (100–120°). A similar study of fiber angle distributions in the rabbit left and right ventricles has recently been reported [12]. For the most part, fiber angles in the rabbit heart were very similar to those in the dog, except for on the anterior wall, where average fiber orientations were 20–30° counterclockwise of those in the dog. While the most reliable reconstructions of ventricular myofiber architecture have been made using quantitative histological techniques, diffusion tensor magnetic resonance imaging (DTI) has proven to be a reliable technique for estimating fiber orientation nondestructively in fixed [13,14] and even intact beating human hearts [15].

The locus of fiber orientations at a given depth in the ventricular wall has a spiral geometry that may be modeled as a general helix by simple differential geometry. The position vector $\mathbf{x}$ of a point on a helix inscribed on an ellipsoidal surface that is symmetric about the x_1 axis and has major and minor radii, a and b, is given by the parametric equation

$$\mathbf{x} = a \sin t \, \boldsymbol{e}_1 + b \cos t \sin wt \, \boldsymbol{e}_2 + b \cos t \cos wt \, \boldsymbol{e}_3, \tag{8.4}$$

where the parameter is t and the helix makes $w/4$ full turns between the apex and the equator. A positive w defines a left-handed helix with a positive pitch. The fiber angle or helix pitch angle η varies along the arc length:

$$\sin \eta = \sqrt{\frac{a^2 \cos^2 t + b^2 \sin^2 t}{(a^2 + b^2 w^2)\cos^2 t + b^2 \sin^2 t}}. \tag{8.5}$$

If another deformed configuration $\hat{\mathbf{x}}$ is defined in the same way as Equation 8.4, the fiber segment extension ratio $d\hat{s}/ds$ associated with a change in the ellipsoid geometry [16] can be derived from

$$\frac{d\hat{s}}{ds} = \frac{\dfrac{d\hat{s}}{dt}}{\dfrac{ds}{dt}} = \frac{\left|\dfrac{d\hat{\mathbf{x}}}{dt}\right|}{\left|\dfrac{d\mathbf{x}}{dt}\right|}. \tag{8.6}$$

Epicardium

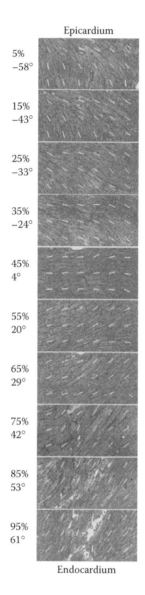

5%
−58°

15%
−43°

25%
−33°

35%
−24°

45%
4°

55%
20°

65%
29°

75%
42°

85%
53°

95%
61°

Endocardium

FIGURE 8.2 Cardiac muscle fiber orientations vary continuously through the left ventricular wall from a negative angle at the epicardium (0%) to near zero (circumferential) at the midwall (50%) and to increasing positive values toward the endocardium (100%). (Micrographs of murine myocardium from the author's laboratory, courtesy of Jyoti Rao.)

Although the traditional notion of discrete myofiber bundles has been revised in view of the continuous transmural variation of muscle fiber angle in the plane of the wall, there is a transverse laminar structure in the myocardium that groups fibers together in sheets at an average of 4 ± 2 myocytes thick (48 ± 20 μm) separated by histologically distinct cleavage planes [17–19]. LeGrice and colleagues investigated these structures in a detailed morphometric study of four dog hearts [19]. They describe an ordered laminar arrangement of myocytes with extensive cleavage planes running approximately radially from the endocardium toward the epicardium in transmural section. Like the fibers, the sheets also have a branching pattern with the number of branches varying considerably through the wall thickness. Recent reports suggest that, in addition to fiber orientations, DTI may be able to detect laminar sheet orientations [20]. The tensor of diffusion coefficients in the myocardium detected by DTI has been shown to be orthotropic, and the principal axis of slowest diffusion was seen to coincide with the direction normal to the sheet planes.

The fibrous architecture of the myocardium has motivated models of myocardial material symmetry as transversely isotropic. The transverse laminae are the first structural evidence for material orthotropy and have motivated the development of models describing the variation of fiber, sheet, and sheet-normal axes throughout the ventricular wall [21]. This has led to the idea that the laminar architecture of the ventricular myocardium affects the significant transverse shears [22] and myofiber rearrangement [18] described in the intact heart during systole. By measuring three-dimensional distributions of strain across the wall thickness using biplane radiography of radiopaque markers, LeGrice and colleagues [23] found that the cleavage planes coincide closely with the planes of maximum shearing during ejection, and that the consequent reorientation of the myocytes may contribute 50% or more of normal systolic wall thickening. Arts et al. [24] showed that the distributions of sheet orientations measured within the left ventricular wall of the dog heart coincided closely with those predicted from observed three-dimensional wall strains using the assumption that laminae are oriented in planes that contain the muscle fibers and maximize interlaminar shearing. This assumption also leads to the conclusion that two families of sheet orientations may be expected. Indeed, a retrospective analysis of the histology supported this prediction and more recent observations confirm the presence of two distinct populations of sheet plane in the inner half of the ventricular wall.

A detailed description of the morphogenesis of the muscle fiber system in the developing heart is not available but there is evidence of an organized myofiber pattern by day 12 in the fetal mouse heart that is similar to that seen at birth (day 20) [25]. Abnormalities of cardiac muscle fiber patterns have been described in some disease conditions. In hypertrophic cardiomyopathy, which is often familial, there is substantial myofiber disarray, typically in the interventricular septum [10,26].

8.2.3 Extracellular Matrix Organization

The cardiac extracellular matrix primarily consists of the fibrillar collagens, type I (85%) and III (11%), synthesized by the cardiac fibroblasts, the most abundant cell type in the heart. Collagen is the major structural protein in connective tissues, but only comprises 2–5% of the myocardium by weight, compared with the myocytes, which make up 90% [27]. The collagen matrix has a hierarchical organization (Figure 8.3), and has been classified according to conventions established for skeletal muscle into endomysium, perimysium, and epimysium [28,29]. The endomysium is associated with individual cells and includes a fine weave surrounding the cell and transverse structural connections 120–150 nm long connecting adjacent myocytes, with attachments localized near the z-line of the sarcomere. The primary purpose of the endomysium is probably to maintain registration between adjacent cells. The perimysium groups cells together and includes the collagen fibers that wrap bundles of cells into the laminar sheets described above as well as large coiled fibers typically 1–3 μm in diameter composed of smaller collagen fibrils (40–50 nm) [30]. The helix period of the coiled perimysial fibers is about 20 μm and the convolution index (ratio of fiber arc length to midline length) is approximately 1.3 in the unloaded state of the ventricle [31,32]. These perimysial fibers are most likely to be the major structural elements of the collagen extracellular matrix though they probably contribute to myocardial strain energy by uncoiling rather than stretching [31]. Finally, a thick epimysial collagen sheath surrounds the entire myocardium forming the protective epicardium (visceral pericardium) and endocardium.

Collagen content, organization, cross-linking, and ratio of types I to III change with age and in various disease conditions, including myocardial ischemia and infarction, hypertension, and hypertrophy (Table 8.4). Changes in myocardial collagen content and organization coincide with alterations in diastolic myocardial stiffness [33]. Collagen intermolecular cross-linking is mediated by two separate mechanisms. The formation of enzymatic hydroxylysyl pyridinoline cross-links is catalyzed by lysyl oxidase, which requires copper as a cofactor. Nonenzymatic collagen cross-links known as advanced

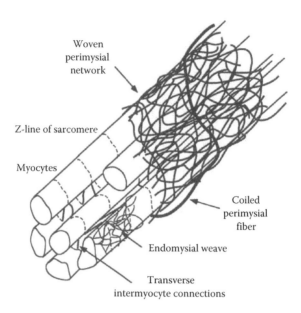

FIGURE 8.3 Schematic representation of cardiac tissue structure showing the association of endomysial and perimysial collagen fibers with cardiac myocytes. (Courtesy of Dr. Deidre MacKenna.)

TABLE 8.4 Changes in Ventricular Collagen Structure and Mechanics with Age and Disease

Condition	Collagen Morphology	Types and Cross-Linking	Passive Stiffness	Others
Pressure overload hypertrophy	[Hydroxyproline]: ↑-↑↑↑↑ [147,148] Area fraction: ↑↑↑↑ [148,149]	Type III: ↑[150] Cross-links: No change [151]	Chamber: ↑-↑↑↑ [148,149] Tissue: ↑↑↑ [152]	Perivascular fibrosis: ↑↑↑ [148] Focal scarring: [153,154]
Volume overload hypertrophy	[Hydroxyproline]: No change-↓: [155,156] Area fraction: No change [147,157]	Cross-links: ↑ [151,156] Type III/I: ↑ [156]	Chamber: ↓[158] Tissue: No change/↑ [158]	Parallel changes
Acute ischemia/ stunning	[Hydroxyproline]: ↓ [180] Light microscopy: No change/↓ [159] ↓↓ endomysial fibers [160]		↓ early [161] ↑ late [162]	Collagenase activity: ↑ [163,164]
Chronic myocardial infarction	[Hydroxyproline]: ↑↑↑ [165,166] Loss of birefringence [167]	Type III: ↑[168]	Chamber: ↑ early [169] Chamber: ↓ late [169]	Organization: ↑-↑↑↑↑ [170,171]
Age	[Hydroxyproline]: ↑-↑↑↑↑ [163,172] Collagen fiber diameter ↑[172]	Type III/I: ↓[173] Cross-links: ↑[173]	Chamber: ↑ [174] Papillary muscle: ↑[175]	Light microscopy: fibril diameter ↑ [172]

glycation end products can be formed in the presence of reducing sugars. This mechanism has been seen to significantly increase ventricular wall stiffness independent of changes in tissue collagen content, not only in diabetics but also in an animal model of volume overload hypertrophy [34]. Hence, the collagen matrix plays an important role in determining the elastic material properties of the ventricular myocardium.

8.3 Cardiac Pump Function

8.3.1 Ventricular Hemodynamics

The most basic mechanical parameters of the cardiac pump are blood pressure and volume flow rate, especially in the major pumping chambers, the ventricles. From the point of view of wall mechanics, the ventricular pressure is the most important boundary condition. Schematic representations of the time courses of pressure and volume in the left ventricle are shown in Figure 8.4. Ventricular filling immediately following mitral valve opening (MVO) is initially rapid because the ventricle produces a diastolic suction as the relaxing myocardium recoils elastically from its compressed systolic configuration below the resting chamber volume. The later slow phase of ventricular filling (diastasis) is followed finally by atrial contraction. The deceleration of the inflowing blood reverses the pressure gradient across the mitral valve leaflets and causes them to close (MVC). Valve closure may not, however, be completely passive because the atrial side of the mitral valve leaflets, which, unlike the pulmonic and aortic valves, are cardiac in embryological origin, have muscle [35] and nerve cells, and are electrically coupled to atrial conduction [36].

Ventricular contraction is initiated by excitation, which is almost synchronous (the duration of the QRS complex of the ECG is only about 60 ms in the normal adult) and begins about 0.1–0.2 s after atrial depolarization. Pressure rises rapidly during the isovolumic contraction phase (about 50 ms in adult humans), and the aortic valve opens (AVO) when the developed pressure exceeds the aortic pressure (afterload). Most of the cardiac output is ejected within the first quarter of the ejection phase before the pressure has peaked. The aortic valve closes (AVC) 200–300 ms after AVO when the ventricular pressure falls below the aortic pressure owing to the deceleration of the ejecting blood. The dichrotic notch, a characteristic feature of the aortic pressure waveform and a useful marker of aortic valve closure, is caused by pulse wave reflections in the aorta. Since the pulmonary artery pressure against which the

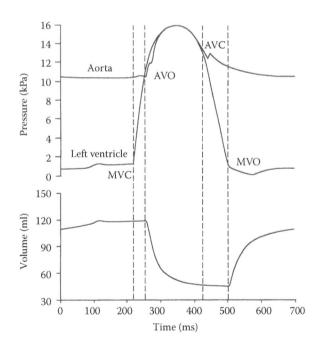

FIGURE 8.4 Left ventricular pressure, aortic pressure, and left ventricular volume during a single cardiac cycle showing the times of mitral valve closure (MVC), aortic valve opening (AVO), aortic valve closure (AVC), and mitral valve opening (MVO).

right ventricle pumps is much lower than the aortic pressure, the pulmonic valve opens before and closes after the aortic valve. The ventricular pressure falls during isovolumic relaxation, and the cycle continues. The rate of pressure decay from the value P_0 at the time of the peak rate of pressure fall until MVO is commonly characterized by a single exponential time constant, that is

$$P(t) = P_0\, e^{-t/\tau} + P_\infty, \tag{8.7}$$

where P_∞ is the (negative) baseline pressure to which the ventricle would eventually relax if MVO were prevented [37]. In dogs and humans, τ is normally about 40 ms, but it is increased by various factors, including elevated afterload, asynchronous contraction associated with abnormal activation sequence or regional dysfunction, and slowed cytosolic calcium reuptake to the sarcoplasmic reticulum associated with cardiac hypertrophy and failure. The pressure and volume curves for the right ventricle look essentially the same; however, the right ventricular and pulmonary artery pressures are only about a fifth of the corresponding pressures on the left side of the heart. The intraventricular septum separates the right and left ventricles and can transmit forces from one to the other. An increase in right ventricular volume may increase the left ventricular pressure by deformation of the septum. This direct interaction is most significant during filling [38].

The phases of the cardiac cycle are customarily divided into systole and diastole. The end of diastole—the start of systole—is generally defined as the time of mitral valve closure. Mechanical end-systole is usually defined as the end of ejection, but Brutsaert and colleagues proposed extending systole until the onset of diastasis (see the review by Brutsaert and Sys [39]) since there remains considerable myofilament interaction and active tension during relaxation. The distinction is important from the point of view of cardiac muscle mechanics: the myocardium is still active for much of diastole and may never be fully relaxed at sufficiently high heart rates (over 150 beats per minute). Here, we will retain the traditional definition of diastole, but consider the ventricular myocardium to be "passive" or "resting" only in the final slow-filling stage of diastole.

8.3.2 Ventricular Pressure–Volume Relations and Energetics

A useful alternative to Figure 8.4 for displaying ventricular pressure and volume changes is the pressure–volume loop shown in Figure 8.5a. During the last 20 years, the ventricular pressure–volume relationship has been explored extensively, particularly by Sagawa, Suga, and colleagues, who wrote a comprehensive book on the approach [40]. The isovolumic phases of the cardiac cycle can be recognized as the vertical segments of the loop, the lower limb represents ventricular filling, and the upper segment is the ejection phase. The difference on the horizontal axis between the vertical isovolumic segments is the stroke volume, which expressed as a fraction of the end-diastolic volume is the ejection fraction. The effects of altered loading on the ventricular pressure–volume relation have been studied in many preparations, but the best controlled experiments have used the isolated cross-circulated canine heart in which the ventricle fills and ejects against a computer-controlled volume servo-pump.

Changes in the filling pressure of the ventricle (preload) move the end-diastolic point along the unique end-diastolic pressure–volume relation (EDPVR), which represents the passive filling mechanics of the chamber that are determined primarily by the thick-walled geometry and nonlinear elasticity of the resting ventricular wall. Alternatively, if the afterload seen by the left ventricle is increased, stroke volume decreases in a predictable manner. The locus of end-ejection points (AVC) forms the end-systolic pressure–volume relation (ESPVR), which is approximately linear in a variety of conditions and also largely independent of the ventricular load history. Hence, the ESPVR is almost the same for isovolumic beats as for ejecting beats, although consistent effects of ejection history have been well characterized [41]. Connecting pressure–volume points at corresponding times in the cardiac cycle also results in a relatively linear relationship throughout systole with the intercept on the volume axis V_0 remaining nearly constant (Figure 8.5b). This leads to the valuable approximation that the ventricular

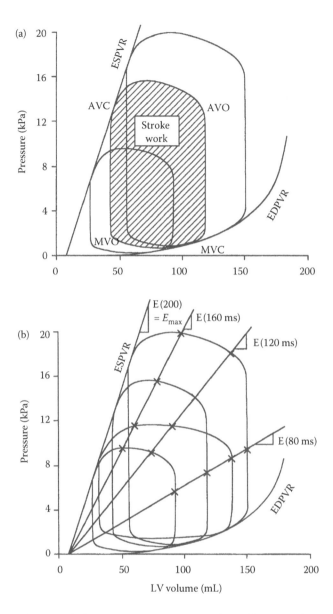

FIGURE 8.5 Schematic diagram of left ventricular pressure–volume loops: (a) end-systolic pressure–volume relation (ESPVR), end-diastolic pressure–volume relation (EDPVR), and stroke work. The three P–V loops show the effects of changes in preload and afterload. (b) Time-varying elastance approximation of ventricular pump function (see text).

volume $V(t)$ at any instance during systole is simply proportional to the instantaneous pressure $P(t)$ through a time-varying elastance $E(t)$:

$$P(t) = E(t)\{V(t) - V_0\}. \tag{8.8}$$

The maximum elastance E_{max}, the slope of the ESPVR, has acquired considerable significance as an index of cardiac contractility that is independent of ventricular loading conditions. As the inotropic state of the myocardium increases, for example, with catecholamine infusion, E_{max} increases, and with a negative inotropic effect such as a reduction in coronary artery pressure, it decreases.

The area of the ventricular pressure–volume loop is the external work (EW) performed by the myocardium on the ejecting blood:

$$EW = \int_{EDV}^{ESV} P(t)dV \qquad (8.9)$$

Plotting this stroke work against a suitable measure of preload gives a ventricular function curve, which illustrates the single most important intrinsic mechanical property of the heart pump. In 1914, Patterson and Starling [42] performed detailed experiments on the canine heart–lung preparation, and Starling summarized their results with his famous "Law of the Heart," which states that the work output of the heart increases with ventricular filling. The so-called Frank–Starling mechanism is now well recognized to be an intrinsic mechanical property of the cardiac muscle (see Section 8.4).

External stroke work is closely related to cardiac energy utilization. Since myocardial contraction is fueled by ATP, 90–95% of which is normally produced by oxidative phosphorylation, cardiac energy consumption is often studied in terms of myocardial oxygen consumption, VO_2 (mL O_2 g^{-1} beat^{-1}). Since energy is also expended during nonworking contractions, Suga and colleagues [43] defined the pressure–volume area (PVA) (J g^{-1} beat^{-1}) as the loop area (external stroke work) plus the end-systolic potential energy (internal work), which is the area under the ESPVR left of the isovolumic relaxation line (Figure 8.5a)

$$PVA = EW + PE. \qquad (8.10)$$

The PVA has strong linear correlation with VO_2 independent of ejection history. Equation 8.11 has typical values for the dog heart:

$$VO_2 = 0.12(PVA) + 2.0 \times 10^{-4}. \qquad (8.11)$$

The intercept represents the sum of the oxygen consumption for basal metabolism and the energy associated with the activation of the contractile apparatus, which is primarily used to cycle intracellular Ca^{2+} for excitation–contraction coupling [43]. The reciprocal of the slope is the contractile efficiency [44,45]. The VO_2–PVA relation shifts its elevation but not its slope with increments in E_{max} with most positive and negative inotropic interventions [44,46–49]. However, ischemic–reperfused viable but "stunned" myocardium has a smaller O_2 cost of PVA [50].

Although the PVA approach has also been useful in many settings, it is fundamentally phenomenological. Because the time-varying elastance assumptions ignores the well-documented load-history dependence of cardiac muscle tension [51–53], theoretical analyses that attempt to reconcile PVA with cross-bridge mechanoenergetics [54] are usually based on isometric or isotonic contractions. So that regional oxygen consumption in the intact heart can be related to myofiber biophysics, regional variations on the PVA have been proposed, such as the tension–area area [55], normalization of E_{max} [56], and the fiber stress–strain area [57].

In mammals, there are characteristic variations in cardiac function with heart size. In the power law relation for heart rate as a function of body mass (analogous to Equation 8.3), the coefficient k is 241 beats min^{-1} and the power α is −0.25 [5]. In the smallest mammals, like soricine shrews that weigh only a few grams, maximum heart rates exceeding 1000 beats min^{-1} have been measured [58]. Ventricular cavity volume scales linearly with heart weight, and ejection fraction and blood pressure are reasonably invariant from rats to horses. Hence, stroke work also scales directly with heart size [59], and thus work rate and energy consumption would be expected to increase with decreased body size in the same manner as heart rate. However, careful studies have demonstrated only a twofold increase in myocardial heat production as body mass decreases in mammals ranging from humans to rats, despite a 4.6-fold increase in heart rate [60]. This suggests that cardiac energy expenditure does not scale in proportion to heart rate and that cardiac metabolism is a lower proportion of total body metabolism in the smaller species.

The primary determinants of the EDPVR are the material properties of resting myocardium, the chamber dimensions and wall thickness, and the boundary conditions at the epicardium, endocardium, and valve annulus [61]. The EDPVR has been approximated by an exponential function of volume (see, e.g., Chapter 9 in Reference 62), though a cubic polynomial also works well. Therefore, the passive chamber stiffness dP/dV is approximately proportional to the filling pressure. Important influences on the EDPVR include the extent of relaxation, ventricular interaction and pericardial constraints, and coronary vascular engorgement. The material properties and boundary conditions in the septum are important since they determine how the septum deforms [63,64]. Through septal interaction, the end-diastolic pressure–volume relationship of the left ventricle may be directly affected by changes in the hemodynamic loading conditions of the right ventricle. The ventricles also interact indirectly since the output of the right ventricle is returned as the input to the left ventricle via the pulmonary circulation. Slinker and Glantz [65], using pulmonary artery and venae caval occlusions to produce direct (immediate) and indirect (delayed) interaction transients, concluded that the direct interaction is about half as significant as the indirect coupling. The pericardium provides a low friction mechanical enclosure for the beating heart that constrains ventricular overextension [66]. Since the pericardium has stiffer elastic properties than the ventricles [67], it contributes to direct ventricular interactions. The pericardium also augments the mechanical coupling between the atria and ventricles [68]. Increasing coronary perfusion pressure has been seen to increase the slope of the diastolic pressure–volume relation (an "erectile" effect) [69,70].

8.4 Myocardial Material Properties

8.4.1 Muscle Contractile Properties

Cardiac muscle mechanics testing is far more difficult than skeletal muscle testing mainly owing to the lack of ideal test specimens like the long single fiber preparations that have been so valuable for studying the mechanisms of skeletal muscle mechanics. Moreover, under physiological conditions, cardiac muscle cannot be stimulated to produce sustained tetanic contractions due to the absolute refractory period of the myocyte cell membrane. Cardiac muscle also exhibits a mechanical property analogous to the relative refractory period of excitation. After a single isometric contraction, some recovery time is required before another contraction of equal amplitude can be activated. The time constant for this mechanical restitution property of cardiac muscle is about 1 s [71].

Unlike skeletal muscle, in which maximal active force generation occurs at a sarcomere length that optimizes myofilament overlap (~2.1 μm), the isometric twitch tension developed by isolated cardiac muscle continues to rise with increased sarcomere length in the physiological range (1.6–2.4 μm). Early evidence for a descending limb of the cardiac muscle isometric length–tension curve was found to be caused by shortening in the central region of the isolated muscle at the expense of stretching at the damaged ends where specimen was tethered to the test apparatus. If muscle length is controlled so that sarcomere length in the undamaged part of the muscle is indeed constant, or if the developed tension is plotted against the instantaneous sarcomere length rather than the muscle length, the descending limb is eliminated [72]. Thus, the increase with chamber volume of end-systolic pressure and stroke work is reflected in isolated muscle as a monotonic increase in peak isometric tension with sarcomere length. Unlike in skeletal muscle, resting tension becomes very significant at sarcomere lengths over 2.3 μm. The increase in slope of the ESPVR associated with increased contractility is mirrored by the effects of increased calcium concentration in the length–tension relation. The duration as well as the tension developed in the active cardiac twitch also increases substantially with sarcomere length.

The relationship between cytosolic calcium concentration and isometric muscle tension has mostly been investigated in muscle preparations in which the sarcolemma has been chemically permeabilized.

Because there is evidence that this chemical "skinning" alters the calcium sensitivity of myofilament interaction, recent studies have also investigated myofilament calcium sensitivity in intact muscles tetanized by high-frequency stimulation in the presence of a compound such as ryanodine that open calcium release sites in the sarcoplasmic reticulum. Intracellular calcium concentration was estimated using calcium-sensitive optical indicators such as Fura. The myofilaments are activated in a graded manner by micromolar concentrations of calcium, which binds to troponin-C according to a sigmoidal relation [73]. Half-maximal tension in cardiac muscle is developed at intracellular calcium concentrations of 10^{-6} to 10^{-5} M (the C_{50}) depending on factors such as species and temperature [71]. Hence, relative isometric tension $T_0/T_{\max}$ may be modeled using [74,75].

$$\frac{T_0}{T_{\max}} = \frac{[Ca]^n}{[Ca]^n + C_{50}^n}.$$ (8.12)

The Hill coefficient (n) governs the steepness of the sigmoidal curve. A wide variety of values have been reported but most have been in the range 3–6 [76–79]. The steepness of the isometric length–tension relation, compared with that of skeletal muscle is due to length-dependent calcium sensitivity. That is, the C_{50} (M) changes with sarcomere length, L (μm). Kentish et al. [77] also reported a dependence of the Hill coefficient n on sarcomere length, but this was probably due to shortening during contraction of their specimens. In experiments in which sarcomere length was tightly controlled, no length dependence of n was found [80]. Niederer et al. [181] used a Hill coefficient of 5 for intact rat preparations at room temperature and the following approximation for C_{50} to fit the data of skinned rat cardiac muscle:

$$C_{50} = 4.72\left(1 - 4.0\left(\frac{L}{L_{\text{ref}} - 1}\right)\right),$$ (8.13)

where the reference sarcomere length L_{ref} was taken to be 2.0 μm.

The isotonic force–velocity relation of cardiac muscle is similar to that of skeletal muscle, and A. V. Hill's well-known hyperbolic relation is a good approximation except at larger forces greater than about 85% of the isometric value. The maximal (unloaded) velocity of shortening is essentially independent of preload, but does change with time during the cardiac twitch and is affected by factors that affect contractile ATPase activity and hence cross-bridge cycling rates. De Tombe and colleagues [81], using sarcomere length-controlled isovelocity release experiments, found that viscous forces impose a significant internal load opposing sarcomere shortening. If the isotonic shortening response is adjusted for the confounding effects of passive viscoelasticity, the underlying cross-bridge force–velocity relation is found to be linear.

Cardiac muscle contraction also exhibits other significant length-history-dependent properties. An important example is "deactivation" associated with length transients. Following a brief length transient that dissociates cross-bridges, the tension that is redeveloped reaches the original isometric value when the transient is imposed early in the twitch before peak tension is reached. But, following transients applied at times after the peak twitch tension has occurred, the fraction of tension redeveloped declines progressively since the activator calcium has fallen to levels below that necessary for all crossbridges to reattach [82].

There have been many model formulations of cardiac muscle contractile mechanics, too numerous to summarize here. In essence, they may be grouped into three categories. Time-varying elastance models include the essential dependence of cardiac active force development on muscle length and time. These models would seem to be well suited to create EDPVR and ESPVR curves in the continuum analysis of whole heart mechanics [1,83,84] by virtue of the success of the time-varying elastance concept of ventricular function (see Section 8.3.2 above). However, to obtain more realistic flow and pressure waveforms when a whole-heart model is coupled to an afterload, or in the presence of an asynchronous ventricular activation pattern, contractile models that incorporate a force–velocity relation are more appropriate. In

"Hill" models, the active fiber stress development is modified by shortening or lengthening according to the force–velocity relation, so that fiber tension is reduced by increased shortening velocity [85,86]. Fully history-dependent models are more complex and are generally based on A. F. Huxley's cross-bridge theory [53,87–89]. A statistical approach known as the distribution moment model has also been shown to provide an excellent approximation to cross-bridge theory [90]. Alternative, more phenomenological approaches are Hunter's fading memory theory [75]—which captures the complete length-history dependence of cardiac muscle contraction—and Markov models of myofilament activation [91–93] without requiring all the biophysical complexity of cross-bridge models.

Recently, Campbell et al. proposed a mechanistic Markov model of cardiac thin filament activation in which emphasis was put on interactions among nearest-neighbor regulatory units (RUs) [94]. In the model, RUs are composed of seven actin monomers, troponin C, troponin I, and tropomyosin, together with the S1 region of myosin (Figure 8.6) [95]. Interactions were assumed to arise from structural coupling of adjacent tropomyosins, such that tropomyosin shifting within each RU was influenced by the tropomyosin status of its neighbors. Model results suggested that this single mechanism was capable of producing cooperative activation of force-Ca^{2+} dynamics in intact cardiac muscle (Figure 8.7).

The appropriate choice of model will depend on the purpose of the analysis. For many models of global ventricular function, a time-varying elastance or Hill-type model will suffice, but for an analysis of sarcomere dynamics in isolated muscle or the ejecting heart, a history-dependent analysis is more appropriate.

Although Hill's basic assumption that resting and active muscle fiber tensions are additive is axiomatic in one-dimensional tests of isolated cardiac mechanics, there remains little experimental information on how the passive and active material properties of myocardium superpose in two dimensions or three. The simplest and commonest assumption is that active stress is strictly one-dimensional and adds to the fiber component of the three-dimensional passive stress. However, even this addition will indirectly affect all the other components of the stress response, since myocardial elastic deformations are finite, nonlinear, and approximately isochoric (volume conserving). In an interesting and important new development, biaxial testing of tetanized and barium-contracted ventricular myocardium has shown that the developed systolic stress also has a large component in directions transverse to the mean myofiber axis that can exceed 50% of the axial fiber component [96]. The magnitude of this transverse active stress depended significantly on the biaxial loading conditions. Moreover, evidence from osmotic swelling and other studies suggests that transverse strain can affect contractile tension development along the fiber axis by altering myofibril lattice spacing [97,98]. The mechanisms of transverse active stress development

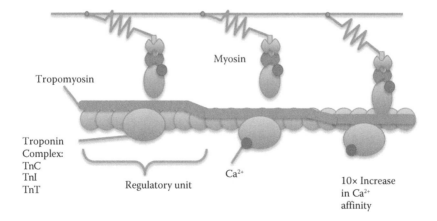

FIGURE 8.6 Diagram of myofilament Ca^{2+} activation. This depiction is based on concepts reviewed in Reference 95. (Reproduced with permission from S. G. Campbell, *The Role of Regulatory Light Chain Phosphorylation in Left Ventricular Function*, La Jolla: University of California, San Diego, 2010, p. 215.)

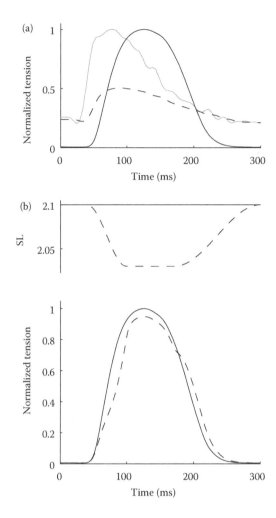

FIGURE 8.7 Twitches simulated with a Markov model of myofilament activation that properly accounts for structural interactions among regulatory proteins [176]. (a) Twitch tension was simulated in response to an intra-cellular Ca^{2+} transient measured in mouse papillary muscle (gray trace in background). In the absence of coopera-tive interactions between neighboring tropomyosin molecules along the length of actin filaments, diastolic tension is high, and the time course of twitch very nearly follows that of the driving Ca^{2+} transient (dashed trace). When neighboring tropomyosin molecules interact (solid trace), the cooperative effects can be seen as low diastolic ten-sion (cooperative inhibition) as well as enhanced peak tension (cooperative activation). (b) An illustration of length and velocity dependence in the same model, responding to isometric (solid traces) and nonisometric (dashed traces) conditions. (Courtesy of Dr. Stuart Campbell.)

remain unclear but two possible contributors are the geometry of the cross-bridge head itself, which is oriented oblique to the myofilament axis [99], and the dispersion of myofiber orientation [10].

8.4.2 Resting Myocardial Properties

Since, by the Frank–Starling mechanism, end-diastolic volume directly affects systolic ventricular work, the mechanics of resting myocardium also have fundamental physiological significance. Most biomechanics studies of passive myocardial properties have been conducted in isolated, arrested whole-heart or tissue preparations. Passive cardiac muscle exhibits most of the mechanical properties characteristic of soft tissues in general [100]. In cyclic uniaxial loading and unloading, the stress–strain relationship is nonlinear with small but significant hysteresis. Depending on the preparation used, resting cardiac muscle typically requires 2–10 repeated loading cycles to achieve a reproducible (preconditioned) response. Intact cardiac muscle experiences finite deformations during the normal cardiac cycle, with maximum Lagrangian strains (which are generally radial and endocardial) that may easily exceed 0.5 in magnitude. Hence, the classical linear theory of elasticity is quite inappropriate for resting myocardial mechanics. The hysteresis of the tissue is consistent with a viscoelastic response, which is undoubtedly related to the substantial water content of the myocardium (about 80% by mass). Changes in water content, such as edema, can cause substantial alterations in the passive stiffness and viscoelastic properties of myocardium. The viscoelasticity of passive cardiac muscle has been characterized in creep and relaxation studies of papillary muscle from cat and rabbit. In both species, the tensile stress in response to a step in strain relaxes 30–40% in the first 10 s [101,102]. The relaxation curves exhibit a short exponential time constant (<0.02 s) and a long one (about 1000 s), and are largely independent of the strain magnitude, which supports the approximation that myocardial viscoelasticity is quasilinear. Myocardial creep under isotonic loading is 2–3% of the original length after 100 s of isotonic loading and is also quasilinear with an exponential time course. There is also evidence that passive ventricular muscle exhibits other anelastic properties such as maximum-strain-dependent "strain softening" [103,104], a well-known property in elastomers first described by Mullins [105].

Since the hysteresis of passive cardiac muscle is small and only weakly affected by changes in strain rate, the assumption of pseudoelasticity [100] is often appropriate. That is, the resting myocardium is considered to be a finite elastic material with different elastic properties in loading versus unloading. Although various preparations have been used to study resting myocardial elasticity, the most detailed and complete information has come from biaxial and multiaxial tests of isolated sheets of cardiac tissue, mainly from the dog [106–108]. These experiments have shown that the arrested myocardium exhibits significant anisotropy with substantially greater stiffness in the muscle fiber direction than transversely. In equibiaxial tests of muscle sheets cut from planes parallel to the ventricular wall, fiber stress was greater than the transverse stress (Figure 8.8) by an average factor of close to 2.0 [109]. Moreover, because of the structural organization of the myocardium described in Section 8.2, there is also significant anisotropy

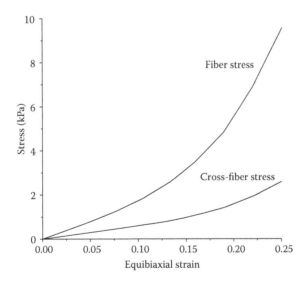

FIGURE 8.8 Representative stress–strain curves for passive rat myocardium computed using Equations 8.17 and 8.19. Fiber and cross-fiber stresses are shown for equibiaxial strain. (Courtesy of Dr. Jeffrey Omens.)

in the plane of the tissue transverse to the fiber axis, with the fiber direction being the stiffest, followed by the cross-fiber direction within a sheet, with the direction normal to a sheet being the softest [110]. Dokos and coworkers [110] have demonstrated that myocardial shear properties are also anisotropic.

The biaxial stress–strain properties of passive myocardium display some heterogeneity. Recently, Novak et al. [111] measured regional variations of biaxial mechanics in the canine left ventricle. Specimens from the inner and outer thirds of the left ventricular free wall were stiffer than those from the midwall and interventricular septum, but the degree of anisotropy was similar in each region. Significant species variations in myocardial stiffness have also been described. Using measurements of two-dimensional regional strain during left ventricular inflation in the isolated whole heart, a parameter optimization approach showed that canine cardiac tissue was several times stiffer than that of the rat, though the nonlinearity and anisotropy were similar [112]. Biaxial testing of the collagenous parietal pericardium and epicardium has shown that these tissues have distinctly different properties than the myocardium being very compliant and isotropic at low biaxial strains (<0.1–0.15) but rapidly becoming very stiff and anisotropic as the strain is increased [67,107].

Various constitutive models have been proposed for the elasticity of passive cardiac tissues. Because of the large deformations and nonlinearity of these materials, the most useful framework has been provided by the pseudostrain-energy formulation for hyperelasticity. For a detailed review of the material properties of passive myocardium and approaches to constitutive modeling, the reader is referred to Chapters 1 through 6 of Reference 113. In hyperelasticity, the components of the stress* are obtained from the strain energy W as a function of the Lagrangian (Green's) strain E_{RS}.

The myocardium is generally assumed to be an incompressible material, which is a good approximation in the isolated tissue, although in the intact heart there can be significant redistribution of tissue volume associated with phasic changes in regional coronary blood volume. Incompressibility is included as a kinematic constraint in the finite elasticity analysis, which introduces a new pressure variable that is added as a Lagrange multiplier in the strain energy. The examples that follow are various strain-energy functions, with representative parameter values (for W in kPa, i.e., mJ mL^{-1}), that have been suggested for cardiac tissues. For the two-dimensional properties of canine myocardium, Yin and colleagues [109] obtained reasonable fits to experimental data with an exponential function

$$W = 0.47e^{(35E_{11}^{1.2}+20E_{22}^{1.2})},\tag{8.14}$$

where E_{11} is the fiber strain and E_{22} is the cross-fiber in-plane strain. Humphrey and Yin [114] proposed a three-dimensional form for W as the sum of an isotropic exponential function of the first principal invariant I_1 of the right Cauchy–Green deformation tensor and another exponential function of the fiber stretch ratio λ_F:

$$W = 0.21(e^{9.4(I_1-3)} - 1) + 0.35(e^{66(\lambda_F-1)^2} - 1),\tag{8.15}$$

The isotropic part of this expression has also been used to model the myocardium of the embryonic chick heart during the ventricular looping stages, with coefficients of 0.02 kPa during diastole and 0.78 kPa at end-systole, and exponent parameters of 1.1 and 0.85, respectively [115]. Another transversely related isotropic strain-energy function was used by Guccione et al. [116] and Omens et al. [117] to model material properties in the isolated mature rat and dog hearts:

$$W = 0.6 \, (e^Q - 1),\tag{8.16}$$

---

* In a hyperelastic material, the *second Piola Kirchhoff* stress tensor is given by $P_{RS} = \dfrac{1}{2}\left(\dfrac{\partial W}{\partial E_{RS}} + \dfrac{\partial W}{\partial E_{SR}}\right)$.

where, in the dog

$$Q = 26.7E_{11}^2 + 2.0(E_{22}^2 + E_{33}^2 + E_{23}^2 + E_{32}^2) + 14.7(E_{12}^2 + E_{21}^2 + E_{13}^2 + E_{31}^2), \tag{8.17}$$

and, in the rat

$$Q = 9.2E_{11}^2 + 2.0(E_{22}^2 + E_{33}^2 + E_{23}^2 + E_{32}^2) + 3.7(E_{12}^2 + E_{21}^2 + E_{13}^2 + E_{31}^2). \tag{8.18}$$

In Equations 8.17 and 8.18, normal and shear strain components involving the radial (x_3) axis are included. Humphrey and colleagues [118] determined a new polynomial form directly from biaxial tests. Novak et al. [111] gave representative coefficients for canine myocardium from three layers of the left ventricular free wall. For the outer third, they obtained

$$W = 4.8(\lambda_F - 1)^2 + 3.4(\lambda_F - 1)^3 + 0.77(I_1 - 3) - 6.1(I_1 - 3)(\lambda_F - 1) + 6.2(I_1 - 3)^2, \tag{8.19}$$

for the midwall region

$$W = 5.3(\lambda_F - 1)^2 + 7.5(\lambda_F - 1)^3 + 0.43(I_1 - 3) - 7.7(I_1 - 3)(\lambda_F - 1) + 5.6(I_1 - 3)^2, \tag{8.20}$$

and for the inner layer of the wall

$$W = 0.51(\lambda_F - 1)^2 + 27.6(\lambda_F - 1)^3 + 0.74(I_1 - 3) - 7.3(I_1 - 3)(\lambda_F - 1) + 7.0(I_1 - 3)^2. \tag{8.21}$$

A power law strain-energy function expressed in terms of circumferential, longitudinal, and transmural extension ratios (λ_1, λ_2, and λ_3) was used [119] to describe the biaxial properties of sheep myocardium 2 weeks after experimental myocardial infarction, in the scarred infarct region:

$$W = 0.36\left(\frac{\lambda_1^{32}}{32} + \frac{\lambda_2^{30}}{30} + \frac{\lambda_3^{31}}{31} - 3\right), \tag{8.22}$$

and in the remote, noninfarcted tissue:

$$W = 0.11\left(\frac{\lambda_1^{22}}{22} + \frac{\lambda_2^{26}}{26} + \frac{\lambda_3^{24}}{24} - 3\right), \tag{8.23}$$

Based on the observation that resting stiffness rises steeply at strains that extend coiled collagen fibers to the limit of uncoiling, Hunter and colleagues have proposed a pole-zero constitutive relation in which the stresses rise asymptotically as the strain approaches a limiting elastic strain [75].

Recently, Holzapfel and Ogden [120] proposed a convex, strong elliptic and stable orthotropic strain-energy law for the myocardium:

$$W = \frac{a}{2b}\exp[b(I_1 - 3)] + \sum_{i=f,s}\frac{a_i}{2b_i}(\exp[b_i(I_{4i} - 1)^2] - 1) + \frac{a_{fs}}{2b_{fs}}(\exp[b_{fs}I_{8fs}^2] - 1) \tag{8.24}$$

consisting of an isotropic term in I_1, transversely isotropic terms in I_{4f} and I_{4s} and an orthotropic term in I_{8fs}. Here, f, s, and n refer to fiber, cross-fiber within the sheet, and sheet-normal directions. The a parameters have unit of stress, whereas the b parameters are dimensionless. The quasi-invariant I_4 is a right Cauchy–Green strain in a preferred direction and I_{8fs} is the right Cauchy–Green fiber-sheet shear strain. Special care was taken to fit this model with data from Yin et al. [109] and Dokos et al. [110].

The strain in the constitutive equation must generally be referred to the stress-free state of the tissue. However, the unloaded state of the passive left ventricle is not stress-free; residual stress exists in the intact, unloaded myocardium, as shown by Omens and Fung [121]. Cross-sectional equatorial rings from potassium-arrested rat hearts spring open elastically when the left ventricular wall is resected radially. The average opening angle of the resulting curved arc is $45 \pm 10°$ in the rat. Subsequent radial cuts produce no further change. Hence, a slice with one radial cut is considered to be stress-free, and there is a nonuniform distribution of residual strain across the intact wall, being compressive at the endocardium and tensile at the epicardium, with some regional differences. Stress analyses of the diastolic left ventricle have shown that residual stress acts to minimize the endocardial stress concentrations that would otherwise be associated with diastolic loading [116]. An important physiological consequence of residual stress is that the sarcomere length is nonuniform in the unloaded resting heart. Rodriguez et al. [122] showed that sarcomere length is about 0.13 µm greater at the epicardium than the endocardium in the unloaded rat heart, and this gradient vanishes when residual stress is relieved. Three-dimensional studies have also revealed the presence of substantial transverse residual shear strains [123]. Residual stress and strain may have an important relationship to cardiac growth and remodeling. Theoretical studies have shown that residual stress in tissues can arise from growth fields that are kinematically incompatible [124,125].

8.5 Regional Ventricular Mechanics: Stress and Strain

Although ventricular pressures and volumes are valuable for assessing the global pumping performance of the heart, myocardial stress and strain distributions are needed to characterize regional ventricular function, especially in pathological conditions, such as myocardial ischemia and infarction, where profound localized changes may occur. The measurement of stress in the intact myocardium involves resolving the local forces acting on defined planes in the heart wall. Attempts to measure local forces [126,127] have had limited success because of the large deformations of the myocardium and the uncertain nature of the mechanical coupling between the transducer elements and the tissue. Efforts to measure intramyocardial pressures using miniature implanted transducers have been more successful but have also raised a controversy over the extent to which they accurately represent changes in interstitial fluid pressure. In all cases, these methods provide an incomplete description of three-dimensional wall stress distributions. Therefore, the most common approach for estimating myocardial stress distributions is the use of mathematical models based on the laws of continuum mechanics. Although there is no room to review these analyses here, the important elements of such models are the geometry and structure, boundary conditions, and material properties, described in the foregoing sections. An excellent review of ventricular wall stress analysis is given by Yin [128]. The most versatile and powerful method for ventricular stress analysis is the finite element method, which has been used in cardiac mechanics for over 20 years [129]. However, models must also be validated with experimental measurements. Since the measurement of myocardial stresses is not yet reliable, the best experimental data for model validation are measurements of strains in the ventricular wall.

The earliest myocardial strain gauges were mercury-in-rubber transducers sutured to the epicardium. These days, local segment length changes are routinely measured with various forms of the piezoelectric crystal sonomicrometer. However, since the ventricular myocardium is a three-dimensional continuum, the local strain is only fully defined by all the normal and shear components of the myocardial strain tensor. Villarreal et al. [130] measured two-dimensional midwall strain components by arranging three piezoelectric crystals in a small triangle so that three segment lengths could be measured simultaneously. They showed that the principal axis of greatest shortening is not aligned with circumferential midwall fibers, and that this axis changes with altered ventricular loading and contractility. Therefore, uniaxial segment measurements do not reveal the full extent of alterations in regional function caused by an experimental intervention. Another approach to measuring regional myocardial strains is the use of clinical imaging techniques, such as magnetic resonance imaging tagging [4] with sophisticated strain analyses like HARP [131] and two- and three-dimensional speckle tracking echocardiography [132]. In unusual circumstances, radiopaque markers are implanted in the myocardium during cardiac surgery or transplantation [133].

In experimental research, implantable radiopaque markers are used for tracking myocardial motions with high spatial and temporal resolution. Meier et al. [134,135] placed triplets of metal markers 10–15 mm apart near the epicardium of the canine right ventricle and reconstructed their positions from biplane cinéradiographic recordings. By polar decomposition, they obtained the two principal epicardial strains, the principal angle, and the local rotation in the region. The use of radiopaque markers was extended to three dimensions by Waldman and colleagues [22], who implanted three closely separated columns of 5–6 metal beads in the ventricular wall. With this technique, it is possible to find all six components of strain and all three rigid-body rotation angles at sites through the wall. For details of this method, see the review by Waldman in Chapter 7 of Glass et al. [113]. An enhancement to this method uses high-order finite element interpolation of the marker positions to compute continuous transmural distributions of myocardial deformation [136].

Studies and models like these are producing an increasingly detailed picture of regional myocardial stress and strain distributions. Of the many interesting observations, there are some useful generalizations, particularly regarding the strain. Myocardial deformations are large and three-dimensional, and hence the nonlinear finite strain tensors are more appropriate measures than the linear infinitesimal Cauchy strain. During filling in the normal heart, the wall stretches biaxially but nonuniformly in the plane of the wall, and thins in the transmural direction. During systole, shortening is also two-dimensional and the wall thickens. There are substantial regional differences in the time course, magnitude, and pattern of myocardial deformations. In humans and dogs, in-plane systolic myocardial shortening and diastolic lengthening vary with longitudinal position on the left and right ventricular free walls generally increasing in magnitude from base to apex.

During both systole and diastole, there are significant shear strains in the wall. In-plane (torsional) shears are negative during diastole, consistent with a small left-handed torsion of the left ventricle during filling, and positive as the ventricular twist reverses during ejection. Consequently, the principal axes of the greatest diastolic segment lengthening and systolic shortening are not circumferential or longitudinal but at oblique axes, that are typically rotated 10–60° clockwise from circumferential. There are circumferential variations in regional left ventricular strain. The principal axes of greatest diastolic lengthening and systolic shortening tend to be more longitudinal on the posterior wall and more circumferentially oriented on the anterior wall. Perhaps the most significant regional variations are transmural. In-plane and transmural, normal or principal strains, are usually significantly greater in magnitude at the endocardium than at the epicardium, both in filling and ejection. However, when the strain is resolved in the local muscle fiber direction, the transmural variation of fiber strain becomes insignificant. The combination of torsional deformation and the transmural variation in fiber direction means that systolic shortening and diastolic lengthening tend to be maximized in the fiber direction at the epicardium and minimized at the endocardium. Hence, whereas maximum shortening and lengthening are closely aligned with muscle fibers at the subepicardium, they are almost perpendicular to the fibers at the subendocardium. In the left ventricular wall, there are also substantial transverse shear strains (i.e., in the circumferential-radial and longitudinal-radial planes) during systole, though during filling they are smaller. Their functional significance remains unclear, though they change substantially during acute myocardial ischemia or ventricular pacing and are apparently associated with the transverse laminae described earlier [23].

Sophisticated continuum mechanics models are needed to determine the stress distributions associated with these complex myocardial deformations. With modern finite element methods, it is now possible to include in the analysis the three-dimensional geometry and fiber architecture, finite deformations, nonlinear material properties, and muscle contraction of the ventricular myocardium. Some models have included other factors such as viscoelasticity, poroelasticity, coronary perfusion, growth and remodeling, regional ischemia, residual stress, and electrical activation. To date, continuum models have provided some valuable insight into regional cardiac mechanics. These include the importance of muscle fiber orientation, torsional deformations and residual stress, and the substantial inhomogeneities associated with regional variations in geometry and fiber angle or myocardial ischemia and infarction. A new arena in which models promise to make important contributions is the rapidly growing field of cardiac resynchronization therapy [137–139]. The use of biventricular pacing in cases of congestive heart failure that are accompanied by electrical conduction asynchrony has been seen to significantly improve ventricular pump function. However, the improvement in mechanical function is not well predicted by the improvement in electrical synchrony. New electromechanical models promise to provide insights into the mechanisms of cardiac resynchronization therapy and potentially to optimize the pacing protocols used [140–142].

8.6 Patient-Specific Modeling

The maturation of computational biology may lead to a new approach to medicine. During the last decade, there have been many improvements in diagnostic medical technologies such as multislice cardiac CT imaging, three-dimensional electroanatomic mapping, and many types of applications of magnetic resonance imaging (i.e., tagging and DTI). Combined with more powerful computing resources and more accurate predictive computational models, it is feasible to begin developing mechanistic patient-specific models that may help diagnosis, guide therapy or surgery, and predict outcomes of the latter. Indeed, in recent years, there have been successes in patient-specific modeling in various clinical domains such as cardiology, orthopedics, brain surgery, cancer, and periodontia [143]. Of these disciplines, the cardiovascular system is an excellent candidate for patient-specific modeling [144], since cardiac models represent one of the most advanced areas of computational biology, bridging the subcellular level to the circulatory level [145]. Despite the advances in medical technology, patient-specific modeling has not yet become a standard of care in clinical practice because the evaluation of the predictive capability of these models has not yet been performed on a large scale [143,146].

Acknowledgments

We are indebted to many colleagues and students, past and present, for their input and perspective of cardiac biomechanics. Owing to space constraints, we have relied on much of their work without adequate citation, especially in the final section. Special thanks to Drs. Jeffrey Omens, Deidre MacKenna, Stuart Campbell, and Jyoti Rao, who provided illustrations used in this chapter.

References

1. L. A. Taber, On a nonlinear theory for muscle shells. Part II—Application to the beating left ventricle, *ASME J Biomech Eng,* 113, 63–71, 1991.
2. D. D. Streeter, Jr and W. T. Hanna, Engineering mechanics for successive states in canine left ventricular myocardium: I. Cavity and wall geometry, *Circ Res,* 33, 639–655, 1973.
3. P. M. F. Nielsen, I. J. Le Grice, B. H. Smaill, and P. J. Hunter, Mathematical model of geometry and fibrous structure of the heart, *Am J Physiol,* 260, H1365–H1378, 1991.
4. A. A. Young and L. Axel, Three-dimensional motion and deformation in the heart wall: Estimation from spatial modulation of magnetization—A model-based approach, *Radiology,* 185, 241–247, 1992.
5. W. R. Stahl, Scaling of respiratory variable in mammals, *J Appl Physiol,* 22, 453–460, 1967.
6. K. Rakusan, Cardiac growth, maturation and aging, in *Growth of the Heart in Health and Disease,* R. Zak, Ed. New York: Raven Press, 1984, 131–164.
7. D. D. Streeter, Jr, Gross morphology and fiber geometry of the heart, in *Handbook of Physiology, Section 2: The Cardiovascular System, Chapter 4.* vol. I, B. R. M, Ed. Bethesda, MD: American Physiological Society, 1979, pp. 61–112.

8. J. E. Saffitz, H. L. Kanter, K. G. Green, T. K. Tolley, and E. C. Beyer, Tissue-specific determinants of anisotropic conduction velocity in canine atrial and ventricular myocardium, *Circ Res,* 74, 1065–1070, 1994.

9. F. Torrent-Guasp, *The Cardiac Muscle.* Madrid: Juan March Foundation, 1973.

10. W. J. Karlon, J. W. Covell, A. D. McCulloch, J. J. Hunter, and J. H. Omens, Automated measurement of myofiber disarray in transgenic mice with ventricular expression of ras, *Anat Rec,* 252, 612–625, 1998.

11. D. D. Streeter, Jr, H. M. Spotnitz, D. P. Patel, J. Ross, Jr, and E. H. Sonnenblick, Fiber orientation in the canine left ventricle during diastole and systole, *Circ Res,* 24, 339–347, 1969.

12. F. J. Vetter and A. D. McCulloch, Three-dimensional analysis of regional cardiac function: A model of rabbit ventricular anatomy, *Prog Biophys Mol Biol,* 69, 157–183, 1998.

13. E. W. Hsu, A. L. Muzikant, S. A. Matulevicius, R. C. Penland, and C. S. Henriquez, Magnetic resonance myocardial fiber-orientation mapping with direct histological correlation, *Am J Physiol,* 274, H1627–H1634, 1998.

14. D. F. Scollan, A. Holmes, R. Winslow, and J. Forder, Histological validation of myocardial microstructure obtained from diffusion tensor magnetic resonance imaging, *Am J Physiol,* 275, H2308–H2318, 1998.

15. J. Dou, W. Y. Tseng, T. G. Reese, and V. J. Wedeen, Combined diffusion and strain MRI reveals structure and function of human myocardial laminar sheets in vivo, *Magn Reson Med,* 50, 107–113, 2003.

16. A. D. McCulloch, B. H. Smaill, and P. J. Hunter, Regional left ventricular epicardial deformation in the passive dog heart, *Circ Res,* 64, 721–733, 1989.

17. B. H. Smaill and P. J. Hunter, Structure and function of the diastolic heart, in *Theory of Heart,* L. Glass, P. J. Hunter, and A. D. McCulloch, Eds. New York: Springer-Verlag, 1991, pp. 1–29.

18. H. M. Spotnitz, W. D. Spotnitz, T. S. Cottrell, D. Spiro, and E. H. Sonnenblick, Cellular basis for volume related wall thickness changes in the rat left ventricle, *J Mol Cell Cardiol,* 6, 317–331, 1974.

19. I. J. LeGrice, B. H. Smaill, L. Z. Chai, S. G. Edgar, J. B. Gavin, and P. J. Hunter, Laminar structure of the heart: Ventricular myocyte arrangement and connective tissue architecture in the dog, *Am J Physiol,* 269, H571–H582, 1995.

20. W. Y. Tseng, V. J. Wedeen, T. G. Reese, R. N. Smith, and E. F. Halpern, Diffusion tensor MRI of myocardial fibers and sheets: Correspondence with visible cut-face texture, *J Magn Reson Imaging,* 17, 31–42, 2003.

21. I. J. Legrice, P. J. Hunter, and B. H. Smaill, Laminar structure of the heart: A mathematical model, *Am J Physiol,* 272, H2466–H2476, 1997.

22. L. K. Waldman, Y. C. Fung, and J. W. Covell, Transmural myocardial deformation in the canine left ventricle: Normal *in vivo* three-dimensional finite strains, *Circ Res,* 57, 152–163, 1985.

23. I. J. LeGrice, Y. Takayama, and J. W. Covell, Transverse shear along myocardial cleavage planes provides a mechanism for normal systolic wall thickening, *Circ Res,* 77, 182–193, 1995.

24. T. Arts, K. D. Costa, J. W. Covell, and A. D. McCulloch, Relating myocardial laminar architecture to shear strain and muscle fiber orientation, *Am J Physiol Heart Circ Physiol,* 280, H2222–H2229, 2001.

25. M. McLean, M. A. Ross, and J. Prothero, Three-dimensional reconstruction of the myofiber pattern in the fetal and neonatal mouse heart, *Anat Rec,* 224, 392–406, 1989.

26. B. J. Maron, R. O. Bonow, R. O. D. Cannon, M. B. Leon, and S. E. Epstein, Hypertrophic cardiomyopathy. Interrelations of clinical manifestations, pathophysiology, and therapy (1), *N Engl J Med,* 316, 780–789, 1987.

27. K. T. Weber, Cardiac interstituim in health and disease: The fibrillar collagen network, *J Am Coll Cardiol,* 13, 1637–165, 1989.

28. T. F. Robinson, L. Cohen-Gould, and S. M. Factor, Skeletal framework of mammalian heart muscle: Arrangement of inter- and pericellular connective tissue structures, *Lab Invest,* 49, 482–498, 1983.

29. J. B. Caulfield and T. K. Borg, The collagen network of the heart, *Lab Invest,* 40, 364–371, 1979.

30. T. F. Robinson, M. A. Geraci, E. H. Sonnenblick, and S. M. Factor, Coiled perimysial fibers of papillary muscle in rat heart: Morphology, distribution, and changes in configuration, *Circ Res,* 63, 577–592, 1988.

31. D. A. MacKenna, J. H. Omens, and J. W. Covell, Left ventricular perimysial collagen fibers uncoil rather than stretch during diastolic filling, *Basic Res Cardiol,* 91, 111–122, 1996.

32. D. A. MacKenna, S. M. Vaplon, and A. D. McCulloch, Microstructural model of perimysial collagen fibers for resting myocardial mechanics during ventricular filling, *Am J Physiol,* 273, H1576– H1586, 1997.

33. D. A. MacKenna and A. D. McCulloch, Contribution of the collagen extracellular matrix to ventricular mechanics, in *Systolic and Diastolic Function of the Heart,* N. B. Ingels, G. T. Daughters, J. Baan, J. W. Covell, R. S. Reneman, and F. C.-P. Yin, Eds. Amsterdam: IOS Press, 1996, pp. 35–46.

34. K. L. Herrmann, A. D. McCulloch, and J. H. Omens, Glycated collagen cross-linking alters cardiac mechanics in volume-overload hypertrophy, *Am J Physiol Heart Circ Physiol,* 284, H1277–H1284, 2003.

35. A. Itoh, G. Krishnamurthy, J. C. Swanson, D. B. Ennis, W. Bothe, E. Kuhl, M. Karlsson, L. R. Davis, D. C. Miller, and N. B. Ingels, Jr., Active stiffening of mitral valve leaflets in the beating heart, *Am J Physiol Heart Circ Physiol,* 296, H1766–H1773, 2009.

36. E. H. Sonnenblick, L. M. Napolitano, W. M. Daggett, and T. Cooper, An intrinsic neuromuscular basis for mitral valve motion in the dog, *Circ Res,* 21, 9–15, 1967.

37. E. L. Yellin, M. Hori, C. Yoran, E. H. Sonnenblick, S. Gabbay, and R. W. M. Frater, Left ventricular relaxation in the filling and nonfilling intact canine heart, *Am J Physiol,* 250, H620–H629, 1986.

38. J. S. Janicki and K. T. Weber, The pericardium and ventricular interaction, distensibility and function, *Am J Physiol,* 238, H494–H503, 1980.

39. D. L. Brutsaert and S. U. Sys, Relaxation and diastole of the heart, *Physiol Rev,* 69, 1228, 1989.

40. K. Sagawa, L. Maughan, H. Suga, and K. Sunagawa, *Cardiac Contraction and the Pressure-Volume Relationship.* New York: Oxford University Press, 1988.

41. W. C. Hunter, End-systolic pressure as a balance between opposing effects of ejection, *Circ Res,* 64, 265–275, 1989.

42. S. W. Patterson and E. H. Starling, On the mechanical factors which determine the output of the ventricles, *J Physiol,* 48, 357–379, 1914.

43. H. Suga, T. Hayashi, and M. Shirahata, Ventricular systolic pressure-volume area as predictor of cardiac oxygen consumption, *Am J Physiol,* 240, H39–H44, 1981.

44. H. Suga and Y. Goto, Cardiac oxygen costs of contractility (Emax) and mechanical energy (PVA): New key concepts in cardiac energetics, in *Recent Progress in Failing Heart Syndrome,* S. Sasayama and H. Suga, Eds. Tokyo: Springer-Verlag, 1991, pp. 61–115.

45. H. Suga, Y. Goto, O. Kawaguchi, K. Hata, T. Takasago, A. Saeki, and T. W. Taylor, Ventricular perspective on efficiency, *Basic Res Cardiol,* 88 Suppl 2, 43–65, 1993.

46. H. Suga, Ventricular energetics, *Physiol Rev,* 70, 247–277, 1990.

47. H. Suga, Y. Goto, Y. Yasumura, T. Nozawa, S. Futaki, N. Tanaka, and M. Uenishi, O_2 consumption of dog heart under decreased coronary perfusion and propranolol, *Am J Physiol,* 254, H292–H303, 1988.

48. D. D. Zhao, T. Namba, J. Araki, K. Ishioka, M. Takaki, and H. Suga, Nipradilol depresses cardiac contractility and O_2 consumption without decreasing coronary resistance in dogs, *Acta Med Okayama,* 47, 29–33, 1993.

49. T. Namba, M. Takaki, J. Araki, K. Ishioka, and H. Suga, Energetics of the negative and positive inotropism of pentobarbitone sodium in the canine left ventricle, *Cardiovasc Res,* 28, 557–564, 1994.

50. Y. Ohgoshi, Y. Goto, S. Futaki, H. Taku, O. Kawaguchi, and H. Suga, Increased oxygen cost of contractility in stunned myocardium of dog, *Circ Res,* 69, 975–988, 1991.

51. D. Burkhoff, M. Schnellbacher, R. A. Stennett, D. Zwas, K. Ogino, and J. P. Morgan, Explaining load-dependent ventricular performance and energetics based on a model of E-C coupling, in *Cardiac Energetics: From Emax to Pressure-Volume Area*, M. M. LeWinter, H. Suga, and M. W. Watkins, Eds. Boston: Kluwer Academic Publishers, 1995.

52. H. E. ter Keurs and P. P. de Tombe, Determinants of velocity of sarcomere shortening in mammalian myocardium, *Adv Exp Med Biol,* 332, 649–664; discussion 664–665, 1993.

53. J. M. Guccione and A. D. McCulloch, Mechanics of active contraction in cardiac muscle: Part I—Constitutive relations for fiber stress that describe deactivation, *J Biomech Eng,* 115, 72–81, 1993.

54. T. W. Taylor, Y. Goto, and H. Suga, Variable cross-bridge cycling-ATP coupling accounts for cardiac mechanoenergetics, *Am J Physiol,* 264, H994–H1004, 1993.

55. Y. Goto, S. Futaki, O. Kawaguchi, K. Hata, T. Takasago, A. Saeki, T. Nishioka, T. W. Taylor, and H. Suga, Coupling between regional myocardial oxygen consumption and contraction under altered preload and afterload, *J Am Coll Cardiol,* 21, 1522–1531, 1993.

56. M. Sugawara, Y. Kondoh, and K. Nakano, Normalization of Emax and PVA, in *Cardiac Energetics: From Emax to Pressure-Volume Area,* M. M. LeWinter, H. Suga, and M. W. Watkins, Eds. Boston: Kluwer Academic Publishers, 1995, pp. 65–78.

57. T. Delhaas, T. Arts, F. W. Prinzen, and R. S. Reneman, Regional fibre stress-fibre strain area as an estimate of regional blood flow and oxygen demand in the canine heart, *J Physiol (Lond),* 477, 481–496, 1994.

58. M. Vornanen, Maximum heart rate of sorcine shrews: Correlation with contractile properties and myosin composition, *Am J Physiol,* 31, R842–RR851, 1992.

59. J. P. Holt, E. A. Rhode, S. A. Peoples, and H. Kines, Left ventricular function in mammals of greatly different size, *Circ Res,* 10, 798–806, 1962.

60. D. S. Loiselle and C. L. Gibbs, Species differences in cardiac energetics, *Am J Physiol,* 237(1), H90–H98, 1979.

61. J. C. Gilbert and S. A. Glantz, Determinants of left ventricular filling and of the diastolic pressure-volume relation, *Circ Res,* 64, 827–852, 1989.

62. W. H. Gaasch and M. M. LeWinter, *Left Ventricular Diastolic Dysfunction and Heart Failure.* Philadelphia: Lea & Febiger, 1994.

63. S. A. Glantz, G. A. Misbach, W. Y. Moores, D. G. Mathey, J. Lekuen, D. F. Stowe, W. W. Parmley, and J. V. Tyberg, The pericardium substantially affects the left ventricular diastolic pressure-volume relationship in the dog, *Circ Res,* 42, 433–441, 1978.

64. S. A. Glantz and W. W. Parmley, Factors which affect the diastolic pressure-volume curve, *Circ Res,* 42, 171–180, 1978.

65. B. K. Slinker and S. A. Glantz, End-systolic and end-diastolic ventricular interaction, *Am J Physiol,* 251, H1062–H1075, 1986.

66. I. Mirsky and J. S. Rankin, The effects of geometry, elasticity, and external pressures on the diastolic pressure-volume and stiffness-stress relations: How important is the pericardium?, *Circ Res,* 44, 601–611, 1979.

67. M. C. Lee, Y. C. Fung, R. Shabetai, and M. M. LeWinter, Biaxial mechanical properties of human pericardium and canine comparisons, *Am J Physiol,* 253, H75–H82, 1987.

68. C. A. Gibbons-Kroeker, N. G. Shrive, I. Belenkie, and J. V. Tyberg, Pericardium modulates left and right ventricular stroke volumes to compensate for sudden changes in atrial volume, *Am J Physiol Heart Circ Physiol,* 284, H2247–H2254, 2003.

69. K. May-Newman, J. H. Omens, R. S. Pavelec, and A. D. McCulloch, Three-dimensional transmural mechanical interaction between the coronary vasculature and passive myocardium in the dog, *Circ Res,* 74, 1166–1178, 1994.

70. P. F. Salisbury, C. E. Cross, and P. A. Rieben, Influence of coronary artery pressure upon myocardial elasticity, *Circ Res,* 8, 794–800, 1960.

71. D. M. Bers, *Excitation-Contraction Coupling and Cardiac Contractile Force.* Dordrecht: Kluwer, 1991.

72. H. E. D. J. ter Keurs, W. H. Rijnsburger, R. van Heuningen, and M. J. Nagelsmit, Tension development and sarcomere length in rat cardiac trabeculae: Evidence of length-dependent activation, *Circ Res,* 46, 703–713, 1980.

73. J. C. Rüegg, *Calcium in Muscle Activation: A Comparative Approach,* 2nd ed. vol. 19. Berlin: Springer-Verlag, 1988.

74. A. Tözeren, Continuum rheology of muscle contraction and its application to cardiac contractility, *Biophys J,* 47, 303–309, 1985.

75. P. J. Hunter, A. D. McCulloch, and H. E. ter Keurs, Modelling the mechanical properties of cardiac muscle, *Prog Biophys Mol Biol,* 69, 289–331, 1998.

76. P. H. Backx, W. D. Gao, M. D. Azan-Backx, and E. Marban, The relationship between contractile force and intracellular [Ca^{2+}] in intact rat cardiac trabeculae, *J Gen Physiol,* 105, 1–19, 1995.

77. J. C. Kentish, H. E. D. J. Ter Keurs, L. Ricciari, J. J. J. Bucx, and M. I. M. Noble, Comparisons between the sarcomere length-force relations of intact and skinned trabeculae from rat right ventricle, *Circ Res,* 58, 755–768, 1986.

78. D. T. Yue, E. Marban, and W. G. Wier, Relationship between force and intracellular [Ca^{2+}] in tetanized mammalian heart muscle, *J Gen Physiol,* 87, 223–242, 1986.

79. W. D. Gao, P. H. Backx, M. Azan-Backx, and E. Marban, Myofilament Ca^{2+} sensitivity in intact versus skinned rat ventricular muscle, *Circ Res,* 74, 408–415, 1994.

80. D. P. Dobesh, J. P. Konhilas, and P. P. de Tombe, Cooperative activation in cardiac muscle: Impact of sarcomere length, *Am J Physiol Heart Circ Physiol,* 282, H1055–H1062, 2002.

81. P. P. de Tombe and H. E. ter Keurs, An internal viscous element limits unloaded velocity of sarcomere shortening in rat myocardium, *J Physiol (Lond),* 454, 619–642, 1992.

82. H. E. D. J. ter Keurs, W. H. Rijnsburger, and R. van Heuningen, Restoring forces and relaxation of rat cardiac muscle, *Eur Heart J,* 1, 67–80, 1980.

83. T. Arts, R. S. Reneman, and P. C. Veenstra, A model of the mechanics of the left ventricle, *Ann Biomed Eng,* 7, 299–318, 1979.

84. R. S. Chadwick, Mechanics of the left ventricle, *Biophys J,* 39, 279–288, 1982.

85. E. Nevo and Y. Lanir, Structural finite deformation model of the left ventricle during diastole and systole, *J Biomech Eng,* 111, 342–349, 1989.

86. T. Arts, P. C. Veenstra, and R. S. Reneman, Epicardial deformation and left ventricular wall mechanics during ejection in the dog, *Am J Physiol,* 243, H379–H390, 1982.

87. R. B. Panerai, A model of cardiac muscle mechanics and energetics, *J Biomech,* 13, 929–940, 1980.

88. A. Landesberg, V. S. Markhasin, R. Beyar, and S. Sideman, Effect of cellular inhomogeneity on cardiac tissue mechanics based on intracellular control mechanisms, *Am J Physiol,* 270, H1101–H1114, 1996.

89. A. Landesberg and S. Sideman, Coupling calcium binding to troponin C and cross-bridge cycling in skinned cardiac cells, *Am J Physiol,* 266, H1260–H1271, 1994.

90. S. P. Ma and G. I. Zahalak, A distribution-moment model of energetics in skeletal muscle [see comments], *J Biomech,* 24, 21–35, 1991.

91. F. B. Sachse, G. Seemann, K. Chaisaowong, and D. Weiss, Quantitative reconstruction of cardiac electromechanics in human myocardium: Assembly of electrophysiologic and tension generation models, *J Cardiovasc Electrophysiol,* 14, S210–S218, 2003.

92. J. J. Rice, F. Wang, D. M. Bers, and P. P. de Tombe, Approximate model of cooperative activation and crossbridge cycling in cardiac muscle using ordinary differential equations, *Biophys J,* 95, 2368–2390, 2008.

93. A. Landesberg, L. Livshitz, and H. E. Ter Keurs, The effect of sarcomere shortening velocity on force generation, analysis, and verification of models for crossbridge dynamics, *Ann Biomed Eng,* 28, 968–978, 2000.

94. S. G. Campbell, F. V. Lionetti, K. S. Campbell, and A. D. McCulloch, Coupling of adjacent tropomyosins enhances cross-bridge-mediated cooperative activation in a Markov model of the cardiac thin filament, *Biophys J,* 98, 2254–2264, 2010.

95. A. M. Gordon, E. Homsher, and M. Regnier, Regulation of contraction in striated muscle, *Physiol Rev,* 80, 853–924, 2000.

96. D. H. S. Lin and F. C. P. Yin, A multiaxial constitutive law for mammalian left ventricular myocardium in steady-state barium contracture or tetanus, *J Biomech Eng,* 120, 504–517, 1998.

97. M. Schoenberg, Geometrical factors influencing muscle force development. I. The effect of filament spacing upon axial forces, *Biophys J,* 30, 51–67, 1980.

98. G. I. Zahalak, Non-axial muscle stress and stiffness, *J Theor Biol,* 182, 59–84, 1996.

99. M. Schoenberg, Geometrical factors influencing muscle force development. II. Radial forces, *Biophys J,* 30, 69–77, 1980.

100. Y. C. Fung, *Biomechanics: Mechanical Properties of Living Tissues,* 2nd ed. New York: Springer-Verlag Inc., 1993.

101. J. G. Pinto and P. J. Patitucci, Creep in cardiac muscle, *Am J Physiol,* 232, H553–H563, 1977.

102. J. G. Pinto and P. J. Patitucci, Visco-elasticity of passive cardiac muscle, *J Biomech Eng,* 102, 57–61, 1980.

103. J. L. Emery, J. H. Omens, and A. D. McCulloch, Strain softening in rat left ventricular myocardium, *J Biomech Eng,* 119, 6–12, 1997.

104. J. L. Emery, J. H. Omens, and A. D. McCulloch, Biaxial mechanics of the passively overstretched left ventricle, *Am J Physiol,* 272, H2299–H2305, 1997.

105. L. Mullins, Effect of stretching on the properties of rubber, *J Rubber Res,* 16, 275–289, 1947.

106. H. R. Halperin, P. H. Chew, M. L. Weisfeldt, K. Sagawa, J. D. Humphrey, and F. C. P. Yin, Transverse stiffness: A method for estimation of myocardial wall stress, *Circ Res,* 61, 695–703, 1987.

107. J. D. Humphrey, R. K. Strumpf, and F. C. P. Yin, Biaxial mechanical behavior of excised ventricular epicardium, *Am J Physiol,* 259, H101–H108, 1990.

108. L. L. Demer and F. C. P. Yin, Passive biaxial mechanical properties of isolated canine myocardium, *J Physiol,* 339, 615–630, 1983.

109. F. C. P. Yin, R. K. Strumpf, P. H. Chew, and S. L. Zeger, Quantification of the mechanical properties of noncontracting canine myocardium under simultaneous biaxial loading, *J Biomech,* 20, 577–589, 1987.

110. S. Dokos, B. H. Smaill, A. A. Young, and I. J. LeGrice, Shear properties of passive ventricular myocardium, *Am J Physiol Heart Circ Physiol,* 283, H2650–H2659, 2002.

111. V. P. Novak, F. C. P. Yin, and J. D. Humphrey, Regional mechanical properties of passive myocardium, *J Biomech,* 27, 403–412, 1994.

112. J. H. Omens, D. A. MacKenna, and A. D. McCulloch, Measurement of strain and analysis of stress in resting rat left ventricular myocardium, *J Biomech,* 26, 665–676, 1993.

113. L. Glass, P. Hunter, and A. D. McCulloch, Theory of heart: Biomechanics, biophysics and nonlinear dynamics of cardiac function, in *Institute for Nonlinear Science,* H. Abarbanel, Ed. New York: Springer-Verlag, 1991.

114. J. D. Humphrey and F. C. P. Yin, A new constitutive formulation for characterizing the mechanical behavior of soft tissues, *Biophys J,* 52, 563–570, 1987.

115. I.-E. Lin and L. A. Taber, Mechanical effects of looping in the embryonic chick heart, *J Biomech,* 27, 311–321, 1994.

116. J. M. Guccione, A. D. McCulloch, and L. K. Waldman, Passive material properties of intact ventricular myocardium determined from a cylindrical model, *J Biomech Eng,* 113, 42–55, 1991.

117. J. H. Omens, D. A. MacKenna, and A. D. McCulloch, Measurement of two-dimensional strain and analysis of stress in the arrested rat left ventricle, *Adv Bioeng,* BED-20, 635–638, 1991.

118. J. D. Humphrey, R. K. Strumpf, and F. C. P. Yin, Determination of a constitutive relation for passive myocardium: I. A New functional form, *J Biomech Eng,* 112, 333–339, 1990.

119. K. B. Gupta, M. B. Ratcliff, M. A. Fallert, L. H. Edmunds, Jr, and D. K. Bogen, Changes in passive mechanical stiffness of myocardial tissue with aneurysm formation, *Circulation,* 89, 2315–2326, 1994.

120. G. A. Holzapfel and R. W. Ogden, Constitutive modelling of passive myocardium: A structurally based framework for material characterization, *Philos Transact A Math Phys Eng Sci,* 367, 3445–3475, 2009.

121. J. H. Omens and Y. C. Fung, Residual strain in rat left ventricle, *Circ Res,* 66, 37–45, 1990.

122. E. K. Rodriguez, J. H. Omens, L. K. Waldman, and A. D. McCulloch, Effect of residual stress on transmural sarcomere length distribution in rat left ventricle, *Am J Physiol,* 264, H1048–H1056, 1993.

123. K. Costa, K. May-Newman, D. Farr, W. O'Dell, A. McCulloch, and J. Omens, Three-dimensional residual strain in canine mid-anterior left ventricle, *Am J Physiol,* 273, H1968–H1976, 1997.

124. R. Skalak, G. Dasgupta, M. Moss, E. Otten, P. Dullemeijer, and H. Vilmann, Analytical description of growth, *J Theor Biol,* 94, 555–577, 1982.

125. E. K. Rodriguez, A. Hoger, and A. D. McCulloch, Stress-dependent finite growth in soft elastic tissues, *J Biomech,* 27, 455–467, 1994.

126. E. O. Feigl, G. A. Simon, and D. L. Fry, Auxotonic and isometric cardiac force transducers, *J Appl Physiol,* 23, 597–600, 1967.

127. R. M. Huisman, G. Elzinga, N. Westerhof, and P. Sipkema, Measurement of left ventricular wall stress, *Cardiovasc Res,* 14, 142–153, 1980.

128. F. C. P. Yin, Ventricular wall stress, *Circ Res,* 49, 829–842, 1981.

129. F. C. P. Yin, Applications of the finite-element method to ventricular mechanics, *CRC Crit Rev Biomed Eng,* 12, 311–342, 1985.

130. F. J. Villarreal, L. K. Waldman, and W. Y. W. Lew, Technique for measuring regional two-dimensional finite strains in canine left ventricle, *Circ Res,* 62, 711–721, 1988.

131. N. F. Osman and J. L. Prince, Visualizing myocardial function using HARP MRI, *Phys Med Biol,* 45, 1665, 2000.

132. T. Kawagishi, Speckle tracking for assessment of cardiac motion and dyssynchrony, *Echocardiography,* 25, 1167–1171, 2008.

133. N. B. Ingels, Jr, G. T. Daughters, II, E. B. Stinson, and E. L. Alderman, Measurement of midwall myocardial dynamics in intact man by radiography of surgically implanted markers, *Circulation,* 52, 859–867, 1975.

134. G. D. Meier, A. A. Bove, W. P. Santamore, and P. R. Lynch, Contractile function in canine right ventricle, *Am J Physiol,* 239, H794–H804, 1980.

135. G. D. Meier, M. C. Ziskin, W. P. Santamore, and A. A. Bove, Kinematics of the beating heart, *IEEE Trans Biomed Eng,* 27, 319–329, 1980.

136. A. D. McCulloch and J. H. Omens, Non-homogeneous analysis of three-dimensional transmural finite deformations in canine ventricular myocardium, *J Biomech,* 24, 539–548, 1991.

137. C. Leclercq, O. Faris, R. Tunin, J. Johnson, R. Kato, F. Evans, J. Spinelli, H. Halperin, E. McVeigh, and D. A. Kass, Systolic improvement and mechanical resynchronization does not require electrical synchrony in the dilated failing heart with left bundle-branch block, *Circulation,* 106, 1760–1763, 2002.

138. R. C. P. Kerckhoffs, J. Lumens, K. Vernooy, J. H. Omens, L. J. Mulligan, T. Delhaas, T. Arts, A. D. McCulloch, and F. W. Prinzen, Cardiac Resynchronization: Insight from experimental and computational models, *Progr Biophys Mol Biol,* 97, 543–561, 2008.

139. R. C. P. Kerckhoffs, J. H. Omens, A. D. McCulloch, and L. J. Mulligan, Ventricular dilation and electrical dyssynchrony synergistically increase regional mechanical non-uniformity but not mechanical dyssynchrony: A computational model, *Circulation: Heart Fail,* 3, 528–536, 2010.

140. T. P. Usyk and A. D. McCulloch, Electromechanical model of cardiac resynchronization in the dilated failing heart with left bundle branch block, *J Electrocardiol,* 36, 57–61, 2003.

141. R. C. Kerckhoffs, A. D. McCulloch, J. H. Omens, and L. J. Mulligan, Effects of biventricular pacing and scar size in a computational model of the failing heart with left bundle branch block, *Med Image Anal,* 13, 362–369, 2009.

142. V. Gurev, J. Constantino, J. J. Rice, and N. A. Trayanova, Distribution of electromechanical delay in the heart: Insights from a three-dimensional electromechanical model, 99, 745–754, 2010.

143. M. L. Neal and R. Kerckhoffs, Current progress in patient-specific modeling, *Brief Bioinform,* 11, 111–126, 2010.

144. R. C. P. Kerckhoffs, *Patient Specific Modeling of the Cardiovascular System: Technology-Driven Personalized Medicine*, New York, NY: Springer, 2010, p. 265.

145. J. Southern, J. Pitt-Francis, J. Whiteley, D. Stokeley, H. Kobashi, R. Nobes, Y. Kadooka, and D. Gavaghan, Multi-scale computational modelling in biology and physiology, *Prog Biophys Mol Biol,* 96, 60–89, 2008.

146. L. Antiga, M. Piccinelli, L. Botti, B. Ene-Iordache, A. Remuzzi, and D. Steinman, An image-based modeling framework for patient-specific computational hemodynamics, *Med Biol Eng Comput,* 46, 1097–1112, 2008.

147. I. Medugorac, Myocardial collagen in different forms of hypertrophy in the rat, *Res Exp Med (Berl),* 177, 201–211, 1980.

148. K. T. Weber, J. S. Janicki, S. G. Shroff, R. Pick, R. M. Chen, and R. I. Bashey, Collagen remodeling of the pressure-overloaded, hypertrophied nonhuman primate myocardium, *Circ Res,* 62, 757–765, 1988.

149. J. E. Jalil, C. W. Doering, J. S. Janicki, R. Pick, W. A. Clark, C. Abrahams, and K. T. Weber, Structural vs. contractile protein remodeling and myocardial stiffness in hypertrophied rat left ventricle, *J Mol Cell Cardiol,* 20, 1179–1187, 1988.

150. D. Mukherjee and S. Sen, Collagen phenotypes during development and regression of myocardial hypertrophy in spontaneously hypertensive rats, *Circ Res,* 67, 1474–1480, 1990.

151. J. Harper, E. Harper, and J. W. Covell, Collagen characterization in volume-overload- and pressure-overload-induced cardiac hypertrophy in minipigs, *Am J Physiol,* 265, H434–H438, 1993.

152. J. H. Omens, D. E. Milkes, and J. W. Covell, Effects of pressure overload on the passive mechanics of the rat left ventricle, *Ann Biomed Eng,* 23, 152–163, 1995.

153. F. Contard, V. Koteliansky, F. Marotte, I. Dubus, L. Rappaport, and J. L. Samuel, Specific alterations in the distribution of extracellular matrix components within rat myocardium during the development of pressure overload, *Lab Invest,* 64, 65–75, 1991.

154. M. A. Silver, R. Pick, C. G. Brilla, J. E. Jalil, J. S. Janicki, and K. T. Weber, Reactive and reparative fibrillar collagen remodelling in the hypertrophied rat left ventricle: Two experimental models of myocardial fibrosis, *Cardiovasc Res,* 24, 741–747, 1990.

155. J. B. Michel, J. L. Salzmann, M. Ossondo Nlom, P. Bruneval, D. Barres, and J. P. Camilleri, Morphometric analysis of collagen network and plasma perfused capillary bed in the myocardium of rats during evolution of cardiac hypertrophy, *Basic Res Cardiol,* 81, 142–154, 1986.

156. D. S. Iimoto, J. W. Covell, and E. Harper, Increase in crosslinking of type I and type III collagens associated with volume overload hypertrophy, *Circ Res,* 63, 399–408, 1988.

157. K. T. Weber, R. Pick, M. A. Silver, G. W. Moe, J. S. Janicki, I. H. Zucker, and P. W. Armstrong, Fibrillar collagen and remodeling of dilated canine left ventricle, *Circulation,* 82, 1387–401, 1990.

158. W. J. Corin, T. Murakami, E. S. Monrad, O. M. Hess, and H. P. Krayenbuehl, Left ventricular passive diastolic properties in chronic mitral regurgitation, *Circulation,* 83, 97–807, 1991.

159. P. Whittaker, D. R. Boughner, R. A. Kloner, and K. Przyklenk, Stunned myocardium and myocardial collagen damage: Differential effects of single and repeated occlusions, *Am Heart J,* 121, 434–441, 1991.

160. M. Zhao, H. Zhang, T. F. Robinson, S. M. Factor, E. H. Sonnenblick, and C. Eng, Profound structural alterations of the extracellular collagen matrix in postischemic dysfunctional (stunned) but viable myocardium, *J Am Coll Cardiol,* 10, 1322–1334, 1987.

161. J. S. Forrester, G. Diamond, W. W. Parmley, and H. J. C. Swan, Early increase in left ventricular compliance after myocardial infarction, *J Clin Invest,* 51, 598–603, 1972.

162. F. A. Pirzada, E. A. Ekong, P. S. Vokonas, C. S. Apstein, and W. B. Hood, Jr, Experimental myocardial infarction XIII. Sequential changes in left ventricular pressure-length relationships in the acute phase, *Circulation,* 53, 970–975, 1976.

163. S. Takahashi, A. C. Barry, and S. M. Factor, Collagen degradation in ischaemic rat hearts, *Biochem J,* 265, 233–241, 1990.

164. R. H. Charney, S. Takahashi, M. Zhao, E. H. Sonnenblick, and C. Eng, Collagen loss in the stunned myocardium, *Circulation,* 85, 1483–1490, 1992.

165. C. M. Connelly, W. M. Vogel, A. W. Wiegner, E. L. Osmers, O. H. Bing, R. A. Kloner, D. M. Dunn-Lanchantin, C. Franzblau, and C. S. Apstein, Effects of reperfusion after coronary artery occlusion on post-infarction scar tissue, *Circ Res,* 57, 562–77, 1985.

166. B. I. Jugdutt and R. W. Amy, Healing after myocardial infarction in the dog: Changes in infarct hydroxyproline and topography, *J Am Coll Cardiol,* 7, 91–102, 1986.

167. P. Whittaker, D. R. Boughner, and R. A. Kloner, Analysis of healing after myocardial infarction using polarized light microscopy, *Am J Pathol,* 134, 879–893, 1989.

168. L. T. Jensen, K. Hørslev-Petersen, P. Toft, K. D. Bentsen, P. Grande, E. E. Simonsen, and I. Lorenzen, Serum aminoterminal type III procollagen peptide reflects repair after acute myocardial infarction, *Circulation,* 81, 52–57, 1990.

169. J. M. Pfeffer, M. A. Pfeffer, P. J. Fletcher, and E. Braunwald, Progressive ventricular remodeling in rat with myocardial infarction, *Am J Physiol,* 260, H1406–H1414, 1991.

170. P. Whittaker, D. R. Boughner, and R. A. Kloner, Role of collagen in acute myocardial infarct expansion, *Circulation,* 84, 2123–2134, 1991.

171. J. W. Holmes, H. Yamashita, L. K. Waldman, and J. W. Covell, Scar remodeling and transmural deformation after infarction in the pig, *Circulation,* 90, 411–420, 1994.

172. M. Eghbali, T. F. Robinson, S. Seifter, and O. O. Blumenfeld, Collagen accumulation in heart ventricles as a function of growth and aging, *Cardiovasc Res,* 23, 723–729, 1989.

173. I. Medugorac and R. Jacob, Characterisation of left ventricular collagen in the rat, *Cardiovasc Res,* 17, 15–21, 1983.

174. T. K. Borg, W. F. Ranson, F. A. Moslehy, and J. B. Caulfield, Structural basis of ventricular stiffness, *Lab Invest,* 44, 49–54, 1981.

175. P. Anversa, E. Puntillo, P. Nikitin, G. Olivetti, J. M. Capasso, and E. H. Sonnenblick, Effects of age on mechanical and structural properties of myocardium of Fischer 344 rats, *Am J Physiol,* 256, H1440–H1449, 1989.

176. S. G. Campbell, *The Role of Regulatory Light Chain Phosphorylation in Left Ventricular Function,* La Jolla, CA: University of California San Diego, 2010, p. 215.

177. J. Ross Jr, E. H. Sonnenblick, J. W. Covell, G. A. Kaiser, and D. Spiro, The architecture of the heart in systole and diastole: Technique of rapid fixation and analysis of left ventricular geometry, *Circ Res,* 21, 409–421, 1967.

178. W. Grossman, Cardiac hypertrophy: Useful adaptation or pathologic process? *Am J Med,* 69, 576–583, 1980.

179. W. Grossman, D. Jones, and L. P. McLaurin, Wall stress and patterns of hypertrophy in the human left ventricle, *J Clin Invest,* 56, 56–64, 1975.

180. R. H. Charney, S. Takahashi, M. Zhao, E. H. Sonnenblick, and C. Eng, Collagen loss in the stunned myocardium, *Circulation,* 85, 1483–1490, 1992.

181. S. A. Niederer, P. J. Hunter, and N. P. Smith, A quantitative analysis of cardiac myocyte relaxation: A simulation study, *Biophys J* 90, 1697–722, 2000.

9

Heart Valve Dynamics

Choon Hwai Yap
Georgia Institute of Technology

Erin Spinner
Georgia Institute of Technology

Muralidhar Padala
Emory University School of Medicine

Ajit P. Yoganathan
Georgia Institute of Technology

9.1 Introduction

The heart has four valves (Figure 9.1), which maintain unidirectional blood flow through the heart. They are classified as atrioventricular valves or semilunar valves, depending on their location. The atrioventricular valves are the tricuspid and mitral valves, and the semilunar valves are the pulmonary and aortic valves. The atrioventricular valves control the blood flow entering the ventricles from the atria, and the semilunar valves maintain forward flow from the ventricles to the lungs or distal organs. On the right side of the heart, the tricuspid valve (TV) controls the flow of deoxygenated blood from the right atrium into the right ventricle, and the pulmonary valve maintains forward flow from the right ventricle into the lungs. On the left side, the mitral valve (MV) controls the flow of oxygenated blood from the left atrium into the left ventricle, and the aortic valve maintains forward flow from the left ventricle to the distal organs.

Heart valve function is primarily governed by the pressure gradients across the valves during different cardiac phases, although other active mechanisms have been implicated. During diastole, the ventricular filling phase, the mitral and tricuspid valves open due to higher atrial pressure than the pressure in the relaxed ventricle, thus allowing diastolic filling of both the ventricles. The aortic and pulmonary valves are closed in this phase due to higher pressure in the aorta and pulmonary artery, respectively. Next, as the ventricles contract, ventricular pressure builds up, reaching first the pressure required for closing the atrioventricular valves, and then the pressure required to open the semilunar valves. The period of build up between these two pressures is the isovolumetric contraction phase, where all four valves are closed. During systole, high pressures in the ventricles open the aortic and pulmonary valves, allowing ejection of blood into the arterial tree and the lungs, respectively. Following this, the ventricles relax, reducing pressures, first, to that slightly lower than in the arteries, when the semilunar valves close, and then second, to that slightly lower than that in the atria, when the atrioventricular valves open. The period of reduction of pressures between these two points is known as the isovolumetric

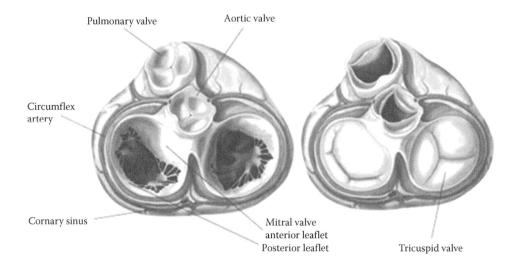

FIGURE 9.1   Superior, short-axis view of the heart showing the heart valves and their anatomies.

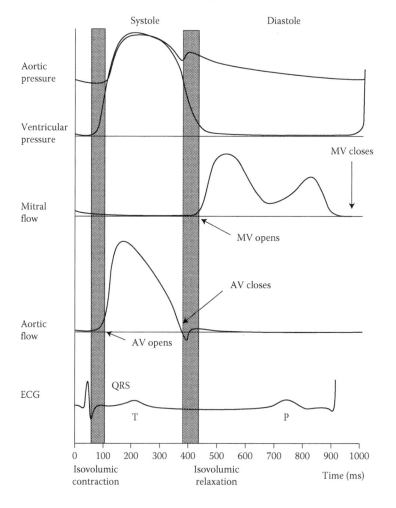

FIGURE 9.2   Typical pressure and flow curve for aortic and mitral valve.

relaxation, when, again, all four valves are closed. The typical pressure and flow curves and the relative durations of all the phases in the cardiac cycle for the aortic and mitral valves are shown in Figure 9.2.

When closed, the pulmonic and tricuspid valves withstand a pressure of approximately 30 mmHg. The closing pressures on the left side of the heart are much higher. The aortic valve withstands pressures of approximately 100 mmHg, while the MV closes against pressures up to 150 mmHg. Diseases of the valves are more prevalent on the left side of the heart than the right side (Lloyd-Jones et al., 2010).

9.2 Aortic Valve

9.2.1 Valve Structure

9.2.1.1 Anatomy

The aortic valve is composed of three semilunar cusps, or leaflets, within the aortic root, which is the base of the aorta abutting the heart. The inferior base of the leaflet is connected to the annulus, which is a fibrous ring embedded in the fibers of the ventricular septum and the anterior leaflet of the MV. The superior base of the leaflet is connected to the valve commissure. The annulus of the aortic valve separates the aorta from the left ventricle, and superior to this ring are bulges in the wall known as the sinuses of Valsalva, or aortic sinuses. Each bulge is aligned with the center of a specific valve leaflet, and the valve leaflets and corresponding sinuses are named according to their anatomical location. The top of the sinus, where it transitions to the tube-like ascending aorta, is termed the sino-tubular junction, and the portion of the aorta between the aortic valve annulus and the sino-tubular junction is known as the aortic root. Two of the aortic sinuses give rise to coronary arteries that branch off the aorta, providing blood flow to the heart itself. The right coronary artery is based at the right or right anterior sinus, the left coronary artery exits the left or left posterior sinus, and the third sinus is called the noncoronary or right posterior sinus. The coronary orifice on the walls of the aortic root has been reported to exhibit variability in location, with a substantial proportion of people having the orifice at or above the sino-tubular junction instead of within the sinus (Muriago et al., 1997). The three valve leaflets are named left coronary leaflet, right coronary leaflet, and noncoronary leaflet due to their anatomical association with the left sinus, the right sinus, and the posterior sinus, and according to the presence or absence of coronaries ostia behind them. Figure 9.3 also shows the configuration of the normal aortic sinuses and valve in the closed position, as well as the average dimensions of various structures in the aortic root, measured from molds of human samples.

The leaflets of the aortic valve show variable dimensions. The posterior leaflet tends to be thicker, have a larger surface area, and weigh more than the right or left coronary leaflets (Silver and Roberts, 1985, Sahasakul et al., 1988), and the average width of the right coronary leaflet is greater than that of the other two (Vollebergh and Becker, 1977). Because the lengths of the aortic valve leaflets are greater than the annular radius, a small overlap of tissue from each leaflet protrudes and forms a coaptation surface within the aorta when the valve is closed (Emery and Arom, 1991). This overlapped tissue, called the lunula, helps to ensure that the valve is sealed.

Each of the aortic valve leaflets is lined with endothelial cells and is composed of collagen, elastin, proteoglycans, protein, polysaccharides, and interstitial cells in a three-layered structure (Figure 9.4). The layer facing the aorta is termed the fibrosa and is the major fibrous layer within the leaflet, and consists mainly of trunk collagen bundle chords in the circumferential direction, interlaced with radially aligned elastin fibers (Vesely and Lozon, 1993). The layer covering the ventricular side of the valve is a thin layer called the ventricularis and is composed of elastin fibers interspersed with some collagen. The ventricularis presents a very smooth surface to the flow of blood (Christie, 1992), while the fibrosa surface is visibly undulating under the microscope. The central portion of the valve, called the spongiosa, contains variable loose connective tissue and proteins, has reduced amount of protein fibers, and is normally not vascularized. It is thought that the semifluid nature of the spongiosa provides the valve leaflet with deformability, allowing the exterior layers of fibers to slide over each other during bending and stretching. Further, the spongiosa layer provides damping to the leaflets to avoid deformation

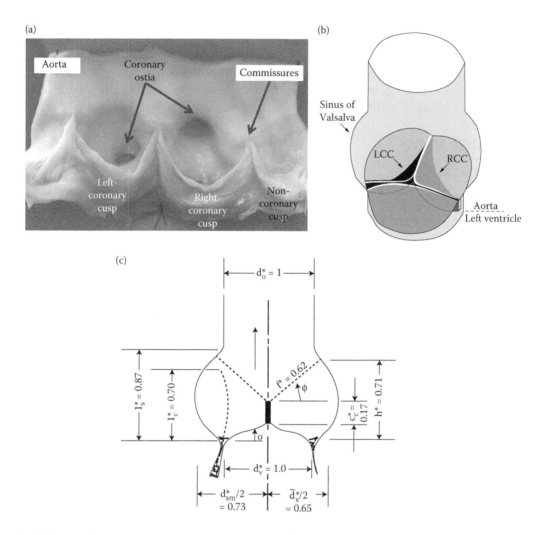

FIGURE 9.3 (a) An excised porcine aortic valve showing (from left to right) the left coronary, right coronary, and noncoronary cusps. The sinuses of Valsalva and the ostia leading to the coronary arteries are also visible. (b) The aortic sinus and valve in the closed position. (c) Dimensions of the aortic valve measured from mold of human samples, expressed as ratios of the outflow tract annulus diameter. (Adapted from Swanson, M. and Clark, R. E. 1974. *Circ Res*, 35, 871–882.)

oscillations (Grande-Allen et al., 2001, 2003, 2007). The collagen fibers within the fibrosa and ventricularis are unorganized in the unstressed state, but when a stress is applied, they become oriented primarily in the circumferential (or width) direction (Christie, 1992, Thubrikar, 1990). The amount of transvalvular pressure required to align the collagen fibers from the relaxed state has been reported to be as low as 1 mmHg (Sacks et al., 1998).

9.2.1.2 Mechanical Properties

Like most biological tissues, the aortic valve leaflets are anisotropic, inhomogeneous, and viscoelastic. The collagen fibers within each leaflet are mostly aligned along the circumferential direction. Vesely and Noseworthy found that both the ventricularis and fibrosa were stiffer in the circumferential direction than in the radial direction (Vesely and Noseworthy, 1992). However, the ventricularis was more extensible radially than circumferentially while the fibrosa had uniform extensibility

(a)   (b)

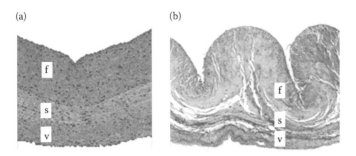

FIGURE 9.4 (a) H&E stain of a cross section of the aortic valve. (Adapted from Hilbert, S. L. et al. 1999. *J Thorac Cardiovasc Surg*, 117, 454–462.) (b) Movat Pentachrome stain of a cross section of the aortic valve showing the three distinct layers with different composition. "f," "s," and "v" indicate fibrosa, spongiosa, and ventricularis, respectively. (Adapted from Schenke-Layland, K. et al. 2009. *Eur Heart J*, 30, 2254–2265.)

in both directions. Elastin fibers are present at a lesser concentration than collagen and are mostly oriented radially. This fiber structure accounts for the anisotropic properties of the valve. The variation in thickness and composition across the leaflets is responsible for their inhomogeneous material properties. Although the aortic valve leaflet as a whole is asymmetric in its distensibility, the basal region tends to be relatively isotropic while the central region shows the greatest degree of anisotropy (Lo and Vesely, 1995). Scott and Vesely (1996) have shown that the elastin in the ventricularis consists of continuous amorphous sheets or compact meshes while elastin in the fibrosa consists of complex arrays of large tubes that extend circumferentially across the leaflet. These tubes may surround the large circumferential collagen bundles in the fibrosa. Mechanical testing of elastin structures from the fibrosa and ventricularis separately have shown that the purpose of elastin in the aortic valve leaflet is to maintain a specific collagen fiber configuration and return the fibers to that state during cyclic loading (Vesely, 1998).

Billiar et al. tested porcine aortic valve leaflets and found that their response curve was similar to those of collagen fibers, with an exponential increase in stress with strain (Billiar and Sacks, 2000). With increasing stress, the leaflets exhibit three distinct responses consecutively, starting a low-stiffness "toe" region, moving on to a transitional "heel" region, and a high-stiffness "linear" region (Figure 9.5). This is in accordance to the fiber architecture of the valve leaflet: the "toe" region represents the uncrimping of the collagen fiber curls and the elastic response of elastins, while the "linear" region represents the stretching of already straightened collagen fibers (Sacks et al., 1998). As expected, the leaflet as a whole was found to have higher stiffness in the circumferential direction than in the radial direction. Further, dynamic testing has revealed that at physiological loading rates, the leaflet material behaves elastically although the leaflets are viscoelastic in nature (Doehring et al., 2004, Stella et al., 2007). The leaflet is capable of undergoing large, rapid anisotropic strains in response to transvalvular pressures and return to its original configuration when unloaded with little hysteresis and creep, leading to its association with the term "quasi-elastic." Performing engineering analysis of the valve structures, Christie et al. concluded that stress in the leaflets in the circumferential direction is the primary load-bearing element, which is in line with the presence of collagen fiber bundles oriented circumferentially (Christie, 1992). Radial stress was found to be small compared to circumferential stress in the closed valve.

In addition to the collagen and elastin, clusters of lipids have been observed in the central spongiosa of porcine aortic valves. Vesely et al. (1994) have shown that the lipids tend to be concentrated at the base of the valve leaflets while the coaptation regions and free edges of the leaflets tend to be devoid of these lipids. In addition, the spatial distribution of the lipids within the spongiosa layer of the aortic leaflets corresponds to areas in which calcification is commonly observed on bioprosthetic valves, suggesting

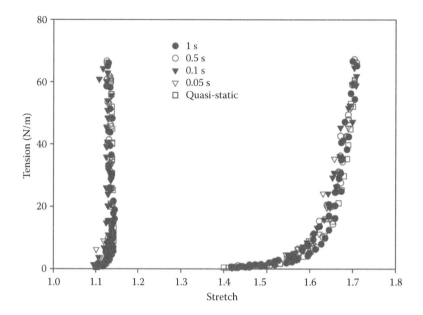

FIGURE 9.5 Mechanical response of fresh aortic valve leaflet to equi-biaxial stress at different loading rates, demonstrating the anisotropy of the tissue as well as the insensitivity of the tissue to loading rates. (Adapted from Stella, J. A., Liao, J., and Sacks, M. S. 2007. *J Biomech*, 40, 3169–3177.)

that these lipid clusters may be potential nucleation sites for calcification. In contrast, pulmonic leaflets showed a substantially lower incidence of lipids (Dunmore-Buyze et al., 1995).

9.2.2 Valve Function

9.2.2.1 Aortic Root Dynamics

During the cardiac cycle, the heart undergoes translation and rotation due to its own contraction pattern. As a result, the base of the aortic valve varies in size and also translates and twists. The dynamics of the aortic root are a result of the combination of passive response to pressures on both sides of the valve as well as active contractions of the muscular shelf on the anterio-medial segment of the annulus. Using marker fluoroscopy in sheeps, Dagum et al. (1999) characterized the aortic root motion. During isovolumetric contraction, the annulus and sino-tubular junction undergo rapid circumferential expansion and the aortic root increases in longitudinal length without shear or torsion. During the ejection phase, the annulus undergoes circumferential contraction whereas the sino-tubular junction continues to expand, and the aortic root undergoes nonuniform shearing, which results in torsional deformation. During the isovolumetric contraction, the aortic root undergoes further circumferential contraction at both the annulus and the sino-tubular junction, and experiences further shearing and torsional deformation, as well as longitudinal compression. During early diastole, the annulus and sino-tubular junction recoils from its dynamically loaded configuration by expanding, and the root is elongated and untwisted from its motion during the other phases. Torsional deformation has been described to be nonuniform over the three sinus segments.

9.2.2.2 Valve Leaflet Dynamics

The systolic motion of the aortic valve can be described in three phases: the rapid opening phase, the slow closing phase, and the rapid closing phase. The rapid opening phase lasts for about 60 ms, when leaflets rapidly open at an average speed of 20 cm/s, the valve opens to the fullest extent, and blood accelerates through the valve. The slow closing phase, which lasts for 330 ms, is when the bulk of ejection occurs, and valve leaflets move approximately 13 mm. The rapid closing phase occurs during late systole, lasts for 40 ms, and witnesses leaflet speed of 26 cm/s (Leyh et al., 1999).

Earlier experiments in measuring the physiologic deformations of the aortic valve leaflets involve using marker fluoroscopy, in which the aortic valve leaflets were surgically tagged with radio-opaque markers and imaged with high-speed x-rays (Thubrikar, 1990). The leaflets were found to be longer during diastole than systole in both the radial and circumferential direction, as is expected due to the high transvalvular pressure across the closed aortic valve stretching the leaflets. Yap et al. (2010) characterized the deformational dynamics of the aortic valve leaflets *in vitro* at high spatial and temporal resolution, and showed the average diastolic stretch ratio of the valve to be 15–18% in the circumferential direction and 45–54% in the radial direction at the base and belly regions of the valve. It was found during diastole that the leaflets rapidly load up to the peak stretch ratios, and plateau at approximately the same stretch ratio until the rapid unloading phase at the end of diastole. During systole, however, the valve stretches slightly in the radial direction (to a lesser extent than during diastole) due to drag forces induced by forward flow, and it compresses slightly in the circumferential direction due to Poisson's effect of radial stretch. It has been reasoned that the stretching of the valve leaflets during diastole is useful in allowing leaflets to come together and achieving proper coaptation, and that the shortening of the leaflets during systole reduces obstruction of the aorta during the ejection of blood (Christie, 1992).

Drastic changes in the valve area described above are results of the valve reacting to the stresses in a passive manner. It is currently unclear if active contractions of aortic valve cells play a role in the deformation dynamics of the leaflets. Active contractions of aortic valve cells have been studied and were found to be able to impart very small forces at physiological biochemical stimulations (Kershaw et al., 2004). On the other hand, stimulants such as serotonin and endothelin were found to alter the stiffness of valve leaflets at the posttransitional zone of the response curve (high-stiffness zone) significantly (El-Hamamsy et al., 2009). It is unclear if the stiffness of the pretransitional zone (low-stiffness zone) is altered, which is the main determinant of the amount of stretch suffered by the leaflets under physiologic loads. Active cell contraction has also been observed to impart additional bending stiffness to the valve leaflet (Merryman et al., 2006). This is an important consideration because the aortic valve leaflet experiences substantial bending during the cardiac cycle: valve leaflet is convex curved toward the ventricle during diastole and curved toward the sinus when open, with the base of the valve leaflet bent to allow the opening. It is hypothesized that leaflet cell contractions is a regulatory mechanism of leaflet kinematics, and biochemical cues are used to control leaflet stiffness tone to influence function.

9.2.2.3 Valve Fluid Dynamics

During the fast opening phase of the valve leaflet, blood is rapidly accelerating through the valve, and peak velocity is reached during the first third of systole. Thereafter, flow begins to decelerate to zero at the end of systole under adverse pressure gradient. The adverse pressure gradient that is developed affects the low momentum fluid near the wall of the aorta more than that at the center; this causes reverse flow into the sinus region (Reul and Talukdar, 1979). The systolic pressure gradient required to accelerate blood through the aortic valve is on the order of a few millimeters of mercury. However, the diastolic pressure difference reaches 80 mmHg across the closed valve in normal individuals.

The aortic valve closes during the end of systole with very little reverse flow through the valve, estimated to be about 2.6 mL per beat (Erasmi et al., 2005). This is often attributed to the influence of the vortical flow in the sinuses behind the leaflets, which is induced by forward flow through the valve during systole. The function of these vortices was first described by Leonardo da Vinci in 1513, and they have been extensively investigated primarily through the use of *in vitro* models (Bellhouse and Reid, 1969, Reul and Talukdar, 1979). More recently, phase contrast magnetic resonance imaging velocity measurements have provided evidence of their presence in humans, as shown in Figure 9.6 (Kvitting et al., 2004, Markl et al., 2005). It has been hypothesized that these vortices create a transverse pressure

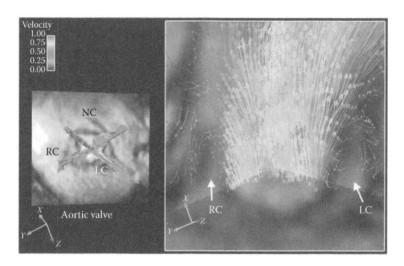

FIGURE 9.6 Three-directional velocity vectors along two-dimensional planes, showing the vortices in the right and left coronary sinuses, obtained through phase contrast magnetic resonance imaging of a healthy subject. (From Markl, M. et al. 2005. *J Thorac Cardiovasc Surg*, 130, 456–463.)

difference that pushes the leaflets toward the center of the aorta and each other at the end of systole, thereby helping with the valve closing process and minimizing regurgitation of blood. However, *in vitro* work showed that the axial pressure difference alone is enough to close the valve (Reul and Talukdar, 1979). Without the sinus vortices, the valve still closes, but the closure is not as quick as when the vortices are present, and the velocity of the leaflet closure motion is not as rapid (Leyh et al., 1999).

The parameters that describe the normal blood flow through the aortic valve are the velocity profile, time course of the blood velocity or flow, and magnitude of the peak velocity. These are influenced in part by the pressure difference between the ventricle and aorta and by the geometry of the aortic valve complex. As seen in Figure 9.7, the velocity profile at the level of the aortic valve annulus is relatively flat. However, there is usually a slight skew toward the septal wall (less than 10% of the center-line velocity), which is caused by the orientation of the aortic valve relative to the long axis of the left ventricle. This skew in the velocity profile has been shown by many experimental techniques, including hot film anemometry, Doppler ultrasound and magnetic resonance imaging (MRI) (Paulsen and Hasenkam, 1983, Rossvoll et al., 1991, Kilner et al., 1993, Sloth et al., 1994). In healthy individuals, blood flows through the aortic valve at the beginning of systole and then rapidly accelerates to its peak value of 1.35 ± 0.35 m/s. For children, this value is slightly higher at 1.5 ± 0.3 m/s (Hatle and Angelsen, 1985). Highly skewed velocity profiles and corresponding helical flow patterns have been observed in the human aortic arch using magnetic resonance phase velocity mapping (Kilner et al., 1993, Markl et al., 2005). The flow patterns just downstream of the aortic valve are of particular interest because of their complexity and relation to valvular and arterial disease. *In vitro* laser Doppler anemometry experiments have shown that these flow patterns are dependent on the valve geometry and thus can be used to evaluate function and performance of the heart valve (Sung and Yoganathan, 1990a).

9.2.3 Valve Disease and Treatment

Diseases of the aortic valve include stenosis, where the valve orifice is narrowed to obstruct blood ejection, and regurgitation, where blood leaks back into the ventricle after valve closure. The leading cause of aortic valve stenosis is the degenerative calcification of the valve leaflets, characterized by lipid accumulation, inflammation, and mineralization. The morphology of such lesions are mostly similar to

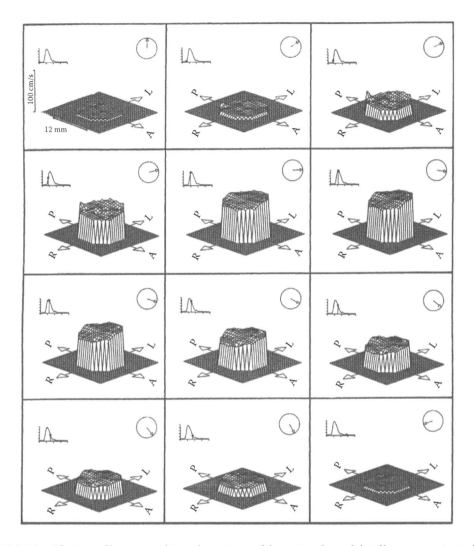

FIGURE 9.7 Velocity profiles measured 2 cm downstream of the aortic valve with hot film anemometry in dogs. The marker on the aortic flow curve shows the timing of the measurements during the cardiac cycle. (From Paulsen, P.K. and Hansenkam, J.M. 1983. *J Biomech.* 16:201–210. With permission.)

that of atherosclerosis, and the two diseases share several common risk factors (Freeman and Otto, 2005), including age, gender, diabetes, hypercholesterolemia, hypertension, rheumatic fever, and congenital malformations such as bicuspid or unicuspid aortic valve (Stewart et al., 1997, Ward, 2000). Rheumatic fever causes scar formation on the valve leaflets, which can independently lead to stenosis, and the scarred surface serves as a calcification site, leading to worsening stenosis. Rheumatic fever is the leading cause of calcific aortic stenosis. Fortunately, in developed countries, the incidences of rheumatic fever have decreased tremendously, and its prevalence is limited to undeveloped countries (Sliwa and Mocumbi, 2010, Lloyd-Jones et al., 2010). Recent studies have shown that the valve responds to mechanical forces and that certain mechanical environment can elicit pathological expressions consistent with native valve degeneration (Butcher et al., 2008). Calcification on the valve leaflet demonstrates specific patterns in most cases. These patterns include calcification only on the aortic surface, along the coaptation line, and at the base of the leaflet (Thubrikar et al., 1986). These patterns have led authors to hypothesize that tissue stress fatigue, such as bending, plays a role in the development of the disease.

The bicuspid aortic valve is a congenital malformation that occurs in 1–2% of the population (Roberts, 1970). This type of valve is highly predisposed to calcification with 50% of aortic stenosis patients having bicuspid aortic valves (Ward, 2000). The predisposition to calcification has been shown to be related to an underlying genetic defect (Garg et al., 2005). However, it is argued that the drastic alteration of geometry and thus mechanical environment in the bicuspid aortic valve is in part responsible for calcification (Robicsek et al., 2004).

Aortic regurgitation may be caused by valve disease or aortic root anomaly. It is commonly associated with aortic stenosis, rheumatic fever, and ascending aorta dilation as seen in patients with bicuspid aortic valve and Marfan syndrome (Tsifansky et al., 2010). The prolapse or the mal-coaptation of the valve is often responsible for regurgitation.

Aortic valve regurgitation is treated with either valve repair or replacement with prosthetic valves, but aortic valve stenosis is typically treated with the replacement of the valve with prosthetic valves due to tissue degeneration. Several prosthetic aortic valve designs are currently available, including fixed xenograft bioprosthetics and mechanical heart valves. These valves however are prone to failure over time, either due to blood damage induced by mechanical valves, or due to structural failure or calcification of xenographic bioprosthetic valves. Tissue engineering of valves appears to be a promising strategy to developing an ideal replacement valves; however, current technology needs to evolve before these valves can be clinically used.

9.3 Pulmonary Valve

9.3.1 Valve Structure

9.3.1.1 Anatomy

The anatomy of the pulmonary valve is similar to that of the aortic valve but the surrounding structure is slightly different. The main differences are that the sinuses are smaller in the pulmonary artery, the pulmonary valve annulus is slightly larger than that of the aortic valve, and the pulmonary valve annulus is entirely muscular in nature while the aortic valve annulus has a fibrous membrane segment where it abuts the MV. An examination of 160 pathologic specimens revealed the aortic valve diameter to be 23.2 ± 3.3 mm, whereas the diameter of the pulmonary valve was measured at 24.3 ± 3.0 mm (Westaby et al., 1984). On average, pulmonary valve leaflets are thinner than aortic valve leaflets: 0.49 mm versus 0.67 mm (Davies, 1980).

The pulmonary valve leaflets have the same structure as that of the aortic valve. The leaflet is composed of three layers, the fibrosa, spongiosa, and ventricularis, with similar composition in each layer (Rabkin-Aikawa et al., 2004), as shown in Figure 9.8. The pulmonary valve has been used as an autograft replacement

(a)   (b)

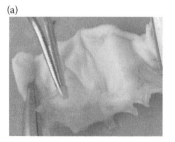
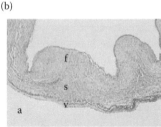

FIGURE 9.8   (a) The fixed pulmonary valve demonstrating the similar valve anatomy to that of the aortic valve. (Adapted from Godart, F. et al. 2009. *J Thorac Cardiovasc Surg*, 137, 1141–1145.) (b) Movat Pentachrom stain of the pulmonary valve leaflet, showing that the three-layered microstructure of the valve similar to that of the aortic valve. (Adapted from Rabkin-Aikawa, E. et al. 2004. *J Thorac Cardiovasc Surg*, 128, 552–561.)

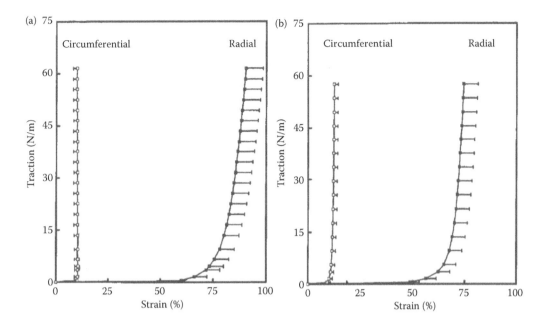

FIGURE 9.9 The mechanical properties of fresh pulmonic valve leaflet (a) versus the aortic valve leaflet (b), from equi-biaxial stress mechanical tests. (Adapted from Christie, G. W. and Barratt-Boyes, B. G. 1995. *Ann Thorac Surg*, 60, S195–S199.)

valve for diseased aortic valve, especially in children, since the valve will remain alive and grows with the patient (Takkenberg et al., 2009). This procedure is commonly known as the Ross procedure after its inventor, and studies on the pulmonary valve is often motivated by this potential use of the valve.

9.3.1.2 Valve Mechanical Properties

The pulmonic valve leaflet has similar mechanical properties as the aortic valve, as shown in Figure 9.9. While the pulmonic valve leaflet is less stiff than the aortic valve in the radial direction, its circumferential direction stiffness is similar to that of the aortic valve, indicating a more pronounced anisotropy (Christie and Barratt-Boyes, 1995). However, the pulmonic valve leaflet has similar extensibilities as the aortic valve leaflet, as well as similar viscoelastic material parameters (Leeson-Dietrich et al., 1995).

9.3.2 Valve Function

9.3.2.1 Valve Dynamics

The pulmonary valve flow behaves similarly to that of the aortic valve but the magnitude of the velocity is smaller. Typical peak velocities for healthy adults are 0.75 ± 0.15 m/s and for children are 0.9 ± 0.2 m/s (Weyman, 1994). As seen in Figure 9.10, a rotation of the peak velocity can be observed in the pulmonary artery velocity profile. During acceleration, the peak velocity is observed inferiorly with the peak rotating counterclockwise throughout the remainder of the ejection phase (Sloth et al., 1994). The mean spatial profile is relatively flat, although there is a region of reverse flow that occurs in late systole, which may be representative of flow separation. Typically, there is only a slight skew in the profile. The peak velocity is generally within 20% of the spatial mean throughout the cardiac cycle. The pulmonary valve is also distinct from the aortic valve in terms of its downstream geometry. The main pulmonary artery splits into the left and right pulmonary artery approximately 5 cm from the pulmonary aortic root, and secondary flow patterns can also be observed in the pulmonary artery and its bifurcation (Sung and Yoganathan, 1990b).

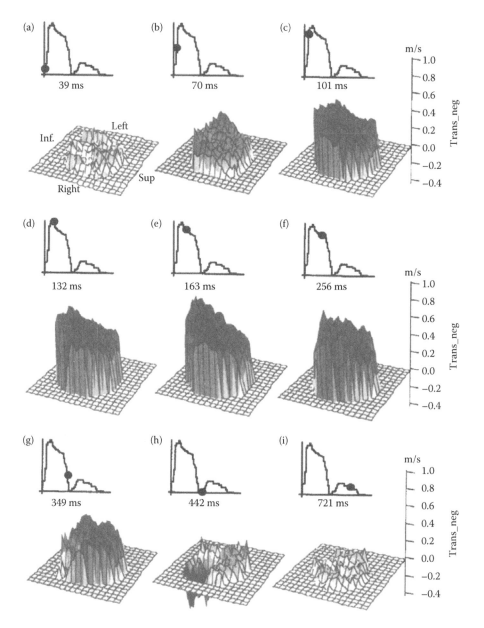

FIGURE 9.10 Velocity profiles downstream of the human pulmonary valve obtained with magnetic resonance phase velocity mapping. The timing of the measurements is shown by the marker on the flow curve. (From Sloth, E. et al. 1994. *Am Heart J.* 128:1130–1138. With permission.)

9.4 Mitral Valve

9.4.1 Valve Structure

9.4.1.1 Anatomy

The MV has a complex geometric structure, with a fibromuscular mitral annulus at the base of the left atrium, two collagenous leaflets, several chordae tendineae, and two papillary muscles (PMs) that emerge from the left ventricular myocardium. Normal MV function requires interplay between the valve's four main components, shown in Figure 9.11. A fibromuscular atrioventricular ring forms the base of the MV at the junction of the left atrium and the left ventricle, with a veil of tissue attached to it along its circumference, which form the mitral leaflets. Fibrous chordae tendineae extend from the ventricular surface of the two leaflets, and extend apically toward the PMs in the left ventricle. These chordae follow a pattern of insertion, such that the leaflets assume an optimal systolic configuration that

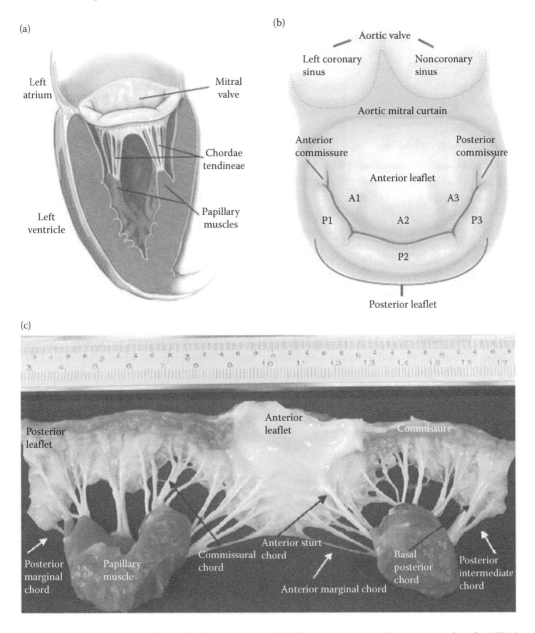

FIGURE 9.11 (a) Schematic of mitral valve structure with different components that constitute the valve. (b) The mitral valve leaflets as located in reference to the aortic valve leaflets with specific distinction between the leaflet cusps. (c) Chordal insertion pattern in an excised porcine mitral valve, depicting the segregation of chordae into primary chordae (inserting into the free edge), secondary (inserting into the base of the leaflet), and tertiary (inserting into the annulus at the commissures).

ensures complete valve competence. Two PMs, antero-lateral and postero-medial, are myocardial structures that extend into the left ventricular cavity (Kalmanson, 1976). Vasculature from the ventricular muscle richly perfuses the PMs, and ensures their contractility during systole.

9.4.1.1.1 Mitral Annulus

The mitral annulus is the anatomical junction between the left atrium and the left ventricle, and serves as the basal insertion site for the MV leaflets. It is an elliptical ring composed of dense collagenous tissue surrounded by muscle. The anterior portion of the annulus is continuous with the base of the noncoronary and left coronary leaflets of the aortic valve. The extremities of this anterior annular section are clearly demarcated by two fibrous protrusions called trigones, from which tendon-like structures extend dorsally along half of the mitral annular ring. The posterior part of the annulus is a nebulous fibrous ring that is not as visually distinct as the anterior annulus. The MV annulus has a three-dimensional saddle shape and is not planar, and dynamically changes its shape over the cardiac cycle (Levine et al., 1987, Glasson et al., 1996).

9.4.1.1.2 Mitral Valve Leaflets

The MV consists of a continuous veil of tissue inserted around the entire circumference of the mitral orifice, which is distinguished into the anterior leaflet and the posterior leaflet. The anterior leaflet has a triangular structure and attaches to the mitral annulus between the trigones, with the greatest leaflet height at the free edge as shown in Figure 9.11. The basal portion of the leaflet is continuous with the aorto-mitral curtain along the noncoronary and left coronary aortic leaflets, while the apical portion of the leaflet forms the free edge of the leaflet that aids coaptation. The posterior leaflet on the other hand covers the entire circumference from one commissure to the other, covering three-fifths of the entire mitral annulus. The leaflet is divided into three individual scallops identified as the P1 (anterior or medial scallop), P2 (the middle scallop), and P3 (posterior or lateral scallop). The height of the posterior leaflet varies from the P1 cusp to the P3 cusp, with P2 cusp having the greatest height from the base to the free edge. The combined area of both leaflets is about twice the size of the mitral orifice; this extra surface area permits a large line of coaptation and ample coverage of the mitral orifice during normal function, and provides compensation during disease (He et al., 1997). The width and height of the anterior leaflet are about 3.3 and 2.3 cm, respectively, and the height of the posterior leaflet is about 1.3 cm, while that of the commissure is about 1.0 cm. The MV tissue can be divided into the rough and smooth zones. The rough zone is defined from the free edge of the valve to the valve's line of closure, and the term rough is used to denote the texture of the leaflet due to the insertion of the chordae tendinae in this area. The smooth zone is thinner and translucent and extends from the line of closure to the annulus in the anterior leaflet and to the basal zone in the posterior leaflet.

Fenoglio and colleagues (Fenoglio et al., 1972) reported that MV leaflets have distinct layers divided by differences in cellularity and collagen density (Figure 9.12). Kunzelman et al. (1993) described the leaflet as consisting of a thick central fibrosa layer, the atrialis or spongiosa layer on the atrial side, and the ventricularis on the ventricular side. The fibrosa has dense collagen fibrils spread in a fan-like arrangement (Figure 9.12), and is thickest near the annulus and thins toward the free edge. The spongiosa has loose collagen with interstitial cells sparsely distributed, extends throughout the entire leaflet, and is the main component of the free edge. Trace randomly oriented collagen and elastin fibers are spread out in the proteoglycan gel in this layer, but elastin and cells diminish toward the free edge. The ventricularis is similar to the spongiosa, but is thinner, rich in elastin, and is continuous with the thin elastin rich layer covering the outer portion of chordae tendinae. This abundance of proteoglycan near the free edge helps sustain the compressive loads during systolic closure, while the abundance of collagen in the other areas helps to sustain tensile load within the leaflet. The atrial and ventricular surfaces of the leaflets are lined with endothelial cells, though of a different morphology on both sides.

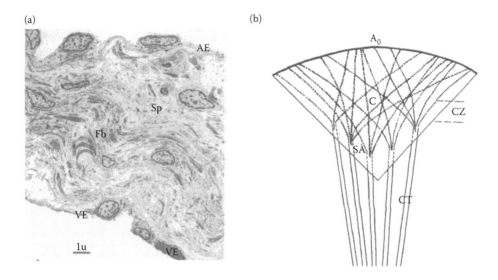

FIGURE 9.12 (a) Histological cross-sectional image of the mitral leaflet showing the atrial and ventricular layers populated with endothelial cells, the fibrosa with collagen fibrils, and spongiosa with interstitial cells. (b) Fan-like arrangement of the collagen fibrils from the region of chordal insertion to the mitral annulus. (From Fenoglio, J. J. et al. 1972. *Circ Res*, 31, 417–430.)

9.4.1.1.3 Chordae Tendineae

The mitral chordae are tendinous structure that arise from the PM tips and insert into the ventricular surface of the anterior and posterior leaflets. They differ in number from valve to valve. However, the chordae can be broadly classified into three classes based on the region of their insertion into the leaflet: Primary or marginal chordae tendineae, secondary or strut chordae tendineae, and tertiary or basal or commissural chordae tendineae. The MV typically consists of 8–12 chordae tendineae, 15–20 mm long, and approximately 0.45 mm in diameter before branching, either at the tip of the PM or at their insertion into the leaflet. The chordae inserting into the anterior leaflet are obliquely aligned along their longitudinal axis, while those on the posterior leaflet insert parallel to each other.

On the anterior leaflet, the marginal chordae that insert into the free edge, the secondary that insert into the belly of the leaflet, and the basal that insert closer to the mitral annulus. The marginal chordae split into three branches soon after their origin from the PM, with one branch inserting into the free margin of the leaflet, one into the intermediate area in the rough zone, and one slightly beyond the line of coaptation. These chords are responsible for the proper coaptation of the MV, since severing them will result in prolapsed leaflet and regurgitation (Obadia et al., 1997). The secondary chordae, which are the thickest chordae, originate from the tips of both the anterior lateral and the posterior medial PMs and insert at the transition from the rough to the smooth zones of the leaflets, where dense collagen networks provides continuity to the fibrous trigones, completed a load-bearing loop between the ventricle and the valve (Cochran et al., 1991). Secondary chordae are the thickest and carry the largest load during systolic loading on the valve and are under continuous tension. It has been speculated that they hold the function of maintaining the normal ventricular size and geometry by pulling the annulus and the PMs toward each other (Silbiger and Bazaz, 2009). The basal chordae insert into the anterior leaflet close to the annulus and toward the commissural sections. Their exact function in the global MV hemodynamic or mechanical function is currently unknown. On the posterior leaflet, the chordal distribution is similar to the anterior with a few exceptions. Posterior basal chordae, which are unique to this leaflet, are a set of chordae that extend directly from the PM to the insertion of the leaflet and do not divide along their entire stem. Additionally, cleft chordae are also seen at the regions dividing the posterior cusp into P1–P2 and P2–P3, where they fan out at the cleft to restrict it from prolapsing into the atrium during systole. Two sets of cleft chordae are observed in humans, which divide the entire posterior leaflet into three scallops.

9.4.1.1.4 Papillary Muscles

There are two PMs arising from the left ventricular myocardium: the antero-lateral PM and the postero-medial PM. The antero-lateral PM often consists of one body or tip and obtains its blood supply from the left anterior descending and the diagonal or a marginal branch of the circumflex artery, while the postero-medial PM consists of two tips and gets its blood supply from the left circumflex or right coronary artery. Because of its single system of blood supply, it is prone to injury from myocardial infarction. The attachment of the PMs to the lateral wall of the left ventricle makes the ventricular wall an integral part of the MV complex. The PMs are active components that contract during systole and maintain a constant distance between the annulus and the PM tip, restricting the prolapse of the mitral leaflets into the atria during systolic closure.

9.4.1.2 Valve Mechanical Properties

Analysis of the two MV leaflets structure indicated that the anterior leaflet is more capable of supporting large tensile loads than the posterior leaflet, since the anterior leaflet has thicker collagen-rich fibrosa layer. This is confirmed by uniaxial tensile testing (Kunzelman and Cochran, 1992). Grashow et al. (2006) performed equi-biaxial mechanical testing of the anterior leaflet. The leaflet was found to exhibit a mechanical response curve similar to that of collagen, with a very long toe region of large strain and slow loading followed by a region of small strain and rapid loading (Figure 9.13). The leaflet exhibits no hysteresis in the circumferential direction, and a very small amount in the radial direction. The valve leaflet was found to be strain rate insensitive over a range of loading rates from 0.07 to 20 Hz, maintaining the same mechanical response and hysteresis.

The mechanical properties of chordae tendineae vary with their type and size. Liao and colleagues reported that chordal grouping based on cross-sectional area demonstrates a stark correlation between the chordal size, type, and mechanical properties (Liao and Vesely, 2003, 2004a, 2004b, 2007, Liao et al., 2009). They reported that the thicker strut chordae are more extensible and less stiff than the thinner marginal chordae. The marginal chordae that are the thinnest had smaller fibril diameters and a greater

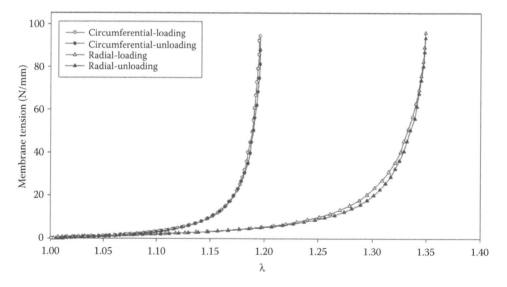

FIGURE 9.13 Mechancial response of the mitral valve anterior leaflet to equibiaxial tensile testing. (Adapted from Grashow, J. S., Yoganathan, A. P., and Sacks, M. S. 2006. *Ann Biomed Eng*, 34, 315–325.)

average fibril density than the other chordae, thus contributing to their stiffness. On the other hand, the extensibility of the chordae seems to increase with increasing chordal diameter or with a reduction in the tensile modulus. In the thicker chordae, the collagen fibrils are extensively crimped and thus allow better elongation than their thinner counterparts.

9.4.2 Valve Function

9.4.2.1 Valve Dynamics

The primary function of the MV is to allow blood flow from the left atrium to the left ventricle during diastole, and prevent the backflow of blood from the left ventricle to the atrium during systole. To perform this physiological function synchronously with the cardiac phase, the MV components works in tandem with one another to ensure proper closure of the leaflets. At the beginning of systole, higher pressure in the left ventricle and lower pressure in the left atrium accelerates the valve leaflets basally toward the mitral annulus. As the leaflets move closer to the mitral annulus, the limited extensibility of the chordae tendineae restricts the leaflets from prolapsing into the atrium. The chordae tendineae are inserted along the leaflet surface such that they not only restrict leaflet prolapse but also impart a curvature to the leaflets that results in good anterior and posterior leaflet overlap and good coaptation. Typically, in humans, the coaptation height measured along the A2–P2 ranges between 5 and 8 mm and varies with the valve size and body surface area. At peak systole, the PMs also contract and transfer an apically directed force to the annulus. This force has been speculated to change the shape of the mitral annulus from a flat diastolic configuration to a three-dimensional systolic saddle shape. Though the exact dynamics and interaction between each MV component are currently unknown, it has been demonstrated to some extent that the transfer of forces from the subannular components to the annular plane plays a critical role in optimizing leaflet coaptation (Nolan et al., 1969). As the ventricular pressure falls during late systole, rapid left atrial filling increases the chamber pressure until an inflection point is reached when the MV opens. The positive pressure gradient between the left atrium and the ventricle displaces the mitral leaflets apically to their completely open position. The strut chordae on the anterior leaflet ensure that the open mitral leaflets do not obstruct the left ventricular outflow tract, and unobstructed left ventricular filling occurs. Figure 9.14a and b depicts the different forces acting on the MV during the systolic and diastolic phase of the cardiac cycle, and

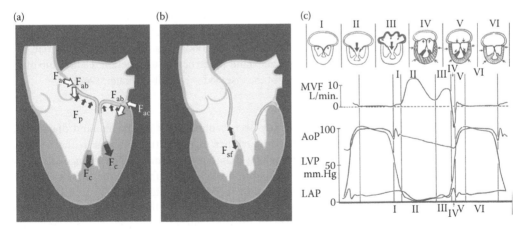

FIGURE 9.14 Forces acting on the mitral valve structure during systolic (a) and diastole (b). F_p: ventricular pressure exerted on the leaflets; F_c: force of systolic papillary muscle contraction; F_{ac}: the annular contraction force; F_{ab}: the annular bending force components; F_{sf}: tension in the strut chordae during diastole preventing systolic anterior motion of the leaflet. (c) Chamber pressures and mitral valve flow recorded during different phases on the cardiac cycle in calves. (Adapted from Nolan, S. P. et al. 1969. *Am Heart J*, 77, 784–791.)

illustrates the structure-to-function relationship between the chamber pressures and the kinematics of the MV components.

Figure 9.14c presents the synchronous recording of the MV flow, and ventricular and atrial chamber pressures in a calf. The duration of the total cardiac cycle is divided into six cardiac phases. Phase I is the period of low flow rate and volume at pre-diastole, when the MV is just about to open. Phase II begins at the time point when the atrioventricular pressure gradient is positive and during this period the flow from the left atrium rapidly accelerates into the left ventricle and slowly declines. Phase III commences at atrial systole, when the left atrium contracts and pushes the fluid volume remaining in the chamber into the left ventricle, creating a second peak in the transmitral flow curve. Phase IV is the only period of flow reversal, occurring during the isovolumetric contraction. This volume could either be slight regurgitation or can be the volume of the fluid displaced by the valve leaflets into the left atrium, termed as the closing volume. Phase V varied between 15 and 40 ms and consisted of minor flow rates related to outflow from the ventricle and motion of the MV. Phase VI extended throughout systole when no MV flow will be detectable for a healthy valve.

9.4.2.1.1 Valve Leaflet Dynamics

The first studies on understanding MV function focused on understanding the opening and closure dynamics of the valve in relevance to the atrial and ventricular hemodynamics. Henderson and Johnson (1912) demonstrated that atrial contraction begins the basal motion of the mitral leaflets toward leaflet closure, with subsequent increase in left ventricular pressure inducing complete valve closure (Henderson and Johnson, 1912). In 1916, Dean repeated the experiments in a perfused cat heart model with a constant atrial pressure head and measured the anterior leaflet mobility using a sensitive lever mechanism with changing left ventricular pressures (Dean, 1916). He observed that with the complete absence of left atrial contraction/systole, the leaflets closed only upon the onset of ventricular contraction and such passive left ventricular pressure-driven closure was associated with large backward flow of blood through the MV into the left atrium. Between 1916 and 1970, a few investigators used large animals to study the role of atrial and ventricular contraction to MV closure, by ablating the left atrial fibers or by inducing a left atrioventricular block (Paravisini, 1953, Brockman, 1962, Sarnoff et al., 1962, Meadows et al., 1963, Braunwald et al., 1966, Williams et al., 1967, 1968, Vandenberg et al., 1969, Zaky et al., 1969, Shah et al., 1970, Bellhouse, 1970b). The conclusion from these studies was that atrial systole contributed to the closure of the mitral leaflets, before the onset of ventricular systole and was necessary for MV closure with limited backflow of blood. In 1962, Salisbury reported *in vivo* force measurements on an anterior strut chord under different drug-induced hemodynamic conditions in anesthetized Mongrel dogs (Salisbury et al., 1963). In the same decade, Frater et al. defined the functional anatomy of the mammalian MV (1961), and developed a systematic approach to understand the structure-to-function relationship of the valve, and proposed principles for plastic surgery of the diseased valve (1964) (Frater, 1964).

9.4.2.1.2 Valve Annulus Dynamics

Though the entire mitral annulus has historically been defined as an incomplete and diaphanous structure, several studies have established the importance of the mitral annulus in the hemodynamic function of the MV. The mitral annulus is a dynamic structure, which changes its shape and size during the cardiac cycle, as demonstrated in animal and human studies (Tsakiris et al., 1971, Levine et al., 1987, 1989). The size of the annulus increased in late diastole until it reached its maximum area. Then, a rapid narrowing of the ring was observed during the atrial and ventricular contractions, followed by a rapid increase in size during ventricular isovolumetric relaxation. Under control conditions in dogs, a decrease in annular area of 19–34% was observed during systole as compared to the diastolic ring size (Tsakiris et al., 1975). The most striking observation was that nearly two-thirds of the annular size reduction occurred during atrial contraction, and the valve annulus was significantly reduced before the onset of ventricular systole as shown in Figure 9.15. A substantial amount of this reduction in annular size is attributable to atrial systole because it is

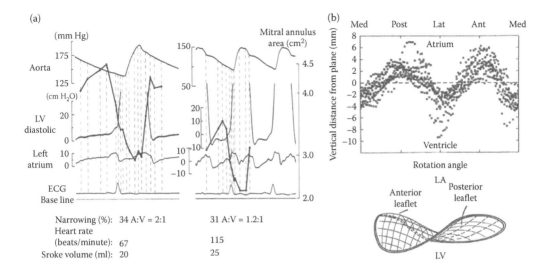

FIGURE 9.15 (a) Temporal contraction of the mitral annulus through the cardiac cycle as measured from fluoroscopic images in anesthetized dogs, with maximal contraction occurring before onset of systole. (Adapted from Tsakiris, A. G. et al. 1971. *J Appl Physiol*, 30, 611–618.) (b) 3D saddle-shaped structure of the mitral annulus as measured from echocardiographic images in normal subjects. (Adapted from Levine, R. A. et al. 1989. *Circulation*, 80, 589–598.)

not seen when atrial activity is absent, such as in the instance of atrial fibrillation (Pai et al., 2003). Further, Tsakiris et al. demonstrated that the mitral annulus moves apically during systole, and toward the left atrium during diastole, with the magnitude and frequency of motion correlating with the left atrial size (Tsakiris et al., 1971).

The mitral annulus in addition also undergoes an apical-basal flexing, imparting it a saddle shape during systole from its flat diastolic configuration, first reported by Levine et al. as shown in Figure 9.15 (Levine et al., 1987, 1988, 1989). When studied *in vitro*, it was found that this saddle shape of the annulus minimizes the stretch of the MV as well as the forces experienced by the chordae as opposed to the flat planar annulus shape (Jimenez et al., 2003, 2007, Padala et al., 2009a).

9.4.2.2 Chordae Tendineae Dynamics

The locations of the chordae tendineae relative to the valve leaflets and papillary muscles are shown in Figure 9.16. Studies on the chordae tendineae mechanics focused on force measurements in the chordae under physiological loading conditions. Chordae forces are elevated during systole but are reduced during diastole. *In vitro* studies using a flexible saddle-shaped annulus revealed that the marginal, secondary, and basal chordae experiences peak systolic forces of approximately 0.2, 1.0, and 0.1 N, respectively (Jimenez et al., 2005b). With the displacement of the PMs, such as in the case of hypertrophy of the ventricle secondary to diseases, it was found that forces in the basal chordae increased significantly while those in the marginal and secondary chordae were unaffected (Jimenez et al., 2005a).

9.4.2.3 Papillary Muscle Dynamics

The locations of the papillary muscles relative to the valve leaflets and chordae tendineae are shown in Figure 9.16. The contraction of the left ventricle is torsional in nature, given that ventricular muscle fibers are arranged helically. This results in the PMs experiencing rotational motion about the long axis of the left ventricle (Gorman et al., 1996). The PMs experiences contractions as well, being muscular in composition. Their shortening coincides with ventricular contraction durations and serves to maintain the distance between the mitral annulus and the tips of the PMs constant (Sanfilippo et al., 1992). The dynamics

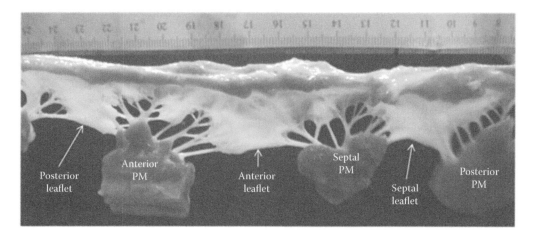

FIGURE 9.16 Explanted porcine valve, showing leaflet and PM locations relative to another.

of the PM aid the formation of ventricular inflow. During diastole, they protrude only minimally into the submitral space, providing room for mitral inflow with reduced resistance. During systole, they bulge into the ventricular cavity, directing flow toward the outflow tract (Armour and Randall, 1970).

9.4.2.4 Valve Fluid Dynamics

In 1971, Bellhouse attempted to explain the movements of the mitral cusps by flow patterns within the left ventricle, and by acceleration and deceleration of blood flow through the MV (Bellhouse, 1970a, 1970b, 1972). He reported stable vortex formation behind the anterior leaflet, which corroborated with previous observations reported in animals by Taylor and Wade, and speculated their role in early diastolic closure of the mitral leaflets (Taylor and Wade, 1969). Even though his model MV did not have chordae tendineae, the diastolic motion of the mitral leaflets matched that measured in animals, challenging existing hypothesis that PM traction governs diastolic opening of valve leaflets (Rushmer et al., 1956). At the same time, using electromagnetic flow probes, Taylor et al. measured the impedance of the MV to transmitral flow, and reported that the MV adapts to changing cardiac output so as to optimize the increase in energy loss (Rushmer et al., 1956, Taylor and Wade, 1969, Taylor, 1972, 1976). At the level of the mitral annulus, the velocity profile was flat and consistent with a plug flow, analogous to the entrance of a pipe. At the free cusp margin, the velocity profile becomes more skewed with higher velocities along the anterior leaflet, with a skewed profile at the free margin outlet; yet the overall profile did not seem to change significantly at higher heart rates.

9.4.3 Disease of the Mitral Valve and Treatment

MV pathologies encompass a spectrum of lesions, which include congenital defects, degeneration of valve tissue, and geometric distortions to the valve secondary to other diseases. Congenital lesions of the MV include annular calcification leading to mitral stenosis, leaflet prolapse due to Marfan syndrome, isolated cleft valve, undivided atrioventricular valve in ostium primum or septum secondum defects, and mitral regurgitation due to congestive heart failure caused by severe stenosis of the left main coronary artery. Though the underlying etiology of each congenital lesion is different, the common manifestations between all the lesions are leaflet and subannular malformations that reduce valve competence. Degenerative MV lesions occur in both children and adults due to genetic mutations such as Marfan syndrome, acquired diseases such as rheumatic heart disease in developing countries, fibroelastic deficiency in adult life due to collagen deficiencies, or Barlow's syndrome speculated to be caused due to genetic and mechanical factors. The last classification of MV lesions, termed as the functional

MV defects, are caused due to perturbations to the MV geometry secondary to other lesions such as ischemic dilated cardiomyopathy or hypertrophic dilated cardiomyopathy.

MV pathologies can be treated with either valve replacement with a prosthetic valve, or surgical repair. The latter is currently the accepted standard of care over valve replacement due to risks associated with anticoagulation therapy, growth of cardiac structure in pediatric patients, and lack of durability of the artificial valves. Surgical therapy for valvular heart disease has seen tremendous progress in the last two decades. In the current era of cardiothoracic surgery, surgical repair of a diseased MV has become a routine procedure that is associated with low mortality rates and excellent acute outcomes. With better understanding of pathological anatomy of MV lesions and increasing surgical experience, several innovative methods for MV repair have been established. However, the long-term durability and chronic outcomes of these techniques are not optimal, with failure rates range from 5% to 40% for the repair of different MV lesions. These disconcerting statistics indicate that MV repair for acute correction of regurgitation or stenosis is achieved, but chronic failure of these repairs is inevitable. The mechanisms of this long-term failure are currently poorly understood. Engineering studies to understand the structural and functional mechanisms of MV dysfunction and recurrent failure of surgical repairs are thus necessary to enable the development of novel MV therapies and devices.

A very common repair technique for mitral regurgitation is the surgical installation of a mitral annuloplasty ring to correct annular dilation. Since its conception in the 1960s (Tsakiris et al., 1967), and made famous by Carpentier in 1983 (Carpentier, 1983), several types of mitral annuloplasty rings have since been developed, and there is a lack of consensus on which ring performs better. Mitral annuloplasty inevitably reduced native annular dynamics, flattened the mitral annular shape, restricted the posterior leaflet mobility (He et al., 1997, Green et al., 1999), and adversely affected ventricular motion (Cheng et al., 2006), although they improve valve coaptation.

In vitro studies have been useful for the evaluation of different surgical repair techniques for prolapsed MV. Padala et al. demonstrated that both resective and nonresective MV repair techniques are effective at acutely eliminating regurgitation, but resective techniques significantly reduce the motion of the resected leaflet and may impact chronic outcomes (Padala et al., 2009a, 2009b). Studies from the same group also demonstrated that the success of percutaneous edge-to-edge repair also largely depends on the size of the mitral annulus and the extent of leaflet distension, and thus indicate proper patient selection for use of this repair (Croft et al., 2007).

9.5 Tricuspid Valve

9.5.1 Valve Structure

9.5.1.1 Anatomy

The TV is located on the right side of the heart between the right atrium and right ventricle. Its perimeter is lined with the septal wall and the right free wall of the heart. The valve consists of an annulus, three leaflets, chordae tendineae, and three PMs. The three leaflets are named according to their position in the heart: anterior, posterior, and septal leaflet. The septal leaflet is located along the septal wall and is attached to the wall with short chordae (Silver et al., 1971). The anterior and posterior leaflets are located along the free wall with the anterior leaflet reported to be the largest (Skwarek et al., 2006, Anwar et al., 2007a, Shah and Raney, 2008). While it is typically accepted that the TV has three main leaflets, numerous studies have reported there to be a variable number of leaflets ranging from 2 up to 7 leaflets (Joudinaud, 2006, Victor and Nayak, 2000). The septal leaflet is always present but the number of leaflets along the free wall can vary.

The annulus is a fibrous ring located on the perimeter of the valve and connects the leaflets to the myocardial wall. The annulus has a complex 3D geometry as seen in Figure 9.17 (Silver et al., 1971, Hiro et al., 2004, Fukuda et al., 2006b, Jouan et al., 2007, Kwan et al., 2007, Anwar et al., 2007b). While some studies have reported the annulus to be oval (Anwar et al., 2007a, 2007b), others report that it

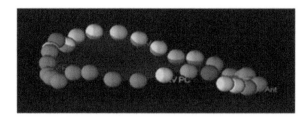

FIGURE 9.17 3D representation of the complex shape of the tricuspid annulus using 3D echocardiography and 3D in house software. (Adapted from Kwan, J. et al. 2007. *Eur J Echocardiogr,* 8, 375–383.)

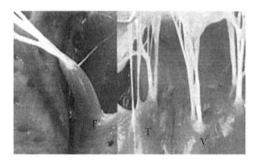

FIGURE 9.18 Classification of the three groups of papillary muscles: F—finger-like, T—tethered, and V—vestigial. Classified using excised porcine hearts by Joudinaud in 2006. (Adapted from Joudinaud, T. M., Flecher, E. M., and Duran, C. M. G. 2006. *J Heart Valve Dis,* 15, 382–388.)

is triangular (Silver et al., 1971). Annulus areas range from 7.6 to 11.2 cm^2 during systole and 11.3 to 18.35 cm^2 during diastole (Tei et al., 1982, Anwar et al., 2007a, Kwan et al., 2007).

There are three PMs located in the right ventricle, which connect to the leaflets via chordae tendineae. The PMs on the right side of the hearts are not as well defined as those seen on the left side of the heart as with the MV (Joudinaud et al., 2006). The PMs are named according to their location in the ventricle: septal, anterior, and posterior. The septal PM is located on the anterior side of the septum between the septal and anterior leaflets, while the posterior PM is located on the posterior side between the septal and posterior leaflets. The anterior PM is located on the free wall between the anterior and posterior leaflets. The PMs are classified into three groups based upon structure: finger-like, with the muscle protruding, tethered, with the muscle imbedded in the wall, and vestigial with the chords attaching directly to the well (Joudinaud et al., 2006) (Figure 9.18). Each PM has several chords that attach to the two corresponding leaflets, for example, the anterior PM has chords that insert into the anterior and posterior leaflets. The chords insert into different locations on the leaflet, including the free-edge, base, and belly of the leaflet, and are classified as marginal/primary, inserting into the free edge of the leaflet, rough zone/ supplemental, inserting between the marginal and intermediate chords, and deep/intermediate, inserting into the belly of the leaflet, respectively. Silver et al. report the deep/strut chordae to be the longest (1.7 ± 0.4 cm). All chords have similar thickness ranging from 0.8 ± 0.3 to 1.1 ± 0.4 cm (Silver et al., 1971).

9.5.2 Valve Function

9.5.2.1 Valve Dynamics

The main function of the TV is to prevent the backflow of blood from the ventricle to the atrium during systole, when blood is being pumped from the right ventricle to the pulmonary artery. The typical pressures on the right side of the heart range from 0 to 5 mmHg for the atrium and from 5 to 40 mmHg for the ventricle as reported using catheter measurements (Hurst and O'Rourke, 2004). The TV closes with

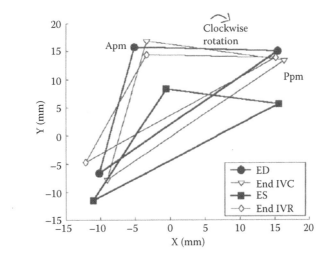

FIGURE 9.19 Results from an *in vivo* sonomicrometry study on sheep show the clockwise rotation motion of the papillary muscles over the cardiac cycle. (Adapted from Jouan, J. et al. 2007. *J Heart Valve Dis*, 16, 511–518.)

the initiation of isovolumetric contraction, and remains closed throughout the systole and isovolumetric relaxation. Once the pressure in the right ventricle is lower than that in the atrium, the valve opens. The valve remains closed for approximately one-third of the cardiac cycle.

The TV annulus area significantly increases from early to late systole in healthy subjects by 5.4 ± 1.6% (Kwan et al., 2007) and experiences differences ranging from 28 to 48% from its minimum to maximum area throughput the cardiac cycle (Tei et al., 1982, Fukuda et al., 2006b, Jouan et al., 2007). The area of the TV annulus is at its maximum during diastole, increasing the efficiency of filling by providing a larger orifice (Jouan et al., 2007) and minimum during systole aiding coaptation of the leaflets. In addition to changes in area throughout the cardiac cycle, the annulus changes its shape as well. The annulus of the TV has a three-dimensional saddle (Hiro et al., 2004, Fukuda et al., 2006b, Kwan et al., 2007), as seen in Figure 9.17, with the annulus becoming more planar during diastole (Hiro et al., 2004).

Juaon et al. (2007) studied the dynamics of the three PMs of the right side of heart during the cardiac cycle and found that the PMs move in a clockwise manner during systole as shown in Figure 9.19. The anterior PM experiences the greatest movement during the cardiac cycle due to the contraction of the myocardium since the PM is located on the free wall. The motion of the PMs has been observed to twist, shift, and bend in relation to the annulus plane, while the distance from the PMs to the annulus plane remains relatively constant (Jouan et al., 2007).

9.5.3 Disease of the Tricuspid Valve and Treatment

Tricuspid regurgitation (TR) is defined as the backflow of blood from the right ventricle to the right atrium through the TV and occurs in 8–35% of the population (Antunes and Barlow, 2007). Commonly, TR occurs in conjunction with MV regurgitation (Antunes and Barlow, 2007). Clinically, small levels of TR are detected by color Doppler imaging in many normal persons (Bonow et al., 1998) and is left untreated as it is not seen as life threatening. TR is commonly secondary to another disease and not due to changes in the natural structure of the valve and its leaflets (King et al., 1984, Matsuyama et al., 2003). Mechanisms of TR include, but are not limited to, changes in preload, afterload, such as in the case of pulmonary hypertension (Abe et al., 1996, Matsuyama et al., 2003), and right ventricular function (Sadeghi et al., 2004, Dreyfus et al., 2005).

Alterations in right ventricular function have detrimental effects on the mechanics of the TV, including less-than-normal systolic reduction in annulus (Tei et al., 1982). Human clinical studies have reported that the tricuspid annulus is twice as large in patients with TR as compared to normal subjects, measuring 35 and 70 mm, respectively (Tei et al., 1982). Studies may have focused on annular dilatation because it is believed to be a better indicator of TV pathology than TR (Dreyfus et al., 2005), since patients with no initial TR and a dilated annulus eventually developed TR. It is important to note that it is believed that only the anterior and posterior segments of the annulus can dilate, since they are the only segments on the free wall (Dreyfus et al., 2005). Right ventricle enlargement also causes tricuspid annulus deformations and displacement of PMs (Tei et al., 1982, Ubago et al., 1983, Gibson et al., 1984, Come and Riley, 1985, Sagie et al., 1994, Hinderliter et al., 2003, Fukuda et al., 2006a), which contributes to TR. It is believed that RV dilatation may affect the anterior PM position (Kim et al., 2006, Anyanwu et al., 2008), while interventricular mechanics have been shown to affect PM positions, with LV dilation significantly displacing the septal PM toward the center of the RV (Spinner et al., 2010). It has also been reported that with RV systolic failure, diastolic pressure rises and the septum moves toward the left side of the heart (Antunes and Barlow, 2007), thus increasing pulmonary pressure, believed to be a factor in TR. It is also believed that TR occurs in conjunction with left-side heart disease and ventricular dysfunction (Fukuda et al., 2006a).

Although little is known about the mechanisms that cause TR, many efforts have been made to correct it. Most recent efforts at correcting TR have been focused on repairing the annulus and reconstructing to its native structure and size, with the use of annuloplasty. Another option for treatment is valve replacement although it is uncommon because functional TR can be repaired with annuloplasty (Chang et al., 2006). It is believed that a complete understanding of valvular and subvalvular mechanics will significantly aid in better treatment options.

References

Abe, T., Tukamoto, M., Yanagiya, M., Morikawa, M., Watanabe, N., and Komatsu, S. 1996. De Vega's annuloplasty for acquired tricuspid disease: Early and late results in 110 patients. *Ann Thorac Surg,* 62, 1876–1877.

Antunes, M. J. and Barlow, J. B. 2007. Management of tricuspid valve regurgitation. *Heart,* 93, 271–276.

Anwar, A. M., Geleijnse, M. L., Soliman, O. I. I., Mcghie, J. S., Frowijn, R., Nemes, A., Van den Bosch, A. E., Galema, T. W., and Ten Cate, F. J. 2007a. Assessment of normal tricuspid valve anatomy in adults by real-time three-dimensional echocardiography. *Int J Cardiovasc Imaging,* 23, 717–724.

Anwar, A. M., Soliman, O. I. I., Nemes, A., Van Geuns, R. J. M., Geleijnse, M. L., and Ten Cate, F. J. 2007b. Value of assessment of tricuspid annulus: Real-time three-dimensional echocardiography and magnetic resonance imaging. *Int J Cardiovasc Imaging,* 23, 701–705.

Anyanwu, A. C., Chikwe, J., and Adams, D. H. 2008. Tricuspid valve repair for treatment and prevention of secondary tricuspid regurgitation in patients undergoing mitral valve surgery. *Curr Cardiol Rep,* 10, 110–117.

Armour, J. A. and Randall, W. C. 1970. Structural basis for cardiac function. *Am J Physiol,* 218, 1517–1523.

Bellhouse, B. J. 1970a. Fluid mechanics of a model mitral valve. *J Physiol,* 207, 72P–73P.

Bellhouse, B. J. 1970b. Mechanism of closure of the mitral valve. *Clin Sci,* 39, 13P–14P.

Bellhouse, B. J. 1972. Fluid mechanics of a model mitral valve and left ventricle. *Cardiovasc Res,* 6, 199–210.

Bellhouse, B. J. and Reid, K. G. 1969. Fluid mechanics of the aortic valve. *Br Heart J,* 31, 391.

Billiar, K. L. and Sacks, M. S. 2000. Biaxial mechanical properties of the natural and glutaraldehyde treated aortic valve cusp—Part I: Experimental results. *J Biomech Eng,* 122, 23–30.

Bonow, R. O., Carabello, B., De Leon, A. C., Edmunds, L. H., Fedderly, B. J., Freed, M. D., Gaasch, W. H. et al. 1998. Acc/Aha guidelines for the management of patients with valvular heart disease—A report of the American College of Cardiology American Heart Association Task Force on practice guidelines (Committee on Management of Patients with Valvular Heart Disease). *J Am Coll Cardiol,* 32, 1486–1582.

Braunwald, E., Rockoff, S. D., Oldham, H. N., Jr., and Ross, J., Jr. 1966. Effective closure of the mitral valve without atrial systole. *Circulation,* 33, 404–409.

Brockman, S. K. 1962. The physiology of closure of the mitral valve. *Surg Forum,* 13, 206–207.

Butcher, J. T., Simmons, C. A., and Warnock, J. N. 2008. Mechanobiology of the aortic heart valve. *J Heart Valve Dis,* 17, 62–73.

Carpentier, A. 1983. Cardiac valve surgery—The "French correction". *J Thorac Cardiovasc Surg,* 86, 323–337.

Chang, B. C., Lim, S. H., Yi, G. Y., Hong, Y. S., Lee, S., Yoo, K. J., Kang, M. S., and Cho, B. K. 2006. Long-term clinical results of tricuspid valve replacement. *Ann Thorac Surg,* 81, 1317–1324.

Cheng, A., Nguyen, T. C., Malinowski, M., Liang, D., Daughters, G. T., Ingels, N. B., Jr., and Miller, D. C. 2006. Effects of undersized mitral annuloplasty on regional transmural left ventricular wall strains and wall thickening mechanisms. *Circulation,* 114, 1600–1609.

Christie, G. W. 1992. Anatomy of aortic heart valve leaflets: The influence of glutaraldehyde fixation on function. *Eur J Cardiothorac Surg,* 6 Suppl 1, S25–S32; discussion S33.

Christie, G. W. and Barratt-Boyes, B. G. 1995. Mechanical properties of porcine pulmonary valve leaflets: How do they differ from aortic leaflets? *Ann Thorac Surg,* 60, S195–S199.

Cochran, R. P., Kunzelman, K. S., Chuong, C. J., Sacks, M. S., and Eberhart, R. C. 1991. Nondestructive analysis of mitral valve collagen fiber orientation. *ASAIO Trans,* 37, M447–M448.

Come, P. C. and Riley, M. F. 1985. Tricuspid anular dilatation and failure of tricuspid leaflet coaptation in tricuspid regurgitation. *Am J Cardiol,* 55, 599–601.

Croft, L. R., Jimenez, J. H., Gorman, R. C., Gorman, J. H. 3rd, and Yoganathan, A. P. 2007. Efficacy of the edge-to-edge repair in the setting of a dilated ventricle: An *in vitro* study. *Ann Thorac Surg,* 84, 1578–1584.

Dagum, P., Green, G. R., Nistal, F. J., Daughters, G. T., Timek, T. A., Foppiano, L. E., Bolger, A. F., Ingels, N. B., Jr., and Miller, D. C. 1999. Deformational dynamics of the aortic root: Modes and physiologic determinants. *Circulation,* 100, II54–II62.

Davies, M. J. 1980. *Pathology of Cardiac Valves,* London, Butterworths.

Dean, A. L. 1916. The movements of the mitral cusps in relation to the cardiac cycle. *Am J Physiol,* 40, 206–217.

Doehring, T. C., Carew, E. O., and Vesely, I. 2004. The effect of strain rate on the viscoelastic response of aortic valve tissue: A direct-fit approach. *Ann Biomed Eng,* 32, 223–232.

Dreyfus, G. D., Corbi, P. J., Chan, J., and Bahrami, T. 2005. Secondary tricuspid regurgitation or dilatation: Which should be the criteria for surgical repair? *Ann Thorac Surg,* 79, 127–132.

Dunmore-Buyze, J., Boughner, D. R., Macris, N., and Vesely, I. 1995. A comparison of macroscopic lipid content within porcine pulmonary and aortic valves. Implications for bioprosthetic valves. *J Thorac Cardiovasc Surg,* 110, 1756–1761.

El-Hamamsy, I., Balachandran, K., Yacoub, M. H., Stevens, L. M., Sarathchandra, P., Taylor, P. M., Yoganathan, A. P., and Chester, A. H. 2009. Endothelium-dependent regulation of the mechanical properties of aortic valve cusps. *J Am Coll Cardiol,* 53, 1448–1455.

Emery, R. W. and Arom, K. V. 1991. *The Aortic Valve,* Philadelphia, Henry & Belfus.

Erasmi, A., Sievers, H. H., Scharfschwerdt, M., Eckel, T., and Misfeld, M. 2005. *In vitro* hydrodynamics, cusp-bending deformation, and root distensibility for different types of aortic valve-sparing operations: Remodeling, sinus prosthesis, and reimplantation. *J Thorac Cardiovasc Surg,* 130, 1044–1049.

Fenoglio, J. J., Jr., Tuan Duc, P., Wit, A. L., Bassett, A. L., and Wagner, B. M. 1972. Canine mitral complex. Ultrastructure and electromechanical properties. *Circ Res,* 31, 417–430.

Frater, R. W. 1964. Anatomical rules for the plastic repair of a diseased mitral valve. *Thorax,* 19, 458–464.

Freeman, R. V. and Otto, C. M. 2005. Spectrum of calcific aortic valve disease: Pathogenesis, disease progression, and treatment strategies. *Circulation,* 111, 3316–3326.

Fukuda, S., Gillinov, A. M., Mccarthy, P. M., Stewart, W. J., Song, J. M., Kihara, T., Daimon, M., Shin, M. S., Thomas, J. D., and Shiota, T. 2006a. Determinants of recurrent or residual functional tricuspid regurgitation after tricuspid annuloplasty. *Circulation,* 114, 1582–1587.

Fukuda, S., Saracino, G., Matsumura, Y., Daimon, M., Tran, H., Greenberg, N. L., Hozumi, T., Yoshikawa, J., Thomas, J. D., and Shiota, T. 2006b. Three-dimensional geometry of the tricuspid annulus in healthy subjects and in patients with functional tricuspid regurgitation—A real-time, 3-dimensional echocardiographic study. *Circulation,* 114, 1492–1498.

Garg, V., Muth, A. N., Ransom, J. F., Schluterman, M. K., Barnes, R., King, I. N., Grossfeld, P. D., and Srivastava, D. 2005. Mutations in NOTCH1 cause aortic valve disease. *Nature,* 437, 270–274.

Gibson, T. C., Foale, R. A., Guyer, D. E., and Weyman, A. E. 1984. Clinical-significance of incomplete tri-cuspid-valve closure seen on two-dimensional echocardiography. *J Am Coll Cardiol,* 4, 1052–1057.

Glasson, J. R., Komeda, M. K., Daughters, G. T., Niczyporuk, M. A., Bolger, A. F., Ingels, N. B., and Miller, D. C. 1996. Three-dimensional regional dynamics of the normal mitral anulus during left ventricu-lar ejection. *J Thorac Cardiovasc Surg,* 111, 574–585.

Godart, F., Bouzguenda, I., Juthier, F., Wautot, F., Prat, A., Rey, C., Corseaux, D., Ung, A., Jude, B., and Vincentelli, A. 2009. Experimental off-pump transventricular pulmonary valve replacement using a self-expandable valved stent: A new approach for pulmonary incompetence after repaired tetralogy of Fallot? *J Thorac Cardiovasc Surg,* 137, 1141–1145.

Gorman, J. H., 3rd, Gupta, K. B., Streicher, J. T., Gorman, R. C., Jackson, B. M., Ratcliffe, M. B., Bogen, D. K., and Edmunds, L. H., Jr. 1996. Dynamic three-dimensional imaging of the mitral valve and left ventricle by rapid sonomicrometry array localization. *J Thorac Cardiovasc Surg,* 112, 712–726.

Grande-Allen, K. J., Cochran, R. P., Reinhall, P. G., and Kunzelman, K. S. 2001. Mechanisms of aortic valve incompetence: Finite-element modeling of Marfan syndrome. *J Thorac Cardiovasc Surg,* 122, 946–954.

Grande-Allen, K. J., Griffin, B. P., Ratliff, N. B., Cosgrove, D. M., and Vesely, I. 2003. Glycosaminoglycan profiles of myxomatous mitral leaflets and chordae parallel the severity of mechanical alterations. *J Am Coll Cardiol,* 42, 271–277.

Grande-Allen, K. J., Osman, N., Ballinger, M. L., Dadlani, H., Marasco, S., and Little, P. J. 2007. Glycosaminoglycan synthesis and structure as targets for the prevention of calcific aortic valve dis-ease. *Cardiovasc Res,* 76, 19–28.

Grashow, J. S., Yoganathan, A. P., and Sacks, M. S. 2006. Biaxial stress-stretch behavior of the mitral valve anterior leaflet at physiologic strain rates. *Ann Biomed Eng,* 34, 315–325.

Green, G. R., Dagum, P., Glasson, J. R., Nistal, J. F., Daughters, G. T., 2nd, Ingels, N. B., Jr., and Miller, D. C. 1999. Restricted posterior leaflet motion after mitral ring annuloplasty. *Ann Thorac Surg,* 68, 2100–2106.

Hatle, L. and Angelsen, B. 1985. *Doppler Ultrasound in Cardiology Physical Principals and Clinical Applications,* Philadelphia, Lea and Febiger.

He, S., Fontaine, A. A., Schwammenthal, E., Yoganathan, A. P., and Levine, R. A. 1997. Integrated mecha-nism for functional mitral regurgitation: Leaflet restriction versus coapting force: *In vitro* studies. *Circulation,* 96, 1826–1834.

Henderson, Y. and Johnson, F.E. 1912. Two modes of closure of the heart valves. *Heart,* 4, 69–82.

Hilbert, S. L., Luna, R. E., Zhang, J., Wang, Y., Hopkins, R. A., Yu, Z. X., and Ferrans, V. J. 1999. Allograft heart valves: The role of apoptosis-mediated cell loss. *J Thorac Cardiovasc Surg,* 117, 454–462.

Hinderliter, A. L., Willis, P. W., Long, W. A., Clarke, W. R., Ralph, D., Caldwell, E. J., Williams, W. et al. 2003. Frequency and severity of tricuspid regurgitation determined by Doppler echocardiography in primary pulmonary hypertension. *Am J Cardiol,* 91, 1033–1037.

Hiro, M. E., Jouan, J., Pagel, M. R., Lansac, E., Lim, K. H., Lim, H. S., and Duran, C. M. G. 2004. Sonometric study of the normal tricuspid valve annulus in sheep. *J Heart Valve Dis,* 13, 452–460.

Hurst, J. W. and O'Rourke, R. A. 2004. *The Heart,* McGraw-Hill Professional.

Jimenez, J. H., Liou, S. W., Padala, M., He, Z., Sacks, M., Gorman, R. C., Gorman, J. H. 3rd, and Yoganathan, A. P. 2007. A saddle-shaped annulus reduces systolic strain on the central region of the mitral valve anterior leaflet. *J Thorac Cardiovasc Surg,* 134, 1562–1568.

Jimenez, J. H., Soerensen, D. D., He, Z., He, S., and Yoganathan, A. P. 2003. Effects of a saddle shaped annulus on mitral valve function and chordal force distribution: An *in vitro* study. *Ann Biomed Eng,* 31, 1171–1181.

Jimenez, J. H., Soerensen, D. D., He, Z., Ritchie, J., and Yoganathan, A. P. 2005a. Effects of papillary muscle position on chordal force distribution: An *in vitro* study. *J Heart Valve Dis,* 14, 295–302.

Jimenez, J. H., Soerensen, D. D., He, Z., Ritchie, J., and Yoganathan, A. P. 2005b. Mitral valve function and chordal force distribution using a flexible annulus model: An *in vitro* study. *Ann Biomed Eng,* 33, 557–566.

Jouan, J., Pagel, M. R., Hiro, M. E., Lim, K. H., Lansac, E., and Duran, C. M. G. 2007. Further information from a sonometric study of the normal tricuspid valve annulus in sheep: Geometric changes during the cardiac cycle. *J Heart Valve Dis,* 16, 511–518.

Joudinaud, T. M., Flecher, E. M., and Duran, C. M. G. 2006. Functional terminology for the tricuspid valve. *J Heart Valve Dis,* 15, 382–388.

Kalmanson, D. (ed.) 1976. *The Mitral Valve: A Pluridisciplinary Approach,* Acton, MA, Publishing Sciences Group Inc.

Kershaw, J. D., Misfeld, M., Sievers, H. H., Yacoub, M. H., and Chester, A. H. 2004. Specific regional and directional contractile responses of aortic cusp tissue. *J Heart Valve Dis,* 13, 798–803.

Kilner, P. J., Yang, G. Z., Mohiaddin, R. H., Firmin, D. N., and Longmore, D. B. 1993. Helical and retrograde secondary flow patterns in the aortic arch studied by three-directional magnetic resonance velocity mapping. *Circulation,* 88, 2235–2247.

Kim, H. K., Kim, Y. J., Park, J. S., Kim, K. H., Kim, K. B., Ahn, H., Sohn, D. W., Oh, B. H., Park, Y. B., and Choi, Y. S. 2006. Determinants of the severity of functional tricuspid regurgitation. *Am J Cardiol,* 98, 236–242.

King, R. M., Schaff, H. V., Danielson, G. K., Gersh, B. J., Orszulak, T. A., Piehler, J. M., Puga, F. J., and Pluth, J. R. 1984. Surgery for tricuspid regurgitation late after mitral-valve replacement. *Circulation,* 70, 193–197.

Kunzelman, K. S. and Cochran, R. P. 1992. Stress/strain characteristics of porcine mitral valve tissue: Parallel versus perpendicular collagen orientation. *J Card Surg,* 7, 71–78.

Kunzelman, K. S., Cochran, R. P., Murphree, S. S., Ring, W. S., Verrier, E. D., and Eberhart, R. C. 1993. Differential collagen distribution in the mitral valve and its influence on biomechanical behaviour. *J Heart Valve Dis,* 2, 236–244.

Kvitting, J. P., Ebbers, T., Wigstrom, L., Engvall, J., Olin, C. L., and Bolger, A. F. 2004. Flow patterns in the aortic root and the aorta studied with time-resolved, 3-dimensional, phase-contrast magnetic resonance imaging: Implications for aortic valve-sparing surgery. *J Thorac Cardiovasc Surg,* 127, 1602–1607.

Kwan, J., Kim, G. C., Jeon, M. J., Kim, D. H., Shiota, T., Thomas, J. D., Park, K. S., and Lee, W. H. 2007. 3D geometry of a normal tricuspid annulus during systole: A comparison study with the mitral annulus using real-time 3D echocardiography. *Eur J Echocardiogr,* 8, 375–383.

Leeson-Dietrich, J., Boughner, D., and Vesely, I. 1995. Porcine pulmonary and aortic valves: A comparison of their tensile viscoelastic properties at physiological strain rates. *J Heart Valve Dis,* 4, 88–94.

Levine, R. A., Handschumacher, M. D., Sanfilippo, A. J., Hagege, A. A., Harrigan, P., Marshall, J. E., and Weyman, A. E. 1989. Three-dimensional echocardiographic reconstruction of the mitral valve, with implications for the diagnosis of mitral valve prolapse. *Circulation,* 80, 589–598.

Levine, R. A., Stathogiannis, E., Newell, J. B., Harrigan, P., and Weyman, A. E. 1988. Reconsideration of echocardiographic standards for mitral valve prolapse: Lack of association between leaflet displacement isolated to the apical four chamber view and independent echocardiographic evidence of abnormality. *J Am Coll Cardiol,* 11, 1010–1019.

Levine, R. A., Triulzi, M. O., Harrigan, P., and Weyman, A. E. 1987. The relationship of mitral annular shape to the diagnosis of mitral valve prolapse. *Circulation,* 75, 756–767.

Leyh, R. G., Schmidtke, C., Sievers, H. H., and Yacoub, M. H. 1999. Opening and closing characteristics of the aortic valve after different types of valve-preserving surgery. *Circulation,* 100, 2153–2160.

Liao, J., Priddy, L. B., Wang, B., Chen, J., and Vesely, I. 2009. Ultrastructure of porcine mitral valve chordae tendineae. *J Heart Valve Dis,* 18, 292–299.

Liao, J. and Vesely, I. 2003. A structural basis for the size-related mechanical properties of mitral valve chordae tendineae. *J Biomech,* 36, 1125–1133.

Liao, J. and Vesely, I. 2004a. Relationship between collagen fibrils, glycosaminoglycans, and stress relaxation in mitral valve chordae tendineae. *Ann Biomed Eng,* 32, 977–983.

Liao, J. and Vesely, I. 2004b. Skewness angle of interfibrillar proteoglycan increases with applied load on chordae tendineae. *Conf Proc IEEE Eng Med Biol Soc,* 5, 3741–3744.

Liao, J. and Vesely, I. 2007. Skewness angle of interfibrillar proteoglycans increases with applied load on mitral valve chordae tendineae. *J Biomech,* 40, 390–398.

Lloyd-Jones, D., Adams, R. J., Brown, T. M., Carnethon, M., Dai, S., De Simone, G., Ferguson, T. B. et al. 2010. Heart disease and stroke statistics—2010 update: A report from the American Heart Association. *Circulation,* 121, e46–e215.

Lo, D. and Vesely, I. 1995. Biaxial strain analysis of the porcine aortic valve. *Ann Thorac Surg,* 60, S374–S378.

Markl, M., Draney, M. T., Miller, D. C., Levin, J. M., Williamson, E. E., Pelc, N. J., Liang, D. H., and Herfkens, R. J. 2005. Time-resolved three-dimensional magnetic resonance velocity mapping of aortic flow in healthy volunteers and patients after valve-sparing aortic root replacement. *J Thorac Cardiovasc Surg,* 130, 456–463.

Matsuyama, K., Matsumoto, M., Sugita, T., Nishizawa, J., Tokuda, Y., and Matsuo, T. 2003. Predictors of residual tricuspid regurgitation after mitral valve surgery. *Ann Thorac Surg,* 75, 1826–1828.

Meadows, W. R., Vanpraagh, S., Indreika, M., and Sharp, J. T. 1963. Premature mitral valve closure: A hemodynamic explanation for absence of the first sound in aortic insufficiency. *Circulation,* 28, 251–258.

Merryman, W. D., Huang, H. Y., Schoen, F. J., and Sacks, M. S. 2006. The effects of cellular contraction on aortic valve leaflet flexural stiffness. *J Biomech,* 39, 88–96.

Muriago, M., Sheppard, M. N., Ho, S. Y., and Anderson, R. H. 1997. Location of the coronary arterial orifices in the normal heart. *Clin Anat,* 10, 297–302.

Nolan, S. P., Dixon, S. H., Jr., Fisher, R. D., and Morrow, A. G. 1969. The influence of atrial contraction and mitral valve mechanics on ventricular filing. A study of instantaneous mitral valve flow *in vivo. Am Heart J,* 77, 784–791.

Obadia, J. F., Casali, C., Chassignolle, J. F., and Janier, M. 1997. Mitral subvalvular apparatus: Different functions of primary and secondary chordae. *Circulation,* 96, 3124–3128.

Padala, M., Hutchison, R. A., Croft, L. R., Jimenez, J. H., Gorman, R. C., Gorman, J. H., 3rd, Sacks, M. S., and Yoganathan, A. P. 2009a. Saddle shape of the mitral annulus reduces systolic strains on the P2 segment of the posterior mitral leaflet. *Ann Thorac Surg,* 88, 1499–1504.

Padala, M., Powell, S. N., Croft, L. R., Thourani, V. H., Yoganathan, A. P., and Adams, D. H. 2009b. Mitral valve hemodynamics after repair of acute posterior leaflet prolapse: Quadrangular resection versus triangular resection versus neochordoplasty. *J Thorac Cardiovasc Surg,* 138, 309–315.

Pai, R. G., Varadarajan, P., and Tanimoto, M. 2003. Effect of atrial fibrillation on the dynamics of mitral annular area. *J Heart Valve Dis,* 12, 31–37.

Paravisini, J. 1953. [On the mechanism of the closure of the mitral valve.]. *Rev Esp Fisiol,* 9, 9–13.

Paulsen, P. K. and Hasenkam, J. M. 1983. Three-dimensional visualization of velocity profiles in the ascending aorta in dogs, measured with a hot-film anemometer. *J Biomech,* 16, 201–210.

Rabkin-Aikawa, E., Aikawa, M., Farber, M., Kratz, J. R., Garcia-Cardena, G., Kouchoukos, N. T., Mitchell, M. B., Jonas, R. A., and Schoen, F. J. 2004. Clinical pulmonary autograft valves: Pathologic evidence of adaptive remodeling in the aortic site. *J Thorac Cardiovasc Surg,* 128, 552–561.

Reul, H. and Talukdar, N. 1979. Heart valve mechanics. In: Hwang N. H. C., G. D. R., and Patel D. J. (ed.) *Quantitative Cardiovascular Studies Clinical and Research Applications of Engineering Principles.* Baltimore, University Park Press.

Roberts, W. C. 1970. The congenitally bicuspid aortic valve. A study of 85 autopsy cases. *Am J Cardiol,* 26, 72–83.

Robicsek, F., Thubrikar, M. J., Cook, J. W., and Fowler, B. 2004. The congenitally bicuspid aortic valve: How does it function? Why does it fail? *Ann Thorac Surg*, 77, 177–185.

Rossvoll, O., Samstad, S., Torp, H. G., Linker, D. T., Skjaerpe, T., Angelsen, B. A., and Hatle, L. 1991. The velocity distribution in the aortic annulus in normal subjects: A quantitative analysis of two-dimensional Doppler flow maps. *J Am Soc Echocardiogr*, 4, 367–378.

Rushmer, R. F., Finlayson, B. L., and Nash, A. A. 1956. Movements of the mitral valve. *Circ Res*, 4, 337–342.

Sacks, M. S., Smith, D. B., and Hiester, E. D. 1998. The aortic valve microstructure: Effects of transvalvular pressure. *J Biomed Mater Res*, 41, 131–141.

Sadeghi, H. M., Kimura, B. J., Raisinghani, A., Blanchard, D. G., Mahmud, E., Fedullo, P. F., Jamieson, S. W., and Demaria, A. N. 2004. Does lowering pulmonary arterial pressure eliminate severe functional tricuspid regurgitation? *J Am Coll Cardiol*, 44, 126–132.

Sagie, A., Schwammenthal, E., Padial, L. R., Vazquez, J. A., Weyman, A. E., and Levine, R. A. 1994. Determinants of functional tricuspid regurgitation in incomplete tricuspid-valve closure—Doppler color-flow study of 109 patients. *J Am Coll Cardiol*, 24, 446–453.

Sahasakul, Y., Edwards, W. D., Naessens, J. M., and Tajik, A. J. 1988. Age-related changes in aortic and mitral valve thickness: Implications for two-dimensional echocardiography based on an autopsy study of 200 normal human hearts. *Am J Cardiol*, 62, 424–430.

Salisbury, P. F., Cross, C. E., and Rieben, P. A. 1963. Chorda tendinea tension. *Am J Physiol*, 205, 385–392.

Sanfilippo, A. J., Harrigan, P., Popovic, A. D., Weyman, A. E., and Levine, R. A. 1992. Papillary muscle traction in mitral valve prolapse: Quantitation by two-dimensional echocardiography. *J Am Coll Cardiol*, 19, 564–571.

Sarnoff, S. J., Gilmore, J. P., and Mitchell, J. H. 1962. Influence of atrial contraction and relaxation on closure of mitral valve. Observations on effects of autonomic nerve activity. *Circ Res*, 11, 26–35.

Schenke-Layland, K., Stock, U. A., Nsair, A., Xie, J., Angelis, E., Fonseca, C. G., Larbig, R. et al. 2009. Cardiomyopathy is associated with structural remodelling of heart valve extracellular matrix. *Eur Heart J*, 30, 2254–2265.

Scott, M. J. and Vesely, I. 1996. Morphology of porcine aortic valve cusp elastin. *J Heart Valve Dis*, 5, 464–471.

Shah, P. M., Kramer, D. H., and Gramiak, R. 1970. Influence of the timing of atrial systole on mitral valve closure and on the first heart sound in man. *Am J Cardiol*, 26, 231–237.

Shah, P. M. and Raney, A. A. 2008. Tricuspid valve disease. *Curr Probl Cardiol*, 33, 47–84.

Silbiger, J. J. and Bazaz, R. 2009. Contemporary insights into the functional anatomy of the mitral valve. *Am Heart J*, 158, 887–895.

Silver, M. A. and Roberts, W. C. 1985. Detailed anatomy of the normally functioning aortic valve in hearts of normal and increased weight. *Am J Cardiol*, 55, 454–461.

Silver, M. D., Lam, J. H. C., Ranganat, N., and Wigle, E. D. 1971. Morphology of human tricuspid valve. *Circulation*, 43, 333–334.

Skwarek, M., Hreczecha, J., Dudziak, M., and Grzybiak M. 2006. The morphology of the right atrioventricular valve in the adult human heart. *Folia Morphol*, 65, 200–208.

Sliwa, K. and Mocumbi, A. O. 2010. Forgotten cardiovascular diseases in Africa. *Clin Res Cardiol*, 99, 65–74.

Sloth, E., Houlind, K. C., Oyre, S., Kim, W. Y., Pedersen, E. M., Jorgensen, H. S., and Hasenkam, J. M. 1994. Three-dimensional visualization of velocity profiles in the human main pulmonary artery with magnetic resonance phase-velocity mapping. *Am Heart J*, 128, 1130–1138.

Spinner, E. M., Sundareswaran, K., Dasi, L. P., Thourani, V. H., Oshinski, J., and Yoganathan, A. P. 2010. Altered right ventricular papillary muscle position and orientation in patients with a dilated left ventricle. *J Thorac Cardiovasc Surg*, 744–749.

Stella, J. A., Liao, J., and Sacks, M. S. 2007. Time-dependent biaxial mechanical behavior of the aortic heart valve leaflet. *J Biomech*, 40, 3169–3177.

Stewart, B. F., Siscovick, D., Lind, B. K., Gardin, J. M., Gottdiener, J. S., Smith, V. E., Kitzman, D. W., and Otto, C. M. 1997. Clinical factors associated with calcific aortic valve disease. Cardiovascular Health Study. *J Am Coll Cardiol,* 29, 630–634.

Sung, H. W. and Yoganathan, A. P. 1990a. Axial flow velocity patterns in a normal human pulmonary artery model: Pulsatile *in vitro* studies. *J Biomech,* 23, 201–214.

Sung, H. W. and Yoganathan, A. P. 1990b. Secondary flow velocity patterns in a pulmonary artery model with varying degrees of valvular pulmonic stenosis: Pulsatile *in vitro* studies. *J Biomech Eng,* 112, 88–92.

Swanson, M. and Clark, R. E. 1974. Dimensions and geometric relationships of the human aortic valve as a function of pressure. *Circ Res,* 35, 871–882.

Takkenberg, J. J., Klieverik, L. M., Schoof, P. H., Van Suylen, R. J., Van Herwerden, L. A., Zondervan, P. E., Roos-Hesselink, J. W., Eijkemans, M. J., Yacoub, M. H., and Bogers, A. J. 2009. The Ross procedure: A systematic review and meta-analysis. *Circulation,* 119, 222–228.

Taylor, D. E. 1972. Mitral valve geometry and flow dynamics at varying heart rates in the dog. *J Physiol,* 227, 37P–38P.

Taylor, D. E. 1976. International symposium on the mitral valve. *Biomed Eng,* 11, 59.

Taylor, D. E. and Wade, J. D. 1969. Flow through the mitral valve during diastolic filling of the left ventricle. *J Physiol,* 200, 73P–74P.

Tei, C., Pilgrim, J. P., Shah, P. M., Ormiston, J. A., and Wong, M. 1982. The tricuspid-valve annulus—Study of size and motion in normal subjects and in patients with tricuspid regurgitation. *Circulation,* 66, 665–671.

Thubrikar, M. 1990. *The Aortic Valve,* Boca Raton, FL, CRC Press.

Thubrikar, M. J., Aouad, J., and Nolan, S. P. 1986. Patterns of calcific deposits in operatively excised stenotic or purely regurgitant aortic valves and their relation to mechanical stress. *Am J Cardiol,* 58, 304–308.

Tsakiris, A. G., Gordon, D. A., Mathieu, Y., and Irving, L. 1975. Motion of both mitral valve leaflets: A cineroentgenographic study in intact dogs. *J Appl Physiol,* 39, 359–366.

Tsakiris, A. G., Rastelli, G. C., Banchero, N., Wood, E. H., and Kirklin, J. W. 1967. Fixation of the annulus of the mitral valve with a rigid ring. Hemodynamic studies. *Am J Cardiol,* 20, 812–819.

Tsakiris, A. G., Von Bernuth, G., Rastelli, G. C., Bourgeois, M. J., Titus, J. L., and Wood, E. H. 1971. Size and motion of the mitral valve annulus in anesthetized intact dogs. *J Appl Physiol,* 30, 611–618.

Tsifansky, M., Morell, V. O., and Muñoz, R. 2010. Aortic valve regurgitation. In: Munoz, R., Morell, V., Cruz, E., and Vetterly, C. (eds.) *Critical Care of Children with Heart Disease.* London, Springer.

Ubago, J. L., Figueroa, A., Ochoteco, A., Colman, T., Duran, R. M., and Duran, C. G. 1983. Analysis of the amount of tricuspid-valve anular dilatation required to produce functional tricuspid regurgitation. *Am J Cardiol,* 52, 155–158.

Vandenberg, R. A., Williams, J. C., Sturm, R. E., and Wood, E. H. 1969. Effect of ventricular extrasystoles on closure of mitral valve. *Circulation,* 39, 197–204.

Vesely, I. 1998. The role of elastin in aortic valve mechanics. *J Biomech,* 31, 115–123.

Vesely, I. and Lozon, A. 1993. Natural preload of aortic valve leaflet components during glutaraldehyde fixation: Effects on tissue mechanics. *J Biomech,* 26, 121–131.

Vesely, I., Macris, N., Dunmore, P. J., and Boughner, D. 1994. The distribution and morphology of aortic valve cusp lipids. *J Heart Valve Dis,* 3, 451–456.

Vesely, I. and Noseworthy, R. 1992. Micromechanics of the fibrosa and the ventricularis in aortic valve leaflets. *J Biomech,* 25, 101–113.

Victor, S. and Nayak, V. M. 2000. Tricuspid valve is bicuspid. *Ann Thorac Surg,* 69, 1989–1990.

Vollebergh, F. E. and Becker, A. E. 1977. Minor congenital variations of cusp size in tricuspid aortic valves. Possible link with isolated aortic stenosis. *Br Heart J,* 39, 1006–1011.

Ward, C. 2000. Clinical significance of the bicuspid aortic valve. *Heart,* 83, 81–85.

Westaby, S., Karp, R. B., Blackstone, E. H., and Bishop, S. P. 1984. Adult human valve dimensions and their surgical significance. *Am J Cardiol,* 53, 552–556.

Weyman, A. E. 1994. *Principles and Practices of Echocardiography,* Philadelphia, Lea & Febiger.

Williams, J. C., O'Donovan, T. P., Cronin, L., and Wood, E. H. 1967. Influence of sequence of atrial and ventricular systoles on closure of mitral valve. *J Appl Physiol,* 22, 786–792.

Williams, J. C., Vandenberg, R. A., O'Donovan, T. P., Sturm, R. E., and Wood, E. H. 1968. Roentgen video densitometer study of mitral valve closure during atrial fibrillation. *J Appl Physiol,* 24, 217–224.

Yap, C. H., Kim, H. S., Balachandran, K., Weiler, M., Haj-Ali, R., and Yoganathan, A. P. 2010. Dynamic deformation characteristics of porcine aortic valve leaflet under normal and hypertensive conditions. *Am J Physiol Heart Circ Physiol,* 298, H395–H405.

Zaky, A., Steinmetz, E., and Feigenbaum, H. 1969. Role of atrium in closure of mitral valve in man. *Am J Physiol,* 217, 1652–1659.

10

Arterial Macrocirculatory Hemodynamics

Baruch B. Lieber
*State University of
New York, Stony Brook*

The arterial circulation is a multiply branched network of compliant tubes. The geometry of the network is complex, and the vessels exhibit nonlinear *viscoelastic* behavior. Flow is pulsatile, and the blood flowing through the network is a suspension of red cells and other particles in plasma, which exhibits complex *non-Newtonian* properties. Whereas the development of an exact biomechanical description of arterial hemodynamics is a formidable task, surprisingly useful results can be obtained with greatly simplified models.

The geometrical parameters of the canine *systemic* and *pulmonary* circulations are summarized in Table 10.1. Vessel diameters vary from a maximum of 19 mm in the proximal aorta to 0.008 mm (8 μm) in the capillaries. Because of the multiple branching, the total cross-sectional area increases from 2.8 cm^2 in the proximal aorta to 1357 cm^2 in the capillaries. Of the total blood volume, approximately 83% is in the systemic circulation, 12% is in the pulmonary circulation, and the remaining 5% is in the heart. Most of the systemic blood is in the venous circulation, where changes in compliance are used to control mean circulatory blood pressure. This chapter will be concerned with flow in the larger arteries, classes 1–5 in the systemic circulation and 1–3 in the pulmonary circulation in Table 10.1.

10.1 Blood Vessel Walls

The detailed properties of blood vessels were described earlier in this section, but a few general observations are made here to facilitate the following discussion. Blood vessels are composed of three layers, the intima, media, and adventitia. The inner layer, or intima, is composed primarily of *endothelial* cells, which line the vessel and are involved in control of vessel diameter. The media, composed of *elastin, collagen,* and smooth muscle, largely determines the elastic properties of the vessel. The outer layer, or adventitia, is composed mainly of connective tissue. Unlike in structures composed of passive elastic materials, vessel diameter and elastic modulus vary with smooth-muscle tone. Dilation in response to increases in flow and *myogenic* constriction in response to increases in pressure have been observed in some arteries. Smooth-muscle tone is also affected by circulating vasoconstrictors such as norepinephrine and vasodilators such as nitroprusside. Blood vessels, like other soft biological tissues, generally do

TABLE 10.1   Model of Vascular Dimensions in a Dog Weighing 20 kg

Class	Vessels	Mean Diam. (mm)	Number of Vessels	Mean Length (mm)	Total Cross-Section (cm²)	Total Blood Volume (mL)	Percentage of Total Volume
			Systemic				
1	Aorta	(19–4.5)	1		(2.8–0.2)	60	
2	Arteries	4.000	40	150.0	5.0	75	
3	Arteries	1.300	500	45.0	6.6	30	
4	Arteries	0.450	6000	13.5	9.5	13	11
5	Arteries	0.150	110,000	4.0	19.4	8	
6	Arterioles	0.050	2.8×10^6	1.2	55.0	7	
7	Capillaries	0.008	2.7×10^9	0.65	1357.9	88	5
8	Venules	0.100	1.0×10^7	1.6	785.4	126	
9	Veins	0.280	660,000	4.8	406.4	196	
10	Veins	0.700	40,000	13.5	154.0	208	
11	Veins	1.800	2100	45.0	53.4	240	
12	Veins	4.500	110	150.0	17.5	263	67
13	Venae cavae	(5–14)	2		(0.2–1.5)	92	
Total						1406	
			Pulmonary				
1	Main artery	1.600	1	28.0	2.0	6	
2	Arteries	4.000	20	10.0	2.5	25	3
3	Arteries	1.000	1550	14.0	12.2	17	
4	Arterioles	0.100	1.5×10^6	0.7	120.0	8	
5	Capillaries	0.008	2.7×10^9	0.5	1357.0	68	4
6	Venules	0.110	2.0×10^6	0.7	190.0	13	
7	Veins	1.100	1650	14.0	15.7	22	
8	Veins	4.200	25	100.0		35	5
9	Main veins	8.000	4	30.0		6	
Total						200	
			Heart				
	Atria		2			30	
	Ventricles	2			54	54	
Total						84	
Total circulation						1690	100

Source: Milnor WR. 1989. *Hemodynamics*, 2nd ed., p. 45. Baltimore, Williams and Wilkins. With permission.

not obey Hooke's law, becoming stiffer as pressure is increased. They also exhibit viscoelastic character-istics such as hysteresis and creep. Fortunately, for many purposes a linear elastic model of blood vessel behavior provides adequate results.

10.2 Flow Characteristics

Blood is a complex substance containing water, inorganic ions, proteins, and cells. Approximately 50% is plasma, a nearly Newtonian fluid consisting of water, ions, and proteins. The balance contains erythrocytes (red blood cells), leukocytes (white blood cells), and platelets. Whereas the behavior of blood in vessels smaller than approximately 100 H exhibits significant non-Newtonian effects, flow in larger vessels can be described reasonably accurately using the Newtonian assumption. There is some evidence suggesting that in blood analog fluids wall shear stress distributions may differ somewhat from Newtonian values (Liepsch et al. 1991).

Flow in the arterial circulation is predominantly laminar with the possible exception of the proximal aorta and main pulmonary artery. In steady flow, transition to turbulence occurs at Reynolds numbers (N_R) above approximately 2300.

$$N_R = \frac{2rV}{\nu}$$

where r = vessel radius, V = velocity, ν = kinematic viscosity/density.

Flow in the major systemic and pulmonary arteries is highly pulsatile. Peak-to-mean flow amplitudes as high as 6 to 1 have been reported in both human and dog (Milnor, 1989, p. 149). Womersley's analysis of incompressible flow in rigid and elastic tubes (Womersley 1957) showed that the importance of pulsatility in the velocity distributions depended on the parameter

$$N_W = r\sqrt{\frac{\omega}{\nu}}$$

where ω = frequency.

This is usually referred to as the Womersley number (N_W) or α-parameter. Womersley's original report is not readily available; however, Milnor provides a reasonably complete account (Milnor, 1989, pp. 106–121).

Mean and peak Reynolds numbers in human and dog are given in Table 10.2, which also includes mean, peak, and minimum velocities as well as the Womersley number. Mean Reynolds numbers in the entire systemic and pulmonary circulations are below 2300. Peak systolic Reynolds numbers exceed 2300 in the aorta and pulmonary artery, and some evidence of transition to turbulence has been reported. In dogs, distributed flow occurs at Reynolds numbers as low as 1000, with higher Womersley numbers increasing the transition Reynolds number (Nerem and Seed, 1972). The values in Table 10.2 are typical for individuals at rest. During exercise, cardiac output and hence Reynolds numbers can increase several fold. The Womersley number also affects the shape of the instantaneous velocity profiles as discussed in Table 10.3.

TABLE 10.2 Normal Average Hemodynamics Values in Man and Dog

	Dog (20 kg)			Man (70 kg, 1.8 m²)		
	N_W	Velocity (cm/s)	N_R	N_W	Velocity (cm/s)	N_R
Systemic vessels						
Ascending aorta	16	15.8(89/0)[a]	870(4900)[b]	21	18(112/0)[a]	1500(9400)[a]
Abdominal aorta	9	12(60.0)	370(1870)	12	14(75/0)	640(3600)
Renal artery	3	41(74/26)	440(800)	4	40(73/26)	700(1300)
Femoral artery	4	10(42/1)	130(580)	4	12(52/2)	200(860)
Femoral vein	5	5	92	7	4	104
Superior vena cava	10	8(20/0)	320(790)	15	9(23/0)	550(1400)
Inferior vena cava	11	19(40/0)	800(1800)	17	21(46/0)	1400(3000)
Pulmonary vessels						
Main artery	14	18(72/0)	900(3700)	20	19(96/0)	1600(7800)
Main vein[c]	7	18(30/9)	270(800)	10	19(38/10)	800(2200)

Source: Milnor WR. 1989. *Hemodynamics*, 2nd ed., p. 148, Baltimore, Williams and Wilkins. With permission.

[a] Mean (systolic/diastolic).

[b] Mean (peak).

[c] One of the usually four terminal pulmonary veins.

TABLE 10.3   Pressure Wave Velocities in Arteries

Artery	Species	Wave Velocity (cm/s)
Ascending aorta	Man	440–520
	Dog	350–472
Thoracic aorta	Man	400–650
	Dog	400–700
Abdominal aorta	Man	500–620
	Dog	550–960
Iliac	Man	700–880
	Dog	700–800
Femoral	Man	800–1800
	Dog	800–1300
Popliteal	Dog	1220–1310
Tibial	Dog	1040–1430
Carotid	Man	680–830
	Dog	610–1240
Pulmonary	Man	168–182
	Dog	255–275
	Rabbit	100
	Pig	190

Source: Milnor WR. 1989. *Hemodynamics*, 2nd ed., p. 235, Baltimore, Williams and Wilkins. With permission.

Note: All data are apparent pressure wave velocities (although the average of higher frequency harmonics approximates the true velocity in many cases), from relatively young subjects with normal cardiovascular systems, at approximately normal distending pressures. Ranges for each vessel and species taken from Table 9.1 of source.

10.3 Wave Propagation

The viscodasticity of blood vessels affects the hemodynamics of arterial flow. The primary function of arterial elasticity is to store blood during systole so that forward flow continues when the aortic valve is dosed. Elasticity also causes a finite wave propagation velocity, which is given approximately by the Moens–Korteweg relationship

$$c = \sqrt{\frac{Eh}{2\rho r}}$$

where E = wall elastic modulus, h = wall thickness, ρ = blood density, r = vessel radius.

Although Moens (1878) and Korteweg (1878) are credited with this formulation, Fung (1984, p. 107) has pointed out that the formula was first derived much earlier (Young, 1808). Wave speeds in arterial blood vessels from several species are given in Table 10.3. In general, wave speeds increase toward the periphery as vessel radius decreases and are considerably lower in the main pulmonary artery than in the aorta owing primarily to the lower pressure and consequently lower elastic modulus.

Wave reflections occur at branches where there is no perfect impedance matching of parent and daughter vessels. The input impedance of a network of vessels is the ratio of pressure to flow. For rigid vessels with laminar flow and negligible inertial effects, the input impedance is simply the resistance and is independent of pressure and flow rate. For elastic vessels, the impedance is dependent on the frequency of the fluctuations in pressure and flow. The impedance can be described by a complex function expressing the amplitude ratio of pressure to flow oscillations and the phase difference between the peaks.

$$\bar{Z}_i(\omega) = \frac{\bar{P}(\omega)}{\bar{Q}(\omega)}$$

$$\left|\bar{Z}_i(\omega)\right| = \left|\frac{\bar{P}(\omega)}{\bar{Q}(\omega)}\right|$$

$$\theta_i(\omega) = \theta[\bar{P}(\omega)] - \theta[\bar{Q}(\omega)]$$

where $\bar{Z}_i$ is the complex impedance, $|\bar{Z}_i|$ is the amplitude, and θ_i is the phase.

For an infinitely long straight tube with constant properties, input impedance will be independent of position in the tube and dependent only on vessel and fluid properties. The corresponding value of input impedance is called the *characteristic impedance Z*, given by

$$Z_0 = \frac{\rho c}{A}$$

where A = vessel cross-sectional area.

In general, the input impedance will vary from point to point in the network because of variations in vessel sizes and properties. If the network has the same impedance at each point (perfect impedance matching), there will be no wave reflections. Such a network will transmit energy most efficiently. The reflection coefficient R, defined as the ratio of reflected to incident wave amplitude is related to the relative characteristic impedance of the vessels at a junction. For a parent tube with characteristic impedance Z_0 branching into two daughter tubes with characteristic impedances Z_1 and Z_2, the reflection coefficient is given by

$$R = \frac{Z_0^{-1} - (Z_1^{-1} + Z_2^{-1})}{Z_0^{-1} + (Z_1^{-1} + Z_2^{-1})}$$

and perfect impedance matching requires

$$\frac{1}{Z_0} = \frac{1}{Z_1} + \frac{1}{Z_2}$$

The arterial circulation exhibits partial impedance matching; however, wave reflections do occur. At each branch point, local reflection coefficients typically are less than 0.2. Nonetheless, global reflection coefficients, which account for all reflections distal to a given site, can be considerably higher (Milnor, 1989, p. 217).

In the absence of wave reflections, the input impedance is equal to the characteristic impedance. Womersley's analysis predicts that impedance modulus will decrease monotonically with increasing frequency, whereas the phase angle is negative at low frequency and becomes progressively more positive with increasing frequency. Typical values calculated from Womersley's analysis are shown in Figure 10.1. In the actual circulation, wave reflections cause oscillations in the modulus and phase. Figure 10.2 shows input impedance measured in the ascending aorta of a human. Measurements of input resistance, characteristic impedance, and the frequency of the first minimum in the input impedance are summarized in Table 10.4.

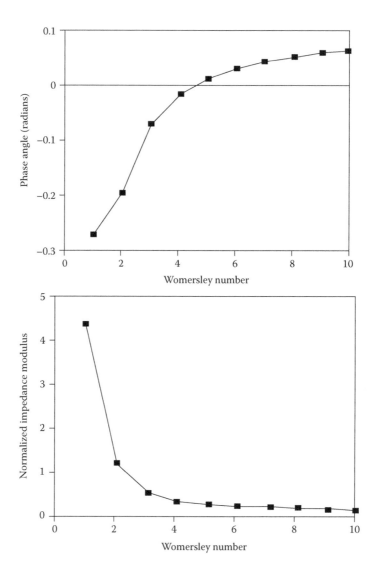

FIGURE 10.1 Characteristic impedance calculated from Womersley's analysis. The top panel contains the phase of the impedance and the bottom panel the modulus, both plotted as a function of the Womersley number N_W, which is promotional to frequency. The curves shown are for an unconstrained tube and include the effects of wall viscosity. The original figure has an inverted phase ordinate. (From Milnor, W.R. 1989. *Hemodynamics*, 2nd ed., p. 172, Baltimore, Williams and Wilkins. With permission.)

Typical pressure and velocity fluctuations throughout the cardiac cycle in man are shown in Figure 10.3. Although mean pressure decreases slightly toward the periphery due to viscous effects, peak pressure shows small increases in the distal aorta due to wave reflection and vessel taper. A rough estimate of mean pressure can be obtained as 1/3 of the sum of systolic pressure and twice the diastolic pressure. Velocity peaks during systole, with some backflow observed in the aorta early in diastole. Flow in the aorta is nearly zero through most of the diastole; however, more peripheral arteries such as the iliac and renal show forward flow throughout the cardiac cycle. This is a result of capacitive discharge of the central arteries as arterial pressure decreases.

Velocity varies across the vessel due to viscous and inertial effects as mentioned earlier. The velocities in Figure 10.3 were measured at one point in the artery. Velocity profiles are complex because the flow is

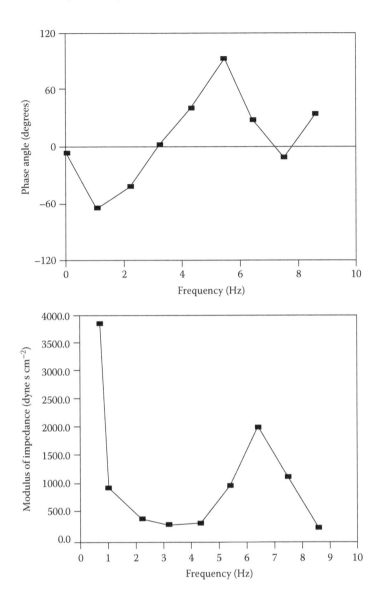

FIGURE 10.2 Input impedance derived from the pressure and velocity data in the ascending aorta of the pig. The top panel contains the phase and the bottom panel the modulus, both plotted as functions of frequency. The peripheral resistance (DC impedance) for this plot was 16,470 dyne s/cm². (From Mills CJ et al. 1970. Pressure–flow relationships and vascular impedance in man. *Cardiovasc Res* 4:405. With permission.)

pulsatile and vessels are elastic, curved, and tapered. Profiles measured in the thoracic aorta of a dog at normal arterial pressure and cardiac output are shown in Figure 10.4. Backflow occurs during diastole, and profiles are flattened even during peak systolic flow. The shape of the profiles varies considerably with mean aortic pressure and cardiac output (Ling et al., 1973).

In more peripheral arteries the profiles resemble parabolic ones as in fully developed laminar flow. The general features of these fully developed flow profiles can be modeled using Womersley's approach, although nonlinear effects may be important in some cases. The qualitative features of the profile depend on the Womersley number N_W. Unsteady effects become more important as N_W increases. Below a value

TABLE 10.4   Characteristic Arterial Impedances in Some Mammals: Average (±SE)

Species	Artery	R_m	Z_0	F_{min}
Dog	Aorta	2809–6830	125–288	6–8
Dog	Pulmonary	536–807	132–295	2–3.5
Dog	Femoral	110–162[a]	4.5–15.8[a]	8–13
Dog	Carotid	69[a]	7.0–9.4[a]	8–11
Rabbit	Aorta	20–50[a]	1.8–2.1[a]	4.5–9.8
Rabbit	Pulmonary		1.1[a]	3.0
Rat	Aorta	153[a]	11.2[a]	12

Source: Milnor WR. 1989. *Hemodynamics*, 2nd ed., p. 183, Baltimore, Williams and Wilkins. With permission.

Note: R_{in}, input resistance (mean arterial pressure/flow) in dyn s/cm⁵. Z_0 characteristic impedance, in dyn s/cm⁵, estimated by averaging high-frequency input impedances in aorta and pulmonary artery; value at 5 Hz for other arteries, f_{min}, frequency of first minimum of Z_i. Values estimated from published figures if averages were not reported. Ranges for each species and vessel taken from values in Table 7.2 of source.

[a] 10^3 dyn s/cm⁵.

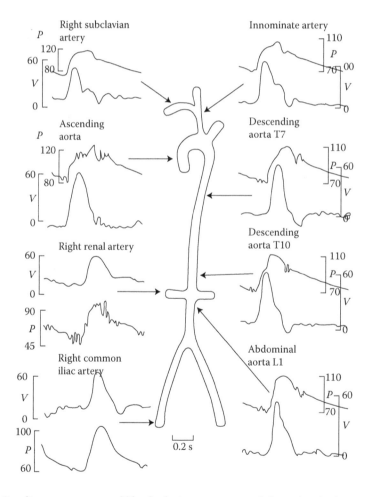

FIGURE 10.3   Simultaneous pressure and blood velocity patterns recorded at points in the systemic circulation of a human. Velocities were recorded with a catheter-tip electromagnetic flowmeter probe. The catheter included a lumen for simultaneous pressure measurement. *V* = velocity (cm/s), *P* = pressure (mm Hg). (From Mills CJ et al. 1970. *Cardiovac Res* 40:405. With permission.)

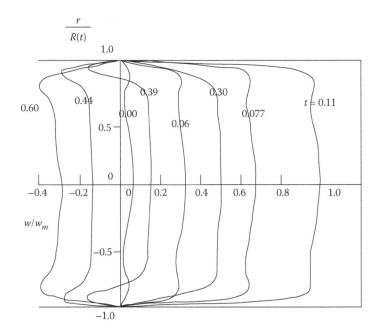

FIGURE 10.4 Velocity profiles obtained with a hot-film anemometer probe in the descending thoracic aorta of a dog at normal arterial pressure and cardiac output. The velocity at t = time/(cardiac period) is plotted as a function of radial position. Velocity w is normalized by the maximum velocity w_m and radial position at each time by the instantaneous vessel radius $R(t)$. The aortic valve opens at $t = 0$. Peak velocity occurs 11% of the cardiac period after aortic valve opening. (From Ling SC et al. 1973. *Circ Res* 33:198. With permission.)

of about 2 the instantaneous profiles are close to the steady parabolic shape. Profiles in the aortic arch are skewed due to curvature of the arch.

10.4 Pathology

Atherosclerosis is a disease of the arterial wall which appears to be strongly influenced by hemodynamics. The disease begins with a thickening of the intimal layer in locations which correlate with the shear stress distribution on the endothelial surface (Friedman et al., 1993). Over time the lesion continues to grow until a significant portion of the vessel lumen is occluded. The peripheral circulation will dilate to compensate for the increase in resistance of the large vessel, compromising the ability of the system to respond to increases in demand during exercise. Eventually the circulation is completely dilated, and resting flow begins to decrease. A blood clot may form at the site or lodge in a narrowed segment, causing an acute loss of blood flow. The disease is particularly dangerous in the coronary and carotid arteries due to the critical oxygen requirements of the heart and brain.

In addition to intimal thickening, the arterial wall properties also change with age. Most measurements suggest that arterial elastic modulus increases with age (hardening of the arteries); however, in some cases arteries do become more compliant (inverse of elasticity) (Learoyd and Taylor, 1966). Local weakening of the wall may also occur, particularly in the descending aorta, giving rise to an aneurysm, which, if ruptures, can cause sudden death.

Defining Terms

Aneurysm: A ballooning of a blood vessel wall either involving the whole circumference or only part of the circumference caused by weakening of the elastic material in the wall.

Atherosclerosis: A disease of the blood vessel characterized by thickening of the vessel wall and eventual occlusion of the vessel.

Collagen: A protein found in blood vessels which is much stiffer than elastin.

Elastin: A very elastic protein found in blood vessels.

Endothelial: The inner lining of blood vessels.

Impedance: A (generally) complex number expressing the ratio of pressure to flow.

Myogenic: A change in smooth-muscle tone due to stretch or relaxation, causing a blood vessel to resist changes in diameter.

Newtonian: A fluid whose stress-rate-of-strain relationship is linear, following Newton's law. The fluid will have a viscosity whose value is independent of rate of strain.

Pulmonary: The circulation which delivers blood to the lungs for reoxygenation and carbon dioxide removal.

Systemic: The circulation which supplies oxygenated blood to the tissues of the body.

Vasoconstrictor: A substance which causes an increase in smooth-muscle tone, thereby constricting blood vessels.

Vasodilator: A substance which causes a decrease in smooth-muscle tone, thereby dilating blood vessels.

Viscoelastic: A substance which exhibits both elastic (solid) and viscous (liquid) characteristics.

References

Chandran KB, Yoganathan AP, and Rittgers SE. 2007 *Biofluid Mechanics, the Human Circulation*. Taylor & Francis, Boca Raton, FL.

Friedman MH, Brinkman AM, Qin JJ, and Seed WA. 1993. Relation between coronary artery geometry and the distribution of early sudanophilic lesions. *Atherosclerosis* 98:193.

Fung YC. 1984. *Biodynamics: Circulation*. Springer-Verlag, New York.

Korteweg DJ. 1878. Uber die Fortpflanzungsgeschwindigkeit des Schalles in elastischen. *Rohren. Ann Phys Chem (NS)* 5:525.

Learoyd BM and Taylor MG. 1966. Alterations with age in the viscoelasdc properties of human arterial walls. *Circ Res* 18:278.

Liepsch D, Thurston G, and Lee M. 1991. Studies of fluids simulating blood-like rheological properties and applications in models of arterial branches. *Biorheology* 28:39.

Ling SC, Atabek WG, Letzing WG, and Patel DJ. 1973. Nonlinear analysis of aortic flow in living dogs. *Circ Res* 33:198.

Mills CJ, Gabe IT, Gault JN et al. 1970. Pressure–flow relationships and vascular impedance in man. *Cardiovasc Res* 4:405.

Milnor WR. 1989. *Hemodynamics*, 2nd ed. Baltimore, Williams and Wilkins.

Moens AI. 1878. *Die Pulskurve*, Leiden, E.J. Brill.

Nerem RM and Seed WA. 1972. An in-vivo study of aortic flow disturbances. *Cardiovasc Res* 6:1.

Womersley JR. 1957. The mathematical analysis of the arterial circulation in a state of oscillatory motion. Wright Air Development Center Technical Report WADC-TR-56-614.

Young T. 1808. Hydraulic investigations, subservient to an intended Croonian lecture on the motion of the blood. *Philos Trans Roy Soc London* 98:164.

Further Information

A good introduction to cardiovascular biomechanics, including arterial hemodynamics, is provided by K. B. Chandran et al. in *Biofluid Mechanics, the Human Circulation*. Y. C. Rung's *Biodynamics—Circulation* is also an excellent starting point, somewhat more mathematical than Chandran. Perhaps the most complete treatment of the subject is in *Hemodynamics* by W. R. Milnor, from which much of this chapter was taken. Milnor's book is quite mathematical and may be difficult for a novice to follow.

Current work in arterial hemodynamics is reported in a number of engineering and physiological journals, including the *Annals of Biomedical Engineering, Journal of Biomechanical Engineering, Circulation Research*, and *The American Journal of Physiology, Heart and Circulatory Physiology*. Symposia sponsored by the American Society of Mechanical Engineers, Biomedical Engineering Society, American Heart Association, and the American Physiological Society contain reports of current research.

11

Mechanics of Blood Vessels

Thomas R. Canfield
Argonne National Laboratory

Philip B. Dobrin
Hines VA Hospital and Loyola University Medical Center

11.1 Assumptions

This chapter is concerned with the mechanical behavior of blood vessels under static loading conditions and the methods required to analyze this behavior. The assumptions underlying this discussion are for *ideal* blood vessels that are at least regionally homogeneous, incompressible, elastic, and cylindrically orthotropic. Although physiologic systems are *nonideal*, much understanding of vascular mechanics has been gained through the use of methods based upon these ideal assumptions.

11.1.1 Homogeneity of the Vessel Wall

On visual inspection, blood vessels appear to be fairly homogeneous and distinct from the surrounding connective tissue. The inhomogeneity of the vascular wall is realized when one examines the tissue under a low-power microscope, where one can easily identify two distinct structures: the media and adventitia. For this reason, the assumption of vessel wall homogeneity is applied cautiously. Such an assumption may be valid only within distinct macroscopic structures. However, few investigators have incorporated macroscopic inhomogeneity into studies of vascular mechanics [1].

11.1.2 Incompressibility of the Vessel Wall

Experimental measurement of wall compressibility of 0.06% at 270 cm of H_2O indicates that the vessel can be considered incompressible when subjected to physiologic pressure and load [2]. In terms of the mechanical behavior of blood vessels, this is small relative to the large magnitude of the distortional strains that occur when blood vessels are deformed under the same conditions. Therefore, vascular compressibility may be important to understand other physiologic processes related to blood vessels, such as the transport of interstitial fluid.

11.1.3 Inelasticity of the Vessel Wall

That blood vessel walls exhibit inelastic behavior such as length–tension and pressure–diameter hysteresis, stress relaxation, and creep has been reported extensively [3,4]. However, blood vessels are able to maintain stability and contain the pressure and flow of blood under a variety of physiologic conditions. These conditions are dynamic but slowly varying with a large static component.

11.1.4 Residual Stress and Strain

Blood vessels are known to retract both longitudinally and circumferentially are excision. This retraction is caused by the relief of distending forces resulting from internal pressure and longitudinal tractions. The magnitude of retraction is influenced by several factors. Among these factors are growth, aging, and hypertension. Circumferential retraction of medium-caliber blood vessels, such as the carotid, iliac, and bracheal arteries, can exceed 70% following reduction of internal blood pressure to zero. In the case of the carotid artery, the amount of longitudinal retraction tends to increase during growth and to decrease in subsequent aging [5]. It would seem reasonable to assume that blood vessels are in a nearly stress-free state when they are fully retracted and free of external loads. This configuration also seems to be a reasonable choice for the reference configuration. However, this ignores residual stress and strain effects that have been the subject of current research [6–11].

Blood vessels are formed in a dynamic environment that gives rise to imbalances between the forces that tend to extend the diameter and length and the internal forces that tend to resist the extension. This imbalance is thought to stimulate the growth of elastin and collagen and to effectively reduce the stresses in the underlying tissue. Under these conditions, it is not surprising that a residual stress state exists when the vessel is fully retracted and free of external tractions. This process has been called *remodeling* [7]. Striking evidence of this remodeling is found when a cylindrical slice of the fully retracted blood vessel is cut longitudinally through the wall. The cylinder springs open, releasing bending stresses kept in balance by the cylindrical geometry [11].

11.2 Vascular Anatomy

A blood vessel can be anatomically divided into three distinct cylindrical sections when viewed under the optical microscope. Starting at the inside of the vessel, they are the intima, the media, and the adventitia. These structures have distinct functions in terms of the blood vessel physiology and mechanical properties.

The intima consists of a thin monolayer of endothelial cells that line the inner surface of the blood vessel. The endothelial cells have little influence on blood vessel mechanics but do play an important role in hemodynamics and transport phenomena. Because of their anatomical location, these cells are subjected to large variations in stress and strain as a result of pulsatile changes in blood pressure and flow.

The media represents the major portion of the vessel wall and provides most of the mechanical strength necessary to sustain structural integrity. The media is organized into alternating layers of interconnected smooth muscle cells and elastic lamellae. There is evidence of collagen throughout the media. These small collagen fibers are found within the bands of smooth muscle and may participate in the transfer of forces between the smooth muscle cells and the elastic lamellae. The elastic lamellae are principally composed of the fibrous protein elastin. The number of elastic lamellae depends upon the wall thickness and the anatomical location [12]. In the case of the canine carotid, the elastic lamellae account for a major component of the static structural response of the blood vessel [13]. This response is modulated by the smooth muscle cells, which have the ability to actively change the mechanical characteristics of the wall [14].

The adventitia consists of loose, more disorganized fibrous connective tissue, which may have less influence on mechanics.

11.3 Axisymmetric Deformation

In the following discussion, we will concern ourselves with the deformation of cylindrical tubes (see Figure 11.1). Blood vessels tend to be nearly cylindrical *in situ* and tend to remain cylindrical when a cylindrical section is excised and studied *in vitro*. Only when the vessel is dissected further does the geometry begin to deviate from cylindrical. For this deformation, there is a unique coordinate mapping

$$(R,\Theta,Z) \to (r,\theta,z) \qquad (11.1)$$

where the undeformed coordinates are given by (R, Θ, Z) and the deformed coordinates are given by (r, θ, z). The deformation is given by a set of restricted functions

$$r = r(R) \qquad (11.2)$$

$$\theta = \beta\Theta \qquad (11.3)$$

$$z = \mu\, Z + C_1 \qquad (11.4)$$

where the constants μ and β have been introduced to account for a uniform longitudinal strain and a symmetric residual strain that are both independent of the coordinate Θ.

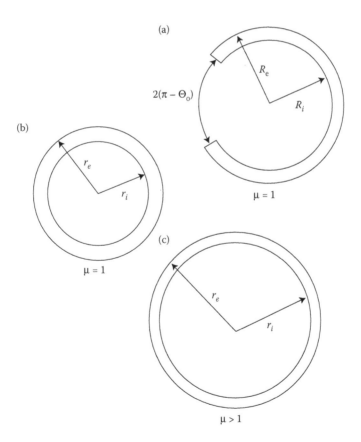

FIGURE 11.1 Cylindrical geometry of a blood vessel. (a) Stress-free reference configuration, (b) fully retracted vessel free of external traction, and (c) vessel *in situ* under longitudinal tether and internal pressurization.

If $\beta = 1$, there is no residual strain. If $\beta \neq 1$, residual stresses and strains are present. If $\beta > 1$, a longitudinal cut through the wall will cause the blood vessel to open up, and the new cross section will form a c-shaped section of an annulus with larger internal and external radii. If $\beta < 1$, the cylindrical shape is unstable, but a thin section will tend to overlap itself. In Choung and Fung's formulation, $\beta = \pi/\Theta_o$, where the angle Θ_o is half the angle spanned by the open annular section [6].

For cylindrical blood vessels, there are two assumed constraints. The first assumption is that the longitudinal strain is uniform through the wall and therefore

$$\lambda_z = \mu = \text{a constant} \tag{11.5}$$

for any cylindrical configuration. Given this, the principal stretch ratios are computed from the above function as

$$\lambda_r = \frac{dr}{dR} \tag{11.6}$$

$$\lambda_\theta = \beta \frac{r}{R} \tag{11.7}$$

$$\lambda_z = \mu \tag{11.8}$$

The second assumption is wall incompressibility, which can be expressed by

$$\lambda_r \lambda_\theta \lambda_z \equiv 1 \tag{11.9}$$

or

$$\beta\mu \frac{r}{R} \frac{dr}{dR} = 1 \tag{11.10}$$

and therefore

$$r\,dr = \frac{1}{\beta\mu} R\,dR \tag{11.11}$$

The integration of this expression yields the solution

$$r^2 = \frac{1}{\beta\mu} R^2 + c_2 \tag{11.12}$$

where

$$c_2 = r_e^2 - \frac{1}{\beta\mu} R_e^2 \tag{11.13}$$

As a result, the principal stretch ratios can be expressed in terms of R as follows:

$$\lambda_r = \frac{R}{\sqrt{\beta\mu(R^2 + \beta\mu c_2)}} \tag{11.14}$$

$$\lambda_\theta = \sqrt{\frac{1}{\beta\mu} + \frac{c_2}{R^2}} \tag{11.15}$$

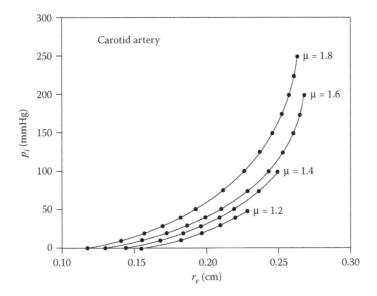

FIGURE 11.2 Pressure–radius curves for the canine carotid artery at various degrees of longitudinal extension.

11.4 Experimental Measurements

The basic experimental setup required to measure the mechanical properties of blood vessels *in vitro* is described in Reference 14. It consists of a temperature-regulated bath of physiologic saline solution to maintain immersed cylindrical blood vessel segments, devices to measure the diameter, an apparatus to hold the vessel at a constant longitudinal extension and to measure longitudinal distending force, and a system to deliver and control the internal pressure of the vessel with 100% oxygen. Typical data obtained from this type of experiment are shown in Figures 11.2 and 11.3.

11.5 Equilibrium

When blood vessels are excised, they retract both longitudinally and circumferentially. Restoration to natural dimensions requires the application of internal pressure, p_i, and a longitudinal tether force, F_T. The internal pressure and longitudinal tether are balanced by the development of forces within the vessel wall. The internal pressure is balanced in the circumferential direction by a wall tension, T. The longitudinal tether force and pressure are balanced by the retractive force of the wall, F_R

$$T = p_i r_i \tag{11.16}$$

$$F_R = F_T + p_i \pi r_i^2 \tag{11.17}$$

The first equation is the familiar law of Laplace for a cylindrical tube with internal radius r_i. It indicates that the force due to internal pressure, p_i, must be balanced by a tensile force (per unit length), T, within the wall. This tension is the integral of the circumferentially directed force intensity (or stress, σ_θ) across the wall

$$T = \int_{r_i}^{r_e} \sigma_\theta dr = \bar{\sigma}_\theta h \tag{11.18}$$

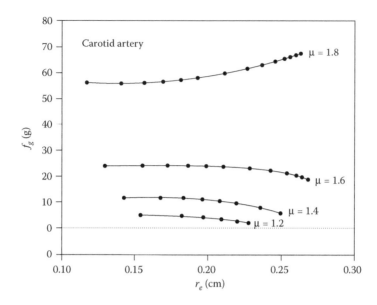

FIGURE 11.3 Longitudinal distending force as a function of radius at various degrees of longitudinal extension.

where $\bar{\sigma}_\theta$ is the mean value of the circumferential stress and h is the wall thickness. Similarly, the longitudinal tether force, F_T, and extending force due to internal pressure are balanced by a retractive internal force, F_R, due to axial stress, σ_z, in the blood vessel wall

$$F_R = 2\pi \int_{r_i}^{r_e} \sigma_z r dr = \bar{\sigma}_z \, \pi h (r_e + r_i) \tag{11.19}$$

where $\bar{\sigma}_z$ is the mean value of this longitudinal stress. The mean stresses are calculated from the above equation as

$$\bar{\sigma}_\theta = p_i \frac{r_i}{h} \tag{11.20}$$

$$\bar{\sigma}_z = \frac{F_T}{\pi h (r_e + r_i)} + \frac{p_i}{2} \frac{r_i}{h} \tag{11.21}$$

The mean stresses are a fairly good approximation for thin-walled tubes where the variations through the wall are small. However, the range of applicability of the thin-wall assumption depends upon the material properties and geometry. In a linear elastic material, the variation in σ_θ is less than 5% for $r/h > 20$. When the material is nonlinear or the deformation is large, the variations in stress can be more severe (see Figure 11.10).

The stress distribution is determined by solving the equilibrium equation

$$\frac{1}{r} \frac{d}{dr} (r\sigma_r) - \frac{\sigma_\theta}{r} = 0 \tag{11.22}$$

This equation governs how the two stresses are related and must change in the cylindrical geometry. For uniform extension and internal pressurization, the stresses must be functions of a single radial coordinate, r, subject to the two boundary conditions for the radial stress:

$$\sigma_r(r_i, \mu) = -p_i \tag{11.23}$$

$$\sigma_r(r_e, \mu) = 0 \tag{11.24}$$

11.6 Strain Energy Density Functions

Blood vessels are able to maintain their structural stability and contain steady oscillating internal pressures. This property suggests a strong elastic component, which has been called *pseudoelasticity* [4]. This elastic response can be characterized by a single potential function called the *strain energy density*. It is a scalar function of the strains that determines the amount of stored elastic energy per unit volume. In the case of a cylindrically orthotropic tube of incompressible material, the strain energy density can be written in the following functional form:

$$W = W^*(\lambda_r, \lambda_\theta, \lambda_z) + \lambda_r \lambda_\theta \lambda_z p \tag{11.25}$$

where p is a scalar function of position, R. The stresses are computed from the strain energy by the following equation:

$$\sigma_i = \lambda_i \frac{\partial W^*}{\partial \lambda_i} + p \tag{11.26}$$

We make the following transformation [15]:

$$\lambda = \frac{\beta r}{\sqrt{\beta \mu (r^2 - c_2)}} \tag{11.27}$$

which upon differentiation gives

$$r \frac{d\lambda}{dr} = \beta^{-1}(\beta \lambda - \mu \lambda^3) \tag{11.28}$$

After these expressions and the stresses in terms of the strain energy density function are introduced into the equilibrium equation, we obtain an ordinary differential equation for p

$$\frac{dp}{d\lambda} = \frac{\beta W^*_{\lambda_\theta} - W^*_{\lambda_r}}{\beta \lambda = \mu \lambda^3} - \frac{d W^*_{\lambda_r}}{d\lambda} \tag{11.29}$$

subject to the boundary conditions

$$p(R_i) = p_i \tag{11.30}$$

$$p(R_e) = 0 \tag{11.31}$$

11.6.1 Isotropic Blood Vessels

A blood vessel generally exhibits anisotropic behavior when subjected to large variations in internal pressure and distending force. When the degree of anisotropy is small, the blood vessel may be treated as isotropic. For isotropic materials, it is convenient to introduce the strain invariants:

$$I_1 = \lambda_r^2 + \lambda_\theta^2 + \lambda_z^2 \tag{11.32}$$

$$I_2 = \lambda_r^2\lambda_\theta^2 + \lambda_\theta^2\lambda_z^2 + \lambda_z^2\lambda_r^2 \tag{11.33}$$

$$I_3 = \lambda_r^2\lambda_\theta^2\lambda_z^2 \tag{11.34}$$

These are measures of strain that are independent of the choice of coordinates. If the material is incompressible

$$I_3 = j^2 \equiv 1 \tag{11.35}$$

and the strain energy density is a function of the first two invariants, then

$$W = W(I_1, I_2) \tag{11.36}$$

The least complex form for an incompressible material is the first-order polynomial, which was first proposed by Mooney to characterize rubber:

$$W^* = \frac{G}{2}[(I_1 - 3) + k(I_2 - 3)] \tag{11.37}$$

It involves only two elastic constants. A special case, where $k = 0$, is the neo-Hookean material, which can be derived from thermodynamics principles for a simple solid. The exact solutions can be obtained for the cylindrical deformation of a thick-walled tube. In the case where there is no residual strain, we have the following equations:

$$P = -G(1 + k\mu^2)\left[\frac{\log\lambda}{\mu} + \frac{1}{2\mu^2\lambda^2}\right] + c_0 \tag{11.38}$$

$$\sigma_r = G\left[\frac{1}{\lambda^2\mu^2} + k\left(\frac{1}{\mu^2} + \frac{1}{\lambda^2}\right)\right] + p \tag{11.39}$$

$$\sigma_\theta = G\left[\lambda^2 + k\left(\frac{1}{\mu^2} + \lambda^2\mu^2\right)\right] + p \tag{11.40}$$

$$\sigma_z = G\left[\mu^2 + k\left(\lambda^2\mu^2 + \frac{1}{\lambda^2}\right)\right] + p \tag{11.41}$$

However, these equations predict stress softening for a vessel subjected to internal pressurization at fixed lengths, rather than the stress stiffening observed in experimental studies on arteries and veins (see Figures 11.4 and 11.5).

An alternative isotropic strain energy density function that can predict the appropriate type of stress stiffening for blood vessels is an exponential where the arguments are a polynomial of the strain invariants. The first-order form is given by

$$W^* = \frac{G_0}{2k_1}\exp[k_1(I_1 - 3) + k_2(I_2 - 3)] \tag{11.42}$$

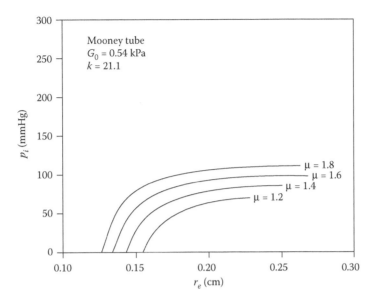

FIGURE 11.4   Pressure–radius curves for a Mooney–Rivlin tube with the approximate dimensions of the carotid.

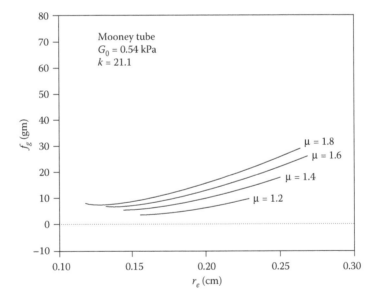

FIGURE 11.5   Longitudinal distending force as a function of radius for the Mooney–Rivlin tube.

This requires the determination of only two independent elastic constants. The third, G_0, is introduced to facilitate scaling of the argument of the exponent (see Figures 11.6 and 11.7). This exponential form is attractive for several reasons. It is a natural extension of the observation that biologic tissue stiffness is proportional to the load in simple elongation. This stress stiffening has been attributed to a statistical recruitment and alignment of tangled and disorganized long chains of proteins. The exponential forms resemble statistical distributions derived from these same arguments.

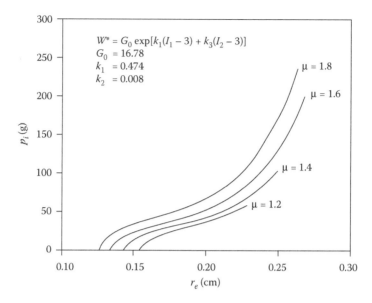

FIGURE 11.6 Pressure–radius curves for the tube with the approximate dimensions of the carotid calculated using an isotropic exponential strain energy density function.

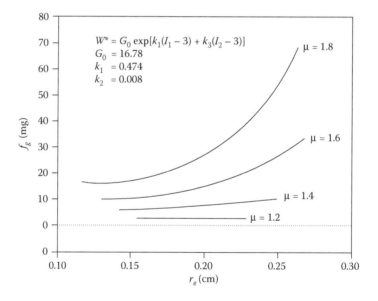

FIGURE 11.7 Longitudinal distending force as a function of radius for the isotropic tube.

11.6.2 Anisotropic Blood Vessels

Studies of the orthotropic behavior of blood vessels may employ polynomial or exponential strain energy density functions that include all strain terms or extension ratios. In particular, the strain energy density function can be of the form

$$W^\star = q_n(\lambda_r, \lambda_\theta, \lambda_z) \tag{11.43}$$

or

$$W^* = e^{q_n(\lambda_r, \lambda_\theta, \lambda_z)} \tag{11.44}$$

where q_n is a polynomial of order n. Since the material is incompressible, the explicit dependence upon λ_r can be eliminated either by substituting $\lambda_r = \lambda_\theta^{-1} \lambda_z^{-1}$ or by assuming that the wall is thin and hence the contribution of these terms is small. Figures 11.8 and 11.9 illustrate how well the experimental data can be fitted to an exponential strain density function whose argument is a polynomial of order $n = 3$.

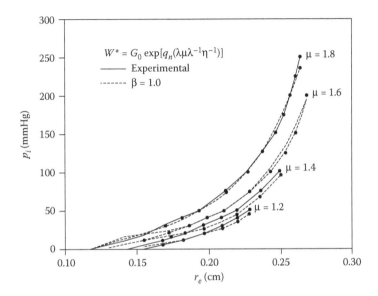

FIGURE 11.8 Pressure–radius curves for a fully orthotropic vessel calculated with an exponential strain energy density function.

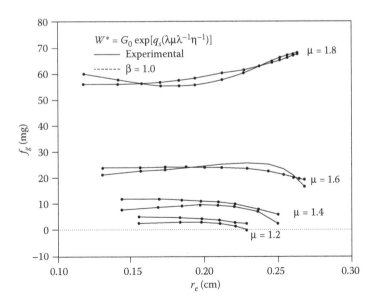

FIGURE 11.9 Longitudinal distending force as a function of radius for the orthotropic vessel.

Care must be taken to formulate expressions that will lead to stresses that behave properly. For this reason, it is convenient to formulate the strain energy density in terms of the Lagrangian strains

$$e_i = 1/2(\lambda_i^2 - 1) \tag{11.45}$$

and in this case, we can consider polynomials of the Lagrangian strains, $q_n(e_r, e_\theta, e_z)$.

Vaishnav et al. [16] proposed using a polynomial of the form

$$W^\star = \sum_{i=2}^{n}\sum_{j=0}^{i} a_{ij-i} e_\theta^{i-j} e_z^j \tag{11.46}$$

to approximate the behavior of the canine aorta. They found better correlation with order-three polynomials over order-two polynomials, but order-four polynomials did not warrant the additional work.

Later, Fung et al. [4] found very good correlation with an expression of the form

$$W - \frac{C}{2}\exp[a_1(e_\theta^2 - e_z^{*2}) + a_2(e_z^2 - e_z^{*2}) + 2a_4(e_\theta e_z - e_\theta^* e_z^*)] \tag{11.47}$$

for the canine carotid artery, where e_θ^* and e_z^* are the strains in a reference configuration at *in situ* length and pressure. Why should this work? One answer appears to be related to residual stresses and strains.

When residual stresses are ignored, large-deformation analysis of thick-walled blood vessels predicts steep distributions in σ_θ and σ_z through the vessel wall, with the highest stresses at the interior. This prediction is considered significant because high tensions in the inner wall could inhibit vascularization and oxygen transport to the vascular tissue.

When residual stresses are considered, the stress distributions flatten considerably and become almost uniform at *in situ* length and pressure. Figure 11.10 shows the radial stress distributions computed for a vessel with $\beta = 1$ and $\beta = 1.11$. Takamizawa and Hayashi [9] have even considered the case where the strain distribution is uniform *in situ*. The physiologic implications are that the vascular tissue

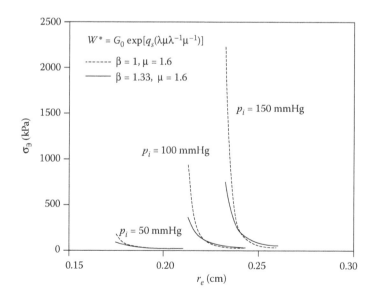

FIGURE 11.10   Stress distributions through the wall at various pressures for the orthotropic vessel.

is in a constant state of flux. The new tissue is synthesized in a state of stress that allows it to redistribute the internal loads more uniformly. There is probably no stress-free reference state [7,8,17]. Continuous dissection of the tissue into smaller and smaller pieces would continue to relieve residual stresses and strains [10].

References

1. Von Maltzahn, W.-W., Desdo, D., and Wiemier, W. 1981. Elastic properties of arteries: A nonlinear two-layer cylindrical model. *J. Biomech.* 4:389.
2. Carew, T.E., Vaishnav, R.N., and Patel, D.J. 1968. Compressibility of the arterial walls. *Circ. Res.* 23:61.
3. Bergel, D.H. 1961. The static elastic properties of the arterial wall. *J. Physiol.* 156:445.
4. Fung, Y.C., Fronek, K., and Patitucci, P. 1979. Pseudoelasticity of arteries and the choice of its mathematical expression. *Am. J. Physiol.* 237:H620.
5. Dobrin, P.B. 1978. Mechanical properties of arteries. *Physiol. Rev.* 58:397.
6. Choung, C.J. and Fung, Y.C. 1986. On residual stresses in arteries. *J. Biomed. Eng.* 108:189.
7. Fung, Y.C., Liu, S.Q., and Zhou, J.B. 1993. Remodeling of the constitutive equation while a blood vessel remodels itself under strain. *J. Biomech. Eng.* 115:453.
8. Rachev, A., Greenwald, S., Kane, T., Moore, J., and Meister, J.-J. 1994. Effects of age-related changes in the residual strains on the stress distribution in the arterial wall. In J. Vossoughi (ed.), *Proceedings of the 13th Society of Biomedical Engineering Recent Developments*, pp. 409–412, Washington DC, University of District of Columbia.
9. Takamizawa, K. and Hayashi, K. 1987. Strain energy density function and the uniform strain hypothesis for arterial mechanics. *J. Biomech.* 20:7.
10. Vassoughi, J. 1992. Longitudinal residual strain in arteries. *Proceedings of the 11th South Biomedical Engineering Conference*, Memphis, TN.
11. Vaishnav, R.N. and Vassoughi, J. 1983. Estimation of residual stresses in aortic segments. In C.W. Hall (ed.), *Biomedical Engineering II, Recent Developments*, pp. 330–333, New York, NY, Pergamon Press.
12. Wolinsky, H. and Glagov, S. 1969. Comparison of abdominal and thoracic aortic media structure in mammals. *Circ. Res.* 25:677.
13. Dobrin, P.B. and Canfield, T.R. 1984. Elastase, collagenase, and the biaxial elastic properties of dog carotid artery. *Am. J. Physiol.* 2547:H124.
14. Dobrin, P.B. and Rovick, A.A. 1969. Influence of vascular smooth muscle on contractile mechanics and elasticity of arteries. *Am. J. Physiol.* 217:1644.
15. Chu, B.M. and Oka, S. 1973. Influence of longitudinal tethering on the tension in thick-walled blood vessels in equilibrium. *Biorheology* 10:517.
16. Vaishnav, R.N., Young, J.T., Janicki, J.S., and Patel, D.J. 1972. Nonlinear anisotropic elastic properties of the canine aorta. *Biophys. J.* 12:1008.
17. Dobrin, P.D., Canfield, T., and Sinha, S. 1975. Development of longitudinal retraction of carotid arteries in neonatal dogs. *Experientia* 31:1295.
18. Doyle, J.M. and Dobrin, P.B. 1971. Finite deformation of the relaxed and contracted dog carotid artery. *Microvasc. Res.* 3:400.

12

The Venous System

Artin A. Shoukas
Johns Hopkins University

Carl F. Rothe
Indiana University

12.1 Introduction

The venous system not only serves as a conduit for the return of blood from the capillaries to the heart but also provides a dynamic, variable blood storage compartment that influences cardiac output. The systemic (noncardiopulmonary) venous system contains more than 75% of the blood volume of the entire systemic circulation. Although the heart is the source of energy for propelling blood throughout the circulation, filling of the right heart before the subsequent beat is primarily passive. The subsequent amount of blood ejected is exquisitely sensitive to the transmural filling pressure (e.g., a change of right heart filling pressure of 1 cm water can cause the cardiac output to change by about 50%).

Because the blood vessels are elastic and have smooth muscle in their walls, contraction or relaxation of the smooth muscle can quickly redistribute blood between the periphery and the heart to influence cardiac filling and thus cardiac output. Even though the right ventricle is not essential for life, its functioning acts to reduce the central venous pressure to facilitate venous return [1]. It largely determines the magnitude of the cardiac output by influencing the degree of filling of the left heart. Dynamic changes in venous tone, by redistributing blood volume, can thus, at rest, change cardiac output over a range of more than ±20%. The dimensions of the vasculature influence both blood flow—by way of their resistive properties—and contained blood volume—by way of their capacitive properties. The arteries have about 10 times the resistance of the veins, and the veins are more than 10 times as compliant as the arteries.

The conduit characteristics of the venous system primarily depend on the anatomy of the system. Valves in the veins of the limbs are crucial for reducing the pressure in dependent parts of the body. Even small movements from skeletal muscle activity tend to compress the veins and move blood toward the heart. A competent valve then blocks back flow, thus relieving the pressure when the movement stops. Even a few steps can reduce the transmural venous pressure in the ankle from as much as 100 mmHg to about 20 mmHg. Without this mechanism, transcapillary movement of fluid into the extravascular spaces results in edema. Varicose (swollen) veins and peripheral pooling of blood can result from damage to the venous valves. During exercise, the rhythmic contraction of the skeletal muscles, in conjunction with venous valves, provides an important mechanism—the skeletal muscle pump—aiding the large increases in blood flow through the muscles without excessive increases in capillary pressure and blood pooling in the veins of the muscles. Without this mechanism, the increase in venous return leading to the dramatic increases in cardiac output would be greatly limited.

12.2 Definitions

12.2.1 Capacitance

Capacitance is a general term that relates the magnitude of contained volume to the transmural pressure across the vessel walls and is defined by the pressure–volume relationship. In living blood vessels, the pressure–volume relationship is complex and nonlinear. At transmural pressure near zero, there is a finite volume within the vessels (see definition of *unstressed volume*). If this volume is then removed from the vessels, there is only a small decrease in transmural pressure as the vessel collapses from a circular cross-section to an elliptical one. This is especially true for superficial or isolated venous vessels. However, for vessels which are tethered or embedded in tissue a negative pressure may result without appreciably changing the shape of the vessels. With increases in contained volume, the vessel becomes distended, and there is a concomitant increase in transmural pressure. The incremental change in volume to incremental change in transmural pressure is often relatively constant. At very high transmural pressures vessels become stiffer, and the incremental volume change to transmural pressure change is small. Because all blood vessels exhibit these nonlinearities, no single parameter can describe capacitance; instead the entire pressure–volume relationship must be considered.

12.2.2 Compliance

Vascular compliance (C) is defined as the slope of the pressure–volume relationship. It is the ratio of the change in incremental volume (ΔV) to a change in incremental transmural pressure (ΔP). Thus, $C = \Delta V/\Delta P$. Because the pressure–volume relationship is nonlinear, the slope of the relationship is not constant over its full range of pressures, and so the compliance should be specified at a given pressure. Units of compliance are those of volume divided by pressure, usually reported in mL/mmHg. Values are typically normalized to wet tissue weight or to total body weight. When the compliance is normalized by the total contained blood volume, it is termed the *vascular distensibility* and represents the fractional change in volume ($\Delta V/V$) per change in transmural pressure; $D = (\Delta V/V)\,\Delta P$, where V is the volume at control or at zero transmural pressure.

12.2.3 Unstressed Volume

Unstressed volume (V_0) is the volume in the vascular system when the transmural pressure is zero. It is a calculated volume obtained by extrapolating the relatively linear segment of the pressure–volume relationship over the normal operating range to zero transmural pressure. Many studies have shown that reflexes and drugs have quantitatively more influence on V_0 than on the compliance.

12.2.4 Stressed Volume

The *stressed volume* (V_s) is the volume of blood in the vascular system that must be removed to change the computed transmural pressure from its prevailing value to zero transmural pressure. It is computed as the product of the vascular compliance and transmural distending pressure: $V_s = V \times P$. The total contained blood volume at a specific pressure (P) is the sum of stressed and unstressed volume. The unstressed volume is then computed as the total blood volume minus the stressed volume. Because of the marked nonlinearity around zero transmural pressure and the required extrapolation, both V_0 and V_s are virtual volumes.

12.2.5 Capacity

Capacity refers to the amount of blood volume contained in the blood vessels at a specific distending pressure. It is the sum of the unstressed volume and the stressed volume, $V = V_0 + V_s$.

12.2.6 Mean Filling Pressure

If the inflow and outflow of an organ are suddenly stopped, and blood volume is redistributed so that all pressures within the vasculature are the same, this pressure is the *mean filling pressure* [2]. This pressure can be measured for the systemic or pulmonary circuits or the body as a whole. The arterial pressure often does not equal the venous pressure as flow is reduced to zero, because blood must move from the distended arterial vessels to the venous beds during the measurement maneuver, and the flow may stop before equilibrium occurs. This is because smooth-muscle activity in the arterial vessels, rheological properties of blood, or high interstitial pressures act to impede the flow. Thus, corrections must often be made [2,3]. The experimentally measured mean filling pressure provides a good estimate of P_v (the pressure in the minute venules), for estimating venous stressed volume.

12.2.7 Venous Resistance

Venous resistance (R) refers to the hindrance to blood flow through the venous vasculature caused by friction of the moving blood along the venous vascular wall. By definition it is the ratio of the pressure gradient between the entrance of the venous circulation, namely the capillaries, and the venous outflow divided by the venous flow rate. Thus,

$$R = \frac{(P_c = P_{ra})}{F} \tag{12.1}$$

where R is the venous resistance, P_c is the capillary pressure, P_{ra} is the right atrial pressure, and F is the venous flow. As flow is decreased to zero, arterial closure may occur, leading to a positive perfusion pressure at zero flow. With partial collapse of veins, a Starling resistor-like condition is present in which an increase in outlet pressure has no influence on flow until the outlet pressure is greater than the "waterfall" pressure.

12.2.8 Venous Inertance

Venous inertance (I_v) is the opposition to a change in flow rate related to the mass of the bolus of blood that is accelerated or decelerated. The inertance I_v for a cylindrical tube with constant cross-sectional area is $I_v = L\rho/A$, where L is the length of the vessel, ρ is the density of the blood, and A is the cross-sectional area [4].

12.3 Methods to Measure Venous Characteristics

Our knowledge of the nature and role of the capacitance characteristics of the venous system has been limited by the difficulty of measuring the various variables needed to compute parameter values. State-of-the-art equipment is often needed because of the low pressures and many disturbing factors present. Many of the techniques that have been used to measure venous capacitance require numerous assumptions that may not be correct or are currently impossible to evaluate [3].

12.3.1 Resistance

For the estimate of vascular resistance, the upstream to outflow pressure gradient across the tissues must be estimated along with a measure of flow. Pressures in large vessels are measured with a catheter connected to a pressure transducer, which typically involves measurement of minute changes in resistance elements attached to a stiff diaphragm which flexes proportionally to the pressure. For the veins in tissue, the upstream pressure, just downstream from the capillaries, is much more difficult to measure because of the minute size (~15 μm) of the vessels. For this a servo-null micropipette technique may be used. A glass micropipette with a tip diameter of about 2 μm is filled with a 1–2 mol saline solution. When the pipette is inserted into a vein, the pressure tends to drive the lower conductance blood plasma into the pipette. The conductance is measured using an AC-driven bridge. A servosystem, driven by the imbalance signal, is used to develop a counter pressure to maintain the interface between the low-conductance filling solution and the plasma near the tip of the pipette. This counter pressure, which equals the intravascular pressure, is measured with a pressure transducer. Careful calibration is essential.

Another approach for estimating the upstream pressure in the veins is to measure the mean filling pressure of the organ (see above) and assume that this pressure is the upstream venous pressure. Because this venous pressure must be less than the capillary pressure and because most of the blood in an organ is in the small veins and venules, this assumption, though tenuous, is not unreasonable. To measure flow many approaches are available, including electromagnetic, transit-time ultrasonic, or Doppler ultrasonic flowmeters. Usually the arterial inflow is measured with the assumption that the outflow is the same. Indicator dilution techniques are also used to estimate average flow. They are based on the principle that the reduction in concentration of infused indicator is inversely proportional to the rate of flow. Either a bolus injection or a continuous infusion may be used. Adequacy of mixing of indicator across the flow stream, lack of collateral flows, and adequately representative sampling must be considered [5].

12.3.2 Capacitance

For estimating the capacitance parameters of the veins, contained volume, rather than flow, and transmural pressure, rather than the longitudinal pressure gradient, must be measured. Pressures are measured as described above. For the desired pressure–volume relationship the total contained volume must be known.

The techniques used to measure total blood volume include *indicator dilution.* The ratio of the integral of indicator concentration time to that of concentration is used to compute the mean transit time (MTT) following the sudden injection of a bolus of indicator [3,5]. The active volume is the product of MTT and flow, with flow measured as outlined above. Scintigraphy provides an image of the distribution of radioactivity in tissues. A radioisotope, such as technetium-99 that is bound to red blood cells which in turn are contained within the vasculature, is injected and allowed to equilibrate. A camera, with many collimating channels sensitive to the emitted radiation, is placed over the tissue. The activity recorded is proportional to the volume of blood. Currently it is not possible to accurately calibrate the systems to provide measures of blood volume because of uncertain attenuation of radiation by the tissue and distance. Furthermore, delimiting a particular organ within the body and separating arterial and venous segments of the circulation are difficult.

12.3.3 Compliance

To estimate compliance, changes in volume are needed. This is generally easier than measuring the total blood volume. Using *plethysmography,* a rigid container is placed around the organ, and a servo system functions to change the fluid volume in the chamber to maintain the chamber pressure constant. The consequent volume change is measured and assumed to be primarily venous, because most of the vascular volume is venous. With a tight system and careful technique, at the end of the experiment both inflow and outflow blood vessels can be occluded and then the contained blood washed out and measured to provide a measure of the total blood volume [6].

12.3.4 Gravimetric Techniques

Gravimetric techniques can be used to measure changes in blood volume. If the organ can be isolated and weighed continuously with the blood vessels intact, changes in volume can be measured in response to drugs or reflexes. With an important modification, this approach can be applied to an organ or the systemic circulation; the tissues are perfused at a constant rate, and the outflow is emptied at a constant pressure into a reservoir. Because the reservoir is emptied at a constant rate for the perfusion, changes in reservoir volume reflect an opposite change in the perfused tissue blood volume [7]. To measure compliance, the outflow pressure is changed (2–5 mmHg) and the corresponding change in reservoir volume noted. With the inflow and outflow pressure held constant, the pressure gradients are assumed to be constant so that 100% of an outflow pressure change can be assumed to be transmitted to the primary capacitance vessels. Any reflex or drug-induced change in reservoir volume may be assumed to be inversely related to an active change in vascular volume [7–9]. If resistances are also changed by the reflex or drug, then corrections are needed and the interpretations are more complex.

12.3.5 Outflow Occlusion

If the outflow downstream from the venous catheter is suddenly occluded, the venous pressure increases, and its rate of increase is measured. The rate of inflow is also measured so that the compliance can be estimated as the ratio flow to rate of pressure rise: Compliance in mL/mmHg = (flow in mL/min)/(rate of venous pressure rise in mmHg/min). The method is predicated on the assumption that the inflow continues at a constant rate and that there is no pressure gradient between the pressure measuring point and the site of compliance for the first few seconds of occlusion when the rate of pressure rise is measured.

12.3.6 Integral of Inflow Minus Outflow

With this technique both inflow and outflow are measured and the difference integrated to provide the volume change during an experimental forcing. If there is a decrease in contained volume, the outflow will be transiently greater than the inflow. The volume change gives a measure of the response to drugs or reflexes. Following a change in venous pressure, the technique can be used to measure compliance. Accurate measures of flow are needed. Serious errors can result if the inflow is not measured but is only assumed to be constant during the experimental protocol. With all methods dependent on measured or controlled flow, small changes in zero offset, which is directly or indirectly integrated, leads to serious error after about 10 min, and so the methods are not useful for long-term or slow responses.

12.4 Typical Values

Cardiac output, the sine qua non of the cardiovascular system, averages about 100 mL/(min-kg). It is about 90 in humans, is over 110 mL/(min-kg) in dogs and cats, and is even higher on a body weight basis in small animals such as rats and mice. The mean arterial blood pressure in relaxed, resting, conscious mammals averages about 90 mmHg. The mean circulatory filling pressure averages about 7 mmHg, and the central venous pressure just outside the right heart about 2 mmHg. The blood volume of the body is about 75 mL/kg, but in humans it is about 10% less, and it is larger in small animals. It is difficult to measure accurately because the volume of distribution of the plasma is about 10% higher than that of the red blood cells.

Vascular compliance averages about 2 mL (mmHg-kg body weight). The majority is in the venules and veins. Arterial compliance is only about 0.05 mL/mmHg-kg. Skeletal muscle compliance is less than that of the body as a whole, whereas the vascular compliance of the liver is about 10 times that of other organs. The stressed volume is the product of compliance and mean filling pressure and so is about 15 mL/kg. By difference, the unstressed volume is about 60 mL/kg.

As flow is increased through a tissue, the contained volume increases even if the outflow pressure is held constant, because there is a finite pressure drop across the veins, which is increased as flow increases. This increase in upstream distending pressure acts to increase the contained blood volume. The volume sensitivity to flow averages about 0.1 mL per 1 mL/min change in flow [10]. For the body as a whole, the sensitivity is about 0.25 mL per 1 mL/min with reflexes blocked, and with reflexes intact it averages about 0.4 mL/min³. Using similar techniques, it appears that the passive compensatory volume redistribution from the peripheral toward the heart during serious left heart failure is similar in magnitude to a reflex-engendered redistribution from activation of venous smooth muscle [6].

The high-pressure carotid sinus baroreceptor reflex system is capable of changing the venous capacitance [9]. Over the full operating range of the reflex it is capable of mobilizing up to 7.5 mL/kg of blood by primarily changing the unstressed vascular volume with little or no changes in venous compliance [7,8]. Although this represents only a 10% change in blood volume, it can cause nearly a 100% change in cardiac output. It is difficult to say with confidence what particular organ and/or tissue is contributing to this blood volume mobilization. Current evidence suggests that the splanchnic vascular bed contributes significantly to the capacitance change, but this also may vary between species [11].

Acknowledgments

This work was supported by the National Heart Lung and Blood Institute grants HL 19039 and HL 07723.

References

1. Furey, S.A.I., Zieske, H., and Levy, M.N. 1984. The essential function of the right heart. *Am. Heart J.* 107: 404.
2. Rothe, C.F. 1993. Mean circulatory filling pressure: its meaning and measurement. *J. Appl. Physiol.* 74: 499.
3. Rothe, C.F. 1983. Venous system: Physiology of the capacitance vessels. In J.T. Shepherd, and F.M. Abboud (Eds.), *Handbook of Physiology: The Cardiovascular System*, sec. 2, Vol. 3, pt 1, pp. 397–452, Bethesda, MD, American Physiology Society.
4. Rose, W. and Shoukas, A.A. 1993. Two-port analysis of systemic venous and arterial impedances. *Am. J. Physiol.* 265 (*Heart Circ. Physiol.* 34): H1577.
5. Lassen, N.A. and Perl, W. 1979. *Tracer Kinetic Methods in Medical Physiology*. New York, Raven Press.
6. Zink, J., Delaive, J., Mazerall, E., and Greenway, C.V. 1976. An improved plethsmograph with servo control of hydrostatic pressure. *J. Appl. Physiol.* 41: 107.
7. Shoukas, A.A. and Sagawa, K. 1973. Control of total systemic vascular capacity by the carotid sinus baroreceptor reflex. *Circ. Res.* 33: 22.
8. Shoukas, A.A., MacAnespie, C.L., Brunner, M.J. et al. 1981. The importance of the spleen in blood volume shifts of the systemic vascular bed caused by the carotid sinus baroreceptor reflex in the dog. *Circ. Res.* 49: 759.
9. Shoukas, A.A. 1993. Overall systems analysis of the carotid sinus baroreceptor reflex control of the circulation. *Anesthesiology* 79: 1402.
10. Rothe, C.F. and Gaddis, M.L. 1990. Autoregulation of cardiac output by passive elastic characteristics of the vascular capacitance system. *Circulation* 81: 360.
11. Haase, E. and Shoukas, A.A. 1991. The role of the carotid sinus baroreceptor reflex on pressure and diameter relations of the microvasculature of the rat intestine. *Am. J. Physiol.* 260: H752.
12. Numao, Y. and Iriuchijima J. 1977. Effect of cardiac output on circulatory blood volume. *Jpn. J. Physiol.* 27: 145.

13

The Microcirculation Physiome

Aleksander S. Popel
Johns Hopkins University

Roland N. Pittman
Virginia Commonwealth University

13.1 Introduction

The microcirculation comprises blood vessels (arterioles, capillaries, and venules) with diameters less than approximately 150 μm. The importance of the microcirculation is underscored by the fact that most of the hydrodynamic resistance of the circulatory system lies in the microvessels (especially in arterioles) and most of the exchange of nutrients and waste products occurs at the level of the smallest microvessels. The subjects of microcirculatory research are blood flow and molecular transport in microvessels, mechanical interactions and molecular exchange between these vessels and the surrounding tissue, and regulation of blood flow, pressure, and molecular transport [43]. This review focuses on quantitative aspects of microvascular research; thus, we frame it in terms of the microcirculation physiome, the quantitative and integrated description of physiological processes that involve the microcirculation in an animal or human, across multiple scales. To achieve a quantitative understanding of the complexity of these processes as well as understanding the relationships between the structure and functional behavior, it is necessary to build experiment-based mathematical and computational models. In addition to describing key experimental findings in the field, we will also review major accomplishments in mathematical and computational modeling and simulations. The experimental and theoretical information on the microcirculation can be organized in the form of databases encompassing anatomical, biophysical, and functional data; gene regulation; signaling and metabolic networks; regulation and control networks at different levels of biological organization; and computational models. This evolving effort is referred to as the Microcirculation Physiome Project, a subset of the Physiome Project [4,5,68].

Quantitative knowledge of microcirculatory blood flow, molecular transport, and their regulation has been accumulated primarily in the past 40 years owing to significant innovations in methods and techniques to measure microcirculatory parameters and analyze microcirculatory data. The development of these methods has required joint efforts of physiologists and biomedical engineers. Key innovations include significant improvements in intravital microscopy, the dual-slit method (Wayland–Johnson) for measuring velocity in microvessels, the servo-null method (Wiederhielm–Intaglietta) for measuring pressure in microvessels, the recessed oxygen microelectrode (Whalen) for polarographic measurements of partial pressure of oxygen, and the microspectrophotometric method (Pittman–Duling) for measuring oxyhemoglobin saturation in microvessels. The single-capillary cannulation method (Landis–Michel) has provided a powerful tool for studies of transport of water and solutes through the capillary endothelium. New experimental techniques have appeared, many adapted from cell biology and modified for *in vivo* studies, that are having a tremendous impact on the field. Examples include confocal and multiphoton microscopy for better three-dimensional resolution of microvascular structures, methods of optical imaging using fluorescent labels (e.g., labeling blood cells for velocity measurements), fluorescent dyes (e.g., calcium ion and nitric oxide sensitive dyes for measuring their dynamics in vascular smooth muscle, endothelium, and surrounding tissue cells *in vivo*), and quantum dots, development of sensors (glass filaments, optical and magnetic tweezers, atomic force microscopy (AFM)) for measuring forces in the nanonewton to piconewton range that are characteristic of cell–cell and molecular interactions, phosphorescence decay measurements as an indicator of oxygen tension and oxygen consumption, and methods of manipulating receptors on the surfaces of blood cells and endothelial cells. In addition to the dramatic developments in experimental techniques, quantitative knowledge and understanding of the microcirculation have been significantly enhanced by theoretical studies, perhaps having a larger impact than in other areas of physiology. Extensive theoretical work has been conducted on the mechanics of the red blood cell (RBC) and leukocyte, from the molecular to the cellular levels, mechanics of blood flow in single microvessels and microvascular networks, oxygen (O_2), carbon dioxide (CO_2), and nitric oxide (NO) exchange between microvessels and surrounding tissue, and water and solute transport through capillary endothelium and the surrounding tissue [81]. These theoretical studies not only aid in the interpretation of experimental data but in many cases also serve as a framework for quantitative testing of working hypotheses and as a guide in designing and conducting further experiments. The accumulated knowledge has led to significant progress in our understanding of mechanisms of regulation of blood flow and molecular exchange in the microcirculation in many organs and tissues under a variety of physiological and pathological conditions (e.g., hypoxia, hypertension, sickle cell anemia, diabetes, inflammation, hemorrhage, ischemia/reperfusion, sepsis, and cancer).

The goal of this chapter is to present an overview of the current status of research on systemic microcirculation. Issues of pulmonary microcirculation are not discussed. Because of space limitations, it is not possible to recognize numerous important contributions to the field of microcirculation. In most cases, we refer to recent reviews, when available, and journal articles where earlier references can be found. We discuss experimental and theoretical findings and point out gaps in our understanding of microcirculatory phenomena.

13.2 Mechanics of Microvascular Blood Flow

Vessel dimensions in the microcirculation are small enough so that the effects of the particulate nature of blood are significant [69]. Blood is a suspension of formed elements (RBCs, white blood cells (leukocytes), and platelets) in plasma. Plasma is an aqueous solution of mostly proteins (albumins, globulins, and fibrinogen) and electrolytes. Under static conditions, human RBCs are biconcave disks with a diameter ~7–9 μm. The main function of the RBC is delivery of O_2 to tissue. Most of the O_2 carried by the blood is chemically bound to hemoglobin inside the RBCs. The mammalian RBC comprises a viscoelastic membrane enveloping a viscous fluid, concentrated hemoglobin solution. The membrane consists of the plasma membrane and underlying cytoskeleton. The membrane can undergo deformations without changing its surface area, which is nearly conserved locally. RBCs are so easily deformable that they can flow through small pores with a diameter <3 μm. Leukocytes (grouped into several categories: granulocytes, monocytes, lymphocytes, macrophages, and phagocytes) are spherical cells with a diameter ~10–20 μm. They are stiffer than RBCs. The main function of these cells is immunologic, that is, protection of the body against microorganisms causing disease. In contrast to mammalian RBCs, leukocytes are nucleated and are endowed with an internal structural cytoskeleton. Leukocytes are capable of active ameboid motion, the property that allows their migration from the blood stream into the tissue. Platelets are disk-shaped blood elements with a diameter ~2–3 μm; they are devoid of a nucleus. Platelets play a key role in thrombogenic processes and blood coagulation. The normal volume fraction (hematocrit) of RBCs in humans is 40–45%. The total volume of RBCs in blood is much greater than the volume of leukocytes and platelets. Rheological properties of blood in arterioles and venules and larger vessels are determined primarily by RBCs; however, leukocytes play an important mechanical role in capillaries and small venules.

Blood plasma is a Newtonian fluid with viscosity of approximately 1.2 cP. The viscosity of whole blood in a rotational viscometer or a large-bore capillary viscometer exhibits shear-thinning behavior, that is, viscosity decreases when shear rate increases. At shear rates >100 s^{-1} and a hematocrit of 40%, typical viscosity values are 3–4 cP. The dominant mechanism of the non-Newtonian behavior is RBC aggregation and the secondary mechanism is RBC deformation under shear forces. The cross-sectional distribution of RBCs in vessels is nonuniform, with a core of concentrated RBC suspension and a cell-free or cell-depleted marginal layer, typically 2–5 μm thick, adjacent to the vessel wall. The nonuniform RBC distribution results in the *Fahraeus effect* (the microvessel hematocrit is smaller than the feed or discharge hematocrit) due to the fact that, on the average, RBCs move with a higher velocity than blood plasma, and the concomitant *Fahraeus–Lindqvist effect* (the apparent viscosity of blood is lower than the bulk viscosity measured with a rotational viscometer or a large-bore capillary viscometer at high shear rate). The *apparent viscosity* of a fluid flowing in a cylindrical vessel of radius R and length L under the influence of a pressure difference ΔP is defined as

$$\eta_a = \frac{\pi \Delta P R^4}{8QL}$$

where Q is the volumetric flow rate. For a Newtonian fluid, the apparent viscosity becomes the dynamic viscosity of the fluid and the above equation represents *Poiseuille's law*. The apparent viscosity is a function of hematocrit, vessel radius, blood flow rate, and other parameters. In the microcirculation, blood flows through a complex branching network of arterioles, capillaries, and venules. Arterioles are typically 10–150 μm in diameter, capillaries are 4–8 μm, and venules are 10–200 μm. Now, we will discuss vascular wall mechanics and blood flow in vessels of different size in more detail.

13.2.1 Mechanics of the Microvascular Wall

The wall of arterioles comprises the intima that contains a single layer of contiguous endothelial cells, the media that contains a single layer of smooth muscle cells in terminal and medium-size arterioles or several layers in the larger arterioles, and the adventitia that contains sympathetic nerve terminals and collagen fibers with occasional fibroblasts and mast cells. Fibers situated between the endothelium and the smooth muscle cells comprise the basement membrane. The single layer of smooth muscle cells terminates at the capillaries and reappears at the level of small venules; the capillary wall is devoid of smooth muscle cells, but instead contains pericytes loosely wrapped around endothelial cells. Venules typically have a larger diameter and smaller wall thickness-to-diameter ratio than arterioles of the corresponding branching order.

Most of our knowledge of the mechanics of the microvascular wall comes from *in vivo* or *in vitro* measurements of vessel diameter as a function of transmural pressure [25]. The development of isolated microvessel preparations has made it possible to precisely control the transmural pressure during experiments. In addition, these preparations allow one to separate the effects of metabolic factors and blood flow rate from the effect of pressure by controlling both the chemical environment and the flow rate through the vessel. Arterioles and venules exhibit vascular tone, that is, their diameter is maximal when smooth muscle is completely relaxed (inactivated). When the vascular smooth muscle is constricted, small arterioles may even completely close their lumen to blood flow, presumably by buckling endothelial cells. Arterioles exhibit a *myogenic response* not observed in other blood vessels, with the exception of cerebral arteries: within a certain physiological pressure range, the vessels constrict in response to elevation of transmural pressure and dilate in response to reduction of transmural pressure; in other words, in a certain range of pressures, the slope of the pressure–diameter relationship is negative [15]. Arterioles of different size exhibit different degrees of myogenic responsiveness. This effect has been documented in many tissues both *in vivo* and *in vitro* (in isolated arterioles) and has been shown to play an important role in the regulation of blood flow and capillary pressure (see Section 13.4 below).

The stress–strain relationship for a thin-walled microvessel can be derived from the experimentally obtained pressure–diameter relationship using the law of Laplace. Stress in the vessel wall can be decomposed into passive and active components. The passive component corresponds to the state of complete vasodilation. The active component determines the vascular tone and the myogenic response. Steady-state stress–strain relationships are, generally, nonlinear. For arterioles, diameter variations of 50% or even 100% under physiological conditions are not unusual, so that finite deformations have to be considered in formulating the constitutive relationship for the wall (relationship between stress, strain, and their temporal derivatives). Experiment-based mathematical models of microvessel mechanics have been formulated [15]. Pertinent to the question of microvascular mechanics is the mechanical interaction of a vessel with its environment, which consists of connective tissue, parenchymal and stromal cells, and extracellular fluid. There is ultrastructural evidence that blood vessels are tethered to the surrounding tissue, so that mechanical forces can be generated when the vessels constrict or dilate, or when the tissue is moving, for example, in contracting striated muscle, myocardium, or intestine. Little quantitative information is currently available about the magnitude of these forces, chiefly because of the difficulty of such measurements. Magnetic tweezers make it possible to probe the mechanics of the microvascular wall *in vivo* and its interaction with the surrounding tissue [38].

Under time-dependent conditions, microvessels exhibit viscoelastic behavior. In response to a stepwise change in the transmural pressure, arterioles typically respond with a fast "passive" change in diameter followed by a slow "active" response with a characteristic time of the order of tens of seconds. For example, when the pressure is suddenly increased, the vessel diameter will quickly increase, with subsequent vasoconstriction that may result in a lower value of steady-state diameter than that prior to the increase in pressure. Therefore, to accurately describe the time-dependent vessel behavior, the constitutive relationship between stress and strain or pressure and diameter must also contain temporal derivatives of these variables. Theoretical analysis of the resulting nonlinear equations shows that such constitutive equations lead to predictions of spontaneous oscillations of vessel diameter (*vasomotion*) under certain conditions [90] that can be characterized theoretically as "deterministic chaos." Theoretical analysis of Ca^{2+} oscillations in vascular smooth muscle cells also predicts spontaneous oscillations [62]. Vasomotion has been observed *in vivo* in various tissues and under various physiological conditions. Whether experimentally observed vasomotion and its effect on blood flow (flow motion) can be quantitatively described by the theoretical studies remains to be established. It should be noted that other mechanisms leading to spontaneous flow oscillations have been reported that are associated with blood rheology and not with vascular wall mechanics [16,48].

For most purposes, capillary compliance is not taken into account. However, in some situations, such as analysis of certain capillary water transport experiments or leukocyte motion in a capillary, this view is not adequate and capillary compliance has to be accounted for. Since the capillary wall is devoid of smooth muscle cells, much of this compliance is passive, and its magnitude is small. However, the presence of contractile proteins in the cytoskeleton of capillary endothelial cells and associated pericytes opens a possibility of active capillary constriction or dilation.

13.2.2 Capillary Blood Flow

Progress in this area is closely related to studies of mechanics of blood cells (described elsewhere in this book). In narrow capillaries, RBCs flow in a single file, separated by gaps of plasma. They deform and assume a parachute-like shape, generally nonaxisymmetric, leaving a submicron plasma sleeve between the RBC and endothelium. In the smallest capillaries, their shape is sausage-like. The hemoglobin solution inside an RBC is a Newtonian fluid. The constitutive relationship for the membrane is often expressed by the Evans–Skalak finite deformations model [69]; molecular-based models considering spectrin, actin, and other RBC cytoskeleton constituents have also been formulated [27,31,52]. The coupled mechanical problem of membrane and fluid motion has been extensively investigated using both analytical and numerical approaches [70]. An important result of the theoretical studies is the prediction of the apparent viscosity of blood. While these predictions are in good agreement with *in vitro* studies in glass tubes, they underestimate a few available *in vivo* capillary measurements of apparent viscosity. In addition, *in vivo* capillary hematocrit is typically lower than predicted from *in vitro* studies with tubes of the same size. To explain the low values of hematocrit, RBC interactions with the endothelial glycocalyx have been implicated [26]. Direct measurements of the glycocalyx thickness and microvascular resistance as well as theoretical analyses elucidate the role of the glycocalyx [93]. The endothelial glycocalyx and its associated macromolecules are often referred to, collectively, as the endothelial surface layer (ESL) [75]. The ESL appears to be exquisitely controlled, and it is affected by a variety of biochemical and mechanical factors [34,58,65].

The motion of leukocytes through blood capillaries has also been studied thoroughly. Because leukocytes are larger and stiffer than RBCs, under normal flow conditions, an increase in capillary resistance caused by a single leukocyte may be orders of magnitude greater than that caused by a single RBC [79]. Under certain conditions, flow stoppage may occur, caused by leukocyte plugging. After a period of ischemia, RBC and leukocyte plugging may prevent tissue reperfusion (ischemia–reperfusion injury) [37]. Chemical bonds between membrane-bound receptors and endothelial adhesion molecules play a crucial role in leukocyte–endothelium interactions. Methods of cell and molecular biology permit manipulation of the receptors and thus make it possible to study leukocyte microcirculatory mechanics at the molecular level; biophysical methods allow force measurements of single adhesion bonds. These methods open new and powerful ways to study cell micromechanics and cell–cell interactions.

13.2.3 Arteriolar and Venular Blood Flow

The cross-sectional distribution of RBCs in arterioles and venules is nonuniform. A concentrated suspension of RBCs forms a core surrounded by a cell-free or cell-depleted layer of plasma. This "lubrication" layer of lower viscosity fluid near the vessel wall results in lower values of the apparent viscosity of blood compared to its bulk viscosity, resulting in the Fahraeus–Lindqvist effect [69,71]. There is experimental evidence that velocity profiles of RBCs are generally symmetric in arterioles, except very close to vascular bifurcations, but may be asymmetric in venules; the profiles are close to parabolic in arterioles at normal flow rates, but are blunted in venules [9,30]. Moreover, flow in the venules may be stratified as the result of converging blood streams that do not mix rapidly. The key to understanding the pattern of arteriolar and venular blood flow is the mechanics of flow at vascular bifurcations, diverging for arteriolar flow and converging for venular flow [23]. An important question is under what physiological or pathological conditions do RBC aggregation affect arteriolar and venular velocity distribution and vascular resistance. Much is known about aggregation *in vitro*, but *in vivo* knowledge is incomplete

[3,12,53,69]. Under pathological conditions, such as sickle cell disease and diabetes, RBCs can interact with the endothelium via adhesion molecules [47].

Owing to recent advancements in computational fluid dynamics, including the application of lattice Boltzmann and dissipative particle dynamics methods, significant progress has been achieved in modeling multiple RBCs in narrow vessels and the formation of cell-free layer with or without the effects of RBC aggregation [32,59,95].

The problems of leukocyte distribution in the microcirculation and their interaction with the microvascular endothelium have attracted considerable attention in recent years [80]. Leukocyte rolling along the walls of venules, but not arterioles, has been demonstrated. This effect results from differences in the microvascular endothelium, mainly attributed to the differential expression of adhesion molecules on the endothelial surface [50]. Platelet distribution in the lumen is important because of platelets' role in blood coagulation. Detailed studies of platelet distribution in arterioles and venules show that the cross-sectional distribution of these disk-shaped blood elements is dependent on the blood flow rate and vessel hematocrit [94]; molecular details of platelet–endothelium interactions are available [86]. Considerable progress has been made in computational modeling of leukocytes in microvessels, and their interactions with the endothelium and with RBCs [13,42,59,61].

13.2.4 Microvascular Networks: Structure and Hemodynamics

Microvascular networks in different organs and tissues differ in their appearance and structural organization. Methods have been developed to quantitatively describe network angioarchitectonics and hemodynamics [69,71]. The microvasculature is an adaptable structure capable of changing its structural and functional characteristics in response to various stimuli [85]. _Angiogenesis_, rarefaction, and microvascular remodeling are important examples of this adaptive behavior that play important physiological and pathophysiological roles. Microvascular hydraulic pressure varies systematically between consecutive branching orders, decreasing from the systemic values down to 20–25 mm Hg in the capillaries and decreasing further by 10–15 mm Hg in the venules. Mean microvascular blood flow rate in arterioles decreases toward the capillaries, in inverse proportion to the number of "parallel" vessels, and increases from capillaries through the venules [53]. In addition to this longitudinal variation of blood flow and pressure among different branching orders, there are significant variations among vessels of the same branching order, referred to as flow heterogeneity. The heterogeneity of blood flow and RBC distribution in microvascular networks has been well documented in a variety of organs and tissues [74]. This phenomenon may have important implications for tissue exchange processes, so significant efforts have been devoted to the quantitative analysis of blood flow in microvascular networks. A mathematical model of blood flow in a network can be formulated as follows. First, network topology or vessel interconnections have to be specified. Second, the diameter and length of every vascular segment have to be known. Alternatively, vessel diameter can be specified as a function of transmural pressure and perhaps some other parameters; these relationships are discussed in the preceding section on wall mechanics. Third, the apparent viscosity of blood has to be specified as a function of vessel diameter, local hematocrit, and shear rate. Fourth, a relationship between RBC flow rates and bulk blood flow rates at diverging bifurcations has to be specified; this relationship is often referred to as the "bifurcation law." Finally, at the inlet vessel branches, boundary conditions have to be specified: bulk flow rate as well as RBC flow rate or hematocrit; alternatively, pressure can be specified at both inlet and outlet branches. This set of generally nonlinear equations can be solved to yield pressure at each bifurcation, blood flow rate through each segment, and discharge or microvessel hematocrit in each segment. These equations also predict vessel diameters if vessel compliance is taken into account. The calculated variables can then be compared with experimental data. Such a detailed comparison was reported for rat mesentery [71,74] and the scheme has been applied by many investigators to different tissues. The empirical relationships reflect the presence of the endothelial glycocalyx and its associated macromolecules, ESL [75]. Predictions of this flow model are also used in models of molecular transport.

13.3 Molecular Transport in the Microcirculation

13.3.1 Transport of Oxygen, Carbon Dioxide, and Nitric Oxide

One of the most important functions of the microcirculation is the delivery of O_2 to tissue and the removal of waste products, particularly of CO_2, from tissue. O_2 is required for aerobic intracellular respiration for the production of adenosine triphosphate (ATP). CO_2 is produced as a by-product of these biochemical reactions. Tissue metabolic rate can change drastically, for example, in aerobic muscle in the transition from rest to exercise, which necessitates commensurate changes in blood flow and O_2 delivery. One of the major issues studied is how O_2 delivery is matched to O_2 demand under different physiological and pathological conditions. This question arises for short-term or long-term regulation of O_2 delivery in an individual organism, organ, or tissue, as well as in the evolutionary sense, in phylogeny. The hypothesis of symmorphosis, a fundamental balance between structure and function, has been formulated for the respiratory and cardiovascular systems and tested in a number of animal species [92].

In the smallest exchange vessels (capillaries and small arterioles and venules), O_2 molecules are released from hemoglobin inside RBCs, diffuse through the plasma, cross the endothelium, the extravascular space, and parenchymal cells until they reach the mitochondria where they are utilized in the process of oxidative phosphorylation. The nonlinear relationship between hemoglobin saturation with O_2 and the local O_2 tension (PO_2) is described by the *oxyhemoglobin dissociation curve* (ODC). The theory of O_2 transport from capillaries to tissue was conceptually formulated by August Krogh in 1918 and it has dominated the thinking of physiologists for nine decades. The model he formulated considered a cylindrical tissue volume supplied by a single central capillary; this element was considered the building block for the entire tissue. A constant metabolic rate was assumed and PO_2 at the capillary–tissue interface was specified. The solution to the corresponding transport equation is the Krogh–Erlang equation describing the radial variation of O_2 tension in tissue. Over the years, the *Krogh tissue cylinder model* has been modified by many investigators to include transport processes in the capillary and PO_2-dependent consumption. However, in the past few years, new conceptual models of O_2 transport have emerged. First, it was discovered experimentally and subsequently corroborated by theoretical analysis that capillaries are not the only source of oxygen, but arterioles (*precapillary* O_2 *transport*) and to a smaller extent venules (postcapillary O_2 transport) also participate in tissue oxygenation; in fact, a complex pattern of O_2 exchange may exist among arterioles, venules, and adjacent capillary networks [64,87]. Second, theoretical analysis of intracapillary transport suggested that a significant part of the resistance to O_2 transport, on the order of 50%, is located within the capillary, primarily due to poor diffusive conductance of the plasma gaps between the erythrocytes; the consequence of this prediction, fluctuations of capillary PO_2, has been confirmed by recent experiments [36]. Third, the effect of *myoglobin-facilitated* O_2 *diffusion* in red muscle fibers and cardiac myocytes has been reevaluated; however, its significance must await additional experimental studies. Fourth, geometric and hemodynamic heterogeneities in O_2 delivery have been quantified experimentally and modeled theoretically. Theoretical analyses of oxygen transport have been applied to a variety of tissues and organs [24,35,67]. One important area of application of this knowledge is artificial oxygen carriers, hemoglobin-based and non-hemoglobin-based [60]; theoretical models of O_2 transport by blood substitutes have been developed [39,89] and used to guide experimental studies.

The transport of CO_2 is coupled to O_2 through the Bohr effect (effect of CO_2 tension on the blood O_2 content) and the Haldane effect (effect of PO_2 on the blood CO_2 content). The diffusion of CO_2 is faster than that of O_2 because CO_2 solubility in tissue is higher; theoretical studies predict that countercurrent exchange of CO_2 between arterioles and venules is of major importance so that equilibration of CO_2 tension with surrounding tissue should occur before capillaries are reached. Experiments are needed to test these theoretical predictions.

Nitric oxide (NO) is a diatomic gas that can be enzymatically synthesized from L-arginine by several isoforms of NO synthase (NOS). There are also nonenzymatic sources of NO. The isoforms of NO synthase are divided into inducible NOS (iNOS or NOS2) and constitutive NOS (cNOS), based on their nondependent and dependent, respectively, control of activity from intracellular calcium/calmodulin. Constitutive NOS are further classified as neuronal NOS (nNOS or NOS1) and endothelial NOS (eNOS or NOS3). Nitric oxide plays an important role in both autocrine and paracrine manners in a myriad of physiological processes, including regulation of blood pressure and blood flow, platelet aggregation, and leukocyte adhesion. In smooth muscle cells, NO activates the enzyme soluble guanylate cyclase (sGC) that catalyzes the conversion of guanosine triphosphate (GTP) to cyclic guanosine monophosphate (cGMP), thus causing vasodilation [8]. Traditionally, eNOS has been considered the principal source of bioavailable microvascular NO under most physiological conditions. Evidence exists that nNOS expressed in nerve fibers, which innervate arterioles, together with nNOS positive mast cells are also major sources of NO [46]. NO produced by endothelial cells diffuses to vascular smooth muscle and to the flowing blood, where it rapidly reacts with hemoglobin in RBCs and free hemoglobin present in pathological conditions, such as sickle cell disease, or during administration of free hemoglobin as a blood substitute. Other nonneuronal cell types, including cardiac and skeletal myocytes, also express nNOS. Direct measurements of NO concentration in the microcirculation with high spatial resolution have been performed with carbon fiber microsensors [10] and optical dyes [46], although recent criticism has been directed to current measurements of NO *in vivo* [40]. In addition to its vasodilatory effect, NO also inhibits mitochondrial respiration by its interaction with cytochrome *c* oxidase [19]. Mathematical models of NO transport have been developed that describe the transport of NO synthesized by eNOS and nNOS in and around microvessels [88]. Other mechanisms have been proposed and are under intense scrutiny, for example, NO reacting with thiols in blood to form long-lived *S*-nitrosothiols (SNOs) with vasodilatory activity [1], and nitrite being a source of NO [91]. There are significant discrepancies between experimental data and theoretical results that await resolution [17,40]; the sources of microvascular bioavailable NO also need to be revealed.

13.3.2 Transport of Solutes and Water

The movement of solute molecules across the capillary wall occurs primarily by two mechanisms: diffusion and solvent drag. Diffusion is the passive mechanism of transport that rapidly and efficiently transports small solutes over the small distances (tens of microns) between the blood supply (capillaries) and tissue cells. Solvent drag refers to the movement of solute that is entrained in the bulk flow of fluid across the capillary wall and is generally negligible, except in cases of large molecules with small diffusivities and high transcapillary fluid flow.

The capillary wall is composed of a single layer of endothelial cells about 1 μm thick. Lipid-soluble substances (e.g., O_2) can diffuse across the entire wall surface, whereas water-soluble substances are restricted to small aqueous pathways equivalent to cylindrical pores 8–9 nm in diameter (e.g., glucose in most capillaries); in capillaries with tight junctions and few fenestrations (brain, testes), glucose moves predominantly by carrier-mediated transport. Total pore area is about 0.1% of the surface area of a capillary. The permeability of the capillary wall to a particular substance depends upon the relative size of the substance and the pore ("restricted" diffusion). The efficiency of diffusive exchange can be increased by increasing the number of perfused capillaries (e.g., heart and muscle tissue from rest to exercise), since this increases the surface area available for exchange and decreases the distances across which molecules must diffuse.

The actual pathways through which small solutes traverse the capillary wall appear to be in the form of clefts between adjacent endothelial cells. Rather than being open slits, these porous channels contain a matrix of small cylindrical fibers (primarily glycosaminoglycans) that occupy about 5% of the volume of these pathways. The permeability properties of the capillary endothelium are modulated by a number of factors, among which are plasma protein concentration and composition, rearrangement of the endothelial cell glycocalyx, calcium influx into the endothelial cell and endothelial cell membrane potential. Many of the studies that have established our current understanding of the endothelial exchange barrier have been carried out on single perfused capillaries in the frog and in mammalian tissues [22,57]. There could be, in addition to the porous pathways, nonporous pathways that involve selective uptake of solutes and subsequent transcellular transport (of particular importance in endothelial barriers). To study such pathways, one must try to minimize the contributions to transcapillary transport from solvent drag.

The processes whereby water passes back and forth across the capillary wall are called filtration and absorption. The flow of water depends upon the relative magnitude of hydraulic and osmotic pressures across the capillary wall and is described quantitatively by the Kedem–Katchalsky equations (the particular form of the equations applied to capillary water transport is referred to as *Starling's law*). Recently, the physical mechanism of Starling's law has been reassessed [41]. Overall, in the steady state, there is an approximate balance between hydraulic and osmotic pressures, which leads to a small net flow of water. Generally, more fluid is filtered than is reabsorbed; the overflow is carried back to the vascular system by the lymphatic circulation. The lymphatic network is composed of a large number of small vessels, the terminal branches of which are closed. Flap valves (similar to those in veins) ensure unidirectional flow of lymph back to the central circulation. The smallest (terminal) vessels are very permeable, even to proteins that occasionally leak from systemic capillaries. Lymph flow is determined by interstitial fluid pressure and the lymphatic "pump" (one–way flap valves and skeletal muscle contraction). The control of interstitial fluid protein concentration is one of the most important functions of the lymphatic system. If more net fluid is filtered than can be removed by the lymphatics, the volume of interstitial fluid increases. This fluid accumulation is called edema. This circumstance is important clinically since solute exchange (e.g., O_2) decreases due to the increased diffusion distances produced when the accumulated fluid pushes the capillaries, tethered to the interstitial matrix, away from each other.

13.4 Regulation of Blood Flow

The cardiovascular system controls blood flow to individual organs (1) by maintaining arterial pressure within narrow limits and (2) by allowing each organ to adjust its vascular resistance to blood flow so that each receives an appropriate fraction of the cardiac output. There are three major mechanisms that control the function of the cardiovascular system: neural, humoral, and local [83]. The sympathetic nervous system and circulating hormones both provide overall vasoregulation, and thus coarse flow control, to all vascular beds. The local mechanisms provide finer regional control within a tissue, usually in response to local changes in tissue activity or local trauma. The three mechanisms can work independently of each other, but there are also interactions among them.

The classical view of blood flow control involved the action of vasomotor influences on a set of vessels called the "resistance vessels," generally arterioles and small arteries smaller than about 100–150 μm in diameter, which controlled flow to and within an organ [82]. The notion of "precapillary sphincters" that control flow in individual capillaries has been abandoned in favor of the current notion that the terminal arterioles control the flow in small capillary networks that branch off of these arterioles. In recent years, it has become clear that the resistance to blood flow is distributed over a wider range of vessel branching orders with diameters up to 500 μm. There are mechanisms to be discussed below that are available for coordinating the actions of local control processes over wider regions.

13.4.1 Neurohumoral Regulation of Blood Flow

The role of neural influences on the vasculature varies greatly from organ to organ. Although all organs receive sympathetic innervation, regulation of blood flow in the cerebral and coronary vascular beds occurs mostly through intrinsic local (metabolic) mechanisms. The circulations in skeletal muscle, skin, and some other organs, however, are significantly affected by the sympathetic nerves. In general, the level of intrinsic myogenic activity and sympathetic discharge sets the state of vascular smooth muscle contraction (basal vascular tone) and hence vascular resistance in organs. This basal tone is modulated by circulating and local vasoactive influences, for example, endothelium–derived relaxing factor (EDRF), identified as nitric oxide, endothelium-derived hyperpolarizing factor (EDHF) [11], prostacyclin (PGI2), endothelin, and vasoactive substances released from parenchymal cells.

13.4.2 Local Regulation of Blood Flow

In addition to neural and humoral mechanisms for regulating the function of the cardiovascular system, there are mechanisms intrinsic to the various tissues that can operate independently of neurohumoral influences. The site of local regulation is the microcirculation. Examples of local control processes are autoregulation of blood flow, reactive hyperemia, and active (or functional) hyperemia. The mechanisms of local regulation have been identified as (1) the myogenic mechanism based on the ability of vascular smooth muscle to actively contract in response to stretch; (2) the metabolic mechanism, based on a link between blood flow and tissue metabolism; and (3) the flow-dependent mechanism, primarily based on the release of NO by endothelial cells in response to shear forces. The effects are coordinated and integrated in the microvascular network via chemical and electrical signals propagating through gap junctions. Experimental evidence and theoretical models are discussed in References 14, 21, 44, 45, 66, 72, 82, and 83.

Cells have a continuous need for O_2 and also continuously produce metabolic wastes, some of which are vasoactive (usually vasodilators). Under normal conditions, there is a balance between O_2 supply and demand, but imbalances give rise to adjustments in blood flow that bring supply back into register with demand. Consider exercising skeletal muscle as an example. With the onset of exercise, metabolite production and O_2 requirements increase. The metabolites diffuse away from their sites of production and reach the vasculature. Vasodilation ensues, lowering resistance to blood flow. The resulting increase in blood flow increases the O_2 supply and finally a new steady state is achieved in which O_2 supply and demand are matched. This scenario operates for other tissues in which metabolic activity changes.

The following O_2–linked metabolites have been implicated as potential chemical mediators in the metabolic hypothesis: adenosine (from ATP hydrolysis: ATP → ADP → AMP → adenosine), H^+, and lactate (from lactic acid generated by glycolysis). Their levels are increased when there is a reduction in O_2 supply relative to demand (i.e., tissue hypoxia). The production of more CO_2 as a result of increased tissue activity (leading to increased oxidative metabolism) leads to vasodilation through increased H^+ concentration. Increased potassium ion and interstitial fluid osmolarity (i.e., more osmotically active particles) transiently cause vasodilation under physiological conditions associated with increased tissue activity.

It has also been established that the RBC itself could act as a mobile sensor for hypoxia [29]. The mechanism works as follows. Under conditions of low oxygen and pH, the RBC releases ATP, which binds to purinergic receptors on the endothelial cells. This leads to the production of the vasodilator NO in the endothelial cells. Since the most likely location for hypoxia would be in or near the venular network, the local vasodilatory response to NO is propagated to upstream vessels causing arteriolar vasodilation (see Section 13.4.3). The phenomenon has been described in a mathematical model [2].

13.4.3 Coordination of Vasomotor Responses

Communication via gap junctions between the two active cell types in the blood vessel wall, smooth muscle and endothelial cells, plays an important role in coordinating the responses among resistance elements in the vascular network [33,82,83]. There is chemical and electrical coupling between the cells of the vessel wall, and this signal, in response to locally released vasoactive substances (e.g., from vessel wall, RBCs, or parenchymal cells), can travel along a vessel in either direction with a length constant of about 2 mm. There are two immediate consequences of this communication. A localized vasodilatory stimulus of metabolic origin will be conducted to contiguous vessels, thereby lowering the resistance to blood flow in a larger region. In addition, this more generalized vasodilation should increase the homogeneity of blood flow in response to the localized metabolic event. The increase in blood flow produced as a result of this vasodilation will also cause flow to increase at upstream sites. The increased shear stress on the endothelium as a result of the flow increase will lead to vasodilation of these larger upstream vessels. Thus, the neurohumoral and local responses are linked together in a complex control system that matches regional perfusion to the local metabolic needs.

13.4.4 Angiogenesis and Vascular Remodeling

In addition to short-term regulation of blood flow operating on the time scale of tens of seconds to minutes, there are mechanisms that operate on the scales of hours, days, and weeks that result in angiogenesis (the capillary growth from preexisting microvessels) and microvascular remodeling or adaptation (structural and geometric changes in the vascular wall) [85]. Stimuli for angiogenesis and microvascular remodeling could be hypoxia, injury, inflammation, or neoplasia. The processes of angiogenesis and vascular remodeling are complex and knowledge at the molecular, cellular, and tissue level is being accumulated at a fast rate. Briefly, it is understood that low cellular oxygen is sensed through a transcription factor HIF1 (hypoxia-inducible factor) pathway, leading to activation of as many as 200 genes [84]. Among them is vascular endothelial growth factor (VEGF)—one of the most potent inducers of angiogenesis. Another VEGF-inducing factor is the transcription coactivator perixosome-proliferator-activated-receptor-gamma coactivator 1α (PGC1α) [49]. VEGF is secreted by parenchymal and stromal cells and diffuses through the extracellular space. Once it reaches endothelial cells, it activates them, causing hyperpermeability and expression of metalloproteinases (MMPs), which then participate in the proteolysis of the extracellular matrix. The activated endothelial cells migrate, proliferate, and differentiate, resulting in the formation of a capillary sprout. Subsequently, the endothelial cells secrete platelet-derived growth factor (PDGF) that participates in recruiting stromal fibroblasts and progenitor cells to the new capillaries. When these cells reach the vessels, they differentiate into pericytes and smooth muscle cells, thus stabilizing the vessels. Many of these processes are poorly understood. Therefore, quantitative computational approaches are particularly useful in gaining a better understanding of these processes; research in this area is rapidly evolving [56,63,77,78]. In parallel to modeling angiogenesis, theoretical models are being developed to describe long-term structural vascular remodeling and adaptation [73].

13.4.5 Enabling Computational Tools and Methodologies for the Microcirculation Physiome Project

Further progress in understanding the microcirculation physiome will benefit from the modeling and simulation infrastructure being developed around the world. These include methods for model development, storage, exchange, and integration. Below, we list some of the important elements of these methods; some of the aspects can be found in Reference 68.

Model types: A growing arsenal of modeling tools is available for building mathematical models: they include algebraic equations, deterministic ordinary and partial differential equations, probabilistic equations and stochastic Monte Carlo simulations, and rule-based agent-based models (ABM). All these tools have been used in describing microcirculatory phenomena.

Multiscale models: Many models span multiple spatial and temporal scales; such models are referred to as *multiscale* [6,31,77,78]. For example, a model of capillary flow (micrometer scale) may include a molecular-detailed model of the RBC membrane (nanometer scale) and endothelial glycocalyx (from nanometer to micrometer scale). A model of capillary sprouting during angiogenesis could include growth factor interactions with receptors (nanometer scale), endothelial cell proliferation, migration, and sprout formation (micrometer scale), and well as whole-body growth factor transport (meter scale);

in the same problem, ligand–receptor interactions occur at seconds to minutes scales, whereas vascular growth occurs at hours to days scale. Creating methodologies for multiscale modeling is an important goal of current research.

Modular design and module integration: Complex models might be composed of multiple modules at the same or different spatial and temporal scales; some of these modules may be commonly used by many investigators (e.g., MAPK—mitogen-activated protein kinases in signal transduction models, or the microcirculatory blood flow model in molecular transport models), whereas others maybe be custom designed for a particular application. These modules may represent different model types (e.g., differential equations versus ABM) and use different programming languages. There are several efforts to integrate multiple modules using a controller/integrator that controls the modules and data exchange between them [54,76]; this is also one of the goals of the Virtual Physiological Human project [20].

Markup languages: To facilitate model exchange among investigators, markup languages have been formulated that abide to the standards accepted by the modeling community. SBML (systems biology markup language) [28] and CellML [7] are the most common for processes described by ordinary differential equations, for example, signaling pathways. For spatial models, FieldML is being developed [18]. Together with modular design, markup languages will also facilitate the creation of public databases of computational models that can be used by different investigators.

Model databases: The BioModels database [51] based primarily on SBML (other formats are also available), and the CellML model repository [55] based on CellML contain hundreds of curated models.

Defining Terms

Angiogenesis: The growth of new capillaries from the preexisting microvessels.
Apparent viscosity: The viscosity of a Newtonian fluid that would require the same pressure difference to produce the same blood flow rate through a circular vessel as the blood.
Fahraeus effect: Microvessel hematocrit is smaller than hematocrit in the feed or discharge reservoir.
Fahraeus–Lindqvist effect: The apparent viscosity of blood in a microvessel is smaller than the bulk viscosity measured with a rotational viscometer or a large-bore capillary viscometer.
Krogh tissue cylinder model: A cylindrical volume of tissue supplied by a central cylindrical capillary.
Multiscale model: A model that considers processes at multiple spatial and/or temporal scales.
Myogenic response: Vasoconstriction in response to elevated transmural pressure and vasodilation in response to reduced transmural pressure.
Myoglobin-facilitated O_2 diffusion: An increase of O_2 diffusive flux as a result of myoglobin molecules acting as a carrier for O_2 molecules.
Oxyhemoglobin dissociation curve: The equilibrium relationship between hemoglobin oxygen saturation and O_2 tension.
Physiome: The quantitative and integrated description of the functional behavior of the physiological state of an animal or human.
Poiseuille's law: The relationship between volumetric flow rate and pressure difference for steady flow of a Newtonian fluid in a long circular tube.
Precapillary O_2 transport: O_2 diffusion from arterioles to the surrounding tissue.
Starling's law: The relationship between water flux through the endothelium and the difference between the hydraulic and osmotic transmural pressures.
Vasomotion: Spontaneous rhythmic variation of microvessel diameter.

Acknowledgments

This work was supported by National Institute of Health grants R01 HL18292, R01 HL101200, and R01 CA138264.

References

1. Allen BW, Stamler JS, and Piantadosi CA. Hemoglobin, nitric oxide and molecular mechanisms of hypoxic vasodilation. *Trends Mol Med* 15: 452–460, 2009.

2. Arciero JC, Carlson BE, and Secomb TW. Theoretical model of metabolic blood flow regulation: Roles of ATP release by red blood cells and conducted responses. *Am J Physiol Heart Circ Physiol* 295: H1562–1571, 2008.

3. Baskurt OK and Meiselman HJ. Blood rheology and hemodynamics. *Semin Thromb Hemost* 29: 435–450, 2003.

4. Bassingthwaighte JB. Microcirculation and the physiome projects. *Microcirculation* 15: 835–839, 2008.

5. Bassingthwaighte JB. Strategies for the physiome project. *Ann Biomed Eng* 28: 1043–1058, 2000.

6. Bassingthwaighte JB, Raymond GM, Butterworth E, Alessio A, and Caldwell JH. Multiscale modeling of metabolism, flows, and exchanges in heterogeneous organs. *Ann N Y Acad Sci* 1188: 111–120, 2009.

7. Beard DA, Britten R, Cooling MT, Garny A, Halstead MD, Hunter PJ, Lawson J et al. CellML metadata standards, associated tools and repositories. *Philos Transact A Math Phys Eng Sci* 367: 1845–1867, 2009.

8. Bian K, Doursout MF, and Murad F. Vascular system: Role of nitric oxide in cardiovascular diseases. *J Clin Hypertens (Greenwich)* 10: 304–310, 2008.

9. Bishop JJ, Nance PR, Popel AS, Intaglietta M, and Johnson PC. Effect of erythrocyte aggregation on velocity profiles in venules. *Am J Physiol Heart Circ Physiol* 280: H222–236, 2001.

10. Bohlen HG, Zhou X, Unthank JL, Miller SJ, and Bills R. Transfer of nitric oxide by blood from upstream to downstream resistance vessels causes microvascular dilation. *Am J Physiol Heart Circ Physiol* 297: H1337–1346, 2009.

11. Busse R, Edwards G, Feletou M, Fleming I, Vanhoutte PM, and Weston AH. EDHF: Bringing the concepts together. *Trends Pharmacol Sci* 23: 374–380, 2002.

12. Cabel M, Meiselman HJ, Popel AS, and Johnson PC. Contribution of red blood cell aggregation to venous vascular resistance in skeletal muscle. *Am J Physiol* 272: H1020–1032, 1997.

13. Caputo KE, Lee D, King MR, and Hammer DA. Adhesive dynamics simulations of the shear threshold effect for leukocytes. *Biophys J* 92: 787–797, 2007.

14. Carlson BE, Arciero JC, and Secomb TW. Theoretical model of blood flow autoregulation: Roles of myogenic, shear-dependent, and metabolic responses. *Am J Physiol Heart Circ Physiol* 295: H1572–1579, 2008.

15. Carlson BE and Secomb TW. A theoretical model for the myogenic response based on the length-tension characteristics of vascular smooth muscle. *Microcirculation* 12: 327–338, 2005.

16. Carr RT, Geddes JB, and Wu F. Oscillations in a simple microvascular network. *Ann Biomed Eng* 33: 764–771, 2005.

17. Chen K, Pittman RN, and Popel AS. Nitric oxide in the vasculature: Where does it come from and where does it go? A quantitative perspective. *Antioxid Redox Signal* 10: 1185–1198, 2008.

18. Christie GR, Nielsen PM, Blackett SA, Bradley CP, and Hunter PJ. FieldML: Concepts and implementation. *Philos Transact A Math Phys Eng Sci* 367: 1869–1884, 2009.

19. Cooper CE, Mason MG, and Nicholls P. A dynamic model of nitric oxide inhibition of mitochondrial cytochrome *c* oxidase. *Biochim Biophys Acta* 1777: 867–876, 2008.

20. Cooper J, Cervenansky F, De Fabritiis G, Fenner J, Friboulet D, Giorgino T, Manos S et al. The Virtual Physiological Human TOOLKIT. *Philos Transact A Math Phys Eng Sci* 368: 3925–3936, 2010.

21. Cornelissen AJ, Dankelman J, VanBavel E, and Spaan JA. Balance between myogenic, flow-dependent, and metabolic flow control in coronary arterial tree: A model study. *Am J Physiol Heart Circ Physiol* 282: H2224–2237, 2002.

22. Curry FR. Microvascular solute and water transport. *Microcirculation* 12: 17–31, 2005.

23. Das B, Enden G, and Popel AS. Stratified multiphase model for blood flow in a venular bifurcation. *Ann Biomed Eng* 25: 135–153, 1997.

24. Dash RK, Li Y, Kim J, Beard DA, Saidel GM, and Cabrera ME. Metabolic dynamics in skeletal muscle during acute reduction in blood flow and oxygen supply to mitochondria: In-silico studies using a multi-scale, top-down integrated model. *PLoS One* 3: e3168, 2008.

25. Davis MJ and Hill MA. Signaling mechanisms underlying the vascular myogenic response. *Physiol Rev* 79: 387–423, 1999.

26. Desjardins C and Duling BR. Heparinase treatment suggests a role for the endothelial cell glycocalyx in regulation of capillary hematocrit. *Am J Physiol* 258: H647–654, 1990.

27. Discher DE. New insights into erythrocyte membrane organization and microelasticity. *Curr Opin Hematol* 7: 117–122, 2000.

28. Drager A, Planatscher H, Motsou Wouamba D, Schroder A, Hucka M, Endler L, Golebiewski M, Muller W, and Zell A. SBML2 L(A)T(E)X: Conversion of SBML files into human-readable reports. *Bioinformatics* 25: 1455–1456, 2009.

29. Ellsworth ML, Ellis CG, Goldman D, Stephenson AH, Dietrich HH, and Sprague RS. Erythrocytes: Oxygen sensors and modulators of vascular tone. *Physiology (Bethesda)* 24: 107–116, 2009.

30. Ellsworth ML and Pittman RN. Evaluation of photometric methods for quantifying convective mass transport in microvessels. *Am J Physiol* 251: H869–879, 1986.

31. Fedosov DA, Caswell B, and Karniadakis GE. A multiscale red blood cell model with accurate mechanics, rheology, and dynamics. *Biophys J* 98: 2215–2225, 2010.

32. Fedosov DA, Caswell B, Popel AS, and Karniadakis GE. Blood flow and cell-free layer in microvessels. *Microcirculation* 17: 615–628, 2010.

33. Figueroa XF, Isakson BE, and Duling BR. Connexins: Gaps in our knowledge of vascular function. *Physiology (Bethesda)* 19: 277–284, 2004.

34. Gao L and Lipowsky HH. Composition of the endothelial glycocalyx and its relation to its thickness and diffusion of small solutes. *Microvasc Res* 80: 394–401, 2010.

35. Goldman D. Theoretical models of microvascular oxygen transport to tissue. *Microcirculation* 15: 795–811, 2008.

36. Golub AS and Pittman RN. Erythrocyte-associated transients in PO_2 revealed in capillaries of rat mesentery. *Am J Physiol Heart Circ Physiol* 288: H2735–2743, 2005.

37. Granger DN, Rodrigues SF, Yildirim A, and Senchenkova EY. Microvascular responses to cardiovascular risk factors. *Microcirculation* 17: 192–20 5, 2010.

38. Guilford WH and Gore RW. The mechanics of arteriole-tissue interaction. *Microvasc Res* 50: 260–287, 1995.

39. Gundersen SI, Chen G, and Palmer AF. Mathematical model of NO and O_2 transport in an arteriole facilitated by hemoglobin based O_2 carriers. *Biophys Chem* 143: 1–17, 2009.

40. Hall CN and Garthwaite J. What is the real physiological NO concentration *in vivo*? *Nitric Oxide* 21: 92–103, 2009.

41. Hu X and Weinbaum S. A new view of Starling's hypothesis at the microstructural level. *Microvasc Res* 58: 281–304, 1999.

42. Jadhav S, Eggleton CD, and Konstantopoulos K. A 3-D computational model predicts that cell deformation affects selectin-mediated leukocyte rolling. *Biophys J* 88: 96–104, 2005.

43. Johnson PC. Overview of the microcirculation. In: *Handbook of Physiology: Microcirculation*, edited by Tuma RF, Duran WN and Ley K: San Diego: Academic Press; 2008, p. xi–xxvi.

44. Kapela A, Bezerianos A, and Tsoukias NM. A mathematical model of vasoreactivity in rat mesenteric arterioles: I. Myoendothelial communication. *Microcirculation*: 16: 694–713, 2009.

45. Kapela A, Nagaraja S, and Tsoukias NM. A mathematical model of vasoreactivity in rat mesenteric arterioles. II. Conducted vasoreactivity. *Am J Physiol Heart Circ Physiol* 298: H52–65, 2010.

46. Kashiwagi S, Kajimura M, Yoshimura Y, and Suematsu M. Nonendothelial source of nitric oxide in arterioles but not in venules: Alternative source revealed *in vivo* by diaminofluorescein microfluorography. *Circ Res* 91: e55–64, 2002.

47. Kaul DK, Finnegan E, and Barabino GA. Sickle red cell-endothelium interactions. *Microcirculation* 16: 97–111, 2009.
48. Kiani MF, Pries AR, Hsu LL, Sarelius IH, and Cokelet GR. Fluctuations in microvascular blood flow parameters caused by hemodynamic mechanisms. *Am J Physiol* 266: H1822–1828, 1994.
49. Leick L, Hellsten Y, Fentz J, Lyngby SS, Wojtaszewski JF, Hidalgo J, and Pilegaard H. PGC-1alpha mediates exercise-induced skeletal muscle VEGF expression in mice. *Am J Physiol Endocrinol Metab* 297: E92–103, 2009.
50. Ley K. The role of selectins in inflammation and disease. *Trends Mol Med* 9: 263–268, 2003.
51. Li C, Donizelli M, Rodriguez N, Dharuri H, Endler L, Chelliah V, Li L et al. BioModels Database: An enhanced, curated and annotated resource for published quantitative kinetic models. *BMC Syst Biol* 4: 92, 2010.
52. Li J, Lykotrafitis G, Dao M, and Suresh S. Cytoskeletal dynamics of human erythrocyte. *Proc Natl Acad Sci USA* 104: 4937–4942, 2007.
53. Lipowsky HH. Microvascular rheology and hemodynamics. *Microcirculation* 12: 5–15, 2005.
54. Liu G, Qutub AA, Vempati P, Mac Gabhann F, and Popel AS. Module-based multiscale simulation of angiogenesis in skeletal muscle. *Theor Biol Med Model.* 8: 6, 2011.
55. Lloyd CM, Lawson JR, Hunter PJ, and Nielsen PF. The CellML model repository. *Bioinformatics* 24: 2122–2123, 2008.
56. Mac Gabhann F and Popel AS. Systems biology of vascular endothelial growth factors. *Microcirculation* 15: 715–738, 2008.
57. Michel CC and Curry FE. Microvascular permeability. *Physiol Rev* 79: 703–761, 1999.
58. Mulivor AW and Lipowsky HH. Inflammation- and ischemia-induced shedding of venular glycocalyx. *Am J Physiol Heart Circ Physiol* 286: H1672–1680, 2004.
59. Munn LL and Dupin MM. Blood cell interactions and segregation in flow. *Ann Biomed Eng* 36: 534–544, 2008.
60. Napolitano LM. Hemoglobin-based oxygen carriers: First, second or third generation? Human or bovine? Where are we now? *Crit Care Clin* 25: 279–301, 2009.
61. Pappu V and Bagchi P. 3D computational modeling and simulation of leukocyte rolling adhesion and deformation. *Comput Biol Med* 38: 738–753, 2008.
62. Parthimos D, Edwards DH, and Griffith TM. Minimal model of arterial chaos generated by coupled intracellular and membrane Ca^{2+} oscillators. *Am J Physiol* 277: H1119–1144, 1999.
63. Peirce SM. Computational and mathematical modeling of angiogenesis. *Microcirculation* 15: 739–751, 2008.
64. Pittman RN. Oxygen transport and exchange in the microcirculation. *Microcirculation* 12: 59–70, 2005.
65. Platts SH and Duling BR. Adenosine A3 receptor activation modulates the capillary endothelial glycocalyx. *Circ Res* 94: 77–82, 2004.
66. Pohl U and de Wit C. A unique role of NO in the control of blood flow. *News Physiol Sci* 14: 74–80, 1999.
67. Popel AS. Theory of oxygen transport to tissue. *Crit Rev Biomed Eng* 17: 257–321, 1989.
68. Popel AS and Hunter PJ. Systems biology and physiome projects. *Wiley Interdisciplinary Reviews: Systems Biology and Medicine* 1: 153–158, 2009.
69. Popel AS and Johnson PC. Microcirculation and hemorheology. *Ann Rev Fluid Mechanics* 37: 43–69, 2005.
70. Pozrikidis C. *Computational Hydrodynamics of Capsules and Biological Cells.* Taylor & Francis, 2010, p. 1–327.
71. Pries AR and Secomb TW. Blood flow in microvascular networks. In: *Handbook of Physiology. Microcirculation.* (2nd Edition ed.), edited by Tuma RF, Duran WN and Ley K: San Diego: Academic Press; 2008, pp. 3–36.
72. Pries AR and Secomb TW. Control of blood vessel structure: Insights from theoretical models. *Am J Physiol Heart Circ Physiol* 288: H1010–1015, 2005.

73. Pries AR and Secomb TW. Modeling structural adaptation of microcirculation. *Microcirculation* 15: 753–764, 2008.

74. Pries AR and Secomb TW. Origins of heterogeneity in tissue perfusion and metabolism. *Cardiovasc Res* 81: 328–335, 2009.

75. Pries AR, Secomb TW, and Gaehtgens P. The endothelial surface layer. *Pflugers Arch* 440: 653–666, 2000.

76. Qutub AA, Liu G, Vempati P, and Popel AS. Integration of angiogenesis modules at multiple scales: From molecular to tissue. *Pac Symp Biocomput* 316–327, 2009.

77. Qutub AA, Mac Gabhann F, Karagiannis ED, and Popel AS. In silico modeling of angiogenesis at multiple scales: From nanoscale to organ system. In: *Multiscale Modeling of Particle Interactions: Applications in Biology and Nanotechnology.* edited by King MR and Gee DJ: Wiley, Hoboken, NJ, 2010, p. 287–320.

78. Qutub AA, Mac Gabhann F, Karagiannis ED, Vempati P, and Popel AS. Multiscale models of angiogenesis. *IEEE Eng Med Biol Mag* 28: 14–31, 2009.

79. Schmid-Schonbein GW. Biomechanics of microcirculatory blood perfusion. *Annu Rev Biomed Eng* 1: 73–102, 1999.

80. Schmid-Schonbein GW and Granger DN. *Molecular Basis for Microcirculatory Disorders.* Springer-Verlag, Paris, France 2003.

81. Secomb TW, Beard DA, Frisbee JC, Smith NP, and Pries AR. The role of theoretical modeling in microcirculation research. *Microcirculation* 15: 693–698, 2008.

82. Segal SS. Integration of blood flow control to skeletal muscle: Key role of feed arteries. *Acta Physiol Scand* 168: 511–518, 2000.

83. Segal SS. Regulation of blood flow in the microcirculation. *Microcirculation* 12: 33–45, 2005.

84. Semenza GL. Hydroxylation of HIF-1: Oxygen sensing at the molecular level. *Physiology (Bethesda)* 19: 176–182, 2004.

85. Skalak TC. Angiogenesis and microvascular remodeling: A brief history and future roadmap. *Microcirculation* 12: 47–58, 2005.

86. Tailor A, Cooper D, and Granger D. Platelet-vessel wall interactions in the microcirculation. *Microcirculation* 12: 275–285, 2005.

87. Tsai AG, Johnson PC, and Intaglietta M. Oxygen gradients in the microcirculation. *Physiol Rev* 83: 933–963, 2003.

88. Tsoukias NM. Nitric oxide bioavailability in the microcirculation: Insights from mathematical models. *Microcirculation* 15: 813–834, 2008.

89. Tsoukias NM, Goldman D, Vadapalli A, Pittman RN, and Popel AS. A computational model of oxygen delivery by hemoglobin-based oxygen carriers in three-dimensional microvascular networks. *J Theor Biol* 248: 657–674, 2007.

90. Ursino M, Colantuoni A, and Bertuglia S. Vasomotion and blood flow regulation in hamster skeletal muscle microcirculation: A theoretical and experimental study. *Microvasc Res* 56: 233–252, 1998.

91. van Faassen EE, Bahrami S, Feelisch M, Hogg N, Kelm M, Kim-Shapiro DB, Kozlov AV et al. Nitrite as regulator of hypoxic signaling in mammalian physiology. *Med Res Rev* 29: 683–741, 2009.

92. Weibel ER and Hoppeler H. Exercise-induced maximal metabolic rate scales with muscle aerobic capacity. *J Exp Biol* 208: 1635–1644, 2005.

93. Weinbaum S, Tarbell JM, and Damiano ER. The structure and function of the endothelial glycocalyx layer. *Annu Rev Biomed Eng* 9: 121–167, 2007.

94. Woldhuis B, Tangelder GJ, Slaaf DW, and Reneman RS. Concentration profile of blood platelets differs in arterioles and venules. *Am J Physiol* 262: H1217–1223, 1992.

95. Zhang J, Johnson PC, and Popel AS. Effects of erythrocyte deformability and aggregation on the cell free layer and apparent viscosity of microscopic blood flows. *Microvasc Res* 77: 265–272, 2009.

Further Information

Handbook of Physiology. Microcirculation (2nd ed.), edited by Tuma RF, Duran WN and Ley K: Elsevier, American Physiological Society, 2008, 949 pp.

Original research articles on microcirculation can be found in academic journals: *Microcirculation*, *Microvascular Research*, *American Journal of Physiology (Heart and Circulatory Physiology)*, *Journal of Vascular Research*, and *Biorheology*.

14

Mechanics and Deformability of Hematocytes

Richard E. Waugh
University of Rochester

Robert M.
Hochmuth
Duke University

14.1 Introduction

The term "hematocytes" refers to the circulating cells of the blood. These are divided into two main classes: erythrocytes, or red cells, and leukocytes, or white cells. In addition to these, there are specialized cell-like structures called platelets. The mechanical properties of these cells are of special interest because of their physiological role as circulating corpuscles in the flowing blood. The importance of the mechanical properties of these cells and their influence on blood flow is evident in a number of hematological pathologies. The properties of the two main types of hematocytes are distinctly different. The essential character of a red cell is that of an elastic bag enclosing a Newtonian fluid of comparatively low viscosity. The essential behavior of leukocytes is that of a highly viscous fluid drop with a more or less constant cortical (surface) tension. Under the action of a given force, red cells deform much more readily than white cells. In this chapter, we focus on descriptions of the behavior of the two cell types separately, concentrating on the viscoelastic characteristics of the red cell membrane and the fluid characteristics of the white cell cytosol.

14.2 Fundamentals

14.2.1 Stresses and Strains in Two Dimensions

The description of the mechanical deformation of the membrane is cast in terms of principal *force resultants* and *principal extension ratios* of the surface. The force resultants, like conventional three-dimensional strain, are generally expressed in terms of a tensorial quantity, the components of which depend on coordinate rotation. For the purposes of describing the constitutive behavior of the surface, it is convenient to express the surface resultants in terms of rotationally invariant quantities. These can be either the principal force resultants N_1 and N_2, or the isotropic resultant $\bar{N}$ and the maximum shear resultant N_s. The surface strain is also a tensorial quantity but may be expressed in terms of the principal extension ratios of the surface λ_1 and λ_2. The *rate* of surface shear deformation is given by (Evans and Skalak 1979)

$$V_s = \left(\frac{\lambda_1}{\lambda_2} \right)^{1/2} \frac{d}{dt} \left(\frac{\lambda_1}{\lambda_2} \right)^{1/2} \tag{14.1}$$

The membrane deformation is calculated from observed macroscopic changes in cell geometry, usually with the use of simple geometric shapes to approximate the cell shape. The membrane force resultants are calculated from force balance relationships. For example, in the determination of the *area expansivity modulus* of the red cell membrane or the *cortical tension* in neutrophils, the force resultants in the plane of the membrane of the red cell or the cortex of a white cell are isotropic. In this case, as long as the membrane surface of the cell does not stick to the pipette, the membrane force resultant can be calculated from the law of Laplace:

$$\Delta P = 2\bar{N} \left(\frac{1}{R_p} - \frac{1}{R_c} \right) \tag{14.2}$$

where R_p is the radius of the pipette, R_c is the radius of the spherical portion of the cell outside the pipette, $\bar{N}$ is the isotropic force resultant (tension) in the membrane, and ΔP is the aspiration pressure in the pipette.

14.2.2 Basic Equations for Newtonian Fluid Flow

The constitutive relations for fluid flow in a sphere undergoing axisymmetric deformation can be written as

$$\sigma_{rr} = -p + 2\eta \frac{\partial V_r}{\partial r} \tag{14.3}$$

$$\sigma_{r\theta} = \eta \left[\frac{1}{r} \frac{\partial V_r}{\partial \theta} + r \frac{\partial}{\partial r} \left(\frac{V_\theta}{r} \right) \right] \tag{14.4}$$

where σ_{rr} and $\sigma_{r\theta}$ are components of the stress tensor, p is the hydrostatic pressure, r is the radial coordinate, θ is the angular coordinate in the direction of the axis of symmetry in spherical coordinates, and V_r and V_θ are components of the fluid velocity vector. These equations effectively define the material viscosity, η. The second term in Equation 14.3 contains the radial strain rate $\dot{\varepsilon}_{rr}$ and the bracketed term in Equation 14.4 corresponds to $\dot{\varepsilon}_{r\theta}$. In general, η may be a function of the strain rate. For the purposes of evaluating this dependence, it is convenient to define the mean shear rate $\dot{\gamma}_m$ averaged over the cell volume and duration of the deformation process t_e:

$$\dot{\gamma}_m = \left(\frac{3}{4} \frac{1}{t_e} \int\limits_{t_e}^{t_e} \int\limits_{0}^{R(t)} \int\limits_{0}^{\pi} \frac{r^2}{R^3} (\dot{\varepsilon}_{ij} \dot{\varepsilon}_{ij}) \sin\theta \ d\theta dr dt \right)^{1/2} \tag{14.5}$$

where repeated indices indicate summation.

14.3 Red Cells

14.3.1 Size and Shape

The normal red cell is a biconcave disk at rest. The average human cell is approximately 7.7 μm in diameter and varies in thickness from ~2.8 μm at the rim to ~1.4 μm at the center (Fung et al. 1981). However, red cells vary considerably in size even within a single individual. The mean surface area is ~130 μm² and the mean volume is 98 μm³ (Table 14.1), but the range of sizes within a population is Gaussian distributed with standard deviations (S.D.) of ~15.8 μm² for the area and ~16.1 μm³ for the volume (Fung et al. 1981). Cells from different species vary enormously in size, and tables for different species have been tabulated elsewhere (Hawkey et al. 1991).

Red cell deformation takes place under two important constraints: fixed surface area and fixed volume. The constraint of fixed volume arises from the impermeability of the membrane to cations. Even though the membrane is highly permeable to water, the inability of salts to cross the membrane prevents significant water loss because of the requirement for colloidal osmotic equilibrium (Lew and Bookchin 1986). The constraint of fixed surface area arises from the large resistance of bilayer membranes to changes in area per molecule (Needham and Nunn 1990). These two constraints place strict limits on the kinds of deformations that the cell can undergo and the size of the aperture that the cell can negotiate. Thus, a major determinant of red cell deformability is its ratio of surface area to volume. One measure of this parameter is the *sphericity*, defined as the dimensionless ratio of the two-thirds power of the cell volume to the cell area times a constant that makes its maximum value 1.0:

$$S = \frac{4\pi}{(4\pi/3)^{2/3}} \cdot \frac{V^{2/3}}{A} \tag{14.6}$$

The mean value of sphericity of a normal population of cells was measured by interference microscopy to be 0.79 with an S.D. of 0.05 at room temperature (Fung et al. 1981). Similar values were obtained using micropipettes: mean = 0.81, S.D. = 0.02 (Waugh and Agre 1988). The membrane area increases with temperature, and the membrane volume decreases with temperature, so the sphericity at physiological temperature is expected to be somewhat smaller. Based on measurements of the thermal area expansivity of 0.12%/°C (Waugh and Evans 1979), and a change in volume of −0.14%/°C (Waugh and Evans 1979), the mean sphericity at 37°C is estimated to be 0.76–0.78 (see Table 14.1).

TABLE 14.1 Parameter Values for a Typical Red Blood Cell (37°C)

Area	132 μm²
Volume	96 μm³
Sphericity	0.77
Membrane area modulus	400 mN/m
Membrane shear modulus	0.006 mN/m
Membrane viscosity	0.00036 mN·s/m
Membrane bending stiffness	0.2×10^{-18} J
Thermal area expansivity	0.12%/°C
$\dfrac{1}{V}\dfrac{dV}{dT}$	−0.14%/°C

TABLE 14.2   Viscosity of Red Cell Cytosol (37°C)

Hemoglobin Concentration (g/L)	Measured Viscosity[a] (mPa · s)	Best Fit Viscosity[b] (mPa · s)
290	4.1–5.0	4.2
310	5.2–6.6	5.3
330	6.6–9.2	6.7
350	8.5–13.0	8.9
370	10.8–17.1	12.1
390	15.0–23.9	17.2

[a] Data taken from Cokelet and Meiselman (1968) and Chien et al. (1970).
[b] Fitted curve from Ross and Minton (1977).

14.3.2 Red Cell Cytosol

The interior of a red cell is a concentrated solution of hemoglobin, the oxygen-carrying protein, and it behaves as a Newtonian fluid (Cokelet and Meiselman 1968). In a normal population of cells, there is a distribution of hemoglobin concentrations in the range of 29–39 g/dl. The viscosity of the cytosol depends on the hemoglobin concentration as well as the temperature (see Table 14.2). Based on theoretical models (Ross and Minton 1977), the temperature dependence of the cytosolic viscosity is expected to be the same as that of water, that is, the ratio of cytosolic viscosity at 37°C to the viscosity at 20°C is the same as the ratio of water viscosity at those same temperatures. In most cases, even in the most dense cells, the resistance to flow of the cytosol is small compared with the viscoelastic resistance of the membrane when membrane deformations are appreciable.

14.3.3 Membrane Area Dilation

The large resistance of the membrane to area dilation has been characterized in micromechanical experiments. The changes in surface area that can be produced in the membrane are small, and so they can be characterized in terms of a simple Hookean elastic relationship between the isotropic force resultant $\overline{N}$ and the fractional change in surface area $\alpha = A/Ao - 1$:

$$\overline{N} = K\alpha \tag{14.7}$$

The proportionality constant K is called the *area compressibility modulus* or the *area expansivity modulus*. Early estimates placed its value at room temperature at ~450 mN/m (Evans and Waugh 1977) and showed a dependence of the modulus on temperature, its value changing from ~300 mN/m at 45°C to a value of ~600 mN/m at 5°C (Waugh and Evans 1979). Subsequently, it was shown that the measurement of this parameter using micropipettes is affected by extraneous electric fields, and the value at room temperature was corrected upward to ~500 mN/m (Katnik and Waugh 1990). The values in Table 14.3 are based on this measurement, and the fractional change in the modulus with temperature is based on the original micropipette measurements (Waugh and Evans 1979).

14.3.4 Membrane Shear Deformation

The shear deformations of the red cell surface can be large, and so a simple linear relationship between force and extension is not adequate for describing the membrane behavior. The large resistance of the membrane composite to area dilation led early investigators to postulate that the membrane maintained constant surface density during shear deformation, that is, the surface was two-dimensionally incompressible. Most of what exists in the literature about the shear deformation of the red cell membrane is based on this assumption. Indeed, even a recent three-dimensional neo-Hookean relationship proposed

TABLE 14.3 Temperature Dependence of Viscoelastic Coefficients of the Red Cell Membrane

Temperature (°C)	K (mN/m)[a]	μ_m (mN/m)[b]	η (mN·s/m)[c]
5	660	0.0078	0.0021
15	580	0.0072	0.0014
25	500	0.0065	0.00074
37	400	0.0058	0.00036
45	340	0.0053	—

[a] Based on a value of the modulus at 25°C of 500 mN/m and the fractional change in modulus with temperature measured by Waugh and Evans (1979).
[b] Based on linear regression to the data of Waugh and Evans (1979).
[c] Data from Hochmuth et al. (1980).

by Dao et al. (2003) applies the constant area constraint in modeling extensional deformation of red cells by optical tweezers. In the mid-1990s, experimental evidence emerged that this assumption is an over-simplification of the true cellular behavior, and that deformation produces changes in the local surface density of the membrane elastic network (Discher et al. 1994). Nevertheless, the older simpler relationships provide a reliable description of the cell behavior that can be useful for many applications, and so the properties of the cell defined under that assumption are summarized here.

For a simple, two-dimensional, incompressible, hyperelastic material, the relationship between the membrane shear force resultant N_s and the material deformation is (Evans and Skalak 1979)

$$N_s = \frac{\mu_m}{2}\left(\frac{\lambda_1}{\lambda_2} - \frac{\lambda_2}{\lambda_1}\right) + 2\eta_m V_s \qquad (14.8)$$

where λ_1 and λ_2 are the principal extension ratios for the deformation and V_s is the rate of surface shear deformation (Equation 14.1). The *membrane shear modulus* μ_m and the *membrane viscosity* η_m are defined by this relationship. Values for these coefficients at different temperatures are given in Table 14.3.

14.3.5 Stress Relaxation and Strain Hardening

Subsequent to these original formulations, a number of refinements to these relationships have been proposed. Observations of persistent deformations after micropipette aspiration for extended periods of time formed the basis for the development of a model for long-term stress relaxation (Markle et al. 1983). The characteristic times for these relaxations were on the order of 1–2 h, and they are thought to correlate with permanent rearrangements of the membrane elastic network.

Another type of stress relaxation is thought to occur over very short times (~0.1 s) after rapid deformation of the membrane either by micropipette (Chien et al. 1978) or in cell extension experiments (Waugh and Bisgrove, unpublished observations). This phenomenon is thought to be due to transient entanglements within the deforming network. Whether or not the phenomenon actually occurs remains controversial. The stresses relax rapidly, and it is difficult to account for inertial effects of the measuring system and to reliably assess the intrinsic cellular response. In a more recent report, magnetic twisting cytometry was used to measure storage and loss moduli over a wide range of frequencies. The strains in these studies were small, and the elastic deformation dominated by bending, so it is unclear if the lack of frequency dependence of the storage modulus observed in that study has implications here, but the membrane behavior at low frequencies was consistent with the moduli determined from cell extension.

Finally, there has been some evidence that the coefficient for shear elasticity may be a function of the surface extension, increasing with increasing deformation. This was first proposed by Fischer in an effort to resolve discrepancies between theoretical predictions and observed behavior of red cells undergoing dynamic deformations in fluid shear (Fischer et al. 1981). Increasing elastic resistance with extension has also been proposed as an explanation for discrepancies between theoretical predictions based on a constant modulus and measurements of the length of a cell projection into a micropipette (Waugh and Marchesi 1990). However, owing to the approximate nature of the mechanical analysis of cell deformation in shear flow, and the limits of optical resolution in micropipette experiments, the evidence for a dependence of the modulus on extension is not clear-cut, and this issue remains unresolved.

14.3.6 New Constitutive Relations for the Red Cell Membrane

More recent descriptions of membrane deformation recognize that the membrane is a composite of two layers with distinct mechanical behavior. The membrane bilayer, composed of phospholipids and integral membrane proteins, exhibits a large elastic resistance to area dilation but is fluid in surface shear. The membrane skeleton, composed of a network of structural proteins at the cytoplasmic surface of the bilayer, is locally compressible and exhibits an elastic resistance to surface shear. The assumption that the membrane skeleton is locally incompressible is no longer applied. This assumption had been challenged over the years on the basis of theoretical considerations, but only very recently has experimental evidence emerged that shows definitively that the membrane skeleton is compressible. This led to a model for membrane behavior (Mohandas and Evans 1994) where the principal stress resultants in the membrane skeleton are related to the membrane deformation by

$$N_1 = \mu_N \left(\frac{\lambda_1}{\lambda_2} - 1 \right) + K_N \left(\lambda_1 \lambda_2 - \frac{1}{(\lambda_1 \lambda_2)^2} \right) \tag{14.9}$$

and

$$N_2 = \mu_N \left(\frac{\lambda_2}{\lambda_1} - 1 \right) + K_N \left(\lambda_1 \lambda_2 - \frac{1}{(\lambda_1 \lambda_2)^2} \right) \tag{14.10}$$

where μ_N and K_N are the shear and isotropic moduli of the membrane skeleton, respectively. Values for the coefficients determined from fluorescence measurements of skeletal density distributions during micropipette aspiration studies are $\mu_N \approx 0.01$ mN/m and $K_N \approx 0.02$ mN/m (Discher et al. 1994). These new concepts for membrane constitutive behavior have yet to be explored thoroughly. The temperature dependence of these moduli is unknown, and the implications such a model will have on interpretation of dynamic deformations of the membrane remain to be resolved.

An important new area of development involves attempts to derive constitutive behavior from molecular-level models of the membrane skeleton. These approaches have led to reliable predictions of cell elastic behavior in micropipette aspiration (Discher et al. 1998) and cell extension using optical tweezers (Li et al. 2005). The most recent models also capture many of the dynamic behaviors of the red cell (Fedesov et al. 2010), although this most recent analysis did not allow for local changes in the density of the elastic network that have been well documented experimentally (Discher et al. 1994). Thus, while there are a number of mathematical descriptions that do an excellent job of capturing the essential characteristics of the cell, one that completely and accurately captures all aspects of the cell behavior remains an unmet goal.

14.3.7 Bending Elasticity

Even though the membrane is very thin, it has a high resistance to surface dilation. This property, coupled with the finite thickness of the membrane gives the membrane a small but finite resistance to bending. This resistance is characterized in terms of the *membrane bending modulus*. The bending resistance of biological membranes is inherently complex because of their lamellar structure. There is a local resistance to bending due to the inherent stiffness of the individual leaflets of the membrane bilayer. (Because the membrane skeleton is compressible, it is thought to contribute little if anything to the membrane bending stiffness.) In addition to this local stiffness, there is a *nonlocal bending resistance* due to the net compression and expansion of the adjacent leaflets resulting from the curvature change. The nonlocal contribution is complicated by the fact that the leaflets may be redistributed laterally within the membrane capsule to equalize the area per molecule within each leaflet. The situation is further complicated by the likely possibility that molecules may exchange between leaflets to alleviate curvature-induced dilation/compression. Thus, the bending stiffness measured by different approaches probably reflects contributions from both local and nonlocal mechanisms, and the measured values may differ because of different contributions from the two mechanisms. Estimates based on buckling instabilities during micropipette aspiration give a value of $\sim 0.18 \times 10^{-18}$ J (Evans 1983), measurements based on the mechanical formation of lipid tubes from the cell surface give a value of $0.2 \pm 0.02 \times 10^{-18}$ J (Butler et al. 2008, Hwang and Waugh 1997), and estimates based on thermal fluctuations of the membrane yield similar values.

14.4 Leukocytes

While red cells account for approximately 40% of the blood volume, leukocytes occupy less than 1% of the blood volume. Yet, because leukocytes are less deformable, they can have a significant influence on blood flow, especially in the microvasculature. Unlike red cells, which are very similar to each other, as are platelets, there are several different kinds of leukocytes. Originally, leukocytes were classified into groups according to their appearance when viewed with the light microscope. Thus, there are *granulocytes*, *monocytes*, and *lymphocytes* (Alberts et al. 2002). The granulocytes with their many internal granules are separated into *neutrophils*, *basophils*, and *eosinophils* according to the way each cell stains. The neutrophil, also called a *polymorphonuclear leukocyte* because of its segmented or "multilobed" nucleus, is the most common white cell in the blood (see Table 14.4). The lymphocytes, which constitute 20–40% of the white cells and which are further subdivided into *B lymphocytes* and *killer* and *helper T lymphocytes*, are the smallest of the white cells. The other types of leukocytes are found with much less frequency. Most of the geometric and mechanical studies of white cells reported below have focused on the neutrophil because it is the most common cell in the circulation, although the lymphocyte has also received attention.

14.4.1 Size and Shape

White cells at rest are spherical. The surfaces of white cells contain many folds, projections, and "microvilli" to provide the cells with sufficient membrane area to deform as they enter capillaries with

TABLE 14.4 Size and Appearance of White Cells in the Circulation

	Occurrence[a] (% of WBCs)	Cell Volume[b] (μm³)	Cell Diameter[b] (μm)	Nucleus[c] % Cell Volume	Cortical Tension (mN/m)
Granulocytes					
Neutrophils	50–70	300–310	8.2–8.4	21	0.024–0.035[d]
Basophils	0–1	—			—
Eosinophils	1–3	—		18	—
Monocytes	1–5	400	9.1	26	0.06[e]
Lymphocytes	20–40	220	7.5	44	0.035[e]

[a] Diggs et al. (1985).
[b] Ting-Beall et al. (1993, 1995).
[c] Schmid-Schönbein et al. (1980).
[d] Evans and Yeung (1989), Needham and Hochmuth (1992), Tsai et al. (1993, 1994).
[e] Hochmuth, Zhelev, and Ting-Beall, unpublished data.

diameters much smaller than the resting diameter of the cell. (Without the reservoir of membrane area in these folds, the constraints of constant volume and membrane area would make a spherical cell essentially undeformable.) The excess surface area of the neutrophil, when measured in a wet preparation, is slightly more than twice the apparent surface area of a smooth sphere with the same diameter (Evans and Yeung 1989, Ting-Beall et al. 1993). It is interesting to note that each type of white cell has its own unique surface topography, which allows one to readily determine if a cell is, for example, a neutrophil or monocyte or lymphocyte (Hochmuth et al. 1994).

The cell volumes listed in Table 14.4 were obtained with the light microscope, either by measuring the diameter of the spherical cell or by aspirating the cell into a small glass pipette with a known diameter and then measuring the resulting length of the cylindrically shaped cell. Other values for cell volume obtained using transmission electron microscopy are somewhat smaller, probably because of cell shrinkage due to fixation and drying prior to measurement (Schmid-Schonbein et al. 1980, Ting-Beall et al. 1995). Although the absolute magnitude of the cell volume measured with the electron microscope may be erroneous, if it is assumed that all parts of the cell dehydrate equally when they are dried in preparation for viewing, then this approach can be used to determine the volume occupied by the nucleus (Table 14.4) and other organelles of various white cells. The volume occupied by the granules in the neutrophil and eosinophil (recall that both are granulocytes) is 15% and 23%, respectively, whereas the granular volume in monocytes and lymphocytes is less than a few percent.

14.4.2 Mechanical Behavior

The early observations of Bagge et al. (1977) led them to suggest that the neutrophil behaves as a simple viscoelastic solid with a Maxwell element (an elastic and viscous element in series) in parallel with an elastic element. This elastic element in the model was thought to pull the unstressed cell into its spherical shape. Subsequently, Evans and colleagues (Evans and Kukan 1984, Evans and Yeung 1989) showed that the cells flow continuously into a pipette, with no apparent approach to a static limit, when a constant suction pressure was applied. Thus, the cytoplasm of the neutrophil should be treated as a liquid rather than a solid, and its surface has a persistent *cortical tension* that causes the cell to assume a spherical shape.

14.4.3 Cortical Tension

Using a micropipette and a small suction pressure to aspirate a hemispherical projection from a cell body into the pipette, Evans and Yeung (1989) measured a value for the cortical tension of 0.035 mN/m. Needham and Hochmuth (1992) measured the cortical tension of individual cells that were driven down a tapered pipette in a series of equilibrium positions. In many cases, the cortical tension increased as the cell moved further into the pipette, which means that the cell has an apparent area expansion modulus (Equation 14.7). They obtained an average value of 0.04 mN/m for the expansion modulus and an extrapolated value for the cortical tension (at zero area dilation) in the resting state of 0.024 mN/m. Herant (Herant et al. 2005) examined cortical tension as a cell engulfed a bead, and found a lower resting value but a much higher dependence on surface dilation. For dilations of the surface up to 25%, they found $T = T_o + k(A - A_o)/A_o$, where $T_o = 0.010$ mN/m and $k = 0.16$ mN/m. The importance of the actin cytoskeleton in maintaining cortical tension was demonstrated by Tsai et al. (1994). The treatment of the cells with a drug that disrupts actin filament structure (CTB = cytochalasin B) resulted in a decrease in cortical tension from 0.027 to 0.022 mN/m at a CTB concentration of 3 μM and to 0.014 mN/m at 30 μM.

Unpublished measurements in one of our laboratories (RMH) indicate that the value for the cortical tension of a monocyte is about double that for a granulocyte, that is, 0.06 mN/m, and the value for a lymphocyte is about 0.035 mN/m.

14.4.4 Apparent Viscosity

Using their model of the neutrophil as a Newtonian liquid drop with a constant cortical tension and (as they showed) a negligible surface viscosity, Yeung and Evans (1989) analyzed the flow of neutrophils into a micropipette and obtained a value for the *cytoplasmic viscosity* of about 200 Pa · s. In their experiments, the aspiration pressures were on the order of 10–1000 Pa. Similar experiments by Needham and Hochmuth (1990) using the same Newtonian model (with a negligible surface viscosity) but using higher aspiration pressures (ranging from 500 to 2000 Pa) gave an average value for the cytoplasmic viscosity of 135 Pa · s for 151 cells from five individuals. The apparent discrepancy between these two sets of experiments was resolved to a large extent by Tsai and colleagues (Tsai et al. 1993), who demonstrated that the neutrophil viscosity decreases with an increasing rate of deformation. They proposed a model of the cytosol as a *power law fluid*:

$$\eta = \eta_c \left(\frac{\dot{\gamma}_m}{\dot{\gamma}_c} \right)^{-b} \tag{14.11}$$

where $b = 0.52$, $\dot{\gamma}_m$ is defined by Equation 14.5, and η_c is a characteristic viscosity of 130 Pa · s when the characteristic mean shear rate, $\dot{\gamma}_c$, is 1 s^{-1}. These values are based on an approximate method for calculating the viscosity from measurements of the total time it takes for a cell to enter a micropipette. Because of different approximations used in the calculations, the values of viscosity reported by Tsai (Tsai et al. 1993) tend to be somewhat smaller than those reported by Evans and coworkers or Hochmuth and coworkers. Nevertheless, the shear rate dependence of the viscosity is the same, regardless of the method of calculation. Values for the viscosity are given in Table 14.5.

In addition to the dependence of the viscosity on shear rate, there is evidence that values estimated using these approximate models also depend on the extent of deformation. In micropipette experiments, the initial rate at which the cell enters the pipette is significantly faster than predicted, even when the shear rate dependence of the viscosity is taken into account. In a separate approach, the cytosolic viscosity was estimated from the observation of the time course of the cell's return to a spherical geometry after expulsion from a micropipette. When the cellular deformations were large, a viscosity of 150 Pa · s was estimated (Tran-Son-Tay et al. 1991), but when the deformations were small, the estimated viscosity was only 60 Pa · s (Dong et al. 1988, Hochmuth et al. 1993). Thus, it appears that the viscosity is smaller when the magnitude of the deformation is small, and increases as deformations become large.

Although it is clear that the essential behavior of the cell is fluid, the simple fluid drop model with a constant and uniform viscosity does not match the observed time course of cell deformation in detail. In addition to variations in viscosity with magnitude and rate of deformation, there is a rapid initial entry phase that is not predicted by the fluid drop model. One approach that was considered to address this was the application of a *Maxwell fluid* model with a constant cortical tension (Dong et al. 1988). While

TABLE 14.5 Viscous Parameters of White Blood Cells

Cell Type	Range of Viscosities (Pa · s)[a]		Characteristic Viscosity (Pa · s)	Shear Rate Dependence (*b*)
	Minimum	Maximum		
Neutrophil	50	500	130[b]	0.52[b]
in 30 µM CTB	41	52	54[b]	0.26[b]
Monocyte	70	1000	—	—
HL60 (G1)	—	—	220[c]	0.53[c]
HL60 (S)	—	—	330[c]	0.56[c]

[a] Evans and Yeung (1989), Needham and Hochmuth (1992), Tsai et al. (1993, 1994).
[b] Tsai et al. (1993, 1994).
[c] Tsai and Waugh (1996a,b).

the model worked well for the shape recovery of neutrophils following small deformations, attempts to apply this model for continuous, finite-deformation flow of a neutrophil into a pipette required continuous adjustment of the material coefficients over time (Dong and Skalak 1992). A more successful approach was taken by Drury and Dembo, who developed a finite element analysis of a cell using a model having substantial cortical dissipation with shear thinning and a shear thinning cytoplasm (Drury and Dembo 2001). Their model matches cellular behavior during micropipette aspiration over a wide range of pipette diameters and entry rates, except for the initial rapid entry phase. To account for this phenomenon, a model was introduced in which the cell interior comprised two distinct phases: the cytoskeleton and the cytosol (Herant et al. 2003). Inclusion of all of these characteristics accurately captures most of the fine details of cell behavior, and has been used in subsequent extensions of this approach to examine phagocytosis (Herant et al. 2006). Unfortunately, these advanced models are complex and not easily summarized, and the reader is referred to the original reports for further details.

Although the mechanical properties of the neutrophil have been studied extensively as discussed above, the other white cells have not been studied in depth. Unpublished results from one of our laboratories (RMH) indicate that monocytes are somewhat more viscous (from roughly 30% to a factor of two) than neutrophils under similar conditions in both recovery experiments and experiments in which the monocyte flows into a pipette. A lymphocyte, when aspirated into a small pipette so that its relatively large nucleus is deformed, behaves as an elastic body in that the projection length into the pipette increases linearly with the suction pressure. This elastic behavior appears to be due to the deformation of the nucleus, which has an apparent area elastic modulus of 2 mN/m. A lymphocyte recovers its shape somewhat more quickly than the neutrophil does, although this recovery process is driven by both the cortical tension and the elastic nucleus. These preliminary results are discussed by Tran-Son-Tay et al. (1994). Finally, the properties of a human myeloid leukemic cell line (HL60) thought to resemble immature neutrophils of the bone marrow have also been characterized, as shown in Table 14.5. The apparent cytoplasmic viscosity varies both as a function of the cell cycle and during maturation toward a more neutrophil-like cell. The characteristic viscosity $\dot{\gamma}_c = 1\,s^{-1}$ is 200 Pa·s for HL60 cells in the G1 stage of the cell cycle. This value increases to 275 Pa·s for cells in the S phase, but decreases with maturation, so that 7 days after induction, the properties approach those of neutrophils (150 Pa·s) (Tsai et al. 1996a,b).

It is important to note in closing that the characteristics described above apply to passive leukocytes. It is the nature of these cells to respond to environmental stimulation and engage in active movements and shape transformations. *White cell activation* produces significant heterogeneous changes in cell properties. The cell projections that form as a result of stimulation (called pseudopodia) are extremely rigid, whereas other regions of the cell may retain the characteristics of a passive cell. In addition, the cell may produce large protrusive or contractile forces. The changes in cellular mechanical properties that result from cellular activation are complex, but are being addressed in computational models of the cell that include cortical dynamics and a multiphase cell interior. Such models have been used to obtain insights into the mechanisms of phagocytosis, and good agreement between model predictions and cell behavior has been demonstrated (Herant et al. 2005, 2006).

14.5 Summary

Constitutive equations that capture the essential features of the responses of red blood cells and passive leukocytes have been formulated, and material parameters characterizing the cellular behavior have been measured. The red cell response is dominated by the cell membrane, which can be described as a hyperviscoelastic, two-dimensional continuum. The passive white cell behaves like a highly viscous fluid drop, and its response to external forces is dominated by the large viscosity of the cytosol. Refinements of these constitutive models and extension of mechanical analysis to activated white cells is anticipated as the ultrastructural events that occur during cellular deformation are delineated in increasing detail.

Definition of Terms

Area expansivity modulus: A measure of the resistance of a membrane to area dilation. It is the proportionality between the isotropic force resultant in the membrane and the corresponding fractional change in membrane area (units: 1 mN/m = 1 dyn/cm = 1000 pN/μm).

Cortical tension: Analogous to surface tension of a liquid drop, it is a persistent contractile force per unit length at the surface of a white blood cell (units: 1 mN/m = 1 dyn/cm).

Cytoplasmic viscosity: A measure of the resistance of the cytosol to flow (units: 1 Pa·s = 10 poise).

Force resultant: The stress in a membrane integrated over the membrane thickness. It is the two-dimensional analog of stress with units of force/length (units: 1 mN/m = 1 dyn/cm = 1000 pN/μm).

Maxwell fluid: A constitutive model in which the response of the material to applied stress includes both an elastic and viscous response in series. In response to a constant applied force, the material will respond elastically at first, then flow. At fixed deformation, the stresses in the material will relax to zero.

Membrane bending modulus: The intrinsic resistance of the membrane to changes in curvature. It is usually construed to exclude nonlocal contributions. It relates the moment resultants (force times length per unit length) in the membrane to the corresponding change in curvature (inverse length) (units: 1 N m = 1 joule = 10^7 erg = 10^{18} pN μm).

Membrane shear modulus: A measure of the elastic resistance of the membrane to surface shear deformation, that is, changes in the shape of the surface at constant surface area (Equation 14.8) (units: 1 mN/m = 1 dyn/cm = 1000 pN/μm).

Membrane viscosity: A measure of the resistance of the membrane to surface shear flow, that is, to the rate of surface shear deformation (Equation 14.8) (units: 1 mN·s/m = 1 mPa·s m = 1 dyn·s/cm = 1 surface poise).

Nonlocal bending resistance: A resistance to bending resulting from the differential expansion and compression of the two adjacent leaflets of a lipid bilayer. It is termed nonlocal because the leaflets can move laterally relative to one another to relieve local strains such that the net resistance to bending depends on the integral of the change in curvature of the entire membrane capsule.

Power law fluid: A model to describe the dependence of the cytoplasmic viscosity on rate of deformation (Equation 14.11).

Principal extension ratios: The ratios of the deformed length and width of a rectangular material element (in principal coordinates) to the undeformed length and width.

Sphericity: A dimensionless ratio of the cell volume (to the 2/3 power) to the cell area. Its value ranges from near zero to one, the maximum value corresponding to a perfect sphere (Equation 14.6).

White cell activation: The response of a leukocyte to external stimuli that involves reorganization and polymerization of the cellular structures and is typically accompanied by changes in cell shape and cell movement.

References

Alberts, B., Johnson, A., Lewis, J., Raff, M., Roberts, K., and Walter, P., 2002. *Molecular Biology of the Cell* Garland Science, New York.

Bagge, U., Skalak, R., and Attefors, R., 1977. Granulocyte rheology, *Adv. Microcirc.* 7, 29–48.

Butler, J., Mohandas, N., and Waugh, R. E., 2008. Integral protein linkage and the bilayer-skeletal separation energy in red blood cells, *Biophys. J.* 95, 1826–1836.

Chien, S., Sung, K. L. P., Skalak, R., and Usami, S., 1978. Theoretical and experimental studies on viscoelastic properties of erythrocyte membrane, *Biophys. J.* 24, 463–487.

Cokelet, G. R. and Meiselman, H. J., 1968. Rheological comparison of hemoglobin solutions and erythro-cyte suspensions, *Science* 162, 275–277.

Dao, M., Lim, C. T., and Suresh, S., 2003. Mechanics of the human red blood cell deformed by optical tweezers, *J. Mech. Phys. Solid* 51, 2259–2280.

Diggs, L. W., Sturm, D., and Bell, A., 1985. *The Morphology of Human Blood Cells.* Abbott Laboratories, Abbott Park, IL.

Discher, D. E., Boal, D. H., and Boey, S. K., 1998. Simulations of the erythrocyte cytoskeleton at large deformation. II. Micropipette aspiration, *Biophys. J.* 75, 1584–1597.

Discher, D. E., Mohandas, N., and Evans, E. A., 1994. Molecular maps of red cell deformation: hidden elasticity and *in situ* connectivity, *Science* 266, 1032–1035.

Dong, C. and Skalak, R., 1992. Leukocyte deformability: Finite element modeling of large viscoelastic deformation, *J. Theor. Biol.* 158, 173–193.

Dong, C., Skalak, R., Sung, K. L. P., Schmid-Schonbein, G. W., and Chien, S., 1988. Passive deformation analysis of human leukocytes, *J. Biomech. Eng.* 110, 27–36.

Drury, J. L. and Dembo, M., 2001. Aspiration of human neutrophils: Effects of shear thinning and cortical dissipation, *Biophys. J.* 81, 3166–3177.

Evans, E. and Kukan, B., 1984. Passive material behavior of granulocytes based on large deformation and recovery after deformation tests, *Blood* 64, 1028–1035.

Evans, E. and Yeung, A., 1989. Apparent viscosity and cortical tension of blood granulocytes determined by micropipet aspiration, *Biophys. J.* 56, 151–160.

Evans, E. A., 1983. Bending elastic modulus of red blood cell membrane derived from buckling instability in micropipet aspiration tests, *Biophys. J.* 43, 27–30.

Evans, E. A. and Skalak, R., 1979. Mechanics and thermodynamics of biomembranes, *CRC Crit. Rev. Bioeng.* 3, 181–418.

Evans, E. A. and Waugh, R., 1977. Osmotic correction to elastic area compressibility measurements on red cell membrane, *Biophys. J.* 20, 307–313.

Fedesov, D. A., Caswell, B., and Karniadakis, G. E., 2010. A multiscale red blood cell model with accurate mechanics, rheology and dynamics, *Biophys. J.* 98, 2215–2225.

Fischer, T. M., Haest, C. W. M., Stohr-Liesen, M., Schmid-Schonbein, H., and Skalak, R., 1981. The stress-free shape of the red blood cell membrane, *Biophys. J.* 34, 409–422.

Fung, Y. C., Tsang, W. C. O., and Patitucci, P., 1981. High-resolution data on the geometry of red blood cells, *Biorheol.* 18, 369–385.

Hawkey, C. M., Bennett, P. M., Gascoyne, S. C., Hart, M. G., and Kirkwood, J. K., 1991. Erythrocyte size, number and haemoglobin content in vertebrates, *Br. J. Haematol.* 77, 392–397.

Herant, M., Heinrich, V., and Dembo, M., 2005. Mechanics of neutrophil phagocytosis: Behavior of the cortical tension, *J. Cell Sci.* 118, 1789–1797.

Herant, M., Heinrich, V., and Dembo, M., 2006. Mechanics of neutrophil phagocytosis: Experiments and quantitative models, *J. Cell Sci.* 119, 1903–1913.

Herant, M., Marganski, W. A., and Dembo, M., 2003. The mechanics of neutrophils: Synthetic modeling of three experiments, *Biophys. J.* 84, 3389–3413.

Hochmuth, R. M., Buxbaum, K. L., and Evans, E. A., 1980. Temperature dependence of the viscoelastic properties of red cell membrane, *Biophys. J.* 29, 177–182.

Hochmuth, R. M., Ting-Beall, H. P., Beaty, B. B., Needham, D., and Tran-Son-Tay, R., 1993. Viscosity of passive human neutrophils undergoing small deformations, *Biophys. J.* 64, 1596–1601.

Hochmuth, R. M., Ting-Beal, H. P., and Zhelev, D. V., 1994. The mechanical properties of individual pas-sive neutrophils *in vitro*, in *Physiology and Pathophysiology of Leukocyte Adhesion*, Granger, D. N. and Schmid-Schoenbein, G. W. Oxford University Press, London.

Hwang, W. C. and Waugh, R. E., 1997. Energy of dissociation of lipid bilayer from the membrane skeleton of red blood cells, *Biophys. J.* 72, 2669–2678.

Katnik, C. and Waugh, R., 1990. Alterations of the apparent area expansivity modulus of red blood cell membrane by electric fields, *Biophys. J.* 57, 877–882.

Lew, V. L. and Bookchin, R. M., 1986. Volume, pH and ion content regulationin human red cells: Analysis of transient behavior with an integrated model, *J. Membr. Biol.* 10, 311–330.

Li, J., Dao, M., Lim, C. T., and Suresh, S., 2005. Spectrin-level modeling of the cytoskeleton and optical tweezers stretching of the erythrocyte, *Biophys. J.* 88, 3707–3719.

Markle, D. R., Evans, E. A., and Hochmuth, R. M., 1983. Force relaxation and permanent deformation of erythrocyte membrane, *Biophys. J.* 42, 91–98.

Mohandas, N. and Evans, E. A., 1994. Mechanical properties of the red cell membrane in relation to molecular structure and genetic defects, *Annu. Rev. Biophys. Biomol. Struct.* 23, 787–818.

Needham, D. and Hochmuth, R. M., 1990. Rapid flow of passive neutrophils into a 4 micron pipet and measurement of cytoplasmic viscosity, *J. Biomech. Eng.* 112, 269–276.

Needham, D. and Hochmuth, R. M., 1992. A sensitive measure of surface stress in the resting neutrophil, *Biophys. J.* 61, 1664–1670.

Needham, D. and Nunn, R. S., 1990. Elastic deformation and failure of lipid bilayer membranes containing cholesterol, *Biophys. J.* 58, 997–1009.

Ross, P. D. and Minton, A. P., 1977. Hard quasispherical model for the viscosity of hemoglobin solutions, *Biochem. Biophys. Res. Commun.* 76, 971–976.

Schmid-Schonbein, G. W., Usami, S., Skalak, R., and Chien, S., 1980. The interaction of leukocytes and erythrocytes in capillary and postcapillary vessels, *Microvasc. Res.* 19, 45–70.

Ting-Beall, H. P., Needham, D., and Hochmuth, R. M., 1993. Volume and osmotic properties of human neutrophils., *Blood* 81, 2774–2780.

Ting-Beall, H. P., Zhelev, D. V., and Hochmuth, R. M., 1995. Comparison of different drying procedures for scanning electron microscopy using human leukocytes, *Microsc. Res. Tech.* 32, 357–361.

Tran-Son-Tay, R., Kirk, T. F., 3rd, Zhelev, D. V., and Hochmuth, R. M., 1994. Numerical simulation of the flow of highly viscous drops down a tapered tube, *J. Biomech. Eng.* 116, 172–177.

Tran-Son-Tay, R., Needham, D., Yeung, A., and Hochmuth, R. M., 1991. Time-dependent recovery of passive neutrophils after large deformation, *Biophys. J.* 60, 856–866.

Tsai, M. A., Frank, R. S., and Waugh, R. E., 1993. Passive mechanical behavior of human neutrophils: Power-law fluid, *Biophys. J.* 65, 2078–2088.

Tsai, M. A., Frank, R. S., and Waugh, R. E., 1994. Passive mechanical behavior of human neutrophils: Effect of cytochalasin B, *Biophys. J.* 66, 2166–2172.

Tsai, M. A., Waugh, R. E., and Keng, P. C., 1996a. Cell cycle-dependence of HL-60 cell deformability, *Biophys. J.* 70, 2023–2029.

Tsai, M. A., Waugh, R. E., and Keng, P. C., 1996b. Changes in HL-60 cell deformability during differentiation induced by DMSO, *Biorheol.* 33, 1–15.

Waugh, R. and Evans, E. A., 1979. Thermoelasticity of red blood cell membrane, *Biophys. J.* 26, 115–132.

Waugh, R. E. and Agre, P., 1988. Reductions of erythrocyte membrane viscoelastic coefficients reflect spectrin deficiencies in hereditary spherocytosis, *J. Clin. Invest.* 81, 133–141.

Waugh, R. E. and Marchesi, S. L., 1990. Consequences of structural abnormalities on the mechanical properties of red blood cell membrane, in *Cellular and Molecular Biology of Normal and Abnormal Erythrocyte Membranes*, Cohen, C. M. and Palek, J. UCLA Symposia, Alan R. Liss, New York, NY, pp. 185–199.

Yeung, A. and Evans, E., 1989. Cortical shell-liquid core model for passive flow of liquid-like spherical cells into micropipets, *Biophys. J.* 56, 139–49.

Further Information

The basic information on the mechanical analysis of biomembrane deformation can be found in Evans and Skalak (1979), which also appeared as a book under the same title (CRC Press, Boca Raton, 1980).

A more recent work that focuses more closely on the structural basis of the membrane properties is Evans and Mohandas, 1994. Mechanical properties of the red cell membrane in relation to molecular structure and genetic defects. *Annual Review of Biophysics & Biomolecular Structure* 23: 787–818. We are unaware of more recent reviews of red cell mechanics, and readers are referred to the primary literature.

The basic information about white blood cell biology can be found in the book by Alberts et al. (1989). A more thorough review of white blood cell structure and response to stimulus can be found in two reviews by T. P. Stossel, one titled "The mechanical response of white blood cells," in the book *Inflammation: Basic Principles and Clinical Correlates*, edited by J. I. Galin et al. Raven Press, New York, 1988, pp. 325–342, and the second titled "The molecular basis of white blood cell motility," in the book *The Molecular Basis of Blood Diseases*, edited by G. Stamatoyannopoulos et al., W. B. Saunders, Philadelphia, 1994, pp. 541–562. Additional information about white cell rheology can be found in the book, *Cell Mechanics and Cellular Engineering*, edited by Van C. Mow et al., Springer Verlag, New York, 1994.

15

Mechanics of Tissue/ Lymphatic Transport

Geert W.
Schmid-Schönbein
*University of California,
San Diego*

Alan R. Hargens
*University of California,
San Diego*

15.1 Introduction

The transport of fluid and metabolites from the blood to the tissue is critically important for maintaining the viability and function of cells within tissues. Similarly, the transport of fluid, biological signaling molecules, microorganisms, and cell disposal products from the tissue to the lymphatic system of vessels and nodes is also crucial to maintain immune surveillance and tissue and organ health. Therefore, it is important to understand the mechanisms for transporting fluid containing micro- and macromolecules or colloidal materials from the blood to the tissue and the drainage of this fluid into the lymphatic system. Because of the abbreviated nature of this chapter, readers are encouraged to consult more complete reviews of blood/tissue/lymphatic transport by Kawai and Ohhashi (2009), Aukland and Reed (1993), Hargens and Akeson (1986), Jain (1987), Lai-Fook (1986), Schmid-Schönbein (1990), Schmid-Schönbein and Zweifach (1994), Staub (1988), Staub et al. (1987), Wei et al. (2003), and Zweifach and Silverberg (1985) and on lymphangiogenesis and its biological and biophysical control factors (Adams and Alitalo, 2007; Swartz and Fleury, 2007; Tammela and Alitalo, 2010). Muthuchamy and Zawieja (2008) have summarized the contractile protein machinery of the lymphatic smooth muscle.

Many previous studies of blood/tissue/lymphatic transport have used isolated organs or whole animals under general anesthesia. Under these conditions, the transport of fluid and metabolites is artificially low in comparison to animals that are actively moving. In some cases, investigators employed passive motion by connecting an animal's limb to a motor to facilitate studies of blood to lymph transport and lymphatic flow. However, new methods and technology allow studies of physiologically active animals so that a better understanding of the importance of transport phenomena in moving tissues is now apparent, especially in the skeletal muscle, skin, and subcutaneous tissue. Therefore, the major focus of this chapter is on the recent developments in the understanding of the mechanics of tissue/lymphatic transport.

The majority of the fluid that is filtered from the microcirculation into the interstitial space is carried out of the tissue via the lymphatic network. This unidirectional transport system originates with a set of blind channels in distal regions of the microcirculation. It carries a variety of interstitial molecules, proteins, metabolites, colloids, and even cells along channels deeply embedded in the tissue parenchyma toward a set of sequential lymph nodes and eventually back into the venous system via the right and left thoracic ducts. The lymphatics are the pathways for immune surveillance and thus, they are one of the important pathways of the immune system (Wei et al., 2003). For example, antigen-presenting dendritic cells, present in small quantities in tissues that are in contact with the external environment (mainly the skin), often acquire foreign antigens. The optimal encounter with naive T cells for presenting these antigens requires that the dendritic cells migrate to draining lymph nodes through lymphatic vessels (Randolph et al., 2005). Their delivery to the lymph nodes depends on the flow into the initial lymphatics (Miteva et al., 2010).

In the following section, we describe basic transport and tissue morphology as related to lymph flow. We also present recent evidence for a two-valve system in lymphatics that offers an updated view of lymph transport.

15.2 Basic Concepts of Tissue/Lymphatic Transport

15.2.1 Transcapillary Filtration

Since lymph is formed from the fluid filtered from the blood, an understanding of transcapillary exchange must be gained first. Usually, pressure parameters favor filtration of the fluid across the capillary wall to the interstitium (J_c) according to the Starling–Landis Equation 15.1:

$$J_c = L_p A[(P_c - P_t) - \sigma_p(\pi_c - \pi_t)] \tag{15.1}$$

where J_c is the net transcapillary fluid transport, L_p is the hydraulic conductivity of the capillary wall, A is the capillary surface area, P_c is the capillary blood pressure, P_t is the interstitial fluid pressure, σ_p is the reflection coefficient for protein, π_c is the capillary blood colloid osmotic pressure, and π_t is the interstitial fluid colloid osmotic pressure.

In the tissue, the fluid transported out of the capillaries is passively carried in the interstitial space via a percolation process around interstitial matrix proteins. According to Darcy's law, the average interstitial fluid velocity

$$q = -(k/\mu) \, \mathrm{grad}(p) \tag{15.2a}$$

where $\mathrm{grad}(p)$ is the pressure gradient, μ is the fluid coefficient of viscosity, and k is an empirical coefficient (it is a tensor in a three-dimensional tissue) whose value depends on the porosity ϕ of the fluid interstitial space. The fluid velocity, v, in the fluid phase around cells and in between solid fibers of the extracellular matrix is related to q by the relation

$$v = q/\phi \tag{15.2b}$$

In the normal tissue (e.g., not swollen), the majority of the fluid that enters the interstitial space is either reabsorbed by the capillary and/or venous vasculature or drained by the initial lymphatic vessels. If all filtered fluid is drained by the lymphatics

$$J_c = J_l \tag{15.3}$$

where J_l is the lymph flow. The fluid flow into the initial lymphatics depends on periodic compression and expansion of the initial lymphatics (microvessels that have a single layer of endothelium with highly specialized cell junctions that form the primary valve system in the lymphatics; see below). The primary valves permit the entry of fluid across the lymphatic endothelium into the initial lymphatics but prevent retrograde flow of fluid back into the interstitial space. Therefore, lymph fluid formation requires that the pressure within the initial lymphatic vessels P_L is lower than the adjacent interstitial fluid pressure P_t for establishing lymph flow:

$$P_t > P_L \tag{15.4}$$

The initial lymphatics have a set of specialized primary valves at the junction between their endothelial cells, so that the fluid can enter if $P_t > P_L$ (which occurs when the initial lymphatic channel expands) but there is no fluid flow when $P_t < P_L$ (when an initial lymphatic vessel is being compressed). The uptake of fluid from the interstitial fluid into the lymphatic channels therefore depends on the periodic mechanical expansion and the expansion of the initial lymphatics and process that is facilitated by a variety of organ-specific intrinsic and extrinsic tissue motions.

Fluid flow inside the lymphatics with Newtonian viscous fluid (which is incompressible at the stresses encountered in the lymphatics) due to low cell concentrations and at low Reynolds number is governed by the Stokes approximation of the equation of motion for incompressible fluid. The fluid is propelled forward by the compression of the initial lymphatics (in the contractile lymphatics by the contraction of the lymphatic smooth muscle), and retrograde flow is prevented by valves.

Each lymphatic compartment (in the initial and the downstream contractile lymphatics) requires a pair of valves to achieve forward flow: one upstream to allow the entry of fluid into the compartment and one downstream to prevent the return of fluid that has been discharged downstream. In the initial lymphatics, the primary valves formed by the endothelial junctions serve as upstream valves, the traditional intraluminal valves serve as secondary downstream valves. In contractile lymphatics, a pair of traditional intraluminal valves, one upstream and one downstream of each lymph compartment ("lymphangion"), serve to provide unidirectional flow toward the lymph nodes.

15.2.2 Starling Pressures and Edema Prevention

Hydrostatic and colloid osmotic pressures within the blood and interstitial fluid primarily govern transcapillary fluid shifts (Figure 15.1). Although input arterial pressure averages about 100 mm Hg at the heart level, capillary blood pressure P_c is significantly reduced due to resistance R, according to the Poiseuille Equation 15.4

$$R = \frac{8\eta l}{\pi r^4} \tag{15.5}$$

where η is the blood viscosity, l is the vessel length between feed artery and capillary, and r is the radius.

Therefore, normally at the heart level, P_c is approximately 30 mm Hg. However, during upright posture, P_c at the foot level is about 90 mm Hg and only about 25 mm Hg at the head level (Parazynski et al., 1991). The differences in P_c between capillaries of the head and feet are due to gravitational variation of the blood pressure such that the pressure $p = \rho g h$. Although myogenic vasoconstriction decreases local capillary pressure below the heart level, volumes of transcapillary filtration and lymph flows are generally higher in tissues of the lower body as compared to those of the upper body. Moreover, one might expect much more sparse distribution of lymphatic vessels in the upper body tissues. The brain has no lymphatics, but most other vascular tissues have lymphatics. In fact, tissues of the lower body of humans and other tall animals have efficient skeletal muscle pumps, prominent lymphatic systems, and noncompliant skin and fascial boundaries to prevent dependent edema (Hargens et al., 1987).

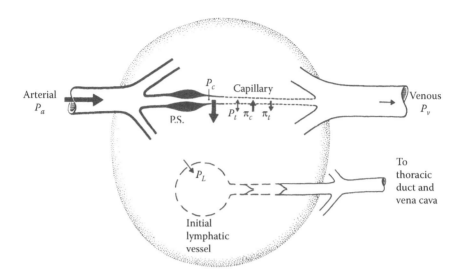

FIGURE 15.1 Starling pressures that regulate transcapillary fluid balance. The pressure parameters that determine the direction and the magnitude of transcapillary exchange include capillary blood pressure P_c, interstitial fluid pressure P_t (directed into the capillary when positive or directed into the tissue when negative), plasma colloidal osmotic pressure π_c, and interstitial fluid colloidal osmotic pressure π_t. Precapillary sphincters (PS) regulate P_c, capillary flow, and capillary surface area A. It is generally agreed that a hydrostatic pressure gradient (P_t > lymph pressure P_l) drains off excess interstitial fluid under conditions of net filtration. The relative magnitudes of pressures are depicted by the size of arrows. (From Hargens AR. 1986. *Handbook of Bioengineering*, vol. 19, pp. 1–35, New York, McGraw-Hill. With permission.)

Other pressure parameters in the Starling–Landis Equation 15.1 such as P_t, π_c, and π_t are not as sensitive to changes in body posture as is P_c. The typical values for P_t range from −2 to 10 mm Hg depending on the tissue or organ under investigation (Wiig, 1990). However, during movement, P_t in the skeletal muscle increases to 150 mm Hg or higher (Murthy et al., 1994), providing a mechanism to promote lymphatic flow and venous return via the skeletal pump (Figure 15.2). Blood colloid osmotic pressure π_c usually ranges between 25 and 35 mm Hg and is the other major force for retaining plasma within the vascular system and preventing edema. Interstitial π_t depends on the reflection coefficient of the capillary wall (σ_p ranges from 0.5 to 0.9 for different tissues) as well as washout of interstitial proteins during high filtration rates (Aukland and Reed, 1993). Typically, π_t ranges between 8 and 15 mm Hg with higher values in the upper body tissues compared to those in the lower body (Aukland and Reed, 1993; Parazynski et al., 1991). Precapillary sphincter activity (see Figure 15.1) also decreases blood flow, decreases capillary filtration area A, and reduces P_c in dependent tissues of the body to help prevent edema during upright posture (Aratow et al., 1991).

The conventional view of Starling's principle should be reconsidered in light of the role of glycocalyx as the semipermeable layer of endothelium. The low rate of transcapillary filtration and lymph formation in many tissues is explained by standing plasma protein gradients within the intercellular cleft of continuous capillaries (glycocalyx model) and around fenestrations (Levick and Michel, 2010). Narrow breaks in the junctional strands of the cleft create high local outward fluid velocities, which may cause a disequilibrium between the subglycocalyx space π and π_t. The recent review of interstitial–lymph transport by Levick and Michel (2010) suggests that the effect of π_t on the filtration of fluid from the capillary to the interstitium (J_c) is less than that predicted by the conventional Starling equation. Hu and Weinbaum (1999) introduced a new analysis of the fluid flow through endothelial gaps by proposing that the glycocalyx serves as the primary molecular sieve required to maintain colloid osmotic pressures. They predict lower filtration rates than predicted by the traditional Starling model.

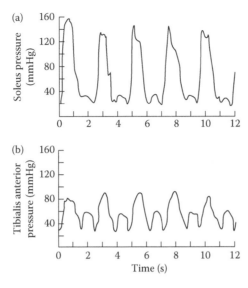

FIGURE 15.2 Simultaneous intramuscular pressure oscillations in the soleus (a) and the tibialis anterior (b) muscles during plantar- and dorsiflexion exercise. Soleus muscle is an integral part of the calf muscle pump. (From Murthy G et al. 1994. *J Appl Physiol* 76:2742. Modified with permission.)

15.2.3 Interstitial Fluid Transport

Interstitial flow of proteins and other macromolecules occurs by two mechanisms: diffusion and convection. During simple diffusion according to Fick's Equation 15.5

$$J_p = -D\frac{\partial c_p}{\partial x}$$

(15.6)

where J_p is the one-dimensional protein flux, D is the diffusion coefficient, and $\partial cp/\partial x$ is the concentration gradient of protein through the interstitial space.

For most macromolecules such as proteins, the diffusional transport is limited. It serves to disperse molecules, but it does not effectively serve to transport large molecules, especially if their diffusion is restricted by interstitial matrix proteins, membrane barriers, or other structures that limit their free thermal motion. Instead, both experimental and theoretical evidence highlights the dependence of volume and solute flows on hydrostatic and osmotic pressure gradients (Hammel, 1994; Hargens and Akeson, 1986) and suggests that convective flow plays the dominating role in interstitial flow and transport of nutrients to tissue cells. For example, in the presence of osmotic or hydrostatic pressure gradients, protein transport J_p is coupled to fluid transport according to

$$J_p = \bar{c}_p J_V$$

(15.7)

where $\bar{c}_p$ is the average protein concentration and J_v is the volume flow of fluid.

The transport of interstitial fluid toward the lymphatics requires convective flow since it depends on relatively few channels in the interstitium. Diffusion cannot serve such a purpose because diffusion merely disperses fluid and proteins. Lymph formation and flow greatly depend upon tissue movement or activity related to muscle contraction and tissue deformations. It is also generally agreed that the formation of the initial lymph depends solely on the composition of nearby interstitial fluid and pressure gradients across the interstitial/lymphatic boundary (Hargens, 1986; Zweifach and Lipowsky, 1984). For this reason, lymph formation and flow can be quantified by measuring the disappearance of isotope-labeled albumin from subcutaneous tissue or skeletal muscle (Reed et al., 1985).

15.2.4 Lymphatic Architecture

To understand lymph transport in engineering terms, it is paramount that we develop a detailed picture of the lymphatic network topology and vessel morphology. This task is facilitated by a number of morphological and ultrastructural studies from past decades that give a general picture of the morphology and location of lymphatic vessels in different tissues. Lymphatics are studied by injections of macroscopic and microscopic contrast media and by light and electron microscopic sections. The display of the lymphatics is organ specific and there are many variations in lymphatic architecture (Schmid-Schönbein, 1990). In this chapter, we will focus our discussion predominantly on skeletal muscle, intestine, and skin. However, the mechanisms outlined below may in part be also relevant to other tissues and organs.

In the skeletal muscle, lymphatics are positioned in the *immediate* proximity of the arterioles. The majority of feeder arteries in the skeletal muscle and most, but not all, of the arcade arterioles are closely accompanied by a lymphatic vessel (Figure 15.3). Lymphatics can be traced along the entire length of the arcade arterioles, but they can be traced only over relatively short distances (less than about 50 μm) into the side branches of the arcades, the transverse (terminal) arterioles that supply the blood into the capillary network. Systematic reconstructions of the lymphatics in skeletal muscle have yielded little evidence for lymphatic channels that enter into the capillary network per se (Skalak et al., 1984). Thus, the network density of lymphatics is quite low compared to the high density of the capillary network in muscle, a characteristic feature of lymphatics in most organs (Skalak et al., 1986). The close association between lymphatics and vasculature is also present in the skin (Ikomi and Schmid-Schönbein, 1995) and in other organs, and may extend into the central vasculature. Saharinen et al. (2004) reviewed

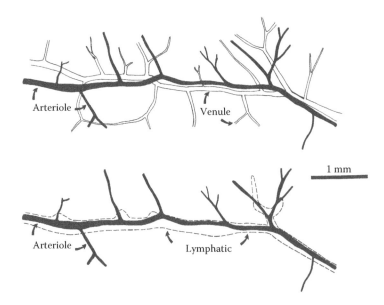

FIGURE 15.3   Tracing of a typical lymphatic channel (bottom panel) in rat spinotrapezius muscle after injection with a micropipette of a carbon contrast suspension. All lymphatics are of the initial type and are closely associated with the arcade arterioles. Few lymphatics follow the path of the arcade venules, or their side branches, the collecting venules, or the transverse arterioles. (With kind permission from Springer Science+Business Media: *Tissue Nutrition and Viability*, Lymph transport in skeletal muscle, 1986, pp. 243–262, Skalak TC, Schmid-Schönbein GW, and Zweifach BW.)

lymphatic vasculature development and molecular regulation in tumor metastasis and inflammation. It is apparent that the current understandings of lymphatic growth factors and strategies to limit lymphatic vessel growth may allow the manipulation of lymphatic growth in disease.

Interstitial fluid flow is itself a major determinant of the growth of lymphatic vessels and their directionality (Boardman and Swartz, 2003; Ng et al., 2004). This consideration is important in the design of tissue engineering approaches for lymphatic vessels (Helm et al., 2007).

15.2.5 Lymphatic Morphology

Histological sections of the lymphatics permit its classification into two distinct subsets: *initial* lymphatics and *collecting* lymphatics. The initial lymphatics (sometimes also denoted as terminal or capillary lymphatics) form a set of blind endings in the tissue that feed into the collecting lymphatics, and that in turn, are the conduits into the lymph nodes. While both initial and collecting lymphatics are lined by a highly attenuated endothelium, only the collecting lymphatics have smooth muscle in their media. In accordance, contractile lymphatics exhibit spontaneous narrowing of their lumen, while there is no evidence for contractility (in the sense of a smooth muscle contraction) in the initial lymphatics. Contractile lymphatics are capable of peristaltic smooth muscle contractions that in conjunction with periodic opening and closing of the intraluminal valves permit unidirectional fluid transport. The lymphatic smooth muscle has adrenergic innervation (Ohhashi et al., 1982), it exhibits myogenic contraction (Hargens and Zweifach, 1977; Mizuno et al., 1997), and it reacts with a variety of vasoactive stimuli (Ohhashi et al., 1978; Benoit, 1997), including signals that involve nitric oxide (Bohlen and Lash, 1992; Ohhashi and Takahashi, 1991; Yokoyama and Ohhashi, 1993). Recently, Kawai and Ohhashi (2009) and Zawieja (2009) reviewed the important intrinsic pump function of the collecting lymphatics with a specialized set of contractile proteins in the smooth muscle.

The lymphatic endothelium has a number of similarities with vascular endothelium. It forms a continuous lining and has typical cytoskeletal fibers such as microtubules, intermediate fibers, and actin in both fiber bundle form and matrix form. There are numerous caveolae, Weibel-Palade bodies, but lymphatic endothelium has fewer interendothelial adhesion complexes and a discontinuous basement membrane. The residues of the basement membrane are attached to interstitial collagen via anchoring filaments (Leak and Burke, 1968) that provide relatively firm attachment of the endothelium to interstitial structures.

15.2.6 Lymphatic Network Display

One of the interesting aspects regarding lymphatic transport in skeletal muscle is the fact that all lymphatics *inside* the muscle parenchyma are of the noncontractile, *initial* type (Skalak et al., 1984). The *collecting* lymphatics can only be observed outside the muscle fibers as conduits to adjacent lymph nodes. The fact that all lymphatics inside the tissue parenchyma are of the initial type is not unique to skeletal muscle, but has been demonstrated in other organs (Unthank and Bohlen, 1988; Yamanaka et al., 1995). The initial lymphatics are positioned in the adventitia of the arcade arterioles surrounded by collagen fibers (Figure 15.4). In this position, they are in immediate proximity to the arteriolar smooth muscle, and adjacent to myelinated nerve fibers and a set of mast cells that accompany the arterioles. The initial lymphatics are frequently sandwiched between arteriolar smooth muscle and their paired venules, and they in turn are embedded between the skeletal muscle fibers (Skalak et al., 1984). The initial lymphatics are firmly attached to the adjacent basement membrane and collagen fibers via anchoring filaments (Leak and Burke, 1968). The basement membrane of the lymphatic endothelium is discontinuous, especially at the interendothelial junctions, so that macromolecules and even cells and particles enter the initial lymphatics (Bach and Lewis, 1973; Bollinger et al., 1981; Casley-Smith, 1962; Ikomi et al., 1996; Strand and Persson, 1979).

The lumen cross section of the initial lymphatics is highly irregular in contrast to the overall circular cross section of the collecting lymphatics (Figure 15.4). The lumen cross section of the initial lymphatics

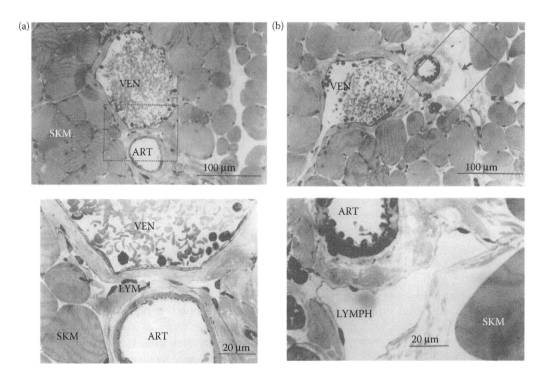

FIGURE 15.4 Histological cross sections of lymphatics (LYM) in rat skeletal muscle before (a) and after (b) contraction of the paired arcade arterioles (ART). The lymphatic channel is of the initial type with a single attenuated endothelial layer (curved arrows). Note that in the dilated arteriole, the lymphatic is essentially compressed (a) whereas the lymphatic is expanded after arteriolar contraction (b) that is noticeable by the folded endothelial cells in the arteriolar lumen. In both cases, the lumen cross-sectional shape of the initial lymphatic channels is highly irregular. All lymphatics in the skeletal muscle have these characteristic features. (Adapted from Skalak TC, Schmid-Schönbein GW, and Zweifach BW. 1984. *Microvasc Res* 28: 95.)

is partially or completely collapsed and may frequently span around the arcade arteriole. In fact, we have documented cases in which the arcade arteriole is completely surrounded by an initial lymphatic channel, highlighting the fact that the activity of the lymphatics is closely linked to that of the arterioles (Ikomi and Schmid-Schönbein, 1995).

Direct labeling of lymphatic and vascular endothelium shows that there exist numerous direct vascular connections between lymphatic and microvascular endothelial vessels with membrane contacts but no detectable fluid exchange between the two systems (Robichaux et al., 2010).

15.2.6.1 Intraluminal (Secondary) Lymphatic Valves

The initial lymphatics in the skeletal muscle have intraluminal valves that consist of bileaflets and a funnel structure (Mazzoni et al., 1987). The leaflets are flexible structures and are opened and closed by a viscous pressure drop along the valve funnel. In the closed position, these leaflets can support considerable pressures (Eisenhoffer et al., 1995; Ikomi et al., 1997). This arrangement preserves normal valve function even in the initial lymphatics with irregularly shaped lumen cross sections.

15.2.6.2 Primary Lymphatic Valves

The lymphatic endothelial cells are attenuated and have many of the morphological characteristics of vascular endothelium, including expression of P-selectin, von Willebrand factor (Di Nucci et al., 1996), and factor VIII (Schmid-Schönbein, 1990). The identity of the lymphatic endothelium involves the transcription factor PROX1 (Johnson et al., 2008). An important difference between vascular and lymphatic endothelium lies in the arrangement of the endothelial junctions. In the initial lymphatics, the endothelial cells lack tight junctions (Schneeberger and Lynch, 1984) and are frequently encountered in an overlapping but open position, so that proteins, large macromolecules, and even chylomicron particles can readily pass through the junctions (Casley-Smith, 1962, 1964; Leak, 1970). Examination of the junctions with scanning electron microscopy shows that there exists a periodic *interdigitating* arrangement of endothelial extensions. Individual extensions are attached via anchoring filaments to the underlying basement membrane and connective tissue, but the two extensions of adjacent endothelial cells resting on top of each other are not attached by interendothelial adhesion complexes. Mild mechanical stretching of the initial lymphatics shows that the endothelial extensions can be separated in part from each other, indicating that the membranes of two neighboring lymphatic endothelial cells are not attached to each other, but are firmly attached to the underlying basement membrane (Castenholz, 1984). Lymphatic endothelium does not exhibit continuous junctional complexes, and instead has a "streak and dot"-like immunostaining pattern of VE-cadherin and associated intracellular proteins desmoplakin and plakoglobulin (Schmelz et al., 1994). VE-cadherin and platelet endothelial cell adhesion molecule (PECAM-1) form an interlaced labeling pattern with minimal overlap, in contrast to vascular endothelium (Baluk et al., 2007; Murfee et al., 2007). But the staining pattern is nonuniform along the initial lymphatics; in larger lymphatics, a more continuous pattern is present. This highly specialized arrangement has been referred to as the *lymphatic endothelial microvalves* (Schmid-Schönbein, 1990) or primary lymphatic valves. They are "*primary*" because fluid from the interstitium must first pass across these valves before entering the lymphatic lumen and then pass across the intraluminal, that is, secondary valves. The particles deposited into the interstitial space adjacent to the initial lymphatics pass across the endothelium of the initial lymphatics. However, once the particles are inside the initial lymphatic lumen, they cannot return back into the interstitial space unless the endothelium is injured. Indeed, the endothelial junctions of the initial lymphatics serve as a functional valve system (Trzewik et al. 2001). Similar to vascular endothelium, the lymphatic endothelial junctions also serve as a signaling mechanism as reviewed by Dejana et al. (2009).

15.2.7 Mechanics of Lymphatic Valves

In contrast to the central large valves in the heart that are closed by inertial fluid forces, the lymphatic valves are small and the fluid Reynolds number is almost zero. Thus, because no inertial forces are available to open and close these valves, a different valve morphology has evolved in these small valves. The valves form long funnel-shaped channels that are inserted into the lymph conduits and attached at their base. The funnel is prevented from inversion by attachment via a buttress to the lymphatic wall. The valve wall structure consists of a collagen layer sandwiched between two endothelial layers and the entire structure is quite deformable under mild physiological fluid pressures. The funnel structure allows a *viscous pressure gradient* that is sufficient to generate a pressure drop during forward fluid motion to open, and upon flow reversal to close the valves (Mazzoni et al., 1987). The primary lymphatic valves also open as passive structures at the peripheral endothelial cell extensions. They require sites where they are free to bend into the lumen of the initial lymphatics and where they are *not* attached by anchoring filaments to the adjacent extracellular matrix (Mendoza and Schmid-Schönbein, 2003).

15.2.8 Lymph Formation and Pump Mechanisms

One of the important questions fundamental to lymphology is: How do fluid and large particles in the interstitium find their way into the initial lymphatics? In light of the relative sparse existence of the initial lymphatics, a directed convective transport is required that can be provided by either a hydrostatic or a colloid osmotic pressure drop (Zweifach and Silberberg, 1979). However, the exact mechanism of this unidirectional flow has remained an elusive target. Several proposals have been advanced and these are discussed in detail in Schmid-Schönbein (1990). Briefly, a number of authors have postulated that there exists a constant pressure drop from the interstitium into the initial lymph, which may support a steady fluid flow into the lymphatics. But repeated measurements with different techniques have uniformly failed to provide supporting evidence for a *steady* pressure drop to transport fluid into the initial lymphatics (Clough and Smaje, 1978; Zweifach and Prather, 1975). Under steady-state conditions, no steady pressure drop exists in the vicinity of the initial lymphatics in skeletal muscle within the resolution of the measurement technique (about 0.2 cm H_2O) (Skalak et al., 1984). An order of magnitude estimate of the pressure drop expected at the relatively slow flow rates of the lymphatics shows, however, that the pressure drop from the interstitium may be significantly lower (Schmid-Schönbein, 1990). Furthermore, the assumption of a *steady* pressure drop is not in agreement with the substantial evidence that lymph flow rate is enhanced under unsteady conditions (see below). Some investigators have postulated an osmotic pressure in the lymphatics to aspirate fluid into the initial lymphatics (Casley-Smith, 1972) due to ultrafiltration across the lymphatic endothelium, a mechanism referred to as "bootstrap effect" (Perl, 1975). Critical tests of this hypothesis, such as the microinjection of hyperosmotic protein solutions, have not led to a uniformly accepted hypothesis for lymph formation involving an osmotic mechanism. Others have suggested a retrograde aspiration mechanism, such that the recoil in the collecting lymphatics serves to lower the pressure in the initial lymphatics upstream of the collecting lymphatics (Reddy, 1986; Reddy and Patel, 1995), or an electric charge difference across the lymphatic endothelium (O'Morchoe et al., 1984).

15.2.9 Tissue Mechanical Motion and Lymphatic Pumping

An intriguing feature is that lymphatic flow rates depend on tissue motion. In a resting tissue, the lymph flow rate is relatively small. But different forms of tissue motion serve to enhance lymph flow. This was originally demonstrated for pulsatile pressures in the rabbit ear. Perfusion of the ear with steady pressure (even at the same mean pressure) stops lymph transport, whereas pulsatile pressures promote lymph transport (Parsons and McMaster, 1938). In light of the paired arrangement of the arterioles and lymphatics, periodic expansion of the arterioles compresses adjacent lymphatics, and vice versa, a reduction of arteriolar diameter during the pressure reduction phase expands adjacent lymphatics (Skalak et al., 1984) (Figure 15.4). Vasomotion, associated with a slower contraction of the arterioles, but with a larger amplitude than pulsatile pressure, increases lymph formation (Colantuoni et al., 1984; Intaglietta and Gross, 1982). In addition, muscle contractions, simple walking (Olszewski and Engeset, 1980), respiration, intestinal peristalsis, skin compression (Ohhashi et al., 1991), and other tissue motions are associated with increased lymph flow rates. Periodic tissue motions are significantly more effective to enhance the lymph flow than elevation of the venous pressure (Ikomi et al., 1996), which is also associated with enhanced fluid filtration (Renkin et al., 1977).

A requirement for lymph fluid flow is the periodic expansion and compression of the initial lymphatics. Since the initial lymphatics do not have their own smooth muscle, the expansion and compression of the initial lymphatics depends on the motion of the tissue in which they are embedded. In skeletal muscle, the strategic location of the initial lymphatics in the adventitia of the arterioles provides the milieu for expansion and compression via several mechanisms: arteriolar pressure pulsations or vasomotion, active or passive skeletal muscle contractions, or external muscle compression. Direct measurements of the cross-sectional area of the initial lymphatics during arteriolar contractions or during skeletal muscle shortening support this hypothesis (Mazzoni et al., 1990; Skalak et al., 1984) (Figure 15.5). The different lymph pump mechanisms are additive. The resting skeletal muscle has much lower lymph flow rates (provided largely by the arteriolar pressure pulsation and vasomotion) than the skeletal muscle during exercise (produced by a combination of intramuscular pressure pulsations and skeletal muscle shortening) (Ballard et al., 1998).

Measurements of lymph flow rates in an afferent lymph vessel (diameter of about 300–500 μm, proximal to the popliteal node) in the hind leg (Ikomi and Schmid-Schönbein, 1996) demonstrate that lymph fluid formation is influenced by passive or active motion of the surrounding tissue. Lymphatics in this tissue region drain the muscle and skin of the hind leg, and the majority is of the *initial* type,

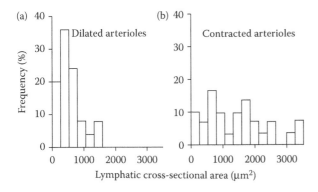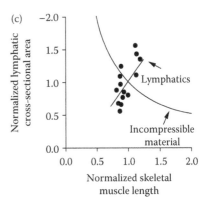

FIGURE 15.5 Histograms of initial lymphatic cross-sectional area in rat spinotrapezius muscle before (a) and after (b) contraction of the paired arteriole with norepinephrine. Lymphatic cross-sectional area as a function of muscle length during active contraction or passive stretch (c). Cross-sectional area and muscle length are normalized with respect to the values *in vivo* in resting muscle. Note the expansion of the initial lymphatics with contraction of the arterioles or muscle stretch. (Adapted from Skalak TC, Schmid-Schönbein GW, and Zweifach BW. 1984. *Microvasc Res* 28: 95; Mazzoni MC, Skalak TC, and Schmid-Schönbein GW. 1990. *Am J Physiol* 259: H1860.)

whereas the collecting lymphatics are detected outside the tissue parenchyma in the fascia proximal to the node. Without whole leg rotation, lymph flow remains at low but nonzero values. If the pulse pressure is stopped, lymph flow falls to values below detectable limits (less than about 10% of the values during pulse pressure). The introduction of whole leg passive movement causes strong, frequency-dependent lymph flow rates that increase linearly with the logarithm of frequency between 0.03 and 1.0 Hz (Figure 15.6). The elevation of venous pressure, which enhances fluid filtration from the vasculature and elevates flow rates, does not significantly alter the dependency of lymph flow on periodic tissue motion (Ikomi et al., 1996).

Similarly, the application of passive tissue compression on the skin elevates the lymph flow rate in a frequency-dependent manner. Lymph flow rates are determined to a significant degree by the *local* action of the lymph pump because the arrest of the heartbeat and the reduction of the central blood pressure to zero do not stop lymph flow. Instead, cardiac arrest reduces lymph flow rate only about 50% during continued leg motion or application of periodic shear stress to the skin for several hours (Ikomi and Schmid-Schönbein, 1996). Periodic compression of the initial lymphatics also enhances proteins and lymphocyte counts in the lymphatics (Ikomi et al., 1996) (Figure 15.7). Thus, either arteriolar smooth muscle or parenchymal skeletal muscle activity expands and compresses the initial lymphatics in skeletal muscle. These mechanisms serve to adjust lymph flow rates according to organ activity such that a resting skeletal muscle has a very low lymph flow rate. During normal daily activity or mild or strenuous exercise, lymph flow rates as well as protein and cell transport into the lymphatics increases (Olszewski et al., 1977).

15.2.9.1 Lymph Pump Mechanism with Primary and Secondary Valves

Regular expansion and compression of the initial lymphatic channels requires a set of valves to achieve unidirectional flow. Such valves open and close with each expansion and compression of the lymphatics to permit entry at the upstream end of the lymphatics and discharge downstream toward the lymph nodes. There is a cycle of valve opening and closing with every expansion and compression of the lymphatic channels. During expansion, the upstream primary lymphatics are open and permit entry of interstitial fluid. The secondary valves are closed to prevent retrograde flow along the lymphatic channels. During compression, the primary valves are closed, whereas the secondary valves are open to permit discharge along the lymphatic channels into the contractile lymphatics and toward the lymph nodes.

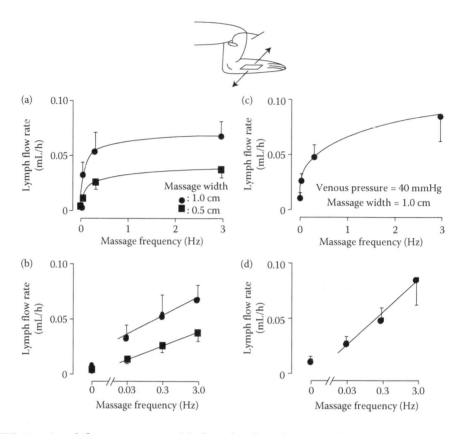

FIGURE 15.6 Lymph flow rates in a prenodal afferent lymphatic draining the hind leg as a function of the frequency of a periodic surface shear motion (massage) without (panels a, b) and with (panels c, d) elevation of the venous pressure by placement of a cuff. Zero frequency refers to a resting leg with a lymph flow rate that depends on pulse pressure. The amplitudes of the tangential skin shear motion were 1 and 0.5 cm (panels a, b) and 1 cm in the presence of the elevated venous pressure (panels c, d). Note that the ordinates in panels c and d are larger than those in panels a and b. (Adapted from Ikomi and Schmid-Schönbein, 1996. *Am J Physiol* 271: H173.)

Thus, we view lymphatic transport as having a robust mechanism that requires the presence of two-valve systems. In fact, all compartments that rely on a repeated cycle of expansion and compression require two-valve systems, the lymphangions along the contractile lymphatics, and even larger structures such as the ventricles of the heart, the blower in the fireplace, or even the shipping locks in the Panama Canal. None of these structures can provide unidirectional transport if one of the valves is removed, irrespective of whether it is located upstream or downstream (Schmid-Schönbein, 2003). In inflammation, the primary lymphatic valves may fail due to apoptosis of the lymphatic endothelium (Lynch et al., 2007). This leads to the failure of the fluid transport into the initial lymphatics and into contractile lymphatics (Zawieja, 1996), eventually forming tissue edema and possibly amplifying the inflammatory process. The strategies to control tissue edema formation need to take into consideration the delicate primary lymphatic endothelium and its specialized junctions by preventing their failure or restoring their function after failure.

15.3 Conclusion

The lymphatic vessels are a unique transport system that is present even in primitive physiological systems. These vessels carry out a multitude of functions, many of which have yet to be discovered.

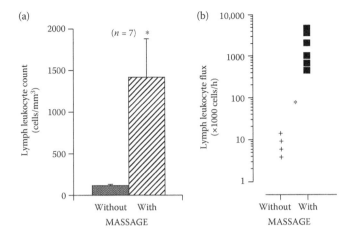

FIGURE 15.7   Lymph leukocyte count (a) and leukocyte flux (b) before and after application of periodic hind leg skin shear motion (massage) at a frequency of about 1 Hz and amplitude of 1 cm. The flux rates were computed from the product of lymph flow rates and the lymphocyte counts. *Statistically significant different from the case without massage. (Adapted from Ikomi and Schmid-Schönbein, 1996. *Am J Physiol* 271: H173.)

Lymphatics have a two-valve system: a primary valve system at the level of the lymphatic endothelium and a secondary valve system in the lumen of the lymphatics, facilitating unidirectional transport toward the lymphatic nodes and thoracic duct. The details of lymphatic growth kinetics are subject to initial molecular analysis designed to identify key growth factors and their molecular control (Lohela et al., 2003). A more detailed bioengineering analysis, especially at the molecular level (Jeltsch et al., 1997), is a fruitful area for future exploration.

Acknowledgments

This work was supported by NASA grants NNX10AM18G and NNX09AP11G as well as NIH grants HL 10881.

Defining Terms

Capillary: The smallest blood vessel of the body that provides oxygen and other nutrients to nearby cells and tissues.

Colloid osmotic pressure: A negative pressure that depends on protein concentration (mainly of albumin and globulins) and prevents excess filtration across the capillary wall.

Edema: Excess fluid or swelling within a given tissue.

Interstitium: The space between cells of various tissues of the body. Normally fluid and proteins within this space are transported from the capillary to the initial lymphatic vessel.

Lymphatic system: The clear network of vessels that return excess fluid and proteins to the blood via the thoracic duct.

References

Adams RH and Alitalo K. 2007. Molecular regulation of angiogenesis and lymphangiogenesis. *Nat Rev Mol Cell Biol* 8: 464–478.

Aratow M, Hargens AR, Meyer J-U et al. 1991. Postural responses of head and foot cutaneous microvascular flow and their sensitivity to bed rest. *Aviat Space Environ Med* 62: 246.

Aukland K and Reed RK. 1993. Interstitial–lymphatic mechanisms in the control of extracellular fluid volume. *Physiol Rev* 73: 1.

Bach C and Lewis GP. 1973. Lymph flow and lymph protein concentration in the skin and muscle of the rabbit hind limb. *J Physiol (Lond)* 235: 477.

Ballard RE, Watenpaugh DE, Breit GA et al. 1998. Leg intramuscular pressures during locomotion in humans. *J Appl Physiol* 84: 1976.

Baluk P, Fuxe J, Hashizume H, Romano T, Lashnits E, Butz S, Vestweber D, Corada M, Molendini C, Dejana E, and McDonald DM. 2007. Functionally specialized junctions between endothelial cells of lymphatic vessels. *J Exp Med* 204: 2349–2362.

Benoit JN. 1997. Effects of alpha-adrenergic stimuli on mesenteric collecting lymphatics in the rat. *Am J Physiol* 273: R331.

Boardman KC and Swartz MA. 2003. Interstitial flow as a guide for lymphangiogenesis. *Circ Res* 92: 801–808.

Bohlen HG and Lash JM. 1992. Intestinal lymphatic vessels release endothelial-dependent vasodilators. *Am J Physiol* 262: H813.

Bollinger A, Jäger K, Sgier F et al. 1981. Fluorescence microlymphography. *Circulation* 64: 1195.

Casley-Smith JR. 1962. The identification of chylomicra and lipoproteins in tissue sections and their passage into jejunal lacteals. *J Cell Biol* 15: 259.

Casley-Smith JR. 1964. Endothelial permeability—The passage of particles into and out of diaphragmatic lymphatics. *Quart J Exp Physiol* 49: 365.

Casley-Smith JR. 1972. The role of the endothelial intercellular junctions in the functioning of the initial lymphatics. *Angiologica* 9: 106.

Castenholz A. 1984. Morphological characteristics of initial lymphatics in the tongue as shown by scanning electron microscopy. *Scanning Electr Microsc* 1984: 1343.

Clough G and Smaje LH. 1978. Simultaneous measurement of pressure in the interstitium and the terminal lymphatics of the cat mesentery. *J Physiol (Lond)* 283: 457.

Colantuoni A, Bertuglia S, and Intaglietta M. 1984. A quantification of rhythmic diameter changes in arterial microcirculation. *Am J Physiol* 246: H508.

Dejana E, Orsenigo F, Molendini C, Baluk P, and McDonald DM. 2009. Organization and signaling of endothelial cell-to-cell junctions in various regions of the blood and lymphatic vascular trees. *Cell Tissue Res* 335: 17–25.

Di Nucci A, Marchetti C, Serafini S et al. 1996. P-selectin and von Willebrand factor in bovine mesenteric lymphatics: An immunofluorescent study. *Lymphology* 29: 25.

Eisenhoffer J, Kagal A, Klein T et al. 1995. Importance of valves and lymphangion contractions in determining pressure gradients in isolated lymphatics exposed to elevations in outflow pressure. *Microvasc Res* 49: 97.

Hammel HT. 1994. How solutes alter water in aqueous solutions. *J Phys Chem* 98: 4196.

Hargens AR. 1986. Interstitial fluid pressure and lymph flow. In: R Skalak, S Chien (eds.), *Handbook of Bioengineering*, 19: pp. 1–35, New York, McGraw-Hill.

Hargens AR and Akeson WH. 1986. Stress effects on tissue nutrition and viability. In: AR Hargens (ed.), *Tissue Nutrition and Viability*, pp. 1–24, New York, Springer-Verlag.

Hargens AR, Millard RW, Pettersson K et al. 1987. Gravitational haemodynamics and oedema prevention in the giraffe. *Nature* 329: 59.

Hargens AR and Zweifach BW. 1977. Contractile stimuli in collecting lymph vessels. *Am J Physiol* 233: H57.

Helm CL, Zisch A, and Swartz MA. 2007. Engineered blood and lymphatic capillaries in 3-D VEGF-fibrin-collagen matrices with interstitial flow. *Biotechnol Bioeng* 96: 167–176.

Hu X and Weinbaum S. 1999. A new view of Starling's hypothesis at the microstructural level. *Microvasc Res* 58: 281–304.

Ikomi F, Hunt J, Hanna G et al. 1996. Interstitial fluid, protein, colloid and leukocyte uptake into interstitial lymphatics. *J Appl Physiol* 81: 2060.

Ikomi F and Schmid-Schönbein GW. 1995. Lymph transport in the skin. *Clin Dermatol* 13(5): 419.

Ikomi F and Schmid-Schönbein GW. 1996. Lymph pump mechanics in the rabbit hind leg. *Am J Physiol* 271: H173.

Ikomi F, Zweifach BW, and Schmid-Schönbein GW. 1997. Fluid pressures in the rabbit popliteal afferent lymphatics during passive tissue motion. *Lymphology* 30: 13.

Intaglietta M and Gross JF. 1982. Vasomotion, tissue fluid flow and the formation of lymph. *Int J Microcirc Clin Exp* 1: 55.

Jain RK. 1987. Transport of molecules in the tumor interstitium: A review. *Cancer Res* 47: 3039.

Jeltsch M, Kaipainen A, Joukov V et al. 1997. Hyperplasia of lymphatic vessels in VEGF-C transgenic mice. *Science* 276: 1423.

Johnson NC, Dillard ME, Baluk P, McDonald DM, Harvey NL, Frase SL, and Oliver G. 2008. Lymphatic endothelial cell identity is reversible and its maintenance requires Prox1 activity. *Genes Dev* 22: 3282–3291.

Kawai Y and Ohhashi T. 2009. Topics of physiological and pathophysiological functions of lymphatics. *Curr Mol Med* 9(8): 942.

Lai-Fook SJ. 1986. Mechanics of lung fluid balance. *Crit Rev Biomed Eng* 13: 171.

Leak LV. 1970. Electron microscopic observations on lymphatic capillaries and the structural components of the connective tissue–lymph interface. *Microvasc Res* 2: 361.

Leak LV and Burke JF. 1968. Ultrastructural studies on the lymphatic anchoring filaments. *J Cell Biol* 36: 129.

Levick JR and Michel CC. 2010. Microvascular fluid exchange and the revised Starling principle. *Cardiovasc Res* 87(2): 198–210.

Lohela M, Saaristo A, Veikkola T, and Alitalo K. 2003. Lymphangiogenic growth factors, receptors and therapies. *Thromb Haemost* 90: 167–184.

Lynch PM, DeLano FA, and Schmid-Schönbein GW. 2007. The primary valves in the initial lymphatics during inflammation. *Lymphat Res Biol* 5: 3–10.

Mazzoni MC, Skalak TC, and Schmid-Schönbein GW. 1987. The structure of lymphatic valves in the spinotrapezius muscle of the rat. *Blood Vessels* 24: 304.

Mazzoni MC, Skalak TC, and Schmid-Schönbein GW. 1990. The effect of skeletal muscle fiber deformation on lymphatic volume. *Am J Physiol* 259: H1860.

Mendoza E and Schmid-Schönbein GW. 2003. A model for mechanics of primary lymphatic valves. *J Biomech Eng* 125: 407–413.

Miteva DO, Rutkowski JM, Dixon JB, Kilarski W, Shields JD, and Swartz MA. 2010. Transmural flow modulates cell and fluid transport functions of lymphatic endothelium. *Circ Res* 106: 920–931.

Mizuno R, Dornyei G, Koller A et al. 1997. Myogenic responses of isolated lymphatics: Modulation by endothelium. *Microcirculation* 4: 413.

Murfee WL, Rappleye JW, Ceballos M, and Schmid-Schönbein GW. 2007. Discontinuous expression of endothelial cell adhesion molecules along initial lymphatic vessels in mesentery: The primary valve structure. *Lymphat Res Biol* 5: 81–90.

Murthy G, Watenpaugh DE, Ballard RE et al. 1994. Supine exercise during lower body negative pressure effectively simulates upright exercise in normal gravity. *J Appl Physiol* 76: 2742.

Muthuchamy M and Zawieja D. 2008. Molecular regulation of lymphatic contractility. *Ann N Y Acad Sci* 1131: 89–99.

Ng CP, Helm CL, and Swartz MA. 2004. Interstitial flow differentially stimulates blood and lymphatic endothelial cell morphogenesis *in vitro*. *Microvasc Res* 68: 258–264.

Ohhashi T, Kawai Y, and Azuma T. 1978. The response of lymphatic smooth muscles to vasoactive substances. *Plügers Arch* 375: 183.

Ohhashi T, Kobayashi S, Tsukahara S et al. 1982. Innervation of bovine mesenteric lymphatics: From the histochemical point of view. *Microvasc Res* 24: 377.

Ohhashi T and Takahashi N. 1991. Acetylcholine-induced release of endothelium-derived relaxing factor from lymphatic endothelial cells. *Am J Physiol* 260: H1172.

Ohhashi T, Yokoyama S, and Ikomi F. 1991. Effects of vibratory stimulation and mechanical massage on micro- and lymph-circulation in the acupuncture points between the paw pads of anesthetized dogs. In: H Niimi, FY Zhuang (eds.), *Recent Advances in Cardiovascular Diseases*, pp. 125–133, National Cardiovascular Center, Osaka.

Olszewski WL and Engeset A. 1980. Intrinsic contractility of prenodal lymph vessels and lymph flow in human leg. *Am J Physiol* 239: H775.

Olszewski WL, Engeset A, Jaeger PM et al. 1977. Flow and composition of leg lymph in normal men during venous stasis, muscular activity and local hyperthermia. *Acta Physiol Scand* 99: 149.

O'Morchoe CCC, Jones WRI, Jarosz HM et al. 1984. Temperature dependence of protein transport across lymphatic endothelium *in vitro*. *J Cell Biol* 98: 629.

Parazynski SE, Hargens AR, Tucker B et al. 1991. Transcapillary fluid shifts in tissues of the head and neck during and after simulated microgravity. *J Appl Physiol* 71: 2469.

Parsons RJ and McMaster PD. 1938. The effect of the pulse upon the formation and flow of lymph. *J Exp Med* 68: 353.

Perl W. 1975. Convection and permeation of albumin between plasma and interstitium. *Microvasc Res* 10: 83.

Randolph GJ, Angeli V, and Swartz MA. 2005. Dendritic-cell trafficking to lymph nodes through lymphatic vessels. *Nat Rev Immunol* 5(8): 617.

Reddy NP. 1986. Lymph circulation: Physiology, pharmacology, and biomechanics. *Crit Rev Biomed Sci* 14: 45.

Reddy NP and Patel K. 1995. A mathematical model of flow through the terminal lymphatics. *Med Eng Phy* 17: 134.

Reed RK, Johansen S, and Noddeland H. 1985. Turnover rate of interstitial albumin in rat skin and skeletal muscle. Effects of limb movements and motor activity. *Acta Physiol Scand* 125: 711.

Renkin EM, Joyner WL, Sloop CH et al. 1977. Influence of venous pressure on plasma–lymph transport in the dog's paw: Convective and dissipative mechanisms. *Microvasc Res* 14: 191.

Robichaux JL, Tanno1 E, Rappleye JW, CeballosM, Schmid-Schönbein GW, and Murfee WL. 2010. Lymphatic/blood endothelial cell connections at the capillary level in the adult rat mesentery. *Anat Rec* 293: 1629–1638.

Saharinen P, Tammela T, Karkkainen MJ, and Alitalo K. 2004. Lymphatic vasculature: Development, molecular regulation and role in tumor metastasis and inflammation. *Trends Immunol* 25: 387.

Schmelz M, Moll R, Kuhn C et al. 1994. Complex adherentes, a new group of desmoplakin-containing junctions in endothelial cells: II. Different types of lymphatic vessels. *Differentiation* 57: 97.

Schmid-Schönbein GW. 1990. Microlymphatics and lymph flow. *Physiol Rev* 70: 987.

Schmid-Schönbein GW. 2003. The second valve system in lymphatics. *Lymphat Res Biol* 1: 25–31.

Schmid-Schönbein GW and Zweifach BW. 1994. Fluid pump mechanisms in initial lymphatics. *News Physiol Sci* 9: 67.

Schneeberger EE and Lynch RD. 1984. Tight junctions: Their structure, composition and function. *Circ Res* 5: 723.

Skalak TC, Schmid-Schönbein GW, and Zweifach BW. 1984. New morphological evidence for a mechanism of lymph formation in skeletal muscle. *Microvasc Res* 28: 95.

Skalak TC, Schmid-Schönbein GW, and Zweifach BW. 1986. Lymph transport in skeletal muscle. In: AR Hargens (ed.), *Tissue Nutrition and Viability*, pp. 243–262, Springer-Verlag, New York.

Staub NC. 1988. New concepts about the pathophysiology of pulmonary edema. *J Thorac Imaging* 3: 8.

Staub NC, Hogg JC, and Hargens AR. 1987. *Interstitial-Lymphatic Liquid and Solute Movement*, pp. 1–290, Basel, Karger.

Strand S-E and Persson BRR. 1979. Quantitative lymphoscintigraphy I: Basic concepts for optimal uptake of radiocolloids in the parasternal lymph nodes of rabbits. *J Nucl Med* 20: 1038.

Swartz MA and Fleury ME. 2007. Interstitial flow and its effects in soft tissues. *Annu Rev Biomed Eng* 9: 229–256.

Tammela T and Alitalo K. 2010. Lymphangiogenesis: Molecular mechanisms and future promise. *Cell* 140: 460–476.

Trzewik J, Mallipattu, SR, Artmann, GM et al. 2001. Evidence for a second valve system in lymphatics: Endothelial microvalves. *FASEB J* 15: 1711.

Unthank JL and Bohlen HG. 1988. Lymphatic pathways and role of valves in lymph propulsion from small intestine. *Am J Physiol* 254: G389.

Wei SH, Parker I, Miller MJ, and Cahalan MD. 2003. A stochastic view of lymphocyte motility and trafficking within the lymph node. *Immunol Rev* 195: 136.

Wiig H. 1990. Evaluation of methodologies for measurement of interstitial fluid pressure (P_i): Physiological implications of recent P_i data. *Crit Rev Biomed Eng* 18: 27.

Yamanaka Y, Araki K, and Ogata T. 1995. Three-dimensional organization of lymphatics in the dog small intestine: A scanning electron microscopic study on corrosion casts. *Arch Hist Cyt* 58: 465.

Yokoyama S and Ohhashi T. 1993. Effects of acetylcholine on spontaneous contractions in isolated bovine mesenteric lymphatics. *Am J Physiol* 264: H1460.

Zawieja DC. 1996. Lymphatic microcirculation. *Microcirculation* 3: 241–243.

Zawieja DC. 2009. Contractile physiology of lymphatics. *Lymphat Res Biol* 7(2): 87–96.

Zweifach BW and Lipowsky HH. 1984. Pressure-flow relations in blood and lymph microcirculation. In: E Renkin and C Michel (eds), *Handbook of Physiology: The Cardiovascular System: Microcirculation*, sec 2, vol. 4, pt 1, pp. 251–307, Bethesda, MD, American Physiological Society.

Zweifach BW and Prather JW. 1975. Micromanipulation of pressure in terminal lymphatics of the mesentary. *J Appl Physiol* 228: 1326.

Zweifach BW and Silberberg A. 1979. The interstitial–lymphatic flow system. In: AC Guyton, DB Young (eds.), *International Review of Physiology—Cardiovascular Physiology III*, pp. 215–260, University Park Press, Baltimore.

Zweifach BW and Silverberg A. 1985. The interstitial–lymphatic flow system. In: MG Johnston, CC Michel (eds.), *Experimental Biology of the Lymphatic Circulation*, pp. 45–79, Elsevier, Amsterdam.

Further Reading

Drinker, C.K. and J.M. Yoffey. 1941. *Lymphatics, Lymph and Lymphoid Tissue: Their Physiological and Clinical Significance.* Harvard University Press, Cambridge, Massachusetts. This is a classic treatment of the lymphatic circulation by two pioneers in the field of lymphatic physiology.

Yoffey, J.M. and F.C. Courtice. 1970. *Lymphatics, Lymph and the Lymphomyeloid Complex.* Academic Press, London, New York. This is a classic book in the field of lymphatic physiology. The book contains a comprehensive review of pertinent literature and experimental physiology on the lymphatic system.

16

Modeling in Cellular Biomechanics

Alexander A.
Spector
Johns Hopkins University

Roger Tran-Son-Tay
University of Florida

16.1 Introduction

Mechanical forces, stresses, strains, and velocities play a critical role in many important aspects of cell physiology, such as adhesion, motility, and signal transduction. Cellular mechanics is now considered an important indicator of pathological conditions, including the state of the disease (e.g., Diez-Silva et al., 2010).

The modeling of cellular mechanics is a challenging task because of the interconnection of mechanical, electrical, and biochemical processes; involvement of different structural cellular components; and multiple timescales. It can involve nonlinear mechanics and thermodynamics, and because of its complexity, it will most likely require the use of computational techniques. Typical requirements in the development of cell models include the constitutive relations describing the state or evolution of the cell and its components, mathematical solution or transformation of the corresponding equations and boundary conditions, and computational implementation of the model.

Modeling is a powerful tool in the simulation of the processes in cells dealing with different temporal and spatial scales. It is effective in the interpretation and design of experiments, as well as in the prediction of new effects and phenomena. It is clear that modeling will play an increased role in improving our understanding of complex cell biology and physiology, under both normal and pathological conditions, and, ultimately, in helping in the treatment of various diseases (Bao and Suresh, 2003; Heidemann and Wirtz, 2004; Kamm and Mofrad, 2006; Discher et al., 2009).

In this chapter, we focus on several important features of cell behavior and cell modeling where cell mechanics plays a crucial role. They include constitutive relationships for the cell and its components (cytoskeleton, nucleus, cellular membrane) and their applications to major experiments to probe cellular mechanical properties. We also consider cell spreading, adhesion, and interaction with the extracellular matrix (ECM). We discuss various forms of cell motility, such as rolling, crawling, swimming, and gliding. Then, we review several forms of mechanotransduction in cells. Finally, we discuss the latest results on the modeling of cells in disease and consider important examples of cancer, malaria, and nuclear envelope deficiency. Some areas where mechanics also plays an important role, such as cell growth and division, are left for further reading.

16.2 Mechanical Properties of the Cell

16.2.1 Constitutive Relations

The basis of the modeling of cell mechanics is the relationships between the applied (internal) forces (stresses) and the corresponding strains or velocities. Under appropriate timescales, cells can be treated as elastic. In this case, the stresses can be expressed in terms of strains (displacement gradients). If a cell undergoes large deformation under physiological or experimental conditions, such as red blood cells (RBCs) in narrow capillaries or cells in the micropipette aspiration experiment (Evans and Skalak, 1980), the corresponding equations become nonlinear. If a cell and the applied forces are such that cellular properties are direction-independent, then the cell can be considered as isotropic. If the properties of the cell or its components are different depending on the direction (e.g., the cylindrical cochlear outer hair cell is softer in the longitudinal direction), then the cell is considered as anisotropic. Cells can acquire anisotropy as a result of structural rearrangements in response to application of certain stimuli (e.g., cytoskeletal reorganization in endothelial cells in response to exposure to blood-related shear stresses or cyclic stretches of the blood vessel). To simulate various time-dependent processes in cells, viscoelastic (viscous) models are used. Although most of the earlier work on cell rheology were focused on RBCs, knowledge of the rheological properties of white blood cells (WBCs) or leukocytes is also important in the comprehension of microcirculation flow dynamics. There are strong evidences (Tran-Son-Tay et al., 1991) that WBCs exhibit behavior similar to liquid drops. However, it is known that they cannot be modeled as simple Newtonian drops because the apparent viscosity of the cells changes with the rate and the extent of deformation. Kan et al. (1999b), using a three-layer model, were able to explain the inconsistencies reported in the literature. In their model, the outer layer is the cortical region surrounding the second layer (cytoplasm), and the third layer is the nucleus. They found that to understand the rheological behavior of WBCs, it is essential to have information on the deformation of the nucleus. Assigning apparent viscosity to cells can be misleading without accounting for the shape of the cell/nucleus under deformation, and can lead to incorrect estimates of the WBC material properties. For example, Kan et al. (1998) found that a compound drop (cell) behaves like a homogeneous simple liquid drop only if the core (nucleus) is sufficiently deformed and the timescale of the core, related to the combination of its viscosity and capillarity, is comparable to that of the shell layer (membrane). In other words, the apparent viscosity depends not only on the rheological properties of the cell but also on the flow dynamics surrounding it. Unless the presence and possible deformation of the nucleus are explicitly accounted for, neither Newtonian nor non-Newtonian models can adequately predict the hydrodynamics of WBCs.

Yamada et al. (2000) developed a method of laser tracking particles embedded in the cytoskeletal components inside living cells. The authors applied this method to measuring the complex modulus of the cellular content within a broad frequency range, and they showed that the frequency dependence of the modulus is close to a power law.

Previously, a number of experiments on adherent cells were interpreted from the standpoint of Maxwell, Voight, and standard linear solid models. More recently, a viscoelastic model with a weak-power dependence of the complex modulus on the frequency (strain rate) was proposed (e.g., Fabry et al., 2001; Lenormand et al., 2007). Like in the engineering structural damping model, the loss tangent in this model is independent of frequency but the weak-power behavior transforms into frequency-linear (fluid-type) behavior for higher frequencies (shorter timescales). The parameters of the power law model have been shown to be applicable to a variety of cells within several orders of the frequency magnitude. It was, however, lately noticed that for slow cellular processes, such as cell differentiation or apoptosis (very low frequencies), the power law changes: thus, there are timescales that are characterized by different power law parameters (Stamenovic et al., 2007).

Purely elastic or viscoelastic models treat the cellular material as a single phase. While the cell has several components, its content can be treated as a biphasic medium where one (solid) phase is associated with the cytoskeleton, and the other (fluid) is related to the cytoplasm. This approach can be further developed to include more phases important to the cell behavior, such as triphasic (solid–fluid–ion) models of cell mechanics (Guilak et al., 2006).

Long molecules that compose the cellular cytoskeleton can be treated from the standpoint of polymer mechanics where the response of the material to the application of a force is associated with changes in entropy (transition from disorder to more order). The cytoskeleton fiber are considered either as chains of segments that are completely free to move in three directions (freely joined chain model) or as flexible slender rods (worm-like chain model).

Similar constitutive relations have been developed for cellular components, such as the cytoskeleton and nucleus. Modeling the cell membrane has the main distinct feature because it has to be treated as an intrinsically two-dimensional (2-D) continuum.

16.2.2 Interpretation of Experiments

There are several major techniques that are used to extract the mechanical properties of cells. The models and experiments are interconnected: the experiments provide free parameters for the models, and, in turn, the models are the basis for the interpretation of the experiments. One of the most common techniques is micropipette aspiration, where a pipette is sealed on the surface of a cell, negative pressure is applied inside the pipette, and a portion of the cell is aspirated inside the pipette (Hochmuth, 2000 for review). The height of the aspirated portion of the cell can be considered as an inverse measure of cell stiffness. The same technique is used to observe the time response of the cell, and in this case, the corresponding relaxation time(s) is a measure of the cell's viscoelastic properties. The experiment with micropipette aspiration of an RBC was interpreted by considering the cell membrane (including the cytoskeleton) as a nonlinear (neo-Hookean) elastic half-space characterized by two parameters, an area expansion modulus and shear modulus. Earlier continuum models of the RBC membrane were summarized in the monograph by Evans and Skalak (1980). Later, Discher et al. (1998) developed an analysis of the micropipette aspiration by considering the RBC cytoskeleton as a polymer network. Each RBC cytoskeletal spectrin was treated as a worm-like chain, and the state of the whole network inside the micropipette was determined by a Monte Carlo simulation (Figure 16.1).

Theret et al. (1988) analyzed the micropipette experiment with endothelial cells. The cell was interpreted as a linear elastic incompressible isotropic half-space, and the pipette was considered as an axisymmetric rigid punch. This approach was later extended (Sato et al., 1990) to consider the cell as a linear viscoelastic incompressible material obeying the standard linear solid model. Haider and Guilak (2002) have applied an axisymmetric boundary integral model to estimate elastic parameters of chondrocytes, assuming the cell to have the shape of a finite sphere. Baaijens et al. (2005) have applied the finite element method to analyze the micropipette aspiration experiment with chondrocytes by assuming them to be nonlinear viscoelastic and biphasic. Zhou et al. (2005) have developed a finite element analysis of the micropipette experiment in the case of large viscoelastic deformations where the cell was treated as a standard neo-Hookean viscoelastic solid. Spector et al. (1998) analyzed the application of the micropipette to a cylindrical cochlear outer hair cell. The cell composite membrane

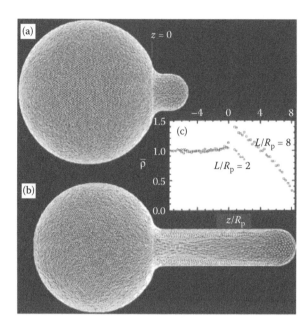

FIGURE 16.1 Simulation of the micropipette aspiration of the red blood cell cytoskeletal network for different ratios, (a) and (b), of the aspiration length, L, to the radius of the pipette, R_p. (c) The profiles of the network element density along the z-axis of the pipette. (From Discher, D.E., Boal, D.H., and Boey, S.K. *Biophys. J.*, 75, 1584, 1998. With permission.)

(wall) was treated as an orthotropic elastic shell, and the corresponding problem was solved by using the Fourier series.

Another technique widely used in the estimation of the properties of cells is atomic force microscopy, where the sample is probed by a rigid tip located at the end of a cantilever of a prescribed stiffness, and the displacement of the tip is tracked with a laser. The cell/tip contact force versus cell deflection characterizes the cell (cellular components) mechanical properties. A traditional interpretation of this experiment is based on the Hertz theory of frictionless contact of a rigid tip with an elastic isotropic half-space (e.g., Radmacher et al., 1996). Mahaffy et al. (2004) have refined this interpretation by interpreting the cell (fibroblast) as a layer of a finite thickness with two types of boundary conditions between the bottom of the cell and the substrate, full slip or full adhesion. The authors applied this approach to capture different properties of different parts of the fibroblast, including the cell's thickest central part as well as thinner areas of the lamellipodia. Unnikrishnan et al. (2007) have used a numerical finite element method to interpret the atomic force microscopy (AFM)-obtained measurements of cellular micromechanical properties.

Magnetocytometry is also a popular method for the characterization of cellular mechanical properties. In this method, a magnetic bead specifically coated to adhere to a targeted area is perturbed by a magnetic field. The properties of the cell are extracted by using the resulting force or torque versus the displacement or rotation angle of the bead. Wang and Ingber (1994) used this technique to analyze how the viscoelastic properties of the cytoskeleton of endothelial cells are controlled by cell shape and the cell's interaction with the ECM. Mijailovich et al. (2002) have developed a finite element interpretation of the experiment. Karcher et al. (2003) considered a bead under the action of a magnetic force on the surface of a cellular monolayer. On the basis of a linear viscoelastic model and finite element solution, the authors found the force/displacement relationship for the bead.

Many methods measure the mechanical properties of cells using probes in contact with the plasma membrane as opposed to probes placed within the cytoplasm. Therefore, these methods assess apparent mechanical properties that are dominated by the cortical cytoskeleton, which is enriched in acto-myosin stress fibers. In contrast, particle tracking microrheology probes the viscoelastic properties of the intracellular milieu by probing the spontaneous displacements of nanoparticles lodged in the cytoplasm of living cells (Wirtz, 2009). This approach allows probing the local, frequency-dependent viscoelastic moduli of cells by analyzing the mean-squared displacements of the cytoplasm-embedded nanoparticles (Tseng et al., 2002).

Other techniques used to probe cellular mechanical properties include laser/optical tweezers, deformation by two plates, and application of shear flow in the microchamber (Van Vilet et al., 2003; Janmey and Schmidt, 2006; Suresh, 2007 for review).

16.2.3 Properties of Cellular Components

There are a number of different approaches to the modeling of the cellular cytoskeleton. The continuum constitutive relations include viscoelastic monophasic, multiphasic, and polymer models (Mofrad et al., 2006). There are also structural models of the cytoskeleton, including an important one that is based on the concept of tensegrity, where the structure is supported by a system of prestressed components balanced by another system whose components are under compression. Ingber (1993, 2003a,b) have proposed to apply this concept to the mechanics of adherent cells, where the prestress is associated with the contractile machinery of actin fibers, and it is balanced by compression in microtubules and traction forces at cellular adhesions. This concept was incorporated into a computational model and applied to the prediction of the rheological behavior of living cells (Sultan et al., 2004). Another example of structural models of the cytoskeleton is the foam-like model proposed by Satcher and Dewey (1996) that was applied to the estimation of the elastic properties of endothelial cell's cytoskeleton. Some cells have naturally anisotropic cytoskeleton; Spector et al. (2001) have considered the 2-D cylindrical cytoskeleton of the cochlear outer hair cell and estimated its anisotropic properties. Fletcher and Mullins (2010) recently reviewed cell mechanics focusing on how the cell cytoskeleton generate, transmit, and respond to mechanical signals for short and long timescales.

The mechanical properties of the nucleus, the stiffest component of the cell, are important for those of the cell as a whole. Also, the mechanotransduction pathway connecting the adhesion sites, the cytoskeleton, and the nucleus results in the alteration of gene expression and protein synthesis. Recently, Lee et al. (2007) and Hale et al. (2008) showed that the molecular interconnections between the nuclear envelope and the cytoskeleton mediated by linkers of nucleus and cytoskeleton (linker nucleoskeleton and cytoskeleton (LINC) complexes) play a critical role in cytoplasmic rheology.

Guilak et al. (2000) have probed the nuclear properties by using the micropipette aspiration experiment and its interpretation on the basis of the standard linear viscoelastic model. Dahl et al. (2005) applied atomic force microscopy and found weak-power law viscoelastic relationships for the nuclear mechanics. Caille et al. (2002) have used two-plate compression of endothelial cells and interpreted the nucleus and cytoplasm as two different hyperelastic materials. Tseng et al. (2004) have applied the particle nanotracking method to estimate the viscoelastic properties of cellular nuclei. A direct force transduction can contribute to the adhesion–cytoskeleton–nucleus mechanotransduction pathway (Maniotis et al., 1997; Thomas et al., 2002). It has also been discovered that there is a mechanism of the cytoskeletal modulation of nuclear shape. In this regard, Jean et al. (2005) have developed a model of force transmission through the cytoskeleton to the nucleus that resulted from endothelial cell rounding. Cell rounding was caused by the alteration of cell adhesion via the application of trypsin. A review of the nuclear mechanics and methods was recently published by Lammerding et al. (2007).

The starting point of modeling cellular membranes is constitutive relations in 2-D space. Some cellular membranes (e.g., the RBC membrane), where the plasma membrane is attached to the underlying 2-D cytoskeleton, can be treated as elastic or viscoelastic solids (Evans and Skalak, 1980). The constitutive relations for the RBC can include bending because this mode of deformation is important to this cell's shape under physiological and experimental conditions (Evans, 1974, 1980). Pure plasma membrane has to be considered as a special liquid whose primary properties are tension and bending.

Helfrich (1973) has proposed energy functional as a function of membrane curvature and its original (spontaneous) curvature. In axisymmetric cases, the Euler–Lagrange equation for the bending energy functional can be explicitly derived in the form of nonlinear fourth-order ordinary differential equation (ODE) and solved by the finite difference method (e.g., Derenyi et al., 2002; Powers et al., 2002; Lim and Huber, 2009). Alternatively, Feng and Klug (2006) have developed a finite element method to directly minimize the bending energy functional. Atilgan and Sun (2007) have developed a coarse-grain triangular element model to analyze membranes and membranes with embedded proteins and found equilibrium states by using the Monte Carlo method. From the standpoint of general continuum mechanics, Steigmann (1999) has shown that the liquid membrane strain energy functional (function) is determined by curvatures and local area compressibility. In many cases, liquid membranes are considered as fully incompressible, and the area preservation condition is introduced via a Lagrange multiplier. Membrane tethers (narrow tubes) are a general phenomenon in liquid membranes. Such tethers can form naturally for cell–cell communication or for the slowing down of moving cells (such as leukocytes). Pulling membrane tethers is also an effective method to probe the local membrane properties. An approach based on thermodynamic balance of the tether system was previously applied to estimate the membrane bending modulus, membrane–cytoskeleton adhesion energy, and tension (e.g., Waugh and Hochmuth, 1987; Bozic et al., 1992; Dai and Sheetz, 1999). The details of the shape of a narrow tether are often unavailable in light microscopy. Alternatively, membrane shape in the whole tether region can be computed from the analysis of the equilibrium (steady-state deformation) of the tether. Calladine and Greenwood (2002) have proposed a version of the shell theory to determine the shape of the membrane in the tether region. Schumacher et al. (2009) have extended this approach and modeled tether shape in different cells, taking into account particular arrangement of bonds between the membrane and the cytoskeleton near the tether.

16.3 Cell Motility

Cell motility refers to the ability of a cell to move spontaneously and actively. All cell movements are a manifestation of mechanical work; they require a fuel (ATP) and proteins that convert the energy stored in ATP into motion. The cytoskeleton plays a critical role in cell motility. It can undergo constant rearrangement, which can produce movements. There are several types of cell motility and some of them are reviewed below.

16.3.1 Cell Spreading and Interaction with the Extracellular Matrix

When a cell is in contact with a proper substrate, it deforms and spreads onto the surface, and this action is called cell spreading. The cell spreading involves many events such as intracellular signaling, reorganization of cytoskeleton, and bond formation among adhesion molecules. In the later stages of cell spreading, actin polymerization pushes the cell membrane outward, making the cell more flattened. Actin polymerization and depolymerization are also responsible for the protrusion and the contraction of lamellipodium in cell crawling.

As an investigation of the early stages of cell spreading, which are considered as a rather passive process, Cuvelier et al. (2007) measured the contact radius with time using reflection interference microscopy for various combinations of cell and substrate types. They observed a universal power law behavior regardless of the experimental conditions, and to explain the behavior, they proposed a model in which a cell is modeled as a viscous adhesive cortical shell enclosing a less viscous interior. They concluded that the cell spreading is limited by its mesoscopic structure and material properties.

Cell spreading (shape), adhesion, and traction force generation as a result of cell interaction with the ECM are critically important for intracellular signaling, cell cycle, and cell fate under normal conditions and in disease. The same factors can determine the lineage commitment of stem cells (Engler et al., 2006; Guilak et al., 2009). Out of the factors determining stem cell lineage commitment, the stiffness of the substrate (ECM) plays an important role. While the physics of this phenomenon has not been fully understood, Walcott and Sun (2010) and Zemel et al. (2010) recently proposed models of this mechanism and related the substrate stiffness to the contractile (traction) forces generated by the cell cytoskeleton. It has also been noticed that the cell interaction with 2-D surfaces (including stem cells) can be quite different from that with three-dimensional (3-D) extracellular matrices (Cukierman et al., 2001; Fraley et al., 2010). Li et al. (2010) proposed a cell spreading model that includes molecular mechanisms of actin polymerization and integrin binding between cell and ECM, and predicted the change of contact radius with time. Their results agree well with experimental data, and confirmed the general power law behavior observed by Cuvelier et al. (2007). Their model also enables the examination of the effects of ECM stiffness and bond density on the cell spreading. Sun et al. (2009) proposed a continuum model of cell spreading in which specific interaction, long-range recruiting interaction, and diffusion of binders are included. The specific interactions between receptors on cell membrane and ligands on substrate surface are described by a chemical reaction equation, and long-range recruiting interactions are simplified by a traction-separation law. Their model identified different stages of cell spreading mediated by different mechanisms. Using a model of evolution of stress fibers and its finite element implementation, McGarry et al. (2009) have simulated the traction forces generated by cells, including fibroblast and mesenchymal stem cells, spread over a system of elastic microposts. Pathak et al. (2008) applied a similar approach to the simulation of cell spreading over a surface micropatterned with ligand-coated patches. Sengers et al. (2007) have presented a review of computational modeling of cell spreading and tissue regeneration in porous scaffolds. Dallon et al. (1999) have developed a model of cells interacting with the ECM where the cells were modeled as discrete objects and the matrix was modeled as a continuum. Using computational simulation, the authors considered the effects of changing cellular properties on fiber alignment.

16.3.2 Cell Rolling and Adhesion

Cell rolling can be described as a decrease in the velocity of cells (occurring only with leukocytes) in preparation to adhere to an endothelial wall. It is an essential part of a larger process of the immune system, which allows leukocytes to travel and bind to trauma-induced tissues. A factor that influences the effectiveness of rolling is cell velocity. As leukocyte velocity decreases (slow rolling), the chance of adhesion rises. Another contributing factor to this phenomenon is time. Leukocytes are viscoelastic bodies, which means that they are susceptible to deformation when a given force is applied over a specific time. As this interval grows, the shape of the leukocyte changes even more, causing an increase in the contact area of the cell. As the contact area increases, so does its chance of adhesion.

As noted earlier, there is much evidence to support the statement that rolling is an absolute prerequisite to leukocyte adhesion. Although this is certainly true for muscle and skin tissue, this is not conclusive for all tissues. The liver, lung, and heart are examples where rolling may not be necessary for leukocyte recruitment. In the lung's alveolar capillaries and the liver's sinusoids, rolling is not observed because the volume of each is extremely small, which allows for adhesion to occur straight from tethering.

The recent cell adhesion paradigm has been developed to emphasize the role of kinetics. Conceptualized by Bell (1978) and refined by several authors (Hammer and Lauffenburger, 1987; Dembo et al., 1988), the reaction kinetics approach integrates the adhesive interaction of the cells with the surface into the adhesion mechanism. Several physicochemical properties can affect the adhesion of a cell, such as rates of reaction, affinity, mechanical elasticity, kinetic response to stress, and length of adhesion molecules.

Several models have been proposed for describing the interaction of the leukocyte with the endothelium cells. Mathematical models of cell rolling/adhesion can be classified into two classes based on equilibrium (Evans, 1985; Alon et al., 1995) and kinetics concepts (Dembo et al., 1988; Alon et al., 1998; Kan et al., 1999a). The kinetic approach is more capable of handling the dynamics of cell adhesion and rolling. In this approach, the formation and dissociation of bonds occur according to the reverse and forward rate constants.

Using this concept, Hammer and Lauffenburger (1987) studied the effect of external flow on cell adhesion. The cell is modeled as a solid sphere, and the receptors at the surface of the sphere are assumed to diffuse and to convect into the contact area. The main finding is that the adhesion parameters, such as the reverse and forward reaction rates and the receptor number, have a strong influence on the peeling of the cell from the substrate.

Dembo et al. (1988) developed a model based on the ideas of Evans (1985) and Bell (1978). In this model, a piece of membrane is attached to the wall, and a pulling force is exerted on one end while the other end is held fixed. The cell membrane is modeled as a thin inextensible membrane. The model of Dembo et al. (1988) was subsequently extended via a probabilistic approach for the formation of bonds by Cozens-Roberts et al. (1990). Other authors used the probabilistic approach and Monte Carlo simulation to study the adhesion process as reviewed by Zhu (2000). Dembo's model has also been extended to account for the distribution of microvilli on the surface of the cell and to stimulate the rolling and the adhesion of a cell on a surface under shear flow. Hammer and Apte (1992) modeled the cell as a microvilli-coated hard sphere covered with adhesive springs. The binding and breakage of bonds and the distribution of the receptors on the tips of the microvilli are computed using a probabilistic approach.

To take into account the cell deformability, which has shown to be necessary for calculating the magnitude of the adhesion force, Dong and Lei (2000) have modeled the cell as a liquid drop encapsulated into an elastic ring. They show how the deformability and the adhesion parameters affect the leukocyte and adhesion process in shear flow. However, only a small portion of the adhesion length is allowed to peel away from the vessel wall. This constraint is not physically sound, and a more sophisticated model was developed by N'Dri et al. (2003).

Chang et al. (2000) used computer simulation of cell adhesion to study the initial tethering and rolling process based on Bell's model, and constructed a state diagram for cell adhesion under viscous flows under an imposed shear rate of 100 s^{-1}. This shear rate corresponds to the experimental value where rolling of the cell occurs. To create the state diagrams, the ratio of rolling velocity V to the hydrodynamic velocity V_H (velocity of nonadherent cells translating near the wall), V/V_H, is computed as a function of the reverse reaction rate, k_{ro}, for a given value of r_o using the Bell equation

$$k_r = k_{ro} \exp\left(\frac{r_o f}{k_B T}\right) \tag{16.1}$$

Here, k_{ro} is the unstressed dissociation rate constant, $k_B T$ the thermal energy, r_o the reactive compliance, and f represents the bond force. From the graph of V/V_H versus k_{ro}, the values of k_{ro} for a given value of r_o are estimated. The estimated values are used to plot k_{ro} as a function of r_o for a given ratio of V/V_H. From these curves, different dynamic states of adhesion can be identified. The first state, where cells move at a velocity greater than 95% of the hydrodynamic velocity V_H, is defined as no adhesion state. The second state, where $0 < V/V_H < 0.5$, is considered as the rolling domain and consists of fast and transient adhesion regimes. The first adhesion state, where $V/V_H = 0.0$ for a given period of time, defines the final state. Figure 16.2 shows the computed values of k_{ro} as a function of r_o.

Adhesion occurs for high values of k_{ro} and low values of r_o, as indicated by the wide area between the no- and firm-adhesion zones in Figure 16.3. As r_o increases, k_{ro} has to decrease for adhesion to take place. In the simulation (Figure 16.3), both association rate k_f and wall shear rate are kept constant. Varying k_f does not change the shape of the state diagram but shifts the location of the rolling envelope in the k_{ro}-r_o plane. The shear rate used in Chang et al. (2000) is in the range of the physiological flow for postcapillary venules and lies between 30 and 400 s^{-1}. They found that as the shear rate increases, there is an abrupt change from firm adhesion to no adhesion without rolling motion. As r_o increases, k_{ro} has to decrease in order for adhesion to take place. In the simulation, both association rate k_f and wall shear rate are kept constant. For values of r_o less than 0.1 Å and high reverse rate constant values k_{ro}, the rolling velocity is independent of the spring constant.

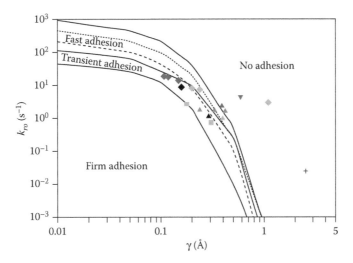

FIGURE 16.2 State diagram for adhesion. Four different states are shown. The dotted curve represents a velocity of 0.3 V_H and the dashed curve represents a velocity of 0.1 V_H. (From Chang, K.C., Tees, D.F.J., and Hammer, D.A., *Proc. Natl. Acad. Sci. USA*, 97, 11262, 2000. With permission.)

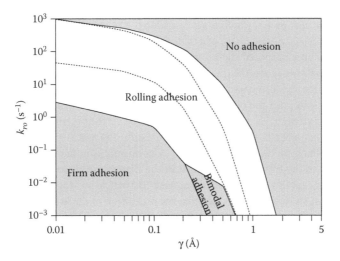

FIGURE 16.3 State diagram for shear rate ranging from 30 to 400 s⁻¹. The dotted curves indicate the boundaries of the rolling state at shear rate $G = 100$ s⁻¹. The rolling adhesion area represents the region where rolling motion occurs over shear rate ranging from 30 to 400 s⁻¹. In the bimodal adhesion regime, cells display either firm adhesion or no adhesion, without rolling motion, as the applied shear rate is altered from 100 to 400 s⁻¹. (From Chang, K.C., Tees, D.F.J., and Hammer, D.A., *Proc. Natl. Acad. Sci. USA*, 97, 11262, 2000. With permission.)

Tees et al. (2002) used the approach described in Chang et al. (2000) to study the effect of particle size on adhesion. They observed that an increase of the particle size raises the rolling velocity. This is consistent with the experimental findings of Shinde Patil et al. (2001). In both studies, the Bell model is used to construct the state diagram but the same results can be achieved using the spring model.

Using leukocytes, Alon et al. (1995) showed that the Bell equation and the spring model both fit the experimental data better than the linear relationship, suggesting an exponential dependence of k_r on f_b.

Chen and Springer (1999) studied the principles that govern the formation of bonds between a cell moving freely over a substrate in shear flow and those governing the bond dissociation due to hydrodynamic forces, and found that bond formation is governed by shear rate whereas bond breakage is governed by shear stress. This experimental data are well described by the Bell equation.

In the study of Smith et al. (1999), a high temporal and spatial resolution microscopy is used to reveal features that previous studies could not capture (Alon et al., 1995). They found that the measured dissociation constants for neutrophil tethering events at 250 pN/bond are lower than the values predicted by the Bell and Hookean spring models. The plateau observed in the graph of the shear stress versus the reaction rate K_r suggests that there is a force value above which the Bell and spring models are not valid. Since the model proposed so far considers the cell as a rigid body, whether the plateau is due to molecular, mechanical, or cell deformation is not clear at this time.

Cell rolling/adhesion has been extensively studied over the years. However, it is clear that much further studies are needed. Table 16.1 summarizes some of the efforts reported in the literature.

16.3.3 Cell Crawling

The process of cell crawling consists of three major stages: (1) pushing the leading edge, (2) establishing new adhesions in the front area and weakening of the exiting adhesions in the trailing area, and (3) pulling the back of the cell. Polymerization of the actin fibers in the protruded area of the crawling cell is considered the main mechanism of pushing the cell ahead. Thus, the modeling of the production of the pushing force is based on the polymerization/depolymerization analysis of actin fibers. There are two main approaches to the modeling of the polymerization-based active forces. In the first approach, the kinetics of a single fiber or array of fibers is considered. In the second, which is the continuum-type model, the fibers are treated as one phase of a two-phase reacting cytosol.

Peskin et al. (1993) have proposed the Brownian Ratchet theory for the active force production. The main component of that theory was the interaction between a rigid protein and a diffusing object in front of it. If the object undergoes a Brownian motion, and the fiber undergoes polymerization, there are rates at which the polymer can push the object and overcome the external resistance. The problem was formulated in terms of a system of reaction–diffusion equations for the probabilities of the polymer to have a certain number of monomers. Two limiting cases, fast diffusion and fast polymerization, were treated analytically that resulted in an explicit force/velocity relationship. This theory was subsequently extended to elastic objects and to the transient attachment of the filament to the object. The correspondence of these models to recent experimental data is discussed in the article by Mogilner and Oster (2003).

Mogilner and Edelstein-Keshet (2002) modeled the protrusion of the leading edge of a cell by considering an array of actin fibers inclined with respect to the cell membrane. The authors have considered the main sequence of events associated with the actin dynamics, including polymerization of the barbed edge of actin polymer and depolymerization at the protein pointed edge. The barbed edges assemble actin monomers with molecules of ATP attached. The new barbed edges are activated by Arp2/3 complexes and they branch to start new actin filaments. The rate of polymerization is controlled by capping of the barbed edges. The problem reduced to a system of reaction–diffusion equations and was solved in the steady-state case. As a result of this solution, the force/velocity relationships corresponding to different regimes were obtained. More recently, Bindschadler et al. (2004) have constructed a comprehensive model of actin cycle that can be used in various problems of cell motility. The authors took into account the major actin-binding protein, regulating actin assembly and disassembly and solved the problem as a steady-state case.

An alternative to the explicit analysis of actin fibers is a continuum approach where the cytoskeletal fibers are treated as one of the two phases of the cytosol. Dembo and Harlow (1986) have proposed a general model of contractile biological polymer networks based on the analysis of reactive interpenetrating flow. In that model, the cytoplasm was viewed as a mixture of a contractile network of randomly oriented cytoskeletal filaments and an aqueous solution. Both phases were treated as homogeneous Newtonian fluids. Alt and Dembo (1999) have applied a similar approach to the modeling of the motion

TABLE 16.1 Overview of Some Fundamental Adhesion Kinetic Models

Kinetic Model	Main Assumptions/Features	Major Findings
Point attachment (Hammer and Lauffenberger, 1987)	Bonds are equally stressed in the contact area (flat)	Adhesion occurrence depends on values of dimensionless quantities that characterize the interaction between the cell and the surface
	Binding and dissociation occur according to characteristic rate constants	
	Receptors diffuse and convect into the binding area of contact	
Peeling (Dembo et al., 1988)	Clamped elastic membrane	Critical tension to overcome the tendency of the membrane to spread over the surface can be calculated
	Bond stress and chemical rate constants are related to bond strain	
	Bonds are linear springs fixed in the plane of the membrane	Predictions of model depend on whether the bonds are catch bonds or slip bonds
	Chemical reaction of bond formation and breakage is reversible	
	Diffusion of adhesion molecules is negligible	If adhesion is mediated by catch bonds, then no matter how much tension is applied, it is impossible to separate the membrane and the surface
Microvilli-coated hard sphere covered with adhesive springs (Hammer and Apte, 1992)	Combined point attachment model with peeling model	Model can describe rolling, transit attachment, and firm adhesion
	Binding determined by a random statistical sampling of a probablility distribution that describes the binding (or unbinding)	A critical adhesion modulator is the spring slippage (it relates the strain of a bond to its rate of breakage; the higher the slippage, the faster the breakage for the same strain)
Two-dimensional elastic ring (Dong et al., 1999)	Bond density related to the kinetics of bond formation	Shear forces acting on the entire cortical shell of the cell are transmitted on a relatively small "peeling zone" at the cell's trailing edge
	Bonds are elastic springs	
	Interaction between moving fluid and adherent cell	
Two-dimensional cell modeled as a liquid and a compound drop (N'Dri et al., 2003)	Cell deforms with nucleus inside	Results compare well with numerical and experimental results found in the literature for simple liquid drop
	Bonds are elastic springs	Cell viscosity and surface tension affect leukocyte rolling velocity
	Macro/micro model for cell deformation	
	Kinetics model based on Dembo (1988). Nanoscale model for ligand–receptor	Nucleus increases the bond lifetime and decreases leukocyte rolling velocity
	Uniform flow at the inlet as in parallel-flow chamber assay	Cell with larger diameter rolls faster. Uniform flow at the inlet as in parallel flow chamber assay

of ameboid cell. The authors paid special attention to the boundary conditions. They introduced three boundary surfaces: the area of contact between the cell and the substrate, the surface separating the cell body and the lamellipodium, and they specified particular boundary conditions along each of these surfaces. The numerical solution of the problem resulted in cellular responses in the form of waves along the direction of the cellular movement. Recently, a two-phase continuum model has been applied to two problems of motility of the active neutrophil. In the first problem, the neutrophil was stimulated with the chemoattractant fMLP and the generation of the pseudopod was modeled, and in the second, the cell moved inside the micropipette toward the same chemoattractant. Two models, a cytoskeletal swelling force and a polymerization force, were used for the active force production. A finite difference method in terms of the time variable and a Galerkin finite element treatment in terms of the special variables were used to obtain numerical solutions.

Bottino et al. (2002) used a version of the continuum two-phase method and studied the crawling of the nematode sperm. This process is also driven by polymerization of another (not actin) protein, called the major sperm protein (MSP). The proposed model considers the major stages of crawling, including filament polymerization and generation of the force for the lamellipodial extension, storage of elastic energy, and finally the production of the contraction that pulls the rear of the cell. The total stresses consisted of two parts, the passive elastic stresses and active tensile stresses. In the acidic environment near the leading edge of the cell, the cytosol solates, and the elastic energy is released to push the cell forward. The solation was modeled by the removal of the active stresses. The solation rate was modeled by a pH gradient with lower pH at the rear part of the cell (Figure 16.4). The finite element method was used in the implementation of a 2-D version of the model.

16.3.4 Cell Swimming and Gliding

Most bacteria move by swimming by which they use helical flagella. In the bacteria with a left-handed helix (e.g., *Escherichia coli* and *Salmonella*), counterclockwise rotation generates a force pushing the cell forward. In contrast, clockwise rotation results in instability of the cell motion: the flagella fly apart, and the cell is not pushed in any particular direction. In the former case, the cell movement looks like smooth swimming, and in the latter case, the cell tumbles. In general, bacteria alternate between these two regimes of movement. The rotation of flagella is controlled by the molecular motor embedded in the bacterial membrane and driven by the transmembrane proton gradient. The movement of the bacterium can be changed by the addition of chemoattractants, which results in the suppression of tumbling and swimming toward a food source.

In contrast to bacterial swimming, many microorganisms, including myxobacteria, cyanobacteria, and flexobacteria, move via gliding. Nozzle-like structures were found in some of these bacteria. Slime is extruded through the nozzle pores, and this fact leads to a hypothesis that bacterial sliding is driven by a slime-related propulsion mechanism. In earlier models of torque and switching in the bacterial flagellar motor, the motor consisted of two, rotating and stationary, parts. The rotating part had tilted positively and negatively charged strips along its surface. The stationary part of the motor included several channels conducting protons. Each channel had two binding sides, and, therefore, could be in four states. The electrostatic energy of the interaction between the charges along the rotation part and protons bound to the channels was converted into the corresponding torque acting on the moving part. Further development and review of the models of this type can be found in Elston and Oster (1996).

CheY is one of the proteins controlling the motor in the flagella in chemotaxis. Phosphorylation of this protein results in tumbling of the bacterium. Mogilner et al. (2002) have modeled the process of switching of the bacterial molecular motor in response to binding CheY. The motor was assumed being in one of the two states that correspond to the two directions of rotation of the flagella. The kinetic equations for the probabilities of the motor being in each state included a rate constant proportional to the concentration of CheY. In addition, the free energy profile with two minima that depends on the CheY concentration was introduced. As a result, the fraction of time that the motor rotates clockwise

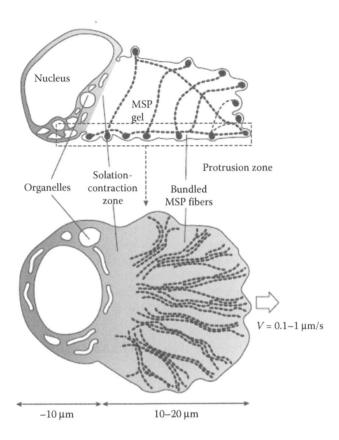

FIGURE 16.4 The model of locomotion of the nematode cell. At the leading edge of the cell, the growing MSP filaments bundle into thick fibers that push the cell front out, and at the same time, store elastic energy. In the acidic environment at the rear part of the cell, the interfilament interaction weakens, the filaments unbundle and contract, providing the contractile force up the cell body. (From Mogilner, A. and Oster, G. *Curr. Biol.*, 13, R721, 2003. With permission.)

was found as a function of the CheY concentration. The function described by a sigmoidal curve was checked against experimental data and good agreement was found. Wolgemuth et al. (2002) have proposed a model of myxobacteria gliding. The authors assumed that the area inside the cell near the nozzle is filled with a polyelectrolyte gel that consists of cross-linked fibers. When the bacterium interacts with its liquid environment, the gel swells and releases from the nozzle. This results in the generation of a propulsive force pushing the bacterium forward. The authors showed that the extrusion of the gel through 50 nozzles produces a force sufficient to drive the bacterium through the viscous environment at velocities observed in the experiment.

16.4 Mechano-, Mechanoelectrical, and Electromechanical Transduction

16.4.1 Mechanotransduction

Cells of all types are constantly exposed to external forces within their physiological environment. In mechanotransduction, cells convert the external mechanical signals into biochemical, morphological, biophysical, and other similar responses. As an example, endothelial cells respond to shear stresses acting on the cell's surface. Under physiological conditions, these stresses are associated with blood flow. In another example, the external stress (compression) causes mechanotransduction in chondrocytes, which is important both for the functioning of natural cartilage and for the design of artificial cartilage. Adhesion (traction) forces along the area of interaction of a cell with ECM determine cell shape, growth, and division (Chen et al., 1997, 2004 for review). General models that include biochemical aspect of signaling are complex, and their philosophy is discussed in the article by Asthagiri and Lauffenburger (2000). Here, we concentrate on some mechanical and mechanoelectrical aspects of the problem. One common phenomenon that accompanies mechanotransduction is a rearrangement of the cellular cytoskeleton in response to external forces. Suciu et al. (1997) have modeled the process of reorientation of the actin filaments in response to shear stresses acting on the membrane of endothelial cells. The authors assumed that the filament angular drift velocity is proportional to the applied shear stress and reduced the problem to a system of integro-differential equations in terms of the partial concentration of actin filaments being in different states (free, attached to the membrane, etc.). The same mathematical approach was later used to model the actin filaments in endothelial cells subjected to a cyclic stretch (simulation of the effect of the circumferential cyclic stretch of blood vessels). Thoumine et al. (1999) have analyzed such changes that occur during fibroblast spreading and they found a significant stiffening of the cell. Sato et al. (2000) have reported significant changes in the viscoelastic properties of endothelial cells as a result of the action of shear stresses. Kaunas et al. (2010) have proposed a kinematic model of fiber dynamics resulting from ECM stretching. Ingber (2006) and Poirier et al. (2007) have presented recent reviews of mechanotransduction and its models.

16.4.2 Mechanoelectrical Transduction, Mechanosensitive Channels, and Electromechanical Transduction

During mechanoelectrical transduction, the mechanical stimuli applied to the cell membrane result in (in-) activation of ionic currents through mechanosensitive channels. In eukaryotic cells, such channels are typically connected to the cell cytoskeleton. In several examples, stretch-activated channels modulate cell volume in cardiac ventricular myocytes, have a functional role in electrical and mechanical activity of smooth muscles, are involved in bone response to mechanical loading, produce a Ca^{2+} influx that leads to waves of calcium-induced calcium release, and so on. One of the features of mechanosensitive channels is the sensing not only of the stimulus itself but also its time history (Sachs and Morris, 1998). The main technique of studying the physiology of mechanosensitive channels is the patch pipette, and it was found that a full opening of the channel requires several cmHg of pressure, or several thousandth of Newton per meter of the equivalent membrane force (resultant). In the modeling of mechanosensitive channels, the channel has several states, and the probability of the channel being open is determined by free energy barriers that depend on the mechanical stimulus. Usually, this stimulus is represented by isotropic tension in the cell membrane, which, in the expression of free energy, is multiplied by a typical change in the area of the channel. Bett and Sachs (2000) have analyzed the mechanosensitive channels in the chick heart, and, to reflect the observed inactivation of ionic current, used a three—closed, open, and inactivated—state model of the channel. The authors have also proposed that inactivation consists of two stages: reorganization of the cytoskeleton and blocking action of an agent released by the cell. A quantitative description of this two-step process was based on a viscoelastic-type model that reflected the mechanical properties of the cortical layer underlying the channel. Auditory hair cells and vestibular cells receive mechanical stimuli and sense them via transducer channels located in the sterocilia bundle on the top of the cell. The channels in hair cells that receive acoustic signals are very fast (Corey and Hudspeth, 1979). A theoretical interpretation of the behavior of these channels is based on gating-spring concept that relates the local tension to the transition probability of the channel to be in open and close states. The latest results on the arrangement of the bundle components involved in mechanotransduction were obtained by Beurg et al. (2009) (also, Gillespie and Muller, 2009 for review). Note that the protein responsible for stereocilia bundle mechanotransduction has not been identified. In was also recently found that, in addition to "passive" mechanotransduction, the stereocilia bundle has active (motor) properties by amplifying input mechanical signals. A mathematical model of such phenomena in the form of dynamical systems was discussed by Nadrowski et al. (2004). One more mode of electromechanical transduction can be found in biological membranes whose curvature is coupled in a bidirectional way to the applied electric field (Petrov, 1999). Physical models of this membrane phenomenon, called flexoelectricity, that related membrane curvature–electric field coupling to a redistribution of electrical charges associated with the bilayer were proposed by Hristova et al. (1991) and, recently, by Harland et al. (2010). Zhang et al. (2001) have explained voltage-induced membrane movement in terms of a redistribution of bilayer charges resulting in changes in membrane tension.

Electromechanical transduction, a special form of signal transduction, was found in outer hair cells in the mammalian cochlea. The hearing process in vertebrates is associated only with the mechano-electric form of transduction via transducer channels in the stereocilia of a single type of sensory cells (see above). However, mammals have a special arrangement with two types of sensory cells, inner and outer hair cells. The outer hair cell provides a positive feedback in the processing of sound where its unique form of motility, called electromotility, plays a critical role. The main features of this phenomenon are cell length (and radius) changes, active force generation, and transfer of an electric charge, all in response to changes in the transmembrane potential. Deformation of the cell causes electric (displacement) current in the cell membrane. These features constitute the direct and converse piezoelectric-like effect. Tolomeo and Steele (1995) have proposed a linear piezoelectric model to describe the outer hair cell mechanics and electromotility. Spector (2001) (also, Spector and Jean, 2004) has proposed a thermo-dynamically based nonlinear model of electromechanical coupling in the outer hair cell. The membrane protein that plays a key role in the outer hair cell electromotility, named prestin, has been identified. Other cells, such as HEK cells, transfected with prestin acquire major features of the outer hair cell electromotility. Thus, modeling piezoelectric cellular membranes is now a more general area where one of the major goals is to combine cellular-level continuous constitutive relations with emerging molecular details of the structure of prestin.

16.5 Modeling Cells in Disease

16.5.1 Cancer

When a normal healthy cell's genetic material is altered, the cell responds differently to the host's growth regulators, leading to an uncontrolled growth of abnormal tumor cells. Like the normal cells, the tumor cells obtain glucose and oxygen and other nourishments, allowing a regular proliferation rate of tumor cells. A solid tumor arises as the growing spheroid of cells expands, making the core region inaccessible to nutrients. Cancer cells have different cytoskeletal structures from those of normal cells after oncogene transformed the normal cell to cancer cell. As a result, cancer cells can have different deformability and motility. Cancer cells have been reported to be more deformable than normal cells (Lee and Lim, 2007).

Individual cancer cell models have been often considered in tumor modeling using cellular automata or agent-based modeling approaches (Hwang et al., 2009). Jiang et al. (2005) used a lattice Monte Carlo model to describe tumor cell dynamics such as proliferation, adhesion, and viability. At the subcellular level, a network model regulates the expression of proteins that control the cell cycle. Their model predicts the microenvironmental conditions required for tumor cell survival and spheroid growth curve under different nutrient supply conditions. Gerlee and Anderson (2007) proposed a cellular automaton model of tumor growth in which each cell is equipped with a microenvironment network that takes environment variables as an input and determines cellular behavior as an output. They found that the tissue oxygen concentration affects the tumor at both the morphological level and the phenotype level. Gerlee and Anderson (2009) also investigated the emergence of a motile invasive phenotype of cancer cell in a tumor using an individual-based modeling approach, and found that a motile subclone can emerge in a wide range of microenvironmental growth conditions.

Tumor often spreads to other parts of the body by metastasis. Cancer cells often leave the tumor, enter into and circulate through the vascular system, leave the circulation, and form another tumor at a location distant from the original site. There have been efforts to model the cancer cell's motility and interactions with tissues during the process of metastasis. Ramis-Conde et al. (2009) presented a mathematical model of cancer cell intravasation. They used an individual force-based multiscale approach for cellular protein pathways and physical properties of the cell. They studied the influence of different protein pathways on transendothelial migration and obtained the simulation results comparable with experimental data. Gerisch and Chaplain (2008) developed a continuum model of cancer cell invasion of tissue in the form of a system of partial differential equations. Their model converges to a system of reaction–diffusion–taxis equations when the sensing radius that cells use to detect their environment goes to zero.

16.5.2 Malaria

Malaria is caused by the infection of RBCs by parasites of which *Plasmodium falciparum* is known to be the deadliest. When RBC is infected by *P. falciparum*, the RBC's biomechanical properties change such that it becomes less deformable and more adhesive. More rigid RBCs tend to block microcirculation, preventing oxygen supply to organs in the body. There have been efforts to model the biomechanical behavior of malaria-infected RBCs. Suresh et al. (2005) incorporated a 3-D hyperelastic constitutive model into a finite element code, and compared with experimental data. They found that the stiffness increases with the maturation of the parasite. By matching the computational model with experimental data, they estimated the shear modulus of RBC infected with different stages of the *P. falciparum* parasite. Jiao et al. (2009) developed a multicomponent model to account for the parasite within the infected RBC. They found that the membrane shear elastic modulus obtained from their multicomponent model is different from the ones obtained from hemispherical cap model and homogeneous half-space model due to the nonnegligible volume occupied by the parasite inside the infected cell. Kondo et al. (2009) developed a numerical model of blood flow with malaria-infected RBCs based on conservation laws of fluid dynamics. They modeled the deformability of infected RBC using springs governed by Hook's law. They simulated the rolling motion resulting from the interactions with endothelial cells and healthy RBCs, which increased the flow resistance. Ferrer et al. (2007) presented an individual-based model of *P. falciparum*-infected erythrocyte *in vitro* cultures. Cells are arranged in a 3-D grid and the rules of behavior are applied to each individual cell and culture medium. They reproduced several published experimental cultures from simulations of the model.

16.5.3 Nuclear Envelope Deficiency

The nucleus in the eukaryotic cell is enclosed by a nuclear envelope that consists of inner and outer nuclear membranes. Beneath the inner nuclear membrane lies the nuclear lamina, which is a network of filaments consisting of lamin proteins. The nuclear lamina is believed to be responsible for the structural integrity of the nucleus. When the genes encoding nuclear envelop proteins are mutated, structural changes occur in the nuclear envelope, which leads to various diseases, such as Emeri–Dreifus muscular dystrophy and Hutchinson–Gilford progeria (early aging) syndrome. Rowat et al. (2005, 2006) used a micropipette aspiration technique and showed that the nuclear envelope undergoes deformations, maintaining structural stability when exposed to mechanical stress. They developed a theory for a 2-D elastic material to characterize the elastic behavior of nuclear membranes. They also found that the nuclear envelopes in mouse embryo fibroblasts lacking the inner nuclear membrane protein, emerin, are more fragile than those in wild-type cells. They presented a model of nucleus stabilization in the pipette, combining their experimental results and theoretical considerations. Yokokawa et al. (2008) characterized the mechanical properties of the nuclear envelope of living HeLa cells in a culture medium by combining AFM imaging and force measurement. Their elasticity measurement showed that the nuclear envelope is soft enough to absorb a large deformation by the AFM probe. Dahl et al. (2004) established swelling conditions that separate the nuclear envelope from the nucleoplasm, and performed micropipette aspiration of swollen and unswollen nuclear envelopes of *Xenopus* oocyte. They measured the network elastic modulus of the nuclear envelope to be 25 mN/m. They found that the nuclear envelope is much stiffer and more resilient than the plasma membranes of cells.

Acknowledgments

The authors are thankful to Drs. Denis Wirtz, Alex Mogilner, and Sean Sun who reviewed the chapter and provided valuable comments. We also acknowledge funding supporting our research, R01 DC 002775 to A.S. and R01 HL 095508 and R01 HL 091005 to R.T.S.T.

References

Alon, R., Chen, S., Fuhlbrigge, R., Puri, K.D., and Springer, T.A. The kinetics and shear threshold of transient and rolling interactions of L-selectin with its ligand on leukocytes, *Proc. Natl. Acad. Sci. USA*, 95, 11631, 1998.

Alon, R., Hammer, D.A., and Springer, T.A. Lifetime of the P-selectin-carbohydrate bond and its response to tensile force in hydrodynamic flow, *Nature (London)*, 374, 539, 1995.

Alt, W. and Dembo, M. Cytoplasm dynamics and cell motion: Two-phase flow model, *Math. Biosci.*, 156, 207, 1999.

Asthagiri, A.R. and Lauffenburger, D.A. Bioengineering models of cell signaling, *Ann. Biomed. Eng.*, 2, 31, 2000.

Atilgan, E. and Sun, S.X. Shape transitions in lipid membranes and protein mediated vesicle fusion and fission, *J. Chem. Phys.*, 126, Art. 095102, 2007.

Baaijens, F.P.T., Triskey, W.R., and Laursen, T.A. Large deformation finite element analysis of micropipette aspiration to determine the mechanical properties of the chondrocyte, *Ann. Biomed. Eng.*, 33, 494, 2005.

Bao, G. and Suresh, S. Cell and molecular mechanics of biological materials, *Nat. Mater.*, 2, 715, 2003.

Bell, G.I. Models for the specific adhesion of cells to cells, *Science*, 200, 618, 1978.

Bett, G.C. and Sachs, F. Activation and inactivation of mechanosensitive currents in the chick heart, *J. Memb. Biol.*, 173, 237, 2000.

Beurg, M., Fettiplace, R., Nam J.H., and Ricci, A.J. Location of inner hair cell mechanotransducer using high-speed calcium imaging, *Nat. Neurosci.*, 12, 553, 2009.

Bindschadler, M., Osborn, E.A., Dewey, C.F. et al. A mechanistic model of the actin cycle, *Biophys. J.*, 86, 2720, 2004.

Bottino, D., Mogilner, A., Roberts, T. et al. How nematode sperm crawl, *Cell Sci.*, 115, 367, 2002.

Bozic, B., Svetina, S., Zeks, B. et al. Role of lamellar membrane structure in tether formation from bilayer vesicles, *Biophys. J.*, 61, 963, 1992.

Caille, N., Thuomine, O., Tardy, Y. et al. Contribution of the nucleus to the mechanical properties of endothelial cells, *J. Biomech.*, 33, 177, 2002.

Calladine, C.R. and Greenwood, J.A. Mechanics of tether formation in liposomes, *J. Biomech. Eng.*, 124, 576, 2002.

Chang, K.C., Tees, D.F.J., and Hammer, D.A. The state diagram for cell adhesion under flow: Leukocyte rolling and firm adhesion, *Proc. Natl. Acad. Sci. USA*, 97, 11262, 2000.

Chen, C.S., Mrksich, M., Huang, S. et al. Geometric control of cell life and death, *Science*, 276, 1425, 1997.

Chen, C.S., Tan, J., and Tien, J. Mechanotransduction of cell-matrix and cell-cell contacts, *Annu. Rev. Biomed. Eng.*, 6, 275, 2004.

Chen, S. and Springer, T.A. An automatic breaking system that stabilizes leukocyte rolling by an increase in selectin bond number with shear, *J. Cell Biol.*, 144, 185, 1999.

Corey, D.P. and Hudspeth, A.J. Response latency of vertebrate hair cells, *Biophys. J.*, 26, 499, 1979.

Cozens-Roberts, C., Lauffenburger, D.A., and Quinn, J.A. A receptor-mediated cell attachment and detachment kinetics; I. Probabilistic model and analysis, *Biophys. J.*, 58, 841, 1990.

Cukierman, E., Pankov, R., Stevens, D.R. et al. Taking cell-matrix adhesions to the third dimension, *Science*, 294, 1708, 2001.

Cuvelier, D., Théry, M., Chu, Y.-S. et al. The universal dynamics of cell spreading, *Curr. Biol.*, 17, 694, 2007.

Dahl, K.N., Engler, A.J., Pajerowski, J.D. et al. Power-law rheology of isolated nuclei with deformation mapping of nuclear substructures, *Biophys. J.*, 89, 2855, 2005.

Dahl, K.N., Kahn, S.M., Wilson, K.L. et al. The nuclear envelope lamina network has elasticity and a compressibility limit suggestive of a molecular shock absorber, *J. Cell. Sci.*, 117, 4779, 2004.

Dai J. and Sheetz, M.P. Membrane tether formation from blebbing cells, *Biophys. J.*, 77, 1999.

Dallon, J.C., Sherratt, J.A., and Maini, P.K. Mathematical modelling of extracellular matrix dynamics using discrete cells: Fiber orientation and tissue regeneration, *J. Theor. Biol.*, 199, 449, 1999.

Dembo, M. and Harlow, F. Cell motility, contractile networks, and the physics of interpenetrating reactive flow, *Biophys. J.*, 50, 109, 1986.

Dembo, M., Torney, D.C., Saxaman, K., and Hammer D. The reaction-limited kinetics of membrane-to-surface adhesion and detachment, *Proc. R. Soc. Lond. B*, 234, 55, 1988.

Derenyi, I., Julecher, F., and Prost, J. Formation and interaction of membrane tubes, *Phys. Rev. E*, 88, Art 238101, 2002.

Diez-Silva, M., Dao, M., Han, J.Y. et al. Shape and biomechanical characteristics of human red blood cells in health and disease, *MRS Bull.*, 35, 382, 2010.

Discher, D., Dong, C., Fredberg, J.J. et al. Biomechanics: Cell research and applications for the next decade, *Ann. Biomed. Eng.*, 37, 847, 2009.

Discher, D.E., Boal, D.H., and Boey, S.K. Simulation of the erythrocyte cytoskeleton at large deformation. II. Micropipette aspiration, *Biophys. J.*, 75, 1584, 1998.

Dong, C. and Lei, X.X. Biomechanics of cell rolling: Shear flow, cell-surface adhesion, and cell deformability, *J. Biomech.*, 33, 35, 2000.

Elston, T.C. and Oster, G. Protein turbines! The bacterial flagellar motor, *Biophys. J.*, 73, 703, 1996.

Engler, A.J., Sen, S., Sweeney, H.L. et al. Matrix elasticity directs stem cell lineage specification, *Cell*, 126, 677, 2006.

Evans, E.A. Bending resistance and chemically induced moments in membrane bilayers, *Biophys. J.*, 14, 923, 1974.

Evans, E.A. Detailed mechanics of membrane-membrane adhesion and separation. I. Continuum of molecular cross-bridges, *Biophys. J.*, 48, 175, 1985.

Evans, E.A. Minimum energy analysis of membrane deformation applied to pipet aspiration and surface adhesion of red blood cells, *Biophys. J.*, 30, 265, 1980.

Evans, E.A. and Skalak, R. *Mechanics and Thermodynamics of Biomembranes*, CRC Press, Boca Raton, FL, 1980.

Fabry, B., Maksym, G.N., Butler, J.P. et al. Scaling the microrheology of living cells, *Physiol. Rev. Lett.*, 87, 148102, 2001.

Feng, F. and Klug, W.S. Finite element modeling of lipid bilayer membranes, *J. Comput. Phys.*, 220, 394, 2006.

Ferrer, J., Vidal, J., Prats, C. et al. Individual-based model and simulation of *Plasmodium falciparum* infected erythrocyte *in vitro* cultures, *J. Theor. Biol.*, 248, 448, 2007.

Fletcher, D.A. and Mullins, R.D. Cell mechanics and the cytoskeleton, *Proc. Natl. Acad. Sci. USA*, 463, 485, 2010.

Fraley, S.I., Feng, Y.F., Krishnamurthy, R. et al. A distinctive role for focal adhesion proteins in three-dimensional cell motility, *Nat. Cell Biol.*, 12, 598, 2010.

Gerisch, A. and Chaplain, M.A.J. Mathematical modeling of cancer cell invasion of tissue: Local and non-local models and the effect of adhesion, *J. Theor. Biol.*, 250, 684, 2008.

Gerlee, P. and Anderson, A.R.A. An evolutionary hybrid cellular automaton model of solid tumour growth, *J. Theor. Biol.*, 246, 583, 2007.

Gerlee, P. and Anderson, A.R.A. Evolution of cell motility in an individual-based model of tumour growth, *J. Theor. Biol.*, 259, 67, 2009.

Gillespie, P.G. and Muller, U. Mechanotransduction by hair cells: Models, molecules, and mechanisms, *Cell*, 139, 33, 2009.

Guilak, F., Cohen, D.M., Estes, B.T. et al. Control of stem cell fate by physical interactions with the extracellular matrix, *Cell Stem Cell*, 5, 17, 2009.

Guilak, F., Haider, M.A., Karcher, E. et al. Mutiphasic models of cell mechanics, In *Cytoskeletal Mechanics. Models and Measurements*, Eds, R. Kamm and Mofrad M.R.K., pp. 84–102, 2006.

Guilak, F., Tedrow, J.R., and Burgkart, R. Viscoelastic properties of the cell nucleus, *Biochem. Biophys. Res. Comm.*, 269, 781, 2000.

Haider M.A. and Guilak, F. An axisymmetric boundary integral model for assessing elastic cell properties in the micropipette aspiration contact problem, *J. Biomech. Eng.*, 124, 586, 2002.

Hale, C.M., Shrestha, A.L., Khatau, S.B. et al. Dysfunctional connections between the nucleus and the actin and microtubule networks in laminopathic models, *Biophys. J.*, 11, 5462, 2008.

Hammer, D.A. and Apte, S.M. Simulation of cell rolling and adhesion on surfaces in shear-flow—General results and analysis of selectin-mediated neutrophil adhesion, *Biophys. J.*, 63, 35, 1992.

Hammer, D.A. and Lauffenburger, D.A. A dynamical model for receptor-mediated cell adhesion to surfaces, *Biophys. J.*, 52, 475, 1987.

Harland, B., Brownell, W.E., Spector, A.A. et al. Voltage-induced bending and electromechanical coupling in lipid bilayers, *Phys. Rev. E*, 81, Art. 031907, 2010.

Heidemann, S.R. and Wirtz, D. Cell and molecular mechanics of biological materials, *Trends Cell Biol.*, 14, 160, 2004.

Helfrich, W. Elastic properties of lipid bilayers: Theory and possible experiments, *Z. Naturforsch.*, C28, 693, 1973.

Hochmuth, R.M. Micropipette aspiration of living cells, *J. Biomech.*, 33, 15, 2000.

Hristova., K. Bivas, I., Petrov, A.G., and Derzanski, A. Influence of the electric double layers of the membrane on the value of its flexoelectric coefficient, *Mol. Cryst. Liq. Cryst.*, 200, 71, 1991.

Hwang, M., Garbey, M., Berceli, S.A. et al. Rule-based simulation of multi-cellular biological systems-A review of modeling techniques, *Cell. Mol. Bioeng.*, 2, 285, 2009.

Ingber, D.E., Cellular mechanotransduction: Putting all the pieces together again, *FASEB J.*, 20, 811, 2006.

Ingber, D.E. Cellular tensegrity-defining new rules of biological design that govern the cytoskeleton, *J. Cell Sci.*, 104, 613, 1993.

Ingber, D.E. Tensegrity I. Cell structure and hierarchical systems biology. *J. Cell Sci.*, 116, 1157, 2003a.

Ingber, D.E. Tensegrity II. How structural networks influence cellular information processing networks, *J. Cell Sci.*, 116, 1397, 2003b.

Janmey, P. and Schmidt, C. Experimental measurements of intracellular mechanics, In *Cytoskeletal Mechanics. Models and Measurements*, Eds, R. Kamm and Mofrad M.R.K., pp. 1–17, Cambridge University Press, Cambridge, 2006.

Jean, R.P., Chen, C.S., and Spector, A.A. Finite-element analysis of the adhesion-cytoskeleton-nucleus mechanotransduction pathway during endothelial cell rounding: Axisymmetric model, *J. Biomech. Eng.*, 127, 594, 2005.

Jiang, Y., Pjesivac-Grbovic, J., Cantrell, C. et al. A multiscale model for avascular tumor growth, *Biophys. J.*, 89, 3884, 2005.

Jiao, G.Y., Tan, K.S.W., Sow, C.H. et al. Computational modeling of the micropipette aspiration of malaria infected erythrocytes, *ICBME 2008, Proceedings*, 23, 1788, 2009.

Kamm, R. and Mofrad, M.R.K. Introduction, with the biological basis for cell mechanics, In *Cytoskeletal Mechanics. Models and Measurements*, Eds, R. Kamm and Mofrad M.R.K., pp. 1–17, Cambridge University Press, Cambridge, 2006.

Kan, H.-C., Udaykumar, H.S., Shyy, W., and Tran-Son-Tay, R. Hydrodynamics of a compound drop with application to leukocyte modeling, *Phys. Fluids*, 10, 760, 1998.

Kan, H.-C., Udaykumar, H.S., Shyy, W., and Tran-Son-Tay, R. Numerical analysis of the deformation of an adherent drop under shear flow, *J. Biomech. Eng.*, 121, 160, 1999a.

Kan, H.-C., Udaykumar H.S., Shyy W. et al. Effects of nucleus on leukocyte recovery, *Ann. Biomed. Eng.*, 27, 648, 1999b.

Karcher, H., Lammerding, J., Huang, H. et al. A three-dimensional viscoelastic model for cell deformation with experimental verification, *Biophys. J.*, 85, 3336, 2003.

Kaunas, R., Huang, Z.Y., and Hahn, J. A kinematic model coupling stress fiber dynamics with JNK activation in response to matrix stretching, *J. Theor. Biol.* 264, 593, 2010.

Kondo, H., Imai, Y., Ishikawa, T. et al. Hemodynamic analysis of microcirculation in malaria infection, *Ann. Biomed. Eng.*, 37, 702, 2009.

Lammerding, J., Dahl, K.N., Discher, D.E. et al. Nuclear mechanics and methods, *Cell Mechanics*, 83, 269, 2007.

Lee, G.Y.H. and Lim, C.T. Biomechanics approaches to studying human diseases, *Trends Biotechnol.*, 25, 111, 2007.

Lee, J.S.H., Hale, C.M., Panorchan, P. et al. Nuclear lamin A/C deficiency induces defects in cell mechanics, polarization, and migration, *Biophys. J*, 93, 2542, 2007.

Lenormand, G., Bursac, P., and Butler, J.P. Out-of-equilibrium dynamics in the cytoskeleton of the living cell, *Phys. Rev. E.*, 76, Art 041901, 2007.

Li, Y., Xu, G.-K., Li, B. et al. A molecular mechanisms-based biophysical model for two-phase cell spreading, *Appl. Phys. Lett.*, 96, 043703, 2010.

Lim, G.H.W. and Huber, G. The tether infinitesimal tori and spheres algorithm: A versatile calculator for axisymmetric problems in equilibrium membrane mechanics, *Biophys. J.*, 96, 2064, 2009.

Mahaffy, R.E., Park, S., Gerde, E. et al. Quantitative analysis of the viscoelastic properties of thin regions of fibroblasts using atomic force microscopy, *Biophys. J.*, 86, 1777, 2004.

Maniotis, A.J., Chen, C.S., and Ingber, D.E. Demonstration of mechanical connections between integrinscy to skeletal filaments, and nucleoplasm that stabilize nuclear structure, *Proc. Natl. Acad. Sci. USA*, 94, 849, 1997.

McGarry, J.P., Fu, J., Yang, M.T. et al. Simulation of the contractile response of cells on an array of microposts, *Phil. Trans. Royal Soc. Phys. Eng Sci.*, 367, 3477, 2009.

Mijailovich, S.M., Kojic, M., Zivkovic, M. et al. A finite element model of cell deformation during magnetic bead twisting, *J. Appl. Physiol*, 93, 1429, 2002.

Mofrad, M.R.K., Karcher, H., and Kamm, R.D. Continuum elastic and viscoelastic models of the cell. In *Cytoskeletal Mechanics. Models and Measurements*, Eds, R. Kamm and Mofrad M.R.K., Cambridge University Press, Cambridge, pp. 71–83, 2006.

Mogilner, A. and Edelstein-Keshet, L. Regulation of actin dynamics in rapidly moving cells: A quantitative analysis, *Biophys. J.*, 83, 1237, 2002.

Mogilner, A., Elston, T.C., Wang, H. et al. Switching in the bacterial flagellar motor, In *Computational Cell Biology*, Fall, C.P., Marland, E.S., Wagner, J.M. et al. Eds. Springer, New York, 2002, chap. 13.

Mogilner, A. and Oster, G. Polymer motors: Pushing out the front and pulling up the back, *Curr. Biol.*, 13, R721, 2003.

Nadrowski, B., Martin, P., and Julicher, F. Active hair-bundle motility harnesses noise to operate near an optimum of mechano sensitivity, *Proc. Natl. Acad. Sci. USA*, 33, 12195, 2004.

N'Dri, N.A., Shyy, W., and Tran-Son-Tay, R., Computational modeling of cell adhesion and movement using a continuum-kinetics approach, *Biophys. J.*, 85, 2273, 2003.

Pathak, A., Deshpande, V.S., McMeeking, R.M., and Evans, A.G.J. The simulation of stress fibre and focal adhesion development in cells on patterned substrates, *Royal Soc. Interface*, 5, 507, 2008.

Peskin, C.S., Odell, G.M., and Oster, G. Cellular motors and thermal fluctuation: The Brownian ratchet, *Biophys. J.*, 65, 316, 1993.

Petrov, A.G. *The Lyotropic State of Matter. Molecular Physics and Living Matter Physics.* Gordon and Breach Publ., Australia, 1999.

Poirier, C.C. and Iglesias, P.A. An integrative approach to understanding mechanosensation. *Brief. Bioinform.*, 8, 258, 2007.

Powers, T.R., Huber, G., Goldstein, R.E. Fluid-membrane tethers: Minimal surfaces and elastic boundary layers, *Phys. Rev. E.*, 65, Art 041901, 2002.

Radmacher, M., Fritz, M., Kacher, C.M. et al. Measuring the viscoelastic properties of human platelets with the atomic force microscope, *Biophys. J.*, 70, 556, 1996.

Ramis-Conde, I., Chaplain M.A.J., Anderson, A.R.A. et al. Multi-scale modeling of cancer cell intravasation: The role of cadherins in metastasis, *Phys. Biol.*, 6, 016008, 2009.

Rowat, A.C., Foster, L.J., Nielsen, M.M. et al. Characterization of the elastic properties of the nuclear envelope, *J. R. Soc. Interface*, 2, 63, 2005.

Rowat, A.C., Lammerding, J., and Ipsen, J.H. Mechanical properties of the cell nucleus and the effect of emerin deficiency, *Biophys. J.*, 91, 4649, 2006.

Sachs, F. and Morris, C.E. Mechanosensitive ion channels in non-specialized cells, In *Reviews of Physiology, Biochemistry, and Pharmacology*, Blausten, M.P. et al., Eds. pp. 1–78, Springer, Berlin, 1998.

Satcher, R.L. and Dewey, C.F. Theoretical estimates of mechanical properties of the endothelial cell cytoskeleton, *Biophys. J.*, 71, 109, 1996.

Sato, M., Nagayama, K., Kataoka, N. et al. Local mechanical properties measured by atomic force microscopy for cultured bovine endothelial cells exposed to shear stress, *J. Biomech.*, 33, 127, 2000.

Sato M., Theret, D.P, Wheeler, L.T. et al. Application of the micropipette technique to the measurement of cultured porcine aortic endothelial cell viscoelastic properties, *J. Biomech. Eng.*, 112, 263, 1990.

Schumacher, K.R., Popel, A.S., Anvari, B. et al. Computational analysis of the tether-pulling experiment to probe plasma membrane-cytoskeleton interaction in cells, *Phys. Rev. E*, 80, Article 041905, 2009.

Sengers, B.G., Taylor, M., Please, C.P. et al. Computational modelling of cell spreading and tissue regeneration in porous scaffolds, *Biomaterials*, 28, 1926, 2007.

Shinde Patil, V.R., Campbell, C.J., Yun, Y.H., Slack, S.M., and Goetz, D.J. Particle diameter influences adhesion under flow, *Biophys. J.*, 80, 1733, 2001.

Smith Mcrae, J., Berg, E.L., and Lawrence, M.B. A direct comparison of selectin-mediated transient, adhesive events using high temporal resolution, *Biophys. J.*, 77, 3371, 1999.

Spector, A.A. A nonlinear electroelastic model of the auditory outer hair cell, *Int. J. Solids Struct.*, 38, 2115, 2001.

Spector, A.A., Ameen, M., and Popel, A.S. Simulation of motor-driven cochlear outer hair cell electromotility, *Biophys. J.*, 81, 11, 2001.

Spector, A.A., Brownell, W.E., and Popel, A.S. Analysis of the micropipette experiment with the anisotropic outer hair cell wall, *J. Acoust. Soc. Am.*, 103, 1001, 1998.

Spector, A.A. and Jean, R.P. Models and balance of energy in the piezoelectric cochlear outer hair cell wall, *J. Biomech. Eng.*, 126, 17, 2004.

Stamenovic, D., Rosenblatt, N., and Montoya-Zavala, M. Rheological behavior of living cells is time scale-dependent, *Biophys. J.*, 93, L39, 2007.

Steigmann, D.J. Fluid films with curvature elasticity, *Arch. Rat. Mech. Anal.*, 150, 127, 1999.

Suciu, A., Civelekoglu, G., Tardy, Y. et al. Model of the alignment of actin filaments in endothelial cells subjected to fluid shear stress, *Bull. Math. Biol.*, 59, 1029, 1997.

Sultan, C., Stamenovic, D., and Ingber, D.E. A computational tensegrity model predicts dynamic rheological behaviors in living cells, *Ann. Biomed. Eng.*, 32, 520, 2004.

Sun, L., Cheng, Q.H., Gao, H.J. et al. Computational modeling for cell spreading on a substrate mediated by specific interactions, long-range recruiting interactions, and diffusion of binders, *Phys. Rev. E*, 79, 061907, 2009.

Suresh, S. Biomechanics and biophysics of cancer cells, *Acta Biomater.*, 3, 413, 2007.

Suresh, S., Spatz, J., Mills, J.P. et al. Connections between single-cell biomechanics and human disease states: Gastrointestinal cancer and malaria, *Acta Biomater.*, 1, 15, 2005.

Tees, D.F.J., Chang, K.C., Rodgers, S.D., and Hammer, D.A. Simulation of cell adhesion to bioreactive surfaces in shear: The effect of cell size, *Ind. Eng. Chem. Res.*, 41, 486, 2002.

Theret, D.P., Levesque, M.J., Sato, M. et al. The application of a homogeneous half-space model in the analysis of endothelial cell micropipette measurements, *J. Biomech. Eng.*, 110, 190, 1988.

Thomas, C.H., Colllier, J.H., Sfeir, C. et al. Engineering gene expression and protein synthesis by modulation of nuclear shape, *Proc. Natl. Acad. Sci. USA*, 99, 1972, 2002.

Thoumine, O., Cardoso, O, and Meister, J.J. Changes in the mechanics of fibroblast during spreading: A micromanipulation study, *Eur. Biophys. J.*, 27, 222, 1999.

Tolomeo, J.A. and Steele, C.R. Orthotropic piezoelectric properties of the cochlear outer hair cell wall. *J. Acoust. Soc. Am.*, 97, 3006, 1995.

Tran-Son-Tay, R., Needham, D., Yeung, A., and Hochmuth, R.M. Time dependent recovery of passive neutrophils after large deformation, *Biophys. J.*, 60, 856, 1991.

Tseng, Y., Kole, T.P., and Wirtz, D. Micro mechanical mapping of live cells by multiple-particle-tracking microrheology, *Biophys. J.*, 83, 3162, 2002.

Tseng, Y., Lee, J.S.H., Kole, T.P. et al. Micro-organization and visco-elasticity of the interphase nucleus revealed by particle nanotracking, *J. Cell Sci.*, 117, 2159, 2004.

Unnikrishnan, G.U., Unnikrishnan, V.U., and Reddy, J.N. Constitutive material modeling of cell: A micromechanics approach, *J. Biomech. Eng.*, 129, 315, 2007.

Van Vilet, K.L., Bao, G., and Suresh, S. The biomechanics toolbox: Experimental approaches for living cells and biomolecules, *Acta Mater.*, 51, 5881, 2003.

Walcott, S. and Sun, S.X. A mechanical model of actin stress fiber formation and substrate elasticity sensing in adherent cells, *Proc. Natl. Acad. Sci. USA*, 107, 7757, 2010.

Wang, N and Ingber, D.E. Control of cytoskeletal mechanics by extracellular matrix, cell shape, and mechanical tension, *Biophys. J.*, 66, 2181, 1994.

Waugh, R.E. and Hochmuth, R.M. Mechanical equilibrium of thick, hollow, liquid membrane cylinders, *Biophys. J.*, 52, 391, 1987.

Wirtz, D. Particle-tracking microrheology of living cells: Principles and applications, *Annu. Rev. Biophys.*, 38, 301, 2009.

Wolgemuth, C., Holczyk, E., Kaiser, D. et al. How Myxobacteria glide, *Curr. Biol.*, 12, 369, 2002.

Yamada, S., Wirtz, D., and Kuo, S.C. Mechanics of living cells measured by laser tracking microrheology, *Biophys. J.*, 78, 1736, 2000.

Yokokawa, M., Takeyasu, K., and Yoshimura S.H. Mechanical properties of plasma membrane and nuclear envelope measured by scanning probe microscope, *J. Microsc.*, 232, 82, 2008.

Zemel, A., Rehfeldt, F., Brown, A.E.X. et al. Optimal matrix rigidity for stress-fibre polarization in stem cells, *Nat. Phys.*, 6, 468, 2010.

Zhang, P.C., Keleshian, A.M., and Sachs, F. Voltage-induced membrane movement, *Nature*, 413, 428, 2001.

Zhou, E.H., Lim, C.T., and Quek, S.T. Finite element simulation of the micropipette aspiration of a living cell under going large viscoelastic deformation, *Mech. Advanced Mater. Struct.*, 12, 501, 2005.

Zhu, C. Kinetics and mechanics of cell adhesion, *J. Biomech.*, 33, 23, 2000.

Further Information

Fall, C.P., Marland, E.S., Wagner, J.M., and Tyson, J.I. Eds. *Computational Cell Biology*, Springer, New York, 2002 (this book consists of several sections written by leading experts in the mathematical and computational analysis of cell physiology; the material includes exercises, necessary mathematics, and software, and it can be used for teaching advanced graduate courses).

Mogilner, A., Wollman, R., Civelekoglu-Scholey, G., and Scholey, J. Modeling mitosis, *Trends Cell Biol.*, 16, 88, 2006.

Zaman, M.H. Ed. *Statistical Mechanics of Cellular Systems and Processes*, Cambridge University Press, Cambridge, 2009 (a collection of chapters on statistical models of molecules, cells, and cellular systems).

17

Cochlear Mechanics

Charles R. Steele
Stanford University

Sunil Puria
Stanford University

The inner ear is a transducer of mechanical force to an appropriate neural excitation. The key element is the receptor cell, or hair cell, which has stereocilia on the apical surface and afferent (and sometimes efferent) neural synapses on the lateral walls and base. Generally, for hair cells, mechanical displacement of the stereocilia in the forward direction toward the tallest stereocilia causes the generation of electrical impulses in the nerves, while backward displacement causes the inhibition of spontaneous neural activity. Displacement in the lateral direction has no effect. For moderate frequencies of sinusoidal stereociliary displacement (20–200 Hz), the neural impulses are in synchrony with the mechanical displacement, one impulse for each cycle of excitation. Such impulses are transmitted to the higher centers of the brain and can be perceived as sound. For lower frequencies, however, neural impulses in synchrony with the excitation are apparently confused with the spontaneous, random firing of the nerves. Consequently, there are three mechanical devices in the inner ear of vertebrates that provide perception in the different frequency ranges. At zero frequency, that is, linear acceleration, the otolithic membrane provides a constant force acting on the stereocilia of hair cells. For low frequencies associated with the rotation of the head, the semicircular canals provide the proper force on the stereocilia. For frequencies in the hearing range, the cochlea provides the proper force on the stereocilia. In nonmammalian vertebrates, the equivalent of the cochlea is a bent tube, and the upper frequency of hearing is at most 12 kHz. For mammals, the upper frequency is considerably higher, 20 kHz for man but extending to almost 200 kHz for toothed whales and some bats. Other creatures, such as certain insects, as well as some frogs and birds living in noisy environments, can perceive high frequencies, but may not have the frequency discrimination of mammals.

Auditory research is a broad field (Keidel and Neff 1976). This chapter provides a brief guide of a restricted view, focusing on the fluid-elastic aspects of the transfer of the input sound pressure into the correct stimulation of hair cell stereocilia in the cochlea. In a general sense, the mechanical functions of the semicircular canals and the otoliths are clear, as are the functions of the outer ear and middle ear; however, the cochlea continues to elude a complete explanation. It is evident that the normal function of the cochlea requires a full integration of mechanical, electrical, and chemical effects on the milli-, micro-, and nanometer scales. Texts that include details of the anatomy are by Pickles (1988), Gulick et al. (1989), and Geisler (1998). Surveys specifically on the cochlea are by Steele (1987), Hudspeth (1989), de Boer (1991), Dallos (1992), Ruggero (1993), and Nobili et al. (1998). Today, many laboratories have excellent websites that contain both introductory information and other details. Nevertheless, because of the immensity of his contributions, Békésy (1960) remains the required reading for anyone embarking on a serious work on the cochlea.

17.1 Anatomy

The cochlea is a coiled tube in the shape of a snail shell (cochlea = schnecke = snail), with a length of about 35 mm and a radius of about 1 mm in human. Figure 17.1 shows a finite element (FE) model that is based entirely on three-dimensional (3D) reconstruction from micro-computed tomography (micro-CT) imaging. This shows the eardrum, middle ear, vestibular canals, as well as the cochlea. Böhnke and Arnold (1999) apparently presented the first construction of an FE model from a CT image. Presently, a number of laboratories possess this capability.

There is not a large size difference across species: the length of the cochlea is 60 mm in elephant and 7 mm in mouse. There are two and a half turns of the coil in man and dolphin, and five turns in guinea pig. There is a correlation of the coiling with the hearing capability of land animals (West 1985). Manoussaki et al. (2008) also consider sea mammals, and find that the ratio of curvature at the base to the curvature at the apex is a feature that correlates strongly with low-frequency hearing limits. However, any benefit of the coiling, which is so striking in mammals, is yet to be found for higher frequency. The default explanation is that the coiling is just for packaging.

Consequently, the cochlea is often modeled as a straight box shown in Figure 17.2, which includes the minimum essential mechanical features. The box is filled with fluid, with mechanical properties close to water. The box is divided into two fluid chambers by a partition, a portion of which, the *basilar membrane* (BM), is thin and tapered. At the left end, representing the basal end of the cochlea, is a piston, the *stapes*, through which sound pressure is applied to the upper fluid chamber. Since the walls

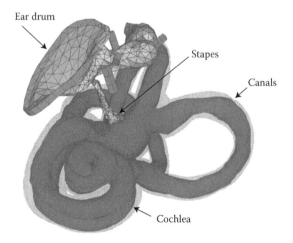

FIGURE 17.1 Finite element model of middle ear, vestibular apparatus, and cochlea. The mesh is generated from a micro-CT image of a human temporal bone.

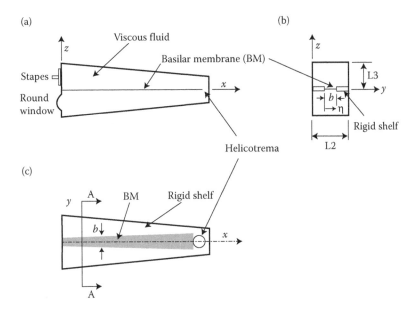

FIGURE 17.2 The standard straight box model of the cochlear with the organ of Corti removed. The Cartesian coordinates {x, y, z} represent the distance from the stapes, the distance across the scala width, and the height above the partition, respectively. (a) Side, (b) cross section (A–A), and (c) top views.

are stiff bone and the fluid is nearly incompressible, there is a relief window, the *round window* (RW), at the basal end of the lower fluid region. At the right end, representing the apex of the cochlea, there is a hole in the partition, the helicotrema, so fluid can flow between the two chambers without obstruction. With realistic physical values for the BM dimensions and elasticity, this box model yields rather good agreement with the cochlear response.

17.1.1 Components

Figure 17.3 shows some details of the BM and the organ of Corti. The partition shown in Figure 17.3 consists of three segments: on the one side, the *bony shelf* (or *primary spiral osseous lamina*), in the middle, the BM, and on the other side, a thick support (*spiral ligament*). A second partition (not shown) is the *Reissner's membrane*, attached at one side above the edge of the bony shelf and attached at the other side to the wall of the cochlea. *Scala media* is the region between the Reissner's membrane and the BM, and is filled with *endolymphatic fluid*. This fluid has an ionic content similar to intracellular fluid, high in potassium and low in sodium, but with a resting positive electrical potential of around +80 mV. The electrical potential is supplied by the *stria vascularis* on the wall in scala media. The region above the Reissner's membrane is *scala vestibuli*, and the region below the main partition is *scala tympani*. Scala vestibuli and scala tympani are connected at the apical end of the cochlea by the *helicotrema*, and are filled with *perilymphatic fluid*. This fluid is similar to extracellular fluid, low in potassium and high in sodium with zero electrical potential. Distributed along the scala media side of the BM is the sensory epithelium, the *organ of Corti*. This contains one row of *inner hair cells* and three rows of *outer hair cells*. In humans, each row contains about 4000 cells. Each of the inner hair cells has about 20 afferent synapses; these are considered to be the primary receptors. In comparison, the outer hair cells are sparsely innervated but have both afferent (5%) and efferent (95%) synapses.

The BM is divided into two sections. Connected to the edge of the bony shelf, on the left in Figure 17.3, is the *arcuate zone,* consisting of a single layer of transverse fibers. Connected to the edge of the spiral

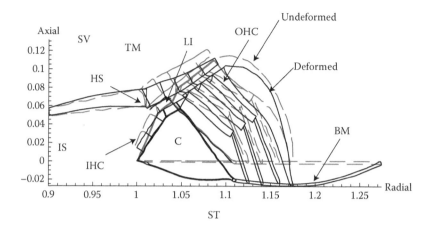

FIGURE 17.3 Shell model for the cross section of cochlea with the organ of Corti in the guinea pig apex (*y–z* plane). The dashed lines show the undeformed configuration, while the solid lines show the deformed configuration due to static pressure loading toward ST, greatly amplified. The radial and axial distances are in millimeters. SV, scala vestibule; ST, scala tympani; IS, inner sulcus; C, cortilymph; TM, tectorial membrane; IP, inner pillar; OP, outer pillar; BM, basilar membrane; IHC, inner hair cells; OHC, outer hair cells; HS, Hensen's stripe; L1, sub-tectorial membrane fluid region. The OHC stereocilia are sheared by the motion of the pillars of Corti and reticular lamina relative to the TM. The basilar membrane is supported on the left by the bony shelf and on the right by the spiral ligament. The IHC are the primary receptors, each with about 20 afferent synapses. The IC is a fluid region in contact with the IHC stereocilia.

ligament, on the right in Figure 17.3, is the *pectinate zone,* consisting of a double layer of transverse fibers in an amorphous ground substance. The *arches of Corti* form a truss over the arcuate zone, which consist of two rows of *pillar cells*. The foot of the inner pillar is attached at the point of connection of the bony shelf to the arcuate zone, while the foot of the outer pillar cell is attached at the common border of the arcuate zone and pectinate zone. The heads of the inner and outer pillars are connected and form the support point for the *reticular lamina*. The other edge of the reticular lamina is attached to the top of *Henson cells,* which have bases connected to the BM. The inner hair cells are attached on the bony shelf side of the inner pillars, while the three rows of outer hair cells are attached to the reticular lamina. The region bounded by the inner pillar cells, the reticular lamina, the Henson cells, and the BM forms another fluid region. This fluid is considered to be perilymph since it appears that ions can flow freely through the arcuate zone of the BM. The stereocilia of the hair cells protrude into the endolymph. Thus, the outer hair cells are immersed in perilymph at 0 mV, have an intracellular potential of −70 mV, and have stereocilia at the upper surface immersed in endolymph at a potential of +80 mV. In some regions of the ears of some vertebrates (Freeman and Weiss 1990), the stereocilia are freestanding. However, mammals always have a *tectorial membrane,* originating near the edge of the bony shelf and overlying the rows of hair cells parallel to the reticular lamina. The tallest rows of stereocilia of the outer hair cells are attached to the tectorial membrane. Under the tectorial membrane and inside the inner hair cells is a fluid space, the *inner sulcus,* filled with endolymph. The stereocilia of the inner hair cells are not attached to the overlying tectorial membrane, so the motion of the fluid in the inner sulcus must provide the mechanical input to these primary receptor cells. Since the inner sulcus is found only in mammals, the fluid motion in this region generated by acoustic input may be crucial to high-frequency discrimination capability.

With a few exceptions of specialization, the dimensions of all the components in the cross section of the mammalian cochlea change smoothly and slowly along the length, in a manner consistent with high stiffness at the base, or input end, and low stiffness at the apical end. For example, in the cat, the BM width increases from 0.1 to 0.4 mm while the thickness of the fiber layers decreases from 13 to 5 μm.

TABLE 17.1   Typical Values and Estimates for Young's Modulus E

Compact bone	20	GPa
Keratin	3	GPa
Basilar membrane fibers	1.9	GPa
Microtubules	1.2	GPa
Actin	1	GPa
Collagen	1	GPa
Reissner's membrane	60	MPa
Red blood cell, extended (assuming thickness = 10 nm)	45	MPa
Rubber, elastin	4	MPa
Basilar membrane ground substance	200	kPa
Tectorial membrane	30	kPa
Jell-O	3	kPa
Henson's cells	1	kPa

The density of transverse collagen fibers decreases more than the thickness, from about 6000 fibers per µm at the base to 500 fibers per µm at the apex (Cabezudo 1978).

17.1.2 Material Properties

Both the perilymph and the endolymph have the viscosity and density of water. The bone of the wall and the bony shelf appear to be similar to a compact bone, with a density approximately twice that of water. The remaining components of the cochlea are a soft tissue with a density near to that of water. The stiffnesses of the components vary over a wide range, as indicated by the values of the Young's modulus listed in Table 17.1. These values are taken directly or estimated from many sources, including the stiffness measurements in the cochlea by Békésy (1960), Gummer et al. (1981), Strelioff and Flock (1984), Miller (1985), Zwislocki and Cefaratti (1989), and Olson and Mountain (1994).

17.2 Passive Models

The anatomy of the cochlea is complex. By modeling, one attempts to isolate and understand the essential features. The following is an indication of proposition and controversy associated with a few such models.

17.2.1 Resonators

The ancient Greeks suggested that the ear consisted of a set of tuned resonant cavities. As each component in the cochlea was discovered subsequently, it was proposed to be the tuned resonator. The most well-known resonance theory is by Helmholtz. According to this theory, the transverse fibers of the BM are under tension and respond like the strings of a piano. The short strings at the base respond to high frequencies and the long strings toward the apex respond to low frequencies. The important feature of the Helmholtz theory is the *place principle,* according to which the receptor cells at a certain *place* along the cochlea are stimulated by a certain frequency. Thus, the cochlea provides a real-time frequency separation (Fourier analysis) of any complex sound input. This aspect of the Helmholtz theory has since been validated, since each of the some 30,000 fibers exiting the cochlea in the auditory nerve is sharply tuned to a particular frequency. A basic difficulty with such a resonance theory is that sharp tuning requires small damping, which is associated with a long ringing after the excitation ceases. Yet the cochlea is remarkable for combining sharp tuning with short time delay for the onset of reception and the same short time delay for the cessation of reception. A particular problem with the

Helmholtz theory arises from the equation for the resonant frequency for a plate consisting of a set of unidirectional fibers (strings) under tension:

$$f = \frac{1}{2b}\sqrt{\frac{T}{\rho_p h}} \tag{17.1}$$

where T is the tensile force per unit width, ρ_p is the density of the plate, b is the length, and h is the thickness of the plate. In man, the frequency range over which the cochlea operates is $f = 200$–$20{,}000$ Hz, a factor of 100, while the change in length b is only a factor of 5 and the thickness of the BM h varies the wrong way by a factor of 2 or so. Thus, to produce the necessary range of frequency, the tension T would have to vary by a factor of about 800. In fact, the spiral ligament, which would supply such tension, varies in area by a factor of only 10.

Instead of the plate under tension, it is better to consider the *bending stiffness* of the BM with the mass from inviscid fluid on both sides. The resonant frequency is

$$f = \frac{1}{2\pi}\sqrt{\frac{4k}{\pi\rho}} \tag{17.2}$$

where ρ is the density of the fluid and k is the volume stiffness (pressure divided by area displacement) of the plate. For a plate with simply supported edges, we have

$$k = \frac{120 c_f EI}{b^5} \approx \frac{10 c_f E t^3}{b^5} \tag{17.3}$$

where c_f is the volume fraction of fibers, E is the Young's modulus, t is the thickness, and b is the width. For a frequency of 1000 Hz, Equation 17.2 indicates the stiffness of $k = 3 \times 10^{10}$ N/m^5, which is within an order of magnitude of values given by Békésy (1960, Figure 12-37) for chicken, mouse, rat, guinea pig, and cow (but not for elephant, which has the specialization of a porous bony shelf). The measurement was on *ex vivo* preparations and it was difficult (no one has attempted to repeat it), and his measured stiffness along the cochlea varies over three orders of magnitude. Consequently, the agreement with Equation 17.2 is considered as reasonable, so Equations 17.2 and 17.3 can be used for an approximation for the location of the maximum amplitude for a given frequency, the best frequency for a point (BF). Table 17.2 shows values at the base and apex of the guinea pig cochlea. The frequency from the tension model (Equation 17.1) and from the bending model (Equations 17.2 and 17.3) show the effectiveness of the bending. For modest ratios of geometry, the variation in frequency is a factor of 400. Of course, in the cochlea, the BF from Equations 17.2 and 17.3 marks not a resonance but rather a transition region.

TABLE 17.2   Frequency Range Capability of BM Pectinate Zone (for Guinea Pig) for Bending Stiffness and Tension Stiffness

	Base	Apex	Ratio
Elastic modulus E	1 GPa	1 GPa	1
BM fiber volume fraction c_f	0.08	0.01	7
BM width b	80 μm	180 μm	0.44
BM fiber layer thickness t	7 μm	1 μm	7
Spiral ligament width c	200 μm	40 μm	5
Frequency tension	247 Hz	130 Hz	1.9
Frequency bending	52,000 Hz	130 Hz	400

17.2.2 Traveling Waves

No theory predicted the actual behavior found in the cochlea in 1928 by Békésy (1960). He observed *traveling waves* moving along the cochlea from the base toward the apex, which have a maximum amplitude at a certain place for a given frequency. The place depends on the frequency, as in the Helmholtz theory, but the amplitude envelope in not very localized. In Békésy's experimental models, and in subsequent mathematical and experimental models, the anatomy of the cochlea is greatly simplified. The coiling, Reissner's membrane, and the organ of Corti are all ignored, so the cochlea is treated as a straight tube with a single partition (Figure 17.2). (An exception is in Fuhrmann et al. 1987.) The gradient in the BM stiffness gives beautiful traveling waves in both experimental and mathematical models.

17.2.3 One-Dimensional Model

A majority of work has been based on the assumption that the fluid motion is one-dimensional (1D). With this simplification, the governing equations are similar to those for an electrical transmission line and for the long wavelength response of an elastic tube containing fluid. The equation for the pressure p in a tube with constant cross-sectional area A and with constant frequency of excitation is

$$\frac{d^2 p}{d^2 x} + \frac{2\rho\omega^2}{AK} p = 0 \tag{17.4}$$

where x is the distance along the tube, and K is the generalized partition stiffness, equal to the net pressure divided by the displaced area of the cross section. The factor of 2 accounts for fluid on both sides of the elastic partition. Often, K is represented in the form of a single-degree-of-freedom oscillator

$$K = k + i\omega d - m\omega^2 \tag{17.5}$$

where k is the static stiffness, d is the damping, and m is the mass density

$$m = \rho_P \frac{h}{b} \tag{17.6}$$

A good approximation is to treat the pectinate zone of the BM as transverse beams with simply supported edges, for which Equation 17.2 gives the stiffness. The solution of Equation 17.4 can be obtained by numerical or asymptotic (called Wentzel-Kramers-Brillouin (WKB) or combined local-global (CLG)) methods. The result is traveling waves for which the amplitude of the BM displacement builds to a maximum and then rapidly diminishes. The parameters of K are adjusted to obtain an agreement with the measurements of the dynamic response in the cochlea. Often, all the material of the organ of Corti is assumed to be rigidly attached to the BM so that h is relatively large and the effect of mass m is large. Then, the maximum response is near the *in vacua* resonance of the partition given by

$$\omega^2 = \frac{bp}{h\rho} \tag{17.7}$$

The following are the objections to the 1D model (e.g., Siebert 1974): (1) The solutions of Equation 17.4 show wavelengths of response in the region of maximum amplitude that are small in comparison with the size of the cross section, violating the basic assumption of 1D fluid flow. (2) In the drained cochlea, Békésy (1960) observed no resonance of the partition, so there is no significant partition mass. The significant mass is entirely from the fluid and therefore Equation 17.7 is not correct. This is consistent with the observations of experimental models. (3) In model studies by Békésy (1960) and others, the localization of response is independent of the area A of the cross section. Thus, Equation 17.4 cannot govern the most interesting part of the response, the region near the maximum amplitude for a given frequency BF. (4) Mechanical and neural measurements in the cochlea show dispersion, which is incompatible with the 1D model (Lighthill 1991). (5) The 1D model fails badly in comparison with experimental measurements in models for which the parameters of geometry, stiffness, viscosity, and density are known. Nevertheless, the simplicity of Equation 17.4 and the analogy with the transmission line have made the 1D model popular. We note that there is interest in utilizing the principles in an analog model built on a silicon chip because of the high performance of the actual cochlea. Watts (1993) reports on the first model with an electrical analog of 2D fluid in the scali. An observation is that the transmission line hardware models are sensitive to failure of one component, while the two-dimensional (2D) model is not. In experimental models, Békésy found that a hole at one point in the membrane had little effect on the response at other points.

17.2.4 Two-Dimensional Model

The pioneering work with 2D fluid motion was begun in 1931 by Ranke, as reported in Ranke (1950) and discussed by Siebert (1974). Analysis of 2D and 3D fluid motion without the *a priori* assumption of long or short wavelengths and for physical values of all parameters is discussed by Steele (1987). The first of the two major benefits derived from the 2D model is the allowance of short-wavelength behavior, that is, the variation in fluid displacement and pressure in the duct height direction. Localized fluid motion near the elastic partition generally occurs near the point of maximum amplitude and the exact value of A becomes immaterial. The second major benefit of a 2D model is the admission of a stiffness-dominated elastic partition (i.e., massless) that better approximates the physiological properties of the BM. The two benefits together address all the objections the 1D model discussed previously. 2D models start with the Navier–Stokes and continuity equations governing the fluid motion, and an anisotropic plate equation governing the elastic partition motion. The displacement potential φ for the incompressible and inviscid fluid must satisfy Laplace's equation:

$$\varphi_{,xx} + \varphi_{,zz} = 0 \tag{17.8}$$

where x is the distance along the partition, z is the distance perpendicular to the partition, and the subscripts with commas denote partial derivatives. The displacement components and pressure are

$$u = \varphi_{,x} \quad w = \varphi_{,z} \quad p = \rho\omega^2\varphi \tag{17.9}$$

The traveling wave solution is assumed in the WKB form:

$$\varphi(x,z,t) \approx \Psi(x)\frac{\cosh n(z-H)}{-n\sinh nH}e^{i\theta} \quad \theta = \omega t - \int_0^x n(x)dx \tag{17.10}$$

where θ is the phase, n is the local wave number, Ψ is the "amplitude" function, and H is the height of the fluid chamber. We use the method of Whitham (Jimenez and Whitham 1976) to obtain the wave number and amplitude function, which has been used on the cochlea (e.g., Taber and Steele 1979, Yoon et al. 2009). Lagrangean density is the difference in the kinetic and potential energy densities:

$$\Lambda = T - V = \rho b \int_0^H (\varphi_{,x}^2 + \varphi_{,z}^2)\,dz - \frac{1}{2}k(bw)^2 \tag{17.11}$$

The kinetic energy is doubled for fluid on both sides of the BM. With the assumed form of Equation 17.10, the time-averaged value becomes

$$\Lambda = \Psi^2(x)F(n,x) \quad F(n,x) = \frac{b}{2}\left(\frac{2\rho\omega^2}{n\tanh nH} - kb \right) \tag{17.12}$$

Then the variational problem yields the Euler equations:

$$\frac{\partial\Lambda}{\partial\Psi} = 0 \tag{17.13}$$

The solution of Equation 17.13 is just

$$F(n,x) = \frac{b}{2}\left(\frac{2\rho\omega^2}{n\tanh nH} - kb \right) = 0 \tag{17.14}$$

which is the eikonal equation, or local dispersion relation. The second Euler equation is

$$\left(\frac{\partial\Lambda}{\partial\theta_{,x}} \right)_{,x} = 0 \tag{17.15}$$

which gives the relation for the amplitude function Ψ:

$$\Psi^2(x)F_{,n}(n,x) = \text{constant} \tag{17.16}$$

For a given frequency, Equation 17.14 must be solved numerically for the wave number n at each point x. The stiffness k, height of the fluid chamber H, and width of the BM b all vary slowly with the distance x. For physiological values of the parameters, the stiffness is large at the stapes $x = 0$, and becomes small toward the apex. Consequently, the wave number is small at the stapes (long wavelength) and becomes large (i.e., short wavelength) as x increases. For small values of the wave number $nH = 1$, the results, Equations 17.14 and 17.16, reduce to the 1D problem, Equation 17.4.

17.2.4.1 Fluid Viscosity

The fluid viscosity is important. There is a viscous boundary layer that is generally smaller than the width of the BM. Taking this into account yields the modified eikonal equation:

$$F(n,x) = \frac{b}{2}\left(\frac{2\rho\omega^2}{n\left[\tanh nH - (1 + (i\omega\rho/\mu n^2))^{-1/2} \right]} - kb \right) = 0 \tag{17.17}$$

where μ is the fluid viscosity. The viscous term produces a small imaginary part of the wave number. This has little effect in the long wavelength region and the location of the peak amplitude, but causes a rapid decrease of the wave amplitude past the peak.

17.2.5 Three-Dimensional Model

A further improvement in the agreement with experimental models can be obtained by adding the component of fluid motion in the direction across the membrane for a full 3D model. The importance

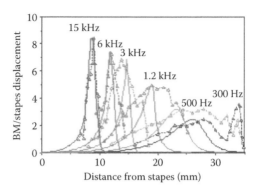

FIGURE 17.4 Comparison of 3D model calculations (solid curves) with experimental results of Zhou et al. (1994) (dashed curves) for the amplitude envelopes for different frequencies. This is the first life-sized model, but with an isotropic BM and fluid viscosity 28 times that of water. The agreement is reasonable for the higher frequencies but rough for the lower frequencies.

of the third dimension is discussed by Kolston (2000). The solution by direct numerical means is computationally intensive, and was first carried out by Raftenberg (1990), who reports a portion of his results for the fluid motion around the organ of Corti. Böhnke et al. (1996) used FE for the most accurate description to date of the structure of the organ of Corti. However, the fluid is not included and only a restricted segment of the cochlea is considered. Both the inviscid fluid and the details of the structure are considered with a simplified element description and simplified geometry by Kolston and Ashmore (1996). Today, a number of laboratories have the capability for treating the actual geometry obtained from micro-CT scans such as shown in Figure 17.1. However, the viscosity of the fluid is not considered, which reduces the computing time with standard FE programs to a reasonable value. Givelberg and Bunn (2003) provide the first numerical solution for a coiled box model with viscous fluid, using forward integration in time. Cheng et al. (2008) use a modified FE approach for the straight box model also with viscous fluid. Computer times are given in hours for the linear response for a single frequency.

An efficient approach for computing the 3D viscous fluid motion is offered by the asymptotic WKB solution, which yields results for computer times of 1 s per frequency. The procedure is the same as for the 2D analysis, except that 10–40 harmonics of motion in the *y*-direction in Figure 17.2 are added. The best verification of the mathematical model and calculation procedure comes from comparison with measurements in experimental models for which the parameters are known (Taber and Steele 1979). Zhou et al. (1994) provide the first life-sized experimental model, designed to be similar to the human cochlea, but with a fluid viscosity 28 times that of water to facilitate optical imaging. Results are shown in Figures 17.4 and 17.5. An improved life-sized model is by White and Grosh (2005), which has fluid on one side of the BM. Fluid is on both sides of the life-sized model by Wittbrodt et al. (2006), and a good agreement was found between the WKB calculation and the experimental measurements. In that model, polyimide is used for the BM, with a layer of 9000 transverse aluminum ribs to achieve a semblance of the orthotropic construction of the actual BM.

As shown by Taber and Steele (1979), the 3D fluid motion has a significant effect on the pressure distribution. This is confirmed by the measurements by Olson (1998) for the pressure at different depths in the cochlea, which show a substantial increase near the partition.

17.3 Active Process

Before around 1980, it was thought that the processing may have two levels. Initially, the BM and the fluid provide the correct place for a given frequency (a purely mechanical "first filter"). Subsequently, the

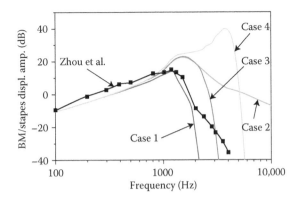

FIGURE 17.5 Comparison of 3D model calculations with experimental results of Zhou et al. (1994) for amplitude at the place $x = 19$ mm as a function of frequency. The scales are logarithmic (20 dB is a factor of 10 in amplitude). Case 1 shows a direct comparison with the physical parameters of the experiment, with isotropic BM and viscosity 28 times that of water. Case 2 is computed for the viscosity reduced to that of water. Case 3 is computed for the BM made of transverse fibers. Case 4 shows the effect of active OHC feed-forward, with the pressure gain $\alpha = 0.21$ and feed-forward distance $\Delta x = 25$ μm. Thus, lower viscosity, BM orthotropy, and active feed-forward all contribute to higher amplitude and increased localization of the response.

micromechanics and electrochemistry in the organ of Corti, with possible neural interactions, perform a further sharpening (a physiologically vulnerable "second filter").

A hint that the two-filter concept had difficulties was in the measurements of Rhode (1971), who found significant nonlinear behavior of the BM in the region of the maximum amplitude at moderate amplitudes of tone intensity. Passive models cannot explain this, since the usual mechanical nonlinearities are significant only at very high intensities, that is, at the threshold of pain. Russell and Sellick (1977) made the first *in vivo* mammalian intracellular hair cell recordings and found that the cells are as sharply tuned as the nerve fibers. Subsequently, improved measurement techniques in several laboratories found that the BM is actually as sharply tuned as the hair cells and the nerve fibers. Thus, the sharp tuning occurs at the BM. No passive cochlear model, even with physically unreasonable parameters, has yielded amplitude and phase response similar to such measurements. Measurements in a damaged or dead cochlea show a response similar to that of a passive model. Further evidence for an active process comes from Kemp (1978), who discovered that sound pulses into the ear caused echoes coming from the cochlea at delay times corresponding to the travel time to the place for the frequency and back. Spontaneous emission of sound energy from the cochlea has now been measured in the external ear canal in all vertebrates (Probst 1990). Some of the emissions can be related to the hearing disability of tinnitus (ringing in the ear). The conclusion drawn from these discoveries is that normal hearing involves an active process in which the energy of the input sound is greatly enhanced. A widely accepted concept is that spontaneous emission of sound energy occurs when the local amplifiers are not functioning properly and enter some sort of limit cycle (Zweig and Shera 1995). However, there remains a doubt about the nature of this process (Allen and Neely 1992, Hudspeth 1989, Nobili et al. 1998).

17.3.1 Outer Hair Cell Electromotility

The hair cell is covered extensively elsewhere in this book. Here, we mention a few important points. Since the outer hair cells have sparse afferent innervation, they have long been suspected of serving a basic motor function, perhaps beating and driving the subtectorial membrane fluid. Nevertheless, it was surprising when Brownell et al. (1985) found that the outer hair cells have *electromotility:* The cell expands and contracts in an oscillating electric field, either extra- or intracellular. The electromotility exists at frequencies far higher than possible for normal contractile mechanisms (Ashmore 1987). The sensitivity is about 20 nm/mV (about 10^5 better than PZT-2, a widely used piezoelectric ceramic). The motility is due to the presence of the protein prestin in the outer hair cell (OHC) plasma membrane, and found nowhere else in the body. Frank et al. (1999) find in the constrained cell that the ratio of axial force generation to transmembrane voltage is constant to nearly 80 kHz. However, it is established that the intracellular voltage change due to the displacement of the stereocilia drops off at a low frequency. Ashmore (2008) provides a comprehensive summary of the topic.

17.3.2 Hair Bundle Transduction Process

A displacement of the stereociliary bundle on a hair cell in the excitatory direction causes an opening of ion channels in the stereocilia, which in turn decreases the intracellular potential. This depolarization causes neural excitation, and in the piezoelectric OHC, a decrease of the cell length. However, in nonmammalian vertebrates, there is no prestin and no electromotility of hair cells. Furthermore, it is well established that the hair bundle can go into spontaneous oscillation. Thus, the resonance of the hair bundle itself can supply energy into the motion. This enhances the reception for sounds of low amplitude. Spontaneous and evoked emissions are similar in character to those from mammalian ears.

Schwander et al. (2010) survey the recent advances in understanding the hair bundle particularly related to the genes linked to deafness. They suggest that both hair bundle motility and somatic electromotility may be needed for mammalian hearing. From a different perspective, Peng and Ricci (2010) also come to this conclusion. It is clear from Dallos et al. (2008) that prestin, which causes the OHC motility, is necessary for normal mammalian hearing. How this operates for high frequencies has been the subject of numerous investigations, including the consideration of the extracellular electrical field by Dallos and Evans (1995), and theoretical treatment of detail of the stereocilia by consideration of Breneman et al. (2009).

17.4 Active Models

De Boer (1991), Geisler (1993), and Hubbard (1993) discuss models in which the electromotility of the outer hair cells feeds energy into the BM. The partition stiffness K is expanded from Equation 17.3 into a transfer function, containing a number of parameters and delay times. These are classed as phenomenological models, for which the physiological basis of the parameters is not of primary concern. The displacement gain may be defined as the ratio of stereociliary shearing displacement to cell expansion. For these models, the gain used is larger by orders of magnitude than the maximum found in laboratory measurements of isolated hair cells.

17.4.1 Push-Forward/Pull-Backward Active Model

Another approach (Steele et al. 1993, Geisler and Sang 1995) appears promising. Because of the inclinations, the OHC, the phalangeal process (PhP), and the reticular lamina form a stiff triangular structure, connected to the BM by Deiters rod (D), as seen in Figure 17.6a. As indicated in Figure 17.6b, a downward force on the BM at the distance x from the stapes causes a shear on the stereocilia at that point. Through the transduction process, the OHC expands, but because of the inclination of the OHC, the push down on the BM occurs at the distance $x + \Delta x_1$. This is the "push-forward" or the "positive feed-forward."

The force of OHC expansion is equal and opposite at the cell ends. The cantilever arrangement of the reticular lamina and the tectorial membrane provides little resistance to this upward force. All that remains to carry this force is the upper end of the PhP. In Figure 17.6b, the shear of the OHC at $x + \Delta x_2$ causes a tension in the PhP connected at that point and an upward force on D located at $x + \Delta x_1$. This is the "pull-backward" or the "negative feed backward." So, the expansion of an OHC causes the push down at the distance Δx_1 in the forward (apical) direction and a pull up at the distance $\Delta x_2 - \Delta x_1$ in the

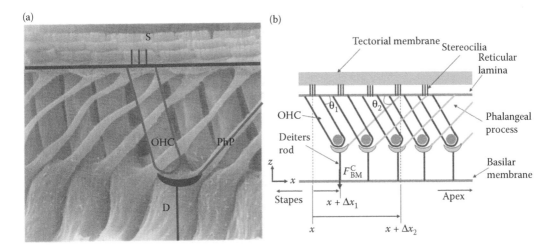

FIGURE 17.6 Scanning electron micrograph (SEM) of the longitudinal view of organ of Corti of the mole rat cochlea (Raphael et al. 1991). Outer hair cell, Deiters cell, phalangeal process, and stereocilia are labeled as OHC, D, PhP, and S, respectively (a). Schematic of the longitudinal view of the organ of Corti (b), showing the tilt of the outer hair cells (OHC) based on SEM image. For one hair cell whose apex lies at a distance x, the base is located at distance $x + \Delta x_1$, while the phalangeal process connected to the base of the hair cell is attached to the upper surface of the reticular lamina at $x + \Delta x_2$. θ_1: the OHC angle with respect to reticular lamina, θ_2: the phalangeal process angle with respect to the reticular laminar. The force on the BM through the Deiters rod is F_{BM}^C, which consists of the downward push due to an expansion of the hair cell at x and an upward pull through the phalangeal process due to an expansion of the hair cell at $x + \Delta x_2$.

backward (basal) direction. There is also a ripple effect, extending in both directions, but we consider only the primary push and pull. Of course, for the response for a given frequency, all the quantities vary sinusoidally, so we refer to this as feed-forward/backward.

The total force acting on the BM (F_{BM}) is twice the fluid force (F_{BM}^f), for fluid on both sides of the BM, plus the OHC force acting through the Deiters rods F_{BM}^C.

$$F_{BM} = 2F_{BM}^f + F_{BM}^C \tag{17.18}$$

The fluid force is the same as for the 3D passive box model. For small amplitudes, the transduction and OHC motility are linear, so the cell force is proportional to the total force on the BM. Thus, the cell force acting on the BM at the point $x + \Delta x_1$ in Figure 17.6b depends on the total force on the BM at x and the total force acting on the BM at $x + \Delta x_2$, as expressed by the difference equation:

$$F_{BM}^C(x + \Delta x_1, t) = \alpha_1 \left[F_{BM}(x,t) \right] - \alpha_2 \left[F_{BM}(x + \Delta x_2, t) \right] \tag{17.19}$$

The constants of proportionality or "gains" from the OHC push and the PhP pull are α_1 and α_2, respectively. The details of OC compliance, OHC transduction, and motility are all lumped into the gains. Because of the small resistance to the vertical force of the reticular lamina and tectorial membrane, the net push and pull must be equal, so $\alpha_1 = \alpha_2 = \alpha$.

With the WKB approximation, all quantities are in the form of an exponential multiplied by a slowly varying function (Equation 17.10). Therefore, the spatial difference can be approximated as

$$F_{BM}^C(x + \Delta x_1, t) = F_{BM}^C(x,t) e^{-in\Delta x_1} \tag{17.20}$$

This is valid when the (complex) wavenumber n does not change significantly in the distance Δx_1. Therefore, the relations Equations 17.18 and 17.19 reduce to

$$F_{BM} = 2F_{BM}^f + F_{BM}^C = \frac{2F_{BM}^f}{1 - \alpha_1 e^{in\Delta x_1} + \alpha_2 e^{-in(\Delta x_2 - \Delta x_1)}} \qquad (17.21)$$

Thus, the box model in Figure 17.2 is used, with the elaborate OC shown in Figures 17.3 and 17.6 represented by the simple terms in the denominator of Equation 17.21. This denominator multiplies the denominator of the fluid term in Equation 17.17 for the 2D model and the equivalent for the 1D or 3D models.

The power series expansion of the denominator of Equation 17.21 is

$$1 - \alpha e^{in\Delta x_1} + \alpha e^{-in(\Delta x_2 - \Delta x_1)} = 1 - \alpha in\Delta x_2 + \cdots \qquad (17.22)$$

which shows that the feed-forward/backward effect is negligible for long wavelengths, when $n\Delta x_2$ is very small. Since the fluid loading in Equation 17.17 is primarily mass-like, the first effect for shorter wavelength in Equation 17.22 is negative damping. For a reversed traveling wave, with n negative, the effect is an increase in the damping.

The full behavior is not transparent from Equation 17.21 but can be seen from the numerical results. For modest values of the gain, $\alpha < 0.2$, the real part of n, which gives the phase, is little affected by the push–pull terms. The imaginary part of n can be substantially modified. Generally, it is determined by the viscosity of the fluid and causes the rapid decrease in amplitude in the region past the maximum response. However, the push–pull terms of Equation 17.21 can overcome the viscosity effect and a region near "best frequency" (BF), where the sign of the imaginary part of n is reversed, that is, a region of "negative damping." Apically, the fluid viscosity resumes dominance and the amplitude decreases exponentially. So, for a given frequency, the push–pull is negligible for a long wavelength (small n) and a very short wavelength (large n) but very significant for a band of wavelengths near BF.

The feed-forward/backward model for the OC involves just the three parameters. Reasonable values for the distances Δx_1 and Δx_2 are used, while the gain α is adjusted for a best fit with the experiments.

The comparison of the 3D calculations and measurements for the (passive) life-sized model in the configuration of Figure 17.2 are shown in Figure 17.4. Various modifications are shown in Figure 17.5 for the frequency response at a particular point. Case 1 is for the experimental situation of an isotropic BM and high fluid viscosity. In Case 2, the viscosity is reduced to that of water, which causes a shift of the peak response to a higher frequency and an increase in peak amplitude. Case 3 shows the effect of reducing the longitudinal stiffness of the BM to zero, corresponding to the transverse fibers in the actual cochlea. The peak amplitude and location do not change, but the high-frequency roll-off is substantially sharper. Finally, Case 4 shows the effect of adding just the feed-forward term of Equation 17.20. The peak amplitude increases by an order of magnitude and the location shifts by an octave, but the high-frequency roll-off remains the same.

A comparison with measurements in the chinchilla cochlea is shown in Figure 17.7, modified from Narayan et al. (1998). In the box model representation of Figure 17.2, the BM properties of width, thickness, elastic modulus, and fiber volume fraction are taken as close as possible to the actual values for the BM pectinate zone. In Figure 17.7a, the amplitude of the BM velocity is normalized to the stapes velocity. So, for a linear system, the response would be independent of input amplitude. Instead, the measured response for a low sound pressure of 20 dB is greater than that for a high sound pressure of 80 dB by two orders of magnitude. This amplification occurs in a narrow frequency band near BF and is due to the active process. When the animal dies, the passive response is close to that for 80 dB. Thus, the active process greatly enhances the response for low sound intensity and is negligible for high intensity. The 3D model results are also shown in Figure 17.7, calculated with values shown in Table 17.3. The simple

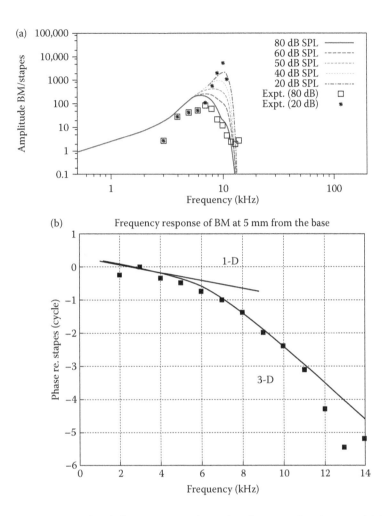

FIGURE 17.7 Experiments in chinchilla (Ruggero et al. 1997) and computed with 3D model (Lim and Steele 2002, modified by Yoon). (a) Amplitude of BM displacement and (b) phase response. The amplitude is normalized to the stapes displacement. Experimental points are shown for 20 and 80 dB SPL. The active process increases the relative amplitude for low-input sound levels.

TABLE 17.3 Properties for Chinchilla Cochlea

Length of the cochlea (mm)	18	Fiber volume fraction (%)	3~0.7
Stapes footplate area (mm²)	0.7	OHC angle (θ_1)	75°
SV area (mm²) (base to apex)	0.6–0.2	Phalangeal process angle (θ_2)	22°
Length of outer hair cell (μm)	25–65	Gain factor (α) for 20 dB SPL	0.11
BM width (mm)	0.15–0.48	Distance from the stapes (x^*) in mm	4
BM thickness (μm)	3–1	Passive best frequency (BF)	7 kHz

push–pull approximation in Equation 17.21 does well in simulating the measurements. The gain varies from 0 for the high intensity to 0.11 for 20 dB. Both the push and the pull are included, which gives a shift of about half an octave of the passive peak to the active, similar to the measurements.

The question remains about how the motion of the BM is transferred to the excitation of the IHC. A remarkable result is by Narayan et al. (1998), who measured the auditory nerve fiber threshold and the BM response in one animal. From the BM measurements, they then determined the fixed amplitude of BM

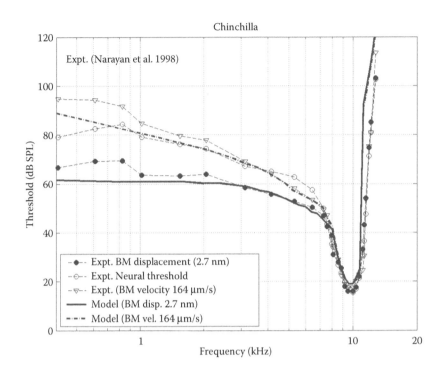

FIGURE 17.8 Comparisons of auditory nerve fiber neural threshold with BM velocity and displacement for chinchilla. The threshold curve for one fiber (open circles connected by a thin solid line) is compared to constant-amplitude BM displacement and velocity reponses as measured in one animal by Narayan et al. (1998). The calculations for the displacement and velocity response of the feed-forward/backward model (thick solid lines and thick dash-dotted lines, respectively) are close to the measurements.

displacement and velocity that most closely matched the auditory nerve threshold. The results are shown in Figure 17.8. The constant BM velocity is close to the neural threshold. Added to Figure 17.8 are the results from the 3D model calculation for constant BM displacement and velocity, which are in good agreement with the measurements. Since the stereocilia of the IHC in Figure 17.3 are not attached to the overlying tectorial membrane, the cells must be excited by the fluid motion. The drag force is due to the fluid velocity. Thus, it is not surprising that there is a better relation of BM velocity, rather than displacement, to neural excitation. In fact, the situation is more complicated. Legan et al. (2005) found that in a mouse mutant, the OHC arrangement is perfectly normal, giving sharp tuning of the BM and normal emissions. The neural threshold is, however, elevated by 60 dB. In this mutant, only the tectorial membrane appears to be altered. In particular, the Hensen stripe that is located near the stereocilia of the IHC is missing. In addition, the outer margin of the tectorial membrane is also missing. Therefore, the proper arrangement of the tectorial membrane is necessary to deliver the proper excitation to the IHC. Steele and Puria (2005) find that the phase of IHC excitation depends on the details of stiffness and geometry of the tectorial membrane.

The significant nonlinear effect is the saturation of the active process at high amplitudes. In Figures 17.7 and 17.8, this is taken into account by letting the gain be a function of the input sound level. It is more realistic to have the gain be a function of the amplitude of the force during the cycle of motion, which introduces substantial nonlinearity (Lim and Steele 2002, 2003). This produces two-tone interaction, the generation of combination tones, and the ringing from a click excitation, all from the simple feed-forward/backward approximation of Equation 17.19. A variety of alternate considerations for the active nonlinear behavior have been proposed. In particular, Dierkes et al. (2008) show that an array of hair cell bundles can provide a substantial sharpening of the response.

17.4.2 Summary of Some Issues

Rapid development in the measurement and computational technique related to auditory biomechanics is ongoing. The following are a few of the open issues.

17.4.2.1 Bone Conduction

Hearing by bone conduction is of high clinical significance. There are many measurements showing that the volume displacements of oval and RW are exactly out of phase for air-conducted acoustic excitation. Because the fluid is nearly incompressible and the walls are stiff bone, the input inward displacement of the stapes in Figure 17.2 will cause a nearly equal volume outward displacement of the RW. All existing theories assume that this is also the case for bone-conducted sound. As shown by Békésy (1960) in models, any sort of excitation, whether through the stapes or through shaking the entire cochlea, will cause the same traveling wave. However, measurements by Stenfeld et al. (2004) indicate that this is not the case for bone conduction. Indeed, for some frequencies, the two windows are in phase. Thus, there must be compliance in the cochlea not yet explained (often referred to as a "third window") that for some reason is more significant for bone conduction.

17.4.3 Traveling Wave

The traveling wave observed in the cochlea by Békésy (1960) was not anticipated by any theoretical consideration. There remain contrary opinions, for example, Sohmer and Freeman (2004) consider their measurements as evidence against the significance of any traveling wave. The traveling wave does not occur in lizards and turtles, but most likely occurs in bird. For mammals, the evidence for the existence and importance of the traveling wave seems overwhelming. We mention the direct *in vivo* observation of waves by Ren (2002), the close relation of BM displacement and neural excitation found in the same animal by Narayan et al. (1998), and the agreement in calculations for the traveling wave and experiment for the BM motion (Figure 17.8). This issue should be at an end.

17.4.4 Motility versus Beating

In nonmammalian hearing organs, there are no pillars, Deiters cells, or inner sulcus as shown in Figure 17.3. Furthermore, the cells similar to OHCs cannot have somatic motility. Nevertheless, in the responsive frequency range, the neural tuning is as sharp as in mammals, and evoked and spontaneous emissions occur very similar to those in mammals (Manley 2006). Crawford and Fettiplace (1985) discovered that the cilia on turtle hair cells have spontaneous activity, that is, they beat without external excitation. This mechanotransducer (MET) channel phenomenon is described as a Hopf bifurcation. In all vertebrates, the cilia and transduction channels are similar. Is the energy of the active process generated by MET instability or somatic motility of the cell, or is it a combination? This is a subject of current investigation. The consensus seems to be building that both are needed for mammalian hearing (Peng and Ricci 2010, Schwander et al. 2010).

17.4.5 OHC Roll-Off

The feed-forward/backward discussed here depends on the force of motility of the OHC to be independent of frequency. However, the electrical properties of the OHC appear to be such that for a fixed amplitude of shear force on the cilia, there is a significant decrease in the intracellular potential at a frequency much less than BF. Several laboratories propose more detailed analysis of intracellular or extracellular behavior that would maintain the effect of the motility for high frequency. Dallos and Evans (1995) find that the extracellular electric field can enhance the motility for high frequency. Another consideration is the stiffness of the OHC, which Zheng et al. (2007) show plays a role. In any case, it is clear that the motility operates at high frequency. Frank et al. (1999) show that the constrained isolated OHC generates force proportional to the transmembrane voltage well past 80 kHz. Grosh et al. (2004) find in the intact guinea pig cochlea, which has an upper limit of hearing of 50 kHz, that mechanical response can be elicited by electrical signals up to 100 kHz. Dallos (2008) provides an overall perspective.

17.4.6 Tectorial Membrane Properties: Resonance?

Many authors have used OC models with a strong resonance of the tectorial membrane (TM), for example, Gummer et al. (1996). It has the effect of overcoming the OHC low-frequency roll-off problem. Several laboratories have measured the properties of the TM, including Gueta et al. (2006), Masaki et al. (2006), and Gavara and Chadwick (2009). Details are different, but the general conclusion is that the TM is a rather soft tissue, with an elastic Young's modulus in the range of 0.5–30 kPa. Different animals have a great difference in TM size. Such a difference for animals that have roughly the same frequency range makes a resonant TM seem to be an unlikely key feature. Nowotny and Gummer (2006) measure the TM response due to electrical stimulation and find no resonance for frequencies well past BF. So, there are indications that the TM does not have a strong resonance.

17.4.7 Multiple Traveling Wave Modes

The box model Figure 17.2 has the traveling wave. In addition, there is a symmetric wave with equal pressure in the fluid regions. Consequently, there is no loading of the BM, so this wave travels with the speed of sound in water. Peterson and Bogert (1950) first formulated the split of the response into the symmetric "fast" wave and asymmetric "slow" wave. The measurements of Olson (1998) confirm the presence of the slow traveling wave and the fast pressure wave in the cochlea. In the cochlea, each of the fluid spaces in the organ of Corti (Figure 17.3) can support an independent wave. Karavitaki (2002) offers measurements of motion of the fluid in the OC that support the notion of multiple waves. As discussed by de Boer (2006), recent models, for example, Mountain and Hubbard (2006), have such capability. The goal remains for a model of the OC with physically realistic geometric and stiffness properties and with 3D viscous fluid, which can simulate the environment of the cilia for all frequencies. The expectation is that additional waves in the inner sulcus (IS) and the fluid spaces of the organ of Corti do play a significant role.

17.4.8 Stiffness Change along the Cochlea

Almost every component of the cochlear cross section has been proposed at one time or another as the fundamental resonance element. Most probably agree with Békésy (1960) that the BM has the strongest stiffness gradient and is the most likely candidate. Modest variation in values of width, thickness, and fiber volume fraction of the pectinate zone work together to explain the frequency range of the Guinea Pig (GP) cochlea. The change in the volume stiffness is five orders of magnitude. The direct measurement of the GP cochlea by Békésy (1960) shows a change of three orders of magnitude, with a reasonable extrapolation to four orders of magnitude. However, Naidu and Mountain (1998) find that the point load stiffness variation is totally inadequate to explain the frequency range in gerbil. With a different preparation, Emadi et al. (2004) find much more compliance in the apical region, which seems to correspond to a reasonable frequency range. This discrepancy in the measurements from the two laboratories has not yet been explained. The gerbil has a very specialized BM. Generally, in mammals, the pectinate zone of the BM in Figure 17.3 consists of two parallel layers of collagen fibers. For gerbil, however, the lower layer is in the form of an arch. It appears that the stiffness measured by both laboratories is in the postbuckling range of this arch. The conclusion is that the soft cells covering the BM make point load or volume compliance measurements difficult to make and interpret. As is often the case, a combination of theoretical mechanics and experimental approaches is needed.

17.5 Concluding Comments

The cochlea (Figure 17.1) is a complex organ with a remarkable capability for the transduction of the input mechanical sound pressure into electrical activity of the auditory nerve fibers. The simple box model (Figure 17.2) represents the passive behavior of the cochlea. Experimental models and 3D calculations based on the physiological values for tissue properties and geometry do well in showing the development of the main traveling wave. The peak of this wave for a particular frequency corresponds to the place of most significant neural excitation. Discrete resonators have the disadvantage that low damping is required for sharp tuning, but high damping is required for quick onset and offset. In contrast, the fluid-elastic behavior of the box in Figure 17.2 provides high frequency selectivity with excellent transient response. A click as well as the onset and offset of a pure tone cause a wave that propagates along the BM with little refection from the far end. So, the basic features of localization and timing are described well by the fluid-elastic response of the box model. A variety of approximations and solution methods have been used. The focus here is on the WKB approach, which is the most efficient method for dealing with the 3D fluid-elastic interaction and has been verified by comparison with experimental models.

Adding to the passive behavior is the active process, which greatly improves the reception of low-intensity sounds for all creatures, including insects. For the mammalian cochlea, this increases the amplitude of response by two orders of magnitude and increases the sharpness of response, without having a big effect on the localization and the phase. In general consideration of dynamic systems, this may seem impossible. A key is the electromotility of the outer hair cells, which can be interpreted as a piezoelectric property of the cell plasma membrane. The active process has been the subject of intense research activity for the last 30 years. A variety of approaches have been developed to explain this phenomenon. The focus here is on the simplest model, based on the geometry of the sensory organ of Corti. This provides a spatial finite difference relation and is referred to as feed-forward/backward. This is not the same as a time delay, and provides a significant input of energy into the traveling wave without disrupting the stability. The rather complex features of the sensory organ make sense with the feed-forward/backward. However, the calculation assumes that the motility persists to frequencies at least for that of the place. How this might occur has not been resolved. Consequently, many consider that the motility may work in combination with the resonance features of the hair bundle. We anticipate that these issues may not be resolved soon.

References

Allen JB and Neely ST. 1992. Micromechanical models of the cochlea. *Phys Today* 45:40–47.

Ashmore J. 2008. Cochlear outer hair cell motility. *Physiol Rev* 88:173–210.

Ashmore JF. 1987. A fast motile response in guinea-pig outer hair cells: The cellular basis of the cochlear amplifier. *J Physiol* 388:323–347.

Békésy G von. 1960. *Experiments in Hearing*. McGraw-Hill, New York.

Böhnke F and Arnold W. 1999. 3D-finite element model of the human Cochlea including fluid-structure couplings. *ORL* 61(5):305–310.

Böhnke F, von Mikusch-Buchberg J, and Arnold W. 1996. 3D finite elemente modell des cochleären Verstärkers. *Biomedizinische Technik* 42:311–312.

Breneman KD, Brownell WE, and Rabbitt RD. 2009. Hair cell bundles: Flexoelectric motors of the inner ear. *PLoS ONE* 4(4):e5201.

Brownell WE, Bader CR, Bertrand D, and de Ribaupierre Y. 1985. Evoked mechanical responses of isolated cochlear outer hair cells. *Science* 227:194–196.

Cabezudo LM. 1978. The ultrastructure of the basilar membrane in the cat. *Acta Otolaryngol* 86:160–175.

Cheng L, White RD, and Grosh K. 2008. Three-dimensional viscous finite element formulation for acoustic fluid–structure interaction. *Comput Methods Appl Mech Eng* 197(49–50):4160–4172.

Crawford AC and Fettiplace R. 1985. The mechanical properties of ciliary bundles of turtle cochlear hair cells. *J Physiol* 364:359–79.

Dallos P. 1992. The active cochlea. *J Neurosci* 12(12):4575–4585.

Dallos P. 2008. Cochlear amplification, outer hair cells and prestin. *Curr Opin Neurobiol* 18(4):370–376.

Dallos P and Evans B. 1995. High-frequency motility of outer hair cells and the cochlear amplifier. *Science* 267:2006–2009.

Dallos P, Wu X, Cheatham MA, Gao J, Zheng J, Anderson CT, Jia S et al. 2008. Prestin-based outer hair cell motility is necessary for Mammalian cochlear amplification. *Neuron* 58(3):333–339.

de Boer E. 1991. Auditory physics. Physical principles in hearing theory. III. *Phys Rep* 203(3):126–231.

de Boer E. 2006. Cochlear activity in perspective. *Auditory Mechanisms, Processes and Models*, Eds. AL Nuttall, T Ren, P Gillespie, K Grosh, and E de Boer, World Scientific, New Jersey, pp. 393–409.

Dierkes K, Lindner B, and Jülicher F. 2008. Enhancement of sensitivity gain and frequency tuning by coupling of active hair bundles. *Proc Natl Acad Sci USA* 105(48):18669–18674.

Emadi G, Richter CP, and Dallos P. 2004. Stiffness of the gerbil basilar membrane: Radial and longitudinal variations. *J Neurophysiol* 91(1):474–488.

Evans BN and Dallos P. 1993. Stereocilia displacement induced somatic motility of cochlear outer hair cells. *Proc Natl Acad Sci* 90:8347–8391.

Frank G, Hemmert W, and Gummer AW. 1999. Limiting dynamics of high-frequency electromechanical transduction of outer hair cells. *Proc Natl Acad Sci USA* 96(8):4420–4425.

Freeman DM and Weiss TF. 1990. Hydrodynamic analysis of a two-dimensional model for micromechanical resonance of free-standing hair bundles. *Hear Res* 48:37–68.

Fuhrmann E, Schneider W, and Schultz M. 1987. Wave propagation in the cochlea (inner ear): Effects of Reissner's membrane and non-rectangular cross section. *Acta Mech* 70:15–30.

Gavara N and Chadwick RS 2009. Collagen-based mechanical anisotropy of the tectorial membrane: Implications for inter-row coupling of outer hair cell bundles. *PLoS ONE* 4(3):e4877.

Geisler CD. 1993. A realizable cochlear model using feedback from motile outer hair cells. *Hear Res* 68:253–262.

Geisler CD. 1998. *From Sound to Synapse: Physiology of the Mammalian Ear*. Oxford University Press, New York.

Geisler CD and C. Sang 1995. A cochlear model using feed-forword outer-hair-cell forces. *Hear Res* 85:132–146.

Givelberg E and Bunn J. 2003. A comprehensive three-dimensional model of the cochlea. *J Comput Phys* 191(2):377–391.

Grosh K, Zheng J, and Zou Y. 2004. High-frequency electromotile responses in the cochlea. *J Acoust Soc Am* 115(5):2178–2184.

Gueta R, Barlam D, Shneck RZ, and Rousso I. 2006. Measurement of the mechanical properties of isolated tectorial membrane using atomic force microscopy. *Proc Natl Acad Sci USA* 103(40):14790–14795.

Gulick WL, Gescheider GA, and Fresina RD 1989. *Hearing: Physiological Acoustics, Neural Coding, and Psychoacoustics*. Oxford University Press, London.

Gummer AW, Hemmert W, and Zenner HP. 1996. Resonant tectorial membrane motion in the inner ear: Its crucial role in frequency tuning. *Proc Natl Acad Sci USA* 93:8727–8732.

Gummer AW, Johnston BM, and Armstrong NJ. 1981. Direct measurements of basilar membrane stiffness in the guinea pig. *J Acoust Soc Am* 70:1298–1309.

Hubbard AE. 1993. A traveling wave-amplifier model of the cochlea. *Science* 259:68–71.

Hudspeth AJ. 1989. How the ear's works work. *Nature* 34:397–404.

Jimenez J and Whitham GB. 1976. An averaged Lagrangian method for dissipative *wavetrains, Proc R Soc Lond A* 349(1658):277–287.

Keidel WD and Neff WD (eds). 1976. *Handbook of Sensory Physiology, Volume V: Auditory System.* Springer-Verlag, Berlin.

Kemp DT. 1978. Stimulated acoustic emissions from within the human auditory system. *J Acoust Soc Am* 64:1386–1391.

Kolston PJ. 2000. The importance of phase data and model dimensionality to cochlear mechanics. *Hear Res* 145(1–2):25–36.

Kolston PJ and Ashmore JF 1996. Finite element micromechanical modeling of the cochlea in three dimensions. *J Acoust Soc Am* 99:455–467.

Karavitaki KD. 2002. Measurements and models of electrically-evoked motion in the gerbil organ of Corti. Boston University. PhD. Thesis.

Legan PK, Lukashkina VA, Goodyear RJ, Lukashkin AN, Verhoeven K, Van Camp G, Russell IJ, and Richardson GP. 2005. A deafness mutation isolates a second role for the tectorial membrane in hearing. *Nat Neurosci* 8(8):1035–1042.

Lighthill J. 1991. Biomechanics of hearing sensitivity. *J Vib Acoust* 113:1–13.

Lim KM and Steele CR. 2002. A three-dimensional nonlinear active cochlear model analyzed by the WKB-numeric method. *Hear Res* 170(1–2):190–205.

Lim KM and Steele CR. 2003. Response suppression and transient behavior in a nonlinear active cochlear model with feed-forward. *Int J Solids Struct* 40(19):5097–5107.

Manley GA. 2006. Spontaneous otoacoustic emissions from free-standing stereovillar bundles of ten species of lizard with small papillae. *Hear Res* 212(1–2):33–47.

Manoussaki D, Chadwick RS, Ketten DR, Arruda J, Dimitriadis EK, and O'Malley JT. 2008. The influence of cochlear shape on low-frequency hearing. *Proc Natl Acad Sci USA* 105(16):6162–6166.

Masaki K, Weiss TF, and Freeman DM. 2006. Poroelastic bulk properties of the tectorial membrane measured with osmotic stress. *Biophys J* 91(6):2356–2370.

Miller CE. 1985. Structural implications of basilar membrane compliance measurements. *J Acoust Soc Am* 77:1465–1474.

Mountain DC and Hubbard AE. 2006. What stimulates the inner hair cell? *Auditory Mechanisms, Processes and Models*, Eds. AL Nuttall, T Ren, P Gillespie, K Grosh, and E de Boer, World Scientific, New Jersey, pp. 466–473.

Naidu RC and Mountain DC. 1998. Measurements of the stiffness map challenge a basic tenet of cochlear theories. *Hear Res* 124:124–131.

Narayan SS, Temchin AN, Recio A, and Ruggero MA. 1998. Frequency tuning of basilar membrane and auditory nerve fibers in the same cochleae. *Science* 282(5395):1882–1884.

Nobili R, Mommano F, and Ashmore J. 1998. How well do we understand the cochlea? *TINS* 21(4):159–166.

Nowotny M and Gummer AW. 2006. Nanomechanics of the subtectorial space caused by electromechanics of cochlear outer hair cells. *Proc Natl Acad Sci USA* 103(7):2120–2125.

Olson ES. 1998. Observing middle and inner ear mechanics with novel intracochlear pressure sensors. *J Acoust Soc Am* 103(6):3445–3463.

Olson ES and Mountain DC. 1994. Mapping the cochlear partition's stiffness to its cellular architecture. *J Acoust Soc Am* 95(1):395–400.

Peng AW and Ricci AJ. 2010. Somatic motility and hair bundle mechanics, are both necessary for cochlear amplification? *Hear Res* 273(1–2):109–122.

Peterson LC and Bogert BP 1950. A dynamical theory of the Cochlea. *J Acoust Soc Am* 22(3):369–381.

Pickles JO. 1988. *An Introduction to the Physiology of Hearing*, 2nd ed. Academic Press, London.

Probst R. 1990. Otoacoustic emissions: An overview. *Adv Oto-Rhino-Laryngol* 44:1–91.

Raftenberg MN. 1990. Flow of endolymph in the inner spiral sulcus and the subtectorial space. *J Acoust Soc Am* 87(6):2606–2620.

Ranke OF. 1950. Theory of operation of the cochlea: A contribution to the hydrodynamics of the cochlea. *J Acoust Soc Am* 22:772–777.

Raphael Y, Lenoir M, Wroblewski R, and Pujol R. 1991. The sensory epithelium and its innervation in the mole rat cochlea. *J Comp Neurol* 314:367–382.

Ren T. 2002. Longitudinal pattern of basilar membrane vibration in the sensitive cochlea. *Proc Natl Acad Sci USA* 99(26):17101–17106.

Rhode WS. 1971. Observations of the vibration of the basilar membrane in squirrel monkeys using the Mössbauer technique. *J Acoust Soc Am* 49:1218–1231.

Ruggero MA. 1993. Distortion in those good vibrations. *Curr Biol* 3(11):755–758.

Ruggero MA, Narayan SS, Temchin AN and Recio A. 2000. Mechanical bases of frequency tuning and neural excitation at the base of the cochlea: Comparison of basilar-membrane vibrations and auditory-nerve-fiber responses in chinchilla. *Proc Natl Acad Sci USA* 97(22):11744–11750.

Ruggero MA, Rich NC, Recio A, Narayan SS, and Robles L. 1997. Basilar-membrane responses to tones at the base of the chinchilla cochlea. *J Acoust Soc Am* 101(4):2151–2163.

Russell IJ and Sellick PM. 1977. Tuning properties of cochlear hair cells. *Nature* 267:858–860.

Schwander M, Kachar B, and Müller U. 2010. The cell biology of hearing. *J Cell Biol* 190(1):9–20.

Siebert WM. 1974. Ranke revisited—A simple short-wave cochlear model. *J Acoust Soc Am* 56(2):594–600.

Sohmer H and Freeman S. 2004. Further evidence for a fluid pathway during bone conduction auditory stimulation. *Hear Res* 193(1–2):105–110.

Steele CR. 1987. Cochlear Mechanics. *Handbook of Bioengineering*, Eds. R Skalak and S Chien, pp. 30.11–30.22, McGraw-Hill, New York.

Steele CR, Baker G, Tolomeo JA, and Zetes DE. 1993. Electro-mechanical models of the outer hair cell, Biophysics of Hair Cell Sensory Systems. Eds. H Duifhuis, JW Horst, P van Dijk, and SM van Netten, World Scientific Press, Singapore, pp. 207–214.

Steele CR and Puria S. 2005. Force on inner hair cell cilia. *Int J Solids Struct* 42(21–22):5887–5904.

Stenfelt S, Hato N, and Goode RL. 2004. Fluid volume displacement at the oval and round windows with air and bone conduction stimulation. *J Acoust Soc Am* 115(2):797–812.

Strelioff D and Flock Å. 1984. Stiffness of sensory-cell hair bundles in the isolated guinea pig cochlea. *Hear Res* 15:19–28.

Taber LA and Steele CR. 1979. Comparison of 'WKB' and experimental results for three-dimensional cochlear models. *J Acoust Soc Am* 65:1007–1018.

Watts L. 1993. *Cochlear Mechanics: Analysis and Analog VLSI*. PhD Thesis, California Institute of Technology.

West CD. 1985. The relationship of the spiral turns of the cochlea and the length of the basilar membrane to the range of audible frequencies in ground dwelling mammals. *J Acoust Soc Am* 77(3):1091–1101.

White RD and Grosh K. 2005. Microengineered hydromechanical cochlear model. *Proc Natl Acad Sci USA* 102(5):1296–1301.

Wittbrodt MJ, Puria S, and Steele CR. 2006. Developing a physical model of the human cochlea using micro-fabrication methods. *Audiol Neurotol* 11:104–112.

Yoon YJ, Puris S, and Steele CR. 2009. A cochlear model using the time-averaged Lagrangean and the push-pull mechanism in the organ of Corti. *J Mechanics Mater Struct* 4(5):977–986.

Zheng J, Deo N, Zou Y, Grosh K, and Nuttall AL. 2007. Alters Cochlear mechanics and amplification: *In vivo* evidence for a role of stiffness modulation in the organ of Corti. *J Neurophysiol* 97:994–1004.

Zhou G, Bintz L, Anderson DZ, and Bright KE. 1994. A life-sized physical model of the human cochlea with optical holographic readout. *J Acoust Soc Am* 93(3):1516–1523.

Zweig G and Shera CA. 1995. The origin of periodicity in the spectrum of evoked otoacoustic emissions. *J Acoust Soc Am* 98(4):2018–2047.

Zwislocki JJ and Cefaratti LK. 1989. Tectorial membrane II: Stiffness measurements *in vivo*. *Hear Res* 42:211–227.

Further Information

The following are workshop proceedings that document many of the developments:

Allen JB, Hall JL, Hubbard A, Neely ST, and Tubis A. (eds). 1985. *Peripheral Auditory Mechanisms*. Springer, Berlin.

Cooper NP and Kemp DT (eds). 2008. *Concepts and Challenges in the Biophysics of Hearing*. World Scientific, Singapore.

Dallos P, Geisler CD, Matthews JW, Ruggero MA, and Steele CR (eds). 1990. *The Mechanics and Biophysics of Hearing*. Springer, Berlin.

De Boer E and Viergever MA (eds). 1983. *Mechanics of Hearing*. Nijhoff, The Hague.

Duifhuis H, Horst JW, van Kijk P, and van Netten SM (eds). 1993. *Biophysics of Hair Cell Sensory Systems*. World Scientific, Singapore.

Gummer AW (ed). 2002. *Biophysics of the Cochlea*. World Scientific, Singapore.

Lewis ER, Long GR, Lyon RF, Narins PM, Steele CR, and Hecht-Poinar E (eds). 1997. *Diversity in Auditory Mechanics*. World Scientific, Singapore.

Nuttal AL, Ren T, Gillespie P, Grosh K, and deBoer E. 2006. *Auditory Mechanismx, Processes and Models*. World Scientific, Singapore.

Wada T, Koike T, Takasada T, Ikeda K, and Ohyama K (eds). 2000. *Recent Developments in Auditory Mechanics*. World Scientific, Singapore.

Wilson JP and Kemp DT (eds). 1988. *Cochlear Mechanisms: Structure, Function, and Models*. Plenum, New York.

18

Inner Ear Hair Cell Bundle Mechanics

Jong-Hoon Nam
University of Rochester

Wally Grant
*Virginia Polytechnic
Institute and State
University*

18.1 Introduction

Hair cells are the sensory receptors in the inner ear. Auditory hair cells in the cochlea detect pressure waves to mediate hearing. Vestibular hair cells in *semicircular canals*, *utricule*, and *saccule* detect head movement and orientation. The hair cells are named so because of their characteristic structure at the apical surface of the cell called the hair bundle (see Figure 18.1). Mechanical stimuli such as sound pressure, acceleration, or gravity arrive through the extracellular structure at the hair bundle where it is turned into neural spike-train signals. How different mechanical stimuli are captured, amplified, and encoded by hair cells is an important question in the inner ear science. The hair bundles have sophisticated structure and characteristic shapes depending on different inner ear organs (Figure 18.1). Even within the same sensory organ, the hair bundle shapes vary considerably and systematically. Considering such diverse and systematically arranged bundle shapes, it is logical to assume that the hair bundle mechanics play a crucial role on the hair cell's function.

18.2 Hair Cell Bundle Structure

Histological studies have enhanced the knowledge on the hair bundle structure. Among the findings are the various linkages that connect the *cilia*, and the more prominent of these are *tip links*. These connect the tip of a *stereocilium* to the shaft of the neighboring stereocilium. Tip links have inspired many biophysical theories (Pickles et al. 1984). Figure 18.2 illustrates structural components of a hair bundle such as stereocilia, *kinocilium*, tip link, and other fine filamentous links.

    A hair cell bundle has dozens of stereocilia, and the numbers range from as few as 10 up to 150. Each stereocilium looks like a sharpened pencil. Its rootlet is inserted into the *cuticular plate*, a dense matrix

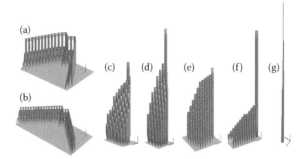

FIGURE 18.1 Various hair bundles from (a) rat cochlea apical turn, (b) rat cochlea basal turn, (c) mouse utricle striolar region, (d) mouse utricle extrastriolar region, (e) turtle utricle striolar region, (f) turtle utricle medial extrastriolar region, and (g) turtle semicircular canal. Scale bars are 1 mm in (a–f) and 5 mm in (g). A hair bundle is composed of hexagonally packed hairs (stereocilia) with unidirectional height gradient. Other than that, the bundles have a great variance in morphology depending on the organ and the location. The consequence of the variance is not yet fully understood.

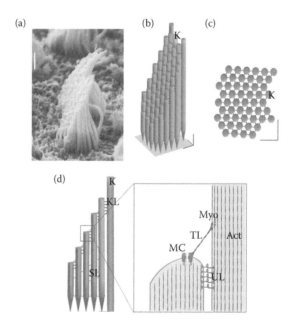

FIGURE 18.2 Structure of a hair bundle. (a) Scanning electron microscopic image of a hair bundle in turtle utricle. Note that wavy-looking stereocilia are preparation artifacts of the SEM; stereocilia *in vivo* are straight. (SEM from E. H. Peterson.) (b) Computer-rendered image of a similar hair bundle in (a). (c) Cross-sectional view of a hair bundle. Kinocilium (K) is at the taller end of bundle. The tip links (TL) are unidirectional along the height gradient of stereocilia. (d) Vertical view of a column of stereocilia, including the kinocilium. A stereocilium is packed with actin fibers (Act), while the kinocilium has a 9 + 2 microtubule structure. The stereocilia are tightly bound by various filaments such as kinocilial link (KL), upper lateral link (UL), tip link (TL), and shaft link (SL). The upper end of the tip link is pulled by myosin motors (Myo) and the bottom end is tethered to mechanotransduction ion channels (MC).

of *actin* fibers in the hair *cell apex*. In the transverse plane, the stereocilia in the bundle are arranged hexagonally (Figure 18.2c). In the sagittal section, stereocilia are arranged in ascending height similar to a staircase (Figure 18.2d). There is one kinocilium at the tallest end of the bundle. The kinocilium in the auditory hair cells disappears as they fully develop while that of vestibular hair cells persists.

Each stereocilium is packed with crystallized *f-actin* fibers. There are 300–400 actin fibers in the shaft region while the number of fibers reduces as the stereocilium tapers into the root (Tilney et al. 1980). The actin fibers are bound together by cross-linking proteins such as *espin* and *fimbrin* (Loomis et al. 2003). The diameter of stereocilia shaft ranges from 200 to 600 nm, and the rootlet of stereocilia is about 50 nm in diameter. The height of stereocilia has a range from 1 to 100 µm. Stereocilia in semicircular canals are approximately 100 µm tall while those in the basal turn of the cochlea are as short as 1 µm.

Various fine filaments tightly bind the stereocilia into a bundle. They are parallel to the cuticular plate and aligned with all three axes of the hexagonal array. In vestibular hair bundles, there are *kinocilial links*, *upper lateral links*, *shaft links*, and *ankle links* (Figure 18.2d). The kinocilial links bind the kinocilium to the rest of the bundle, and like tip links, they are composed of *protocadherin15* and *cadherin23* proteins. The upper lateral links bind the tips of stereocilia, and their molecular identity is unknown. The shaft links and ankle links are found only at the earlier developing stage in the auditory hair cell bundles. Because of their location, which is inefficient as a bundle binder, their mechanical or physiological role is unclear.

Tip links obliquely connect the tips of shorter stereocilia to the shaft of the next taller stereocilia (Figure 18.2d). Unlike other interciliary filaments, the tip links run along the gradient of stereociliary height, which defines the *excitatory–inhibitory* (E–I) direction of the cell. They are 8–11 nm thick and 150–200 nm long (Kachar et al. 2000). The tip link is composed of two proteins, protocadherin15 and cadherin23 (Kazmierczak et al. 2007). The bottom end of a tip link is mechanically coupled to a mechanotransduction ion channel (Beurg et al. 2009). The upper end of a tip link is connected to myosin motors (Holt et al. 2002). The myosin motors run up and down the actin of the stereocilia. Mechanical stimulation is delivered to the transduction channel through tip links and the channel's chance of opening is regulated by the tension maintained by myosin motors at the tip link's upper end. These myosin motors also adjust the tip link tension during the activation process and are responsible for adaptation in the bundle.

18.3 Hair Bundle Mechanical Stiffness

Hair bundles in the inner ear are subject to various mechanical stimuli such as gravity, head acceleration, or sound pressure that produce deflection of the hair bundles. Deflection of a hair bundle results in: stretching of the tip links, opening of the ion channels, that allows a depolarizing inward ion current flow into the hair cell, which in turn initiates neural signals. The study of the transfer function between mechanical stimulus and bundle deformation has centered on hair bundle *mechanical stiffness* (force/unit deflection). Furthermore, the *tonotopic arrangement* (systematic variation of characteristic frequencies along cochlear epithelium) of the hair bundle stiffness together with the mass carried by the bundle can explain its frequency map in lower vertebrates such as a lizard (Manley and Köppl 2008). In mammalian cochlea, the consequence of the variation of bundle stiffness is not yet understood.

The earliest stiffness measurements of hair bundles were made using the guinea pig cochlea (Strelioff and Flock 1984), turtle cochlea (Crawford and Fettiplace 1985), and bullfrog sacculus (Howard and Ashmore 1986). Measured hair bundle stiffness ranges from 0.2 mN/m in bullfrog saccule to 5 mN/m in rat cochlea. Because physiologically meaningful bundle deformation does not exceed 2° in angular rotation of stereocilia, the bundle mechanics was initially assumed to be linear. However, the hair bundle stiffness is nonlinear and it depends on displacement (Howard and Hudspeth 1988), measurement timing (Géléoc et al. 1997), stimulus direction (Szymko et al. 1992), and extracellular calcium concentration (Marquis and Hudspeth 1997, Lumpkin et al. 1997). Among these variations in stiffness, the dependence of the stiffness on the transduction channel activity has provided much insight into inner ear mechano-electric transduction. It was consistently observed across various types of hair cells that the passive hair bundle without transduction channel activity becomes linear in force–displacement relations (bullfrog saccule: Howard and Hudspeth 1988; turtle cochlea: Ricci et al. 2000; mouse cochlea: Russell et al. 1992). Based on this finding, it is now believed that the hair bundle not only receives external stimulus but also provides a mechanical feedback by generating an active force (Kennedy et al. 2005, Chan and Hudspeth 2005). Because this active feedback disappears with the disruption of tip links, or the inactivation of channels, hair bundle force must originate from the transduction channels. This force from the transduction channel has been named the single channel gating force by Howard and Hudspeth (Howard and Hudspeth 1988). The single channel gating force ranges from 0.6 to 3.0 pN. A hair bundle can generate forces up to several hundred pN on a sub-millisecond timescale (Kennedy et al. 2005).

18.4 Analytical Models

A hair cell is most sensitive when the hair bundle deflects along the bilateral symmetric line, called the E–I axis (Shotwell et al. 1981). In other words, it has a primary direction of response. Although under some experimental conditions it has been observed otherwise (Stauffer and Holt 2007, Nam and Fettiplace 2008), stereocilia in a bundle are bound so tightly that they deform in unison (Karavitaki and Corey 2006, Kozlov et al. 2007). This observation has been used as grounds for simplifying the hair bundle mechanics to a *single-degree-of-freedom system*.

A single-degree-of-freedom model (Howard and Hudspeth 1987) for the hair bundle mechanics was represented by two elastic springs and a damper as a Maxwell–Kelvin–Voigt model. The single variable was the displacement of bundle tip along the E–I axis. In the simplest form of bundle mechanics, the force applied to the bundle F_{HB} is expressed as

$$F_{HB} = K_S X - N p_o z + F_0 \tag{18.1}$$

where K_S is the stiffness of the bundle without the tip link additional stiffness included, N is the number of transduction channels in the bundle, p_o is the ratio of open channels to the total number of channels, and z is the single channel gating force. The last term F_0 is a constant to secure $F_{HB} = 0$ at $X = 0$. Without the last two terms, the equation is simply a Hooke's law. The second term in the right-hand side implies the interaction between the transduction channel and the bundle. The channel open probability p_o, is described using first-order Boltzmann relations

$$p_o = \frac{1}{(1 + \exp[(-z(X - X_0)/k_B T)])} \tag{18.2}$$

where k_B is the Boltzmann's constant, T is the absolute temperature, and X_0 is the bundle displacement at 50% open probability. This equation implies that as X increases, the open probability approaches one, and as X decreases, it becomes zero. The single channel gating force z is defined as $z = \gamma k_{GS} b$, where k_{GS} is the spring constant of putative transduction channel complex and b is the gating swing (conformational change of transduction channel between open and closed state). Geometric gain γ is defined as the gating spring elongation divided by the bundle tip displacement and is approximated by the ratio of the interciliary distance and the bundle height. Because of its virtue of simplicity, this single-degree-of-freedom model of hair cell mechanotransduction has been widely adopted and modified for various purposes. For example, Cheung and Corey (2006) compared different adaptation theories of hair cells. Nadrowski and his colleagues (Nadrowski et al. 2004) suggested the positive role of ambient noise to hair cell sensitivity. Martin et al. (2000) explained the spontaneous oscillations of bullfrog saccule hair bundles.

While the single-degree-of-freedom model contributed to the improvement and the understanding of hair cell mechanotransduction, there were approaches more focused on hair bundle mechanics itself. An early study of hair bundles represented the stereocilia by two rigid bars, elastically hinged at their rootlets (Geisler 1993). This model presented ideas on how the stereociliar rotational displacement delivers tension to the tip link by the relative shear between stereocilia. Some studies represent hair bundles as a hinged plate, hemisphere, or array of cylinders, to investigate the fluid mechanics activation of hair bundles (Zetes and Steele 1997, Freeman and Weiss 1988, Shatz 2000). *Finite element* (FE) analysis of hair bundle was first introduced to analyze the mechanical behavior of a single stereocilium (Duncan and Grant 1997). The FE method was further applied to analyze a column of stereocilia (Cotton and Grant 2004) and whole three-dimensional bundles (Silber et al. 2004). This continuum mechanics-based approach was further developed to study hair bundle's dynamic interaction with channel kinetics of utricular hair cell (Nam et al. 2007) and cochlear hair cell (Beurg et al. 2008). The remainder of this chapter introduces the examples of recent progresses in understanding the bundle mechanics and mechanotransduction using the FE method.

18.5 Computational Model

18.5.1 Finite Element Models

The hair bundle is a sophisticated structure, and the geometry of many different hair bundles has been well documented (Duncan et al. 2001, Xue et al. 2005). This information was obtainable with current electron and confocal microscopic techniques. A mechanical consequence of various hair bundle shapes can be better understood with a model that reflects their real structure. The FE method serves such a purpose. It is an efficient and well-established method to analyze the mechanics of complicated structures. Grant and his colleagues introduced the FE methods to analyze hair bundle mechanics (Duncan and Grant 1997, Cotton and Grant 2000, 2004, Nam et al. 2005, 2006, 2007a,b).

The hair bundle FE model is composed of two different element types. Stereocilia and kinocilium are represented by shear deformable Timoshenko beams. For interciliary filaments, link elements were used. Ankle links were neglected in the model as they contribute little structurally. The range of element mesh size for stereocilia was from 0.05 to 1.0 µm, after considering the real geometry of hair bundle, the matrix condition number, and the computational efficiency.

The equation of motion at time t is

$$\mathbf{M}\left[{}^{t+\Delta t}\ddot{\mathbf{U}}^{(k)}\right] + {}^{t}\mathbf{C}\left[{}^{t+\Delta t}\dot{\mathbf{U}}^{(k)}\right] + {}^{t}\mathbf{K}\left[\Delta \mathbf{U}^{(k)}\right] = {}^{t+\Delta t}\mathbf{R} - {}^{t+\Delta t}\mathbf{F}^{(k-1)} \tag{18.3}$$

where $\mathbf{M}$, $\mathbf{C}$, and $\mathbf{K}$ are the mass, damping, and stiffness matrix and $\mathbf{U}$, $\mathbf{R}$, and $\mathbf{F}$ are the displacement, applied force, and internal force vectors. Over-dot variables denote the differentiation with respect to time. Superscripts to the left of the variable t denote time, while those to the right k indicate the iterative step within each time step. For the damping, a proportional damping was used such as

$$^{t}\mathbf{C} = \alpha_{c}\mathbf{M} + \beta_{c}{}^{t}\mathbf{K} \tag{18.4}$$

where α_c and β_c are scalar constants. This relation represents the bundle's internal damping—between stereocilia or within stereocilia. There is another fluid friction caused by the fluid flow on the surface of the hair bundle. This external damping was considered as an external force and included in the external force term $\mathbf{R}$. The damping coefficients α_c and β_c were chosen so that the overall effective damping of the hair bundle matches the experimentally measured values (100–200 nN · s/m).

At each time step, an incremental displacement vector $\Delta \mathbf{U}^{(k)}$ is computed and the displacement updated by

$$^{t+\Delta t}\mathbf{U}^{(k)} = {}^{t+\Delta t}\mathbf{U}^{(k-1)} + \Delta \mathbf{U}^{(k)} \tag{18.5}$$

Iterations of k for that time step continue until the internal force distribution converges.

For the solution of the dynamic structural analysis, the direct Newmark integration method was used. This method was chosen because it is a single-step, implicit method that is unconditionally stable.

The velocity and displacement vectors at time step $t + \Delta t$ are calculated by solving the equations below using two coefficients β and γ:

$$^{t+\Delta t}\dot{\mathbf{U}} = {}^{t}\dot{\mathbf{U}} + \Delta t \left\{ (1-\gamma) {}^{t}\ddot{\mathbf{U}} + \gamma {}^{t+\Delta t}\ddot{\mathbf{U}} \right\} \tag{18.6}$$

$$^{t+\Delta t}\mathbf{U} = {}^{t}\mathbf{U} + {}^{t}\dot{\mathbf{U}}\Delta t + \Delta t^2 \left\{ \left(\frac{1}{2} - \beta \right) {}^{t}\ddot{\mathbf{U}} + \beta {}^{t+\Delta t}\ddot{\mathbf{U}} \right\} \tag{18.7}$$

A typical time step size is 1–10 µs. With a proper choice of Newmark coefficients ($\gamma \geq 0.5$ and $\beta \leq 0.5$), the analysis is stable.

18.5.2 Fluid Flow Stimulation

Fluid mechanics around the hair bundle was considered as follows. For a vestibular hair cell bundle that is subject to relative fluid velocity of less than 1 µm/ms, and a viscosity near 1 mPa-s, results in a Reynolds number range of 10^{-5}–10^{-3}. With such low Reynolds number, the convective terms in the Navier–Stokes equations are eliminated. Nondimensional analysis of the Navier–Stokes equations, for an incompressible fluid, and without body forces, shows that transient effects are small and can be considered negligible (Nam et al. 2005). This same analysis shows that pressure and viscous force effects are important. These are incorporated in Oseen's improvement to Stokes drag at low Reynolds number flow. This drag formulation was used to simulate the drag force acting on individual stereocilia in this work. The Oseen formulation allows for interrupted flow around the cylindrical stereocilia body and is a much better approximation to the actual flow situation encountered by hair cell bundles than Stoke's formulation. The drag formulation used here should be considered as a first-order primary effect, and may underestimate the actual drag force. This underestimation may occur due to the fluid flow encountered after the endolymph flows past the stereocilia.

The drag force D on a cylindrical shape caused by the flow of a viscous fluid is given as

$$D = C_D \frac{1}{2} \rho A |V| V \tag{18.8}$$

where C_D is the drag coefficient, the velocity magnitude V is the relative velocity between the stereocilium and the fluid, A is the projected bundle area normal to the fluid flow, and ρ is the fluid density. Since the stereocilia have long cylindrical shapes and the Reynolds number (Rn) is much less than 1.0, the drag coefficient, C_D, will be approximated by Oseen's drag formulation

$$C_D = \frac{8\pi}{Rn\log(7.4/Rn)} \tag{18.9}$$

The fluid drag on the extracellular links was ignored. Because the hair bundle deflects infinitesimally (angular displacement is less than 2°), no disturbance by the bundle on the fluid flow is considered, that is, the fluid applies force to the bundle, but the bundle does not disturb the fluid. Further details of dynamic analysis and parameter values can be found in Nam et al. (2005).

18.5.3 Transduction Channel Kinetics

The mechanotransduction channel interacts with the hair bundle. In this simulation, the interaction can be achieved by adjusting the original (unstained) length of the tip link. As the channel state changes from closed to open, the length of the tip link was increased by the gating swing and vice versa.

Literature values for the gating swing are estimated between 1 and 10 nm (Cheung and Corey 2006). The upper attachment point of the tip link moves according to the work or myosin, which is termed slow adaptation. Because it is computationally costly to remesh according to the slow adaptation, in the computer model, the slow adaptation was reflected in the length change of the tip link. Therefore, the change of length in the tip link is due to an active process and is described by

$$\Delta x = nb + x_A \qquad (18.10)$$

where b is the gating swing length, n is the channel state (0 when closed, 1 when open), and x_A is the movement of upper attachment due to the slow adaptation.

The transduction channel kinetics is assumed to have four states. This is the minimum number of channel states to consider the calcium effect on channel kinetics. There are open and closed configuration and each configuration has calcium bound and unbound states. Rate coefficients between the states are defined by four rate constants. Two coefficients describe the calcium binding and unbinding rate:

$$k_{01} = k_b C_{FA} \qquad (18.11)$$

$$k_{10} = k_b K_D \qquad (18.12)$$

where k_b is the calcium binding coefficient, C_{FA} is the calcium concentration at the binding site, and K_D is the dissociation constant of calcium. The channel state of opened (k_{CO}) or closed (k_{OC}) is described by the following two expressions, where two additional rate coefficients are utilized

$$k_{CO} = k_F \exp(\eta \Delta E / k_B T) \qquad (18.13)$$

$$k_{OC} = k_R \exp(-(1 - \eta)) \Delta E / k_B T \qquad (18.14)$$

where ΔE is the energy difference between open and closed state of the channel. ΔE is defined by the tension in the tip link f, gating swing b, and calcium-binding modification f_{Ca} such as

$$\Delta E = b(f - f_{ca} - f_0) \qquad (18.15)$$

When positive, f_{Ca} facilitates the channel closure and stabilizes the closed state (Crawford et al. 1989, Cheung and Corey 2006). The myosin motor provided the resting tension of the tip link. Further details of channel kinetics, including the myosin-regulated adaptation, can be found in Beurg et al. (2008).

18.6 Mechanical Properties of Hair Bundle Structures

There are experiments that can be used to arrive at hair bundle mechanical properties. Bashtanov et al. (2004) selectively removed the tip link or shaft links and measured the bundle stiffness by treating hair bundle solutions that contained BAPTA (to remove tip links) or subtilisin (to remove shaft links). They used chicken utricular hair cells for this study. The bundle stiffness was measured by analyzing the frequency of the freely standing bundle's Brownian motion.

Spoon et al. (2007) implemented a similar experiment protocol—removal of tip links or shaft links. Different from Bashtanov et al., they used the glass fiber technique for the stiffness measurement of turtle utricular hair bundles. Computer simulations of similar bundles to those tested complemented the experiment. Simulated bundle is shown in Figure 18.2. The geometric information is from the *striolar region* in the turtle utricle. The striolar region is a narrow crescent-shaped region in the utricular epithelium where the hair bundles' polarity reverses. Like the experiment, four cases were simulated to determine the structural contribution of different link types and to estimate the mechanical properties of the bundle structural components (Figure 18.2d). Link structures of a hair bundle include the tip link assemblies (TLA), the upper lateral links (UL), the kinocilial links (KL), and the shaft links (SL). In addition to these links, the flexibility of stereocilia roots affects the bundle compliance. Here, the TLA includes any proteins in series with the tip link from actin core to actin core, including the tip link itself.

To obtain the stiffness of the hair bundle in a resting state, a small point load of 1.0 pN in the excitatory direction (toward taller edge) is applied at the tip of the kinocilium. The deflection at the tip of the kinocilium is computed and the bundle stiffness is defined as the applied load divided by the tip deflection. The hair bundle without tip links represents the BAPTA-treated hair bundle. The hair bundle missing SL represents the subtilisin-treated hair bundle. A hair bundle washed with BAPTA and subtilisin has no tip or SL.

Four mechanical parameter values were sought in the study: (1) stereocilia Young's modulus E_S, (2) stiffness of the TL k_{TL}, (3) UL stiffness k_{UL}, and (4) SL stiffness k_{SL}. A set of optimal mechanical parameters ($E_S{}^*$, $k_{TL}{}^*$, $k_{UL}{}^*$, and $k_{SL}{}^*$) were found that minimize the difference between the modeled results and the three experimental outcomes (Spoon et al. 2007, namely, 66 ± 9% and 63 ± 10% stiffness reduction after tip and shaft link removal, and the intact bundle stiffness of 42 ± 25 pN/μm ($n = 28$). Initial values of E_S, k_{TL}, k_{UL}, and k_{SL} were taken from the previous study (Nam et al. 2006). Then, three of the parameters were held constant and the value of the fourth was found that minimized the difference. This process was repeated for the other three parameters in turn, and then the entire process was repeated until the values converged. After the optimal mechanical properties were identified ($E_S{}^*$, $k_{TL}{}^*$, $k_{UL}{}^*$, and $k_{SL}{}^*$), a series of parametric studies was performed to observe the effects of each individual mechanical parameter on the whole bundle stiffness. In each of the four parametric studies, three of the optimal mechanical properties were fixed and the remaining parameter varied.

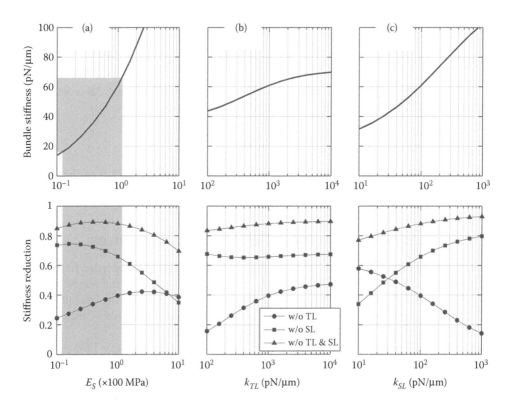

FIGURE 18.3 Identifying the mechanical property of hair bundle structures. The shaded area indicates the measured stiffness range of 42 ± 25 pN/μm ($n = 28$). Top row: stiffness change due to change of (a) Young's modulus of stereocilia E_S, (b) stiffness of tip link k_{TL}, and (c) stiffness of shaft link k_{SL}. Bottom row: fraction of stiffness reduction when TL (circle), SL (square), or both TL and SL (triangle) were removed.

Figure 18.3 shows the simulation results. The shaded area is the range of experimental results. When the Young's modulus of stereocilia $E_S = 100$ MPa, the stiffness of the TLA $k_{TL} = 1000$ pN/μm, and the stiffness of SL $k_{SL} = 100$ pN/μm, the simulated results became close to experimental results. Simulated bundle stiffness was 60 pN/μm. Stiffness reductions due to the removal of TL and SL were 65% and 40%, respectively.

18.7 Hair Bundle Response to Different Types of Stimuli

In experiments, to observe single cell response, the overlying acellular matrix such as *tectorial membrane* in cochlea or otoconial layer in vestibular organs is removed. Then, the mechanical stimulus is delivered by a glass probe or fluid jet. It is unclear how different stimulus types affect a hair cell response. Such different stimulus conditions were simulated using a computer model (Figure 18.4).

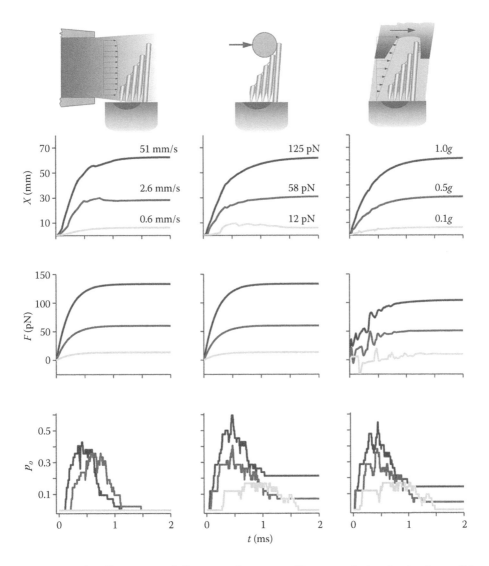

FIGURE 18.4 Hair bundle response to different stimulation types. The top row depicts the stimulus conditions of each column. Below three rows are the time response of hair bundle displacement (X), reaction force at the bundle tip (F), and fraction of open channels (p_o). The columns are the three different stimulus methods: fluid jet, flexible glass fiber, and *in vivo*.

To simulate the flexible glass fiber condition, step forces were applied to the three tallest cilia of the bundle. To simulate the fluid jet condition, the ambient fluid was given velocities ramped from zero to a steady-state value. The time constants and magnitudes of the *in vitro* stimuli were adjusted to achieve $X(t)$ curves similar to the following *in vivo* conditions. To simulate the *in vivo* condition, the bundle was subjected to both a ramped displacement and a shear flow from the ambient fluid. The time course of displacements was selected to match the whole utricle analysis results (Davis et al. 2007). Three stimulus levels were simulated: $0.1g$, $0.5g$, and $1.0g$, where g is the acceleration due to gravity.

18.8 Effect of Different Bundle Shapes

As shown in Figure 18.1, there are strikingly diverse hair bundles. While auditory hair bundles change their height monotonically according to their characteristic frequency, the morphological variation in the vestibular organs is more complex and not well understood. An FE model can help to provide some idea on this matter.

Two hair bundles from different locations in the turtle utricle were chosen. One is from the striolar region (Figure 18.2), where bundles are round shaped with tall stereocilia (up to ~10 μm) and short kinocilium (~10 μm). The other is from the extrastriolar region (outside the striolar region) (Figure 18.1f), where bundles are in elongated oval shape with short stereocilia (up to ~4.5 μm) and tall kinocilium (>10 μm). In the simulation, all other model properties of the two bundles were the same. Even the external force was applied at the same elevation (9 μm). The geometry is the only difference in the simulation. Thus, the results reflect exclusively the effect of different geometry.

Figure 18.5 summarizes the simulation results. The striolar bundle was stiffer than the extrastriolar bundle by five times. A noticeable functional difference is the operating range. The operating range is the bundle displacement required to excite the transduction current from 10% to 90% of its maximum. The operating range of the striolar bundle was 188 nm, while it was 697 nm in extrastriolar bundle. Therefore, the simulation results suggest that the two hair bundles encode a different stimulus range.

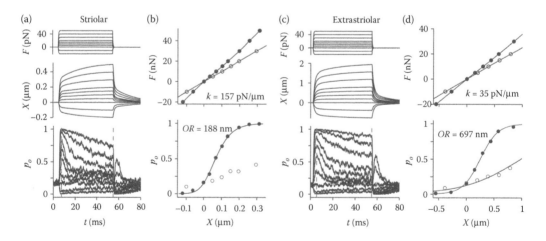

FIGURE 18.5 Comparing different hair bundles from the turtle utricle. (a) Striolar bundle was stimulated with a family of step forces (top). The bundle tip displacement (middle) and the channel open probability were obtained (bottom). (b) F–X relations (top) and p_o–X relations (bottom) of the striolar hair bundle. (c) Extrastriolar bundle was simulated. (d) F–X relations (top) and p_o–X relations (bottom) of the extrastriolar hair bundle. The displacement and the open probability in (b) and (d) were measured at the onset of stimulation (the vertical broken lines in the left of p_o–t plots).

18.9 Concluding Remarks

The understanding of hair cell mechanics, electrophysiology, and the basics of its neural science and mechanical behaviors has made great strides over the past two decades. The interdisciplinary nature of these studies will continue and true hybrid investigators (those with neural, electrophysiology, mechanics backgrounds) will be needed in the future. Biomedical engineers can contribute to this field in two ways. First, their study helps to understand hearing and balancing disorders. Second, their study can provide new insights for the design of biologically inspired mechanotransduction sensors and prosthetics.

References

Bashtanov, M. E., R. J. Goodyear, G. P. Richardson, and I. J. Russell. 2004. The mechanical properties of chick (*Gallus domesticus*) sensory hair bundles: Relative contributions of structures sensitive to calcium chelation and subtilisin treatment. *J Physiol* **559**(Pt 1): 287–99.

Beurg, M., R. Fettiplace, J. H. Nam, and A. J. Ricci. 2009. Localization of inner hair cell mechanotransducer channels using high-speed calcium imaging. *Nat Neurosci* **12**(5): 553–8.

Beurg, M., J. H. Nam, A. Crawford, and R. Fettiplace. 2008. The actions of calcium on hair bundle mechanics in mammalian cochlear hair cells. *Biophys J* **94**(7): 2639–53.

Chan, D. K. and A. J. Hudspeth. 2005. Ca^{2+} current-driven nonlinear amplification by the mammalian cochlea *in vitro*. *Nat Neurosci* **8**(2): 149–55.

Cheung, E. L. and D. P. Corey. 2006. Ca^{2+} changes the force sensitivity of the hair-cell transduction channel. *Biophys J* **90**(1): 124–39.

Cotton, J. and W. Grant. 2004. Computational models of hair cell bundle mechanics: II. Simplified bundle models. *Hear Res* **197**(1–2): 105–11.

Cotton, J. R. and J. W. Grant. 2000. A finite element method for mechanical response of hair cell ciliary bundles. *J Biomech Eng* **122**(1): 44–50.

Crawford, A. C., M. G. Evans, and R. Fettiplace. 1989. Activation and adaptation of transducer currents in turtle hair cells. *J Physiol* **419**: 405–34.

Crawford, A. C. and R. Fettiplace. 1985. The mechanical properties of ciliary bundles of turtle cochlear hair cells. *J Physiol* **364**: 359–79.

Davis, J. L., J. Xue, E. H. Peterson, and J. W. Grant. 2007. Layer thickness and curvature effects on otoconial membrane deformation in the utricle of the red-ear slider turtle: Static and modal analysis. *J Vestib Res* **17**(4): 145–62.

Duncan, R. K. and J. W. Grant. 1997. A finite-element model of inner ear hair bundle micromechanics. *Hear Res* **104**(1–2): 15–26.

Duncan, R. K., K. E. Ile, M. G. Dubin, and J. C. Saunders. 2001. Hair bundle profiles along the chick basilar papilla. *J Anat* **198**(Pt 1): 103–16.

Freeman, D. M. and T. F. Weiss. 1988. The role of fluid inertia in mechanical stimulation of hair cells. *Hear Res* **35**(2–3): 201–7.

Geisler, C. D. 1993. A model of stereociliary tip-link stretches. *Hear Res* **65**(1–2): 79–82.

Geleoc, G. S., G. W. Lennan, G. P. Richardson, and C. J. Kros. 1997. A quantitative comparison of mechanoelectrical transduction in vestibular and auditory hair cells of neonatal mice. *Proc Biol Sci* **264**(1381): 611–21.

Holt, J. R., S. K. Gillespie, and D. W. Provance. 2002. A chemical-genetic strategy implicates myosin-1c in adaptation by hair cells. *Cell* **108**(3): 371–81.

Howard, J. and J. F. Ashmore. 1986. Stiffness of sensory hair bundles in the sacculus of the frog. *Hear Res* **23**(1): 93–104.

Howard, J. and A. J. Hudspeth. 1987. Mechanical relaxation of the hair bundle mediates adaptation in mechanoelectrical transduction by the bullfrog's saccular hair cell. *Proc Natl Acad Sci USA* **84**(9): 3064–8.

Howard, J. and A. J. Hudspeth. 1988. Compliance of the hair bundle associated with gating of mechano-electrical transduction channels in the bullfrog's saccular hair cell. *Neuron* **1**(3): 189–99.

Kachar, B., M. Parakkal, M. Kurc, Y. Zhao, and P. G. Gillespie. 2000. High-resolution structure of hair-cell tip links. *Proc Natl Acad Sci USA* **97**(24): 13336–41.

Karavitaki, K. D. and D. P. Corey. 2006. Hair bundle mechanics at high frequencies: A test of series or parallel transduction. Singapore, World Scientific.

Kazmicrczak, P., H. Sakaguchi, and J. Tokita. 2007. Cadherin 23 and protocadherin 15 interact to form tip-link filaments in sensory hair cells. *Nature* **449**(7158): 87–91.

Kennedy, H. J., A. C. Crawford, and R. Fettiplace. 2005. Force generation by mammalian hair bundles supports a role in cochlear amplification. *Nature* **433**(7028): 880–3.

Kozlov, A. S., T. Risler, and A. J. Hudspeth. 2007. Coherent motion of stereocilia assures the concerted gating of hair-cell transduction channels. *Nat Neurosci* **10**(1): 87–92.

Loomis, P. A., L. Zheng, and G. Sekerkova. 2003. Espin cross-links cause the elongation of microvillus-type parallel actin bundles in vivo. *J Cell Biol* **163**(5): 1045–55.

Lumpkin, E. A., R. E. Marquis, and A. J. Hudspeth. 1997. The selectivity of the hair cell's mechanoelectrical-transduction channel promotes Ca^{2+} flux at low Ca^{2+} concentrations. *Proc Natl Acad Sci USA* **94**(20): 10997–1002.

Manley, G. A. and C. Köppl. 2008. What have lizard ears taught us about auditory physiology? *Hear Res* **238**(1–2): 3–11.

Marquis, R.E. and A. J. Hudspeth. 1997. Effects of extracellular Ca^{2+} concentration on hair-bundle stiffness and gating-spring integrity in hair cells. *Proc Natl Acad Sci USA*. 94(22): 11923–8.

Martin, P., A. D. Mehta, and A. J. Hudspeth. 2000. Negative hair-bundle stiffness betrays a mechanism for mechanical amplification by the hair cell. *Proc Natl Acad Sci USA* **97**(22): 12026–31.

Nadrowski, B., P. Martin, and F. Jülicher. 2004. Active hair-bundle motility harnesses noise to operate near an optimum of mechanosensitivity. *Proc Natl Acad Sci USA* **101**(33): 12195–200.

Nam, J.-H., J. R. Cotton, and J. W. Grant. 2005. Effect of fluid forcing on vestibular hair bundles. *J Vestib Res* **15**(5–6): 263–78.

Nam, J. H., J. R. Cotton, and W. Grant. 2007a. A virtual hair cell, I: addition of gating spring theory into a 3-D bundle mechanical model. *Biophys J* **92**(6): 1918–28.

Nam, J. H., J. R. Cotton, and W. Grant. 2007b. A virtual hair cell, II: evaluation of mechanoelectric transduction parameters. *Biophys J* **92**(6): 1929–37.

Nam, J. H., J. R. Cotton, E. H. Peterson, and W. Grant. 2006. Mechanical properties and consequences of stereocilia and extracellular links in vestibular hair bundles. *Biophys J* **90**(8): 2786–95.

Nam, J. H. and R. Fettiplace. 2008. Theoretical conditions for high-frequency hair bundle oscillations in auditory hair cells. *Biophys J* **95**(10): 4948–62.

Pickles, J. O., S. D. Comis, and M. P. Osborne. 1984. Cross-links between stereocilia in the guinea pig organ of Corti, and their possible relation to sensory transduction. *Hear Res* **15**(2): 103–12.

Ricci, A. J., A. C. Crawford, and R. Fettiplace. 2000. Active hair bundle motion linked to fast transducer adaptation in auditory hair cells. *J Neurosci* **20**(19): 7131–42.

Russell, I. J., M. Kossl, and G. P. Richardson. 1992. Nonlinear mechanical responses of mouse cochlear hair bundles. *Proc Biol Sci* **250**(1329): 217–27.

Shatz, L. F. 2000. The effect of hair bundle shape on hair bundle hydrodynamics of inner ear hair cells at low and high frequencies. *Hear Res* **141**(1–2): 39–50.

Shotwell, S. L., R. Jacobs, and A. J. Hudspeth. 1981. Directional sensitivity of individual vertebrate hair cells to controlled deflection of their hair bundles. *Ann N Y Acad Sci* **374**: 1–10.

Silber, J., J. Cotton, J. H. Nam, E. H. Peterson, and W. Grant. 2004. Computational models of hair cell bundle mechanics: III. 3-D utricular bundles. *Hear Res* **197**(1–2): 112–30.

Spoon C., J. H. Nam, and W. Grant. 2007. Experimental and computational analysis of hair bundle mechanics at different macular locations in the turtle utricle. Abstract No. 736, Association for Research in Otolaryngology 30th Midwinter Meeting, Denver, CO.

Stauffer, E. A. and J. R. Holt. 2007. Sensory transduction and adaptation in inner and outer hair cells of the mouse auditory system. *J Neurophysiol* **98**(6): 3360–9.

Strelioff, D. and A. Flock. 1984. Stiffness of sensory-cell hair bundles in the isolated guinea pig cochlea. *Hear Res* **15**(1): 19–28.

Szymko, Y. M., P. S. Dimitri, and J. C. Saunders. 1992. Stiffness of hair bundles in the chick cochlea. *Hear Res* **59**(2): 241–9.

Tilney, L. G., D. J. Derosier, and M. J. Mulroy. 1980. The organization of actin filaments in the stereocilia of cochlear hair cells. *J Cell Biol* **86**(1): 244–59.

Xue, J. and E. H. Peterson. 2006. Hair bundle heights in the utricle: Differences between macular locations and hair cell types. *J Neurophysiol* **95**: 171–186.

Zetes, D. E. and C. R. Steele. 1997. Fluid-structure interaction of the stereocilia bundle in relation to mechanotransduction. *J Acoust Soc Am* **101**(6): 3593–601.

19

Exercise Physiology

Cathryn R. Dooly
Lander University

Arthur T. Johnson
University of Maryland

19.1 Introduction

The study of exercise physiology should be important to medical and biological engineers because many of the principles and laws of nature are relevant to the homeostasis of the human body. Cognizance of the acute and chronic responses to exercise gives an insight and an understanding of the physiological stresses to which the human body is subjected. To appreciate exercise responses requires a true systems approach to physiology, because during exercise, all physiological responses contribute to a highly integrated and totally supportive mechanism toward the performance of the physical stress of exercise. Unlike the study of pathology and disease, the study of exercise physiology clarifies the way the human body is supposed to function while performing at its healthy best.

For exercise involving resistance, physiological and psychological adjustments begin even before the start of exercise. The central nervous system (CNS) anticipates the task before it, assessing how much muscular force to apply and computing trial limb trajectories to accomplish the required movement. Heart rate, blood pressure, and respiration begin rising in anticipation of increased oxygen demands.

19.2 Muscle Energetics

Human muscle fibers convert chemical energy from the food that we eat into mechanical energy. Energy transfer occurs from the release of energy trapped within chemical bonds. Adenosine triphosphate (ATP), the fundamental energy source for muscle cells, is stored at maximal levels, as well as significant amounts of creatine phosphate (CP) and glycogen, the stored form of glucose.

When the muscle proteins actin and myosin engage in response to high-intensity, short-duration muscular activity, the ATP-CP system (or phosphagan system) is activated in the sarcoplasm of the muscle cell. CP is catabolized by creatine kinase to creatine and inorganic phosphate (Pi), yielding free energy. This energy can be used in turn to generate ATP from adenosine diphosphate (ADP) and Pi. During high-intensity, short-duration muscular activity, as in a one repetition maximum, ATP generation declines rapidly as CP stores are depleted. If physical exertion continues after PC depletion, ATP generation must be accomplished by other pathways, though slower. Maximally contracting skeletal muscle uses approximately 1.7×10^{-5} mole of ATP per gram per second (White et al. 1959). ATP stores in skeletal muscle tissue amount to 5×10^{-6} mole per gram of tissue, or enough to meet muscular energy demands for no longer than 0.5 s. Resting muscle contains 4–6 times as much CP as it does ATP, but the total supply of high-energy phosphate cannot sustain muscular activity for more than a few seconds.

Glycogen is a polysaccharide present in muscle tissue in large amounts. Glycogen is catabolized to glucose and pyruvic acid in the sarcoplasm, which in turn becomes lactic acid in a deoxygenated environment. These reactions, collectively known as *anaerobic* glycolysis, generate ATP in the absence of oxygen.

When sufficient oxygen is available (*aerobic* conditions) in the mitochondria of the muscle cell or other tissues, these processes are reversed. ATP is reformed from ADP and AMP (adenosine monophosphate), CP is reformed from creatine and phosphate, and glycogen is reformed from glucose or lactic acid. Energy to fuel these processes is derived from the complete oxidation of carbohydrates, fatty acids, or amino acids to form carbon dioxide and water. These reactions are summarized by the following equations:

$$ATP \leftrightarrow ADP + P + \text{free energy}$$

$$CP + ADP \leftrightarrow \text{creatine} + ATP$$

$$\text{Glycogen or glucose} + P + ADP \leftrightarrow \text{lactate} + ATP$$

Aerobic:

$$\text{Glycogen or fatty acids} + P + ADP + O_2 \rightarrow CO_2 + H_2O + ATP$$

All conditions:

$$2\,ADP \leftrightarrow ATP + AMP$$

The most intense levels of exercise occur anaerobically (Mole 1983) and can be maintained for only a minute or two (see Figure 19.1).

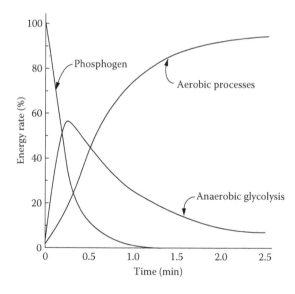

FIGURE 19.1 Energy transfer mechanics. (From Mole, P.A. 1983. Exercise metabolism. In A.A. Bove and D.T. Lowenthal (Eds.), *Exercise Medicine*, pp. 43–48. New York, Academic Press.)

19.3 Cardiovascular Adjustments

Skeletal muscle ergoreceptors and metaboreceptors in muscles, tendons, and joints relay information regarding vibrations and stretch, and the chemical status (O_2, CO_2, electrolytes, glucose, pH) of the muscle, respectively, and relay information to the CNS that the muscles have begun movement (exercise pressor reflex). The CNS processes this information to increase heart rate, stroke volume, and blood pressure via the sympathetic nervous system (SNS). Cardiac output, the amount of blood pumped by the heart per minute, is the product of heart rate and stroke volume (the amount of blood pumped per heart beat). Heart rate increases nearly exponentially at the beginning of exercise with a time constant of about 30 s. Stroke volume does not change immediately but lags a bit until cardiac output completes the loop back to the heart. The increase in stroke volume with exercise is accomplished by Starling's law of the heart, which states that the greater the volume of blood entering the heart during diastole (filling phase), the greater the force of contraction and volume of blood ejected during systole (emptying phase).

At rest, a large volume of blood is stored in the veins, especially in the extremities. When exercise begins, this blood is transferred from the venous side of the heart to the arterial side of the heart. The driving force of blood at the initiation of exercise against the resistance of the arteries causes a rise in both systolic (heart ventricular contraction) and diastolic (the pause between heart contractions when heart chambers fill with blood) blood pressures. These increased blood pressures are detected by cardiac, aortic arch, and carotid arterial baroreceptors (arterial and cardiopulmonary baroreflexes) (see Figure 19.2).

As a consequence, small sphincter muscles encircling the entrance to the arterioles (small arteries) are stimulated to relax via the CNS and locally produced nitric oxide. Using Poiseuille's law, the resistance to blood flow can be calculated as

$$\text{Resistance} = \frac{8\,L\mu}{\pi\,r^4}$$

where R is the resistance of the vessel ($N \cdot s/m^5$), L is the length of the vessel (m), μ is the viscosity of the blood (kg/(m $\cdot$ s) or N s/m^2), and r is the radius of the vessel (m) raised to fourth power.

Blood flow is proportional to the pressure difference across the system, and inversely proportional to resistance. This can be illustrated with the following:

$$\text{Blood flow} = \Delta\text{pressure/resistance}$$

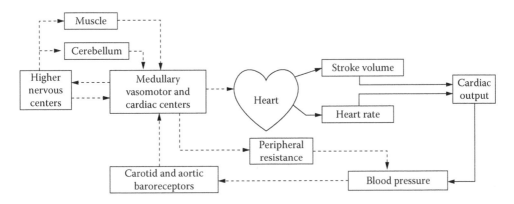

FIGURE 19.2 General scheme for blood pressure regulation. (From Johnson, A.T. 2007. *Biomechanics and Exercise Physiology: Quantitative Modeling*, Taylor & Francis, Boca Raton, FL.)

Note that blood flow can be increased by a change in the pressure difference (Δpressure), a decrease in resistance, or a combination of the two. The most favorable way to increase blood flow is through a change in resistance, since small adjustments in blood vessel radius result in significant changes in resistance (attributed to the relationship between vascular resistance and vessel radius). Change in resistance is largely accomplished by changes in blood vessel radius or diameter, as blood viscosity and vessel length do not change appreciably under normal conditions. Thus, blood flow to the various organs in the body can be regulated by small changes in blood vessel radius via vasoconstriction and vasodilatation. The advantage to this is that blood can be easily diverted to areas where it is needed the most during exercise performance, that is, the exercising muscles.

To meet the oxygen demands of the exercising muscles, blood is diverted away from tissues and organs not directly involved with exercise performance. Blood flow is thus reduced to the gastrointestinal tract and kidneys, and increased not only to exercising skeletal muscle but also to cardiac muscle and the skin. Most resistance to blood flow occurs in the arterioles. These vessels account for as much as 70–80% of the drop in mean arterial pressure across the entire cardiovascular system due to their vasoconstrictive and vasodilatative properties. Increasing the arteriole radius by 19% will decrease the resistance to one-half. Thus, systolic blood pressure returns to baseline, and diastolic blood pressure may actually fall, following recovery from exercise.

The heart operates as two pumping systems in a series. The left heart pumps blood throughout the systemic blood vessels (aorta, arteries, arterioles, capillaries, venules, and veins), whereas the right heart pumps blood throughout the pulmonary blood vessels (pulmonary arteries, veins, capillaries, and venules). Blood pressures in the systemic vessels are higher than blood pressures in the pulmonary system.

Two chambers comprise each pump of the heart. The atria are like an assist device that produces some suction and collects blood from the veins. Their main purpose is to deliver blood to the ventricle of each pump, which is the more powerful chamber that develops blood pressure. The myocardium (middle muscular layer of the heart wall) of the left ventricle is considerably thicker and stronger than the myocardium of the right ventricle. With two pumps and four chambers in a series, matching flow rates among them could be challenging. If the flow rate is not properly matched, blood is at risk of accumulating downstream from the most powerful chamber and upstream from the weakest chamber.

Myocardial tissue exerts a more forceful contraction if it is stretched prior to heart contraction (systole). This property, previously referred to as Starling's law, serves to equalize the flow rates between the two pumps, resulting in a more powerful ejection of blood from the heart during systole, and greater blood volume accumulation during filling (diastole).

19.4 Maximum Oxygen Uptake

The heart has been considered the limiting factor for the delivery of oxygen to the tissues. Increases in heart rate during exercise are achieved primarily through a decrease in the time spent in diastole. Thus, the increase in stroke volume as seen with exercise peaks at about 40–60% of the maximal oxygen consumption, and then plateaus, as filling time is compromised with increased heart rates. As long as the oxygen delivery is sufficient to meet the demands of the working muscles, exercise is considered to be aerobic. When the oxygen delivery is insufficient, anaerobic metabolism will continue to supply the energy needs, but ultimately, lactic acid, a by-product of anaerobiosis, will begin to accumulate in the blood. To remove lactic acid and resynthesize glucose, oxygen is required, which is usually delayed until exercise ceases, or the exercise intensity is substantially reduced to accommodate resynthesis.

The fitness of an individual is characterized by a highly reproducible measure known as maximal oxygen consumption (or VO_2 max). This parameter reflects a person's capacity for aerobic energy transfer as well as the ability to sustain high-intensity exercise for longer than 4 or 5 min (see Figure 19.3). The higher the fitness level, the greater is the VO_2 max. Typical values are 2.5 L/min for young nonathletes, 5.0 L/min for well-trained male athletes, with females having VO_2 max values of 70–80% that of males. Maximal oxygen consumption declines steadily with age at a rate of about 1% per year.

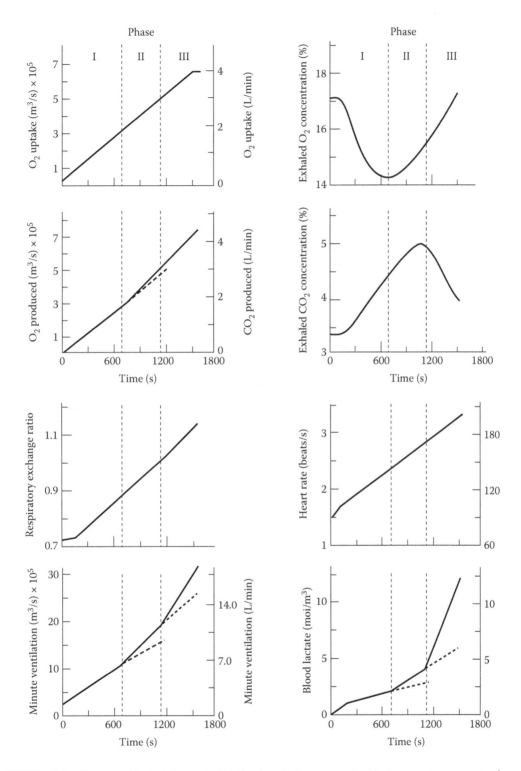

FIGURE 19.3 Concurrent typical changes in blood and respiratory parameters during exercise progressing from rest to maximum. Two transitions shown are the aerobic threshold and the anaerobic threshold. (From Skinner, J.S. and McLellan, T.H. 1980. *Res. Q. Exerc. Sport.* 51: 234.)

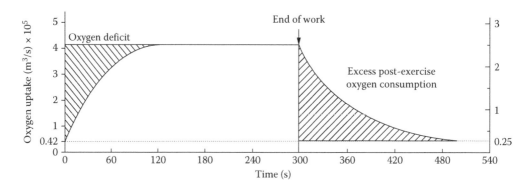

FIGURE 19.4   Oxygen uptake at the beginning and end of exercise. (From Johnson, A.T. 2007. *Biomechanics and Exercise Physiology: Quantitative Modeling*, Taylor & Francis, Boca Raton, FL.)

Exercise levels higher than those that result in VO_2 max can be sustained for various lengths of time. The accumulated difference between the oxygen equivalent of work and VO_2 max is called the oxygen deficit (see Figure 19.4). Oxygen deficit refers to the delay in oxygen consumption at the beginning of exercise, since oxygen consumption does not increase instantaneously to steady-state values. Trained athletes tend to have a smaller oxygen deficit, attributed to an earlier aerobic ATP production at the beginning of exercise, resulting in less lactic acid production, and less dependence on anaerobic metabolism. There is a maximum oxygen deficit that cannot be exceeded by an individual. Once this maximum oxygen deficit has been reached, the individual must cease exercising.

The amount of oxygen used to repay the oxygen deficit is called the excess post-exercise oxygen consumption (EPOC). EPOC is always larger than the oxygen deficit because (1) elevated body temperature immediately following exercise increases the bodily metabolism in general, which requires more than resting oxygen levels to service, (2) increased blood catecholamine (epinephrine and norepinephrine) levels increase the general bodily metabolism, (3) increased respiratory and cardiac muscle activity requires oxygen, and (4) refilling of body oxygen stores. Considering only lactic acid oxygen debt, the total amount of oxygen required to return the body to its normal resting state is about twice the oxygen debt, with the efficiency of anaerobic metabolism at about 50% of aerobic metabolism.

19.5 Respiratory Responses

Respiration also increases when exercise begins, except that the time constant for respiratory responses is about 45 s instead of 30 s for cardiac responses (see Table 19.1). Control of respiration (see Figure 19.5) begins when peripheral chemoreceptors located in the aortic arch, the carotid arteries (in the neck), and the brainstem are stimulated. These specialized receptors are sensitive to changes in oxygen, carbon dioxide, and pH levels but are most sensitive to carbon dioxide and pH. Thus, the primary function of the respiratory system is to remove excess carbon dioxide, and, secondarily, to supply oxygen.

TABLE 19.1   Comparison of Response Time Constants for Four Major Responses of the Body

System	Dominant Time Constant (s)
Heart	30
Respiratory system	45
Oxygen uptake	49
Thermal system	3600

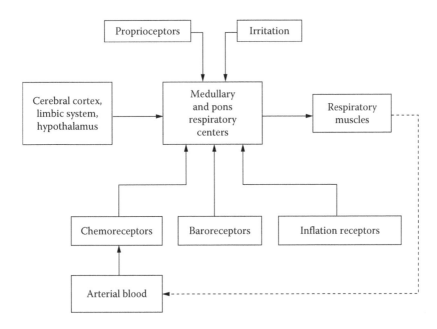

FIGURE 19.5 General scheme of respiratory control. (From Johnson, A.T. 2007. *Biomechanics and Exercise Physiology: Quantitative Modeling*, Taylor & Francis, Boca Raton, FL.)

Perhaps this is because excess carbon dioxide has narcotic effects, but insufficient oxygen does not produce severe reactions until oxygen levels in the inhaled air fall to one-half of normal. However, trained runners have demonstrated exercise-induced hypoxemia (low oxygen levels in the blood) at very high cardiac outputs, resulting in a mismatch in the ventilation–perfusion ratio in the lung, as well as diffusion limitations due to the reduced time red blood cells spend in the pulmonary capillaries.

Oxygen is conveyed by convection (warm air molecules that are replaced by cooler molecules) in the upper airways and by diffusion in the lower airways to the alveoli (air sacs in the lower reaches of the lung where gas is exchanged at the blood–gas barrier). Oxygen must diffuse from the alveoli, through the extremely thin alveolocapillary membrane, composed of a thin layer of endothelial cells, into solution in the blood. Oxygen diffuses further into red blood cells where it is bound chemically to hemoglobin molecules. The order of each of these processes is reversed in the working muscles where the concentration gradient for oxygen is in the opposite direction. The complete transfer of oxygen between alveolar air and pulmonary blood requires about 0.75 s. Carbon dioxide requires somewhat less time, about 0.15 s. Thus, alveolar air more closely reflects the levels of blood carbon dioxide than oxygen.

Both respiration rate and tidal volume (known as ventilation, or the amount of air moved per breath) increase with exercise, but above the lactate threshold, the tidal volume no longer increases (it remains at about 2–2.5 L). From that point, increases in ventilation are accomplished by increases in respiration rate. A similar limitation occurs for stroke volume in the heart (limited to about 120 mL).

The work of respiration, representing only about 1–2% of the body's oxygen consumption at rest increases to 8–10% or more of the body's oxygen consumption during exercise. Contributing greatly to this is the work to overcome resistance to the movement of air in the airways, lung tissue, and chest wall tissue. Turbulent air flow in the upper airways (those nearest and including the mouth and nose) contributes a great deal of pressure drop. The lower airways are not as rigid as the upper airways and are influenced by the stretching and contraction of the lung tissue that surrounds them. High exhalation pressures external to the airways coupled with low static pressures inside (due to high flow rates inside) tend to close these airways somewhat and limit exhalation airflow rates. The resistance of these airways becomes very high, and the respiratory system appears like a flow source, but only during extreme exhalation.

19.6 Optimization

Energy demands during exercise are so great that optimal courses of action are followed for many physiological responses (see Table 19.2). Walking occurs most naturally at a pace that represents the smallest energy expenditure. The transition from walking to running occurs when running expends less energy than walking; ejection of blood from the left ventricle appears to be optimized to minimize energy expenditure; heart rate variation centers around the most efficient rate; and respiratory rate, breathing waveforms, the ratio of inhalation time to exhalation time, airways resistance, tidal volume, and other respiratory parameters all appear to be regulated to minimize energy expenditure (Johnson 1993, 2009).

19.7 Thermoregulatory Response

When exercise is prolonged, heat begins to accumulate in the body. For heat to become stored, exercise must be performed at a relatively low rate. Increased body temperature stimulates neurons in the respiratory center to exert some control over ventilation, but only during prolonged exercise. Acute exercise is too vigorous and ends too abruptly for significant heat accumulation. The energy to fuel muscular activities amounts to, at most, a 20–25% efficiency, and, in general, the smaller the muscle mass, the less efficient it is. Muscle fibers convert chemical energy (from the food we eat) into the mechanical energy required to produce the movement of skeletal muscles. The remaining 75–80% of the total energy expenditure is lost as heat.

The thermal challenges to exercise are met in several ways. Blood sent to the limbs and blood returning from the limbs is normally conveyed by arteries and veins in close proximity deep inside the limb. This tends to conserve heat by countercurrent heat exchange between the arteries and the veins. Thermal stress causes blood to return via surface veins rather than from deep veins. The skin surface temperature increases and the heat loss by convection and radiation (transfer of heat between two objects not in direct contact) also increases. Additionally, vasodilatation of cutaneous blood vessels augments surface heat loss but places an additional burden on the heart to deliver added blood to the skin as well as to the exercising muscles. Plasma volume is thus reduced from excessive sweating to cool the body, and consequently, stroke volume decreases with a concomitant increase in heart rate. Ultimately, cardiac output is reduced since cardiac output equals the product of heart rate and stroke volume. This phenomenon is referred to as the cardiovascular drift.

As the body temperature rises, the hypothalamus stimulates the vasodilatation of skin blood vessels and sweat gland activity to increase evaporative (conversion of a liquid to a gas) heat loss. Different areas of the body begin sweating earlier than others, but eventually the entire body is involved. If the evaporation of sweat occurs on the skin surface, then the full cooling power of evaporating sweat (670 W · h/kg) is felt. If the sweat is absorbed by clothing, then the full benefit of sweat evaporation is not realized at the skin. If the sweat falls from the skin, as is commonly experienced in very humid conditions, no cooling benefit transpires.

Prolonged sweating leads to plasma volume losses, as already stated, with some hemoconcentration (decreased blood volume in relation to number of red blood cells of 2% or more). This increased red cell concentration leads to increased blood viscosity, and cardiac work becomes even greater.

19.8 Applications

The knowledge of exercise physiology imparts to the medical or biological engineer the ability to design devices to be used with or by humans or animals, or to borrow from human physiology to apply to other situations. There is a continual need for engineers to design equipment used by athletes, sports, and health enthusiasts, for diagnostic evaluation, to modify prostheses or devices for the handicapped to allow for performance of greater than light levels of work and exercise, to alleviate physiological stresses caused by personal protective equipment and other occupational ergonometric gear, to design human-powered

TABLE 19.2 Summary of Exercise Responses for a Normal Young Male

	Rest	Light Exercise	Moderate Exercise	Heavy Exercise	Maximal Exercise
Oxygen uptake (L/min)	0.30	0.60	2.2	3.0	3.2
Maximal oxygen uptake (%)	10	20	70	95	100
Physical work rate (W)	0	10	140	240	430
Aerobic fraction (%)	100	100	98	85	50
Performance time (min)	α	480	5	9.3	3.0
Carbon dioxide production (L/min)	0.18	1.5	2.3	2.8	3.7
Respiratory exchange ratio	0.72	0.84	0.94	1.0	1.1
Blood lactic acid (mmol/L)	1.0	1.8	4.0	7.2	9.6
Heart rate (beats/min)	70	130	160	175	200
Stroke volume (L)	0.075	0.100	0.105	0.110	0.110
Cardiac output (L/min)	5.2	13	17	19	22
Minute volume (L/min)	6	22	50	80	120
Tidal volume (L)	0.4	1.6	2.3	2.4	2.4
Respiration rate (breaths/min)	15	26	28	57	60
Peak flow (L/min)	216	340	450	480	480
Muscular efficiency (%)	0	5	18	20	20
Aortic hemoglobin saturation (%)	98	97	94	93	92
Inhalation time (s)	1.5	1.25	1.0	0.7	0.5
Exhalation time (s)	3.0	2.0	1.1	0.75	0.5
Respiratory work rate (W)	0.305	0.705	5.45	12.32	20.03
Cardiac work rate (W)	1.89	4.67	9.61	11.81	14.30
Systolic pressure (mmHg)	120	134	140	162	172
Diastolic pressure (mmHg)	80	85	90	95	100
End-inspiratory lung volume (L)	2.8	3.2	4.6	4.6	4.6
End-expiratory lung volume (L)	2.4	2.2	2.1	2.1	2.1
Gas partial pressures (mmHg)					
Arterial pCO_2	40	41	45	48	50
pO_2	100	98	94	93	92
Venous pCO_2	44	57	64	70	72
pO_2	36	23	17	10	9
Alveolar pCO_2	32	40	28	20	10
pO_2	98	94	110	115	120
Skin conductance [W/(m^2 · °C)]	5.3	7.9	12	13	13
Sweat rate (kg/s)	0.001	0.002	0.008	0.007	0.002
Walking/running speed (m/s)	0	1.0	2.2	6.7	7.1
Ventilation/perfusion of the lung	0.52	0.50	0.54	0.82	1.1
Respiratory evaporative water loss (L/min)	1.02×10^{-5}	4.41×10^{-5}	9.01×10^{-4}	1.35×10^{-3}	2.14×10^{-3}
Total body convective heat loss (W)	24	131	142	149	151
Mean skin temperature (°C)	34	32	30.5	29	28
Heat production (W)	105	190	640	960	1720
Equilibrium rectal temperature (°C)	36.7	38.5	39.3	39.7	500
Final rectal temperature (°C)	37.1	38.26	39.3	37.4	37

machines that are compatible with the capabilities of its operators, and to invent systems to establish and maintain locally benign surroundings in otherwise harsh environments. Recipients of these efforts include athletes, the handicapped, laborers, public safety and military personnel, space and deep sea explorers, farmers, power plant workers, construction workers, and many others where the rate of work is externally imposed or environmentally challenged. The study of exercise physiology, especially in the medical and biological engineer lexicon, can potentially enhance engineering paradigms.

Defining Terms

Anaerobic threshold: The transition between exercise levels that can be sustained through nearly complete aerobic metabolism and those that rely on at least partially anaerobic metabolism. Above the anaerobic threshold, blood lactate increases and the relationship between ventilation and oxygen uptake becomes nonlinear.

Baroreceptors: Stretch receptors located within the cardiovascular system that detect changes in blood pressure.

Cardiovascular drift: Plasma volume losses due to excessive sweating causes an increase in the heart rate during prolonged exercise to compensate for the decrease in stroke volume. This compensation helps to maintain cardiac output.

Chemoreceptors (and metaboreceptors): These sensory organs send information regarding the chemical/metabolic state of muscles (oxygen, carbon dioxide, glucose, electrolytes).

Excess post-exercise oxygen consumption (EPOC): It is the difference between resting oxygen consumption and the accumulated rate of oxygen consumption following exercise termination. EPOC relates to the replacement cost of creatine phosphate, lactic acid resynthesis to glucose, elevated body temperature, catecholamine action, and the cost of elevated heart and breathing rates.

Maximal oxygen consumption: It is the maximum rate of oxygen utilized by the human body during severe dynamic exercise. The amount of oxygen consumed is determined, in part, by age, gender, maximal cardiac output, maximal arterial–mixed venous oxygen difference, and physical condition.

Mechanoreceptors: An end organ that responds to changes in mechanical stress such as stretch, vibration, pressure, compression, or distension.

Oxygen deficit: The accumulated difference between actual oxygen consumption at the beginning of exercise and the rate of oxygen consumption that would exist if oxygen consumption rose immediately to its steady-state level corresponding to exercise level.

References

Johnson, A.T. 1993. How much work is expended for respiration? *Front. Med. Biol. Eng.* 5: 265.
Johnson, A.T. 2007. *Biomechanics and Exercise Physiology: Quantitative Modeling,* Taylor & Francis, Boca Raton, FL.
Mole, P.A. 1983. Exercise metabolism. In A.A. Bove and D.T. Lowenthal (Eds.), *Exercise Medicine*, pp. 43–48. New York, Academic Press.
Skinner, J.S. and McLellan, T. H. 1980. The transition from aerobic to anaerobic metabolism. *Res. Q. Exerc. Sport.* 51: 234.
White, A. Handler, P., Smith, E.L., and Stetten, D. 1959. *Principles of Biochemistry*, New York, McGraw-Hill.

Further Information

Biological Foundations of Biomedical Engineering, edited by J. Kline (Little Brown and Company, 1976) is a very good textbook of physiology written for engineers.

Exercise Physiology: Theory and Application to Fitness and Performance, by S. Powers and E. Howley (McGraw-Hill, 2009) is intended for those persons interested in exercise physiology, clinical exercise physiology, kinesiology, exercise science, and physical therapy. The book contains numerous clinical applications sporting performance and health-related physical fitness.

Physiology of Sport and Exercise, by J. Wilmore, D. Costill and W.L. Kenny (Human Kinetics, 2008) is an excellent additional reference on the physiology of sport and exercise.

Textbook of Work Physiology: Physiological Bases of Exercise by P. O. Astrand, K. Rodahl, H. Dahl and S. Stromme (Human Kinetics, 2003) contains a great deal of updated information on exercise physiology and is generally considered the standard textbook on the subject.

20

Factors Affecting Mechanical Work in Humans

Ben F. Hurley
University of Maryland

Arthur T. Johnson
University of Maryland

High technology has entered our diversions and leisure activities. Sports, exercise, and training are no longer just physical activities but include machines and techniques attuned to individual capabilities and needs. This chapter considers several factors related to exercise and training that help in understanding human performance.

Physiological work performance is determined by energy transformation that begins with the process of photosynthesis and ends with the production of biological work (Figure 20.1). Energy in the form of nuclear transformations is converted into radiant energy, which then transforms the energy from carbon dioxide and water into oxygen and glucose through photosynthesis. In plants, the glucose can also be converted into fats and proteins. Upon ingesting plants or other animals that eat plants, humans convert this energy through cellular respiration (the reverse of photosynthesis) into chemical energy in the form of adenosine triphosphate (ATP). The endergonic reactions (energy absorbed from the surroundings) that produce ATP are followed by exergonic reactions (energy released to the surroundings) that release energy through the breakdown of ATP to produce chemical and mechanical work in the human body. The steps involved in the synthesis and breakdown of carbohydrates, fats, and proteins produce chemical work and provide energy for the mechanical work produced from muscular contractions. The purpose of this chapter is to provide a brief summary of some factors that can affect mechanical work in humans.

20.1 Exercise Biomechanics

20.1.1 Equilibrium

Any body, including the human body, remains in stable equilibrium if the vectorial sum of all forces and torques acting on the body is zero. An unbalanced force results in linear acceleration and an unbalanced torque results in rotational acceleration. Static equilibrium requires that

$$\sum F = 0 \tag{20.1}$$

$$\sum T = 0 \tag{20.2}$$

where F is vectorial forces (N) and T is vectorial torques (N m).

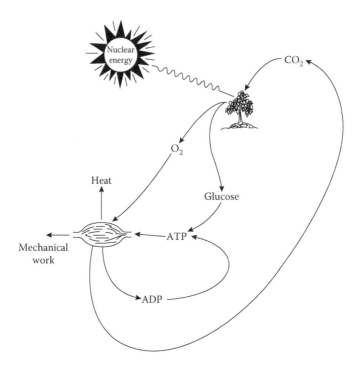

FIGURE 20.1 Schematic of energy transformations leading to muscular mechanical work.

TABLE 20.1 Fraction of Body Weights for Various Parts of the Body

Body Part	Fraction
Head and neck	0.07
Trunk	0.43
Upper arms	0.07
Forearms and hands	0.06
Thighs	0.23
Lower legs and feet	0.14
	1.00

Some sports activities, such as wrestling, weight lifting, and fencing, require stability, whereas other activities, such as running, jumping, and diving, cannot be performed unless there is managed instability. Shifting the body position allows for proper control. The mass of the body is distributed as in Table 20.1, and the center of mass is located at approximately 56% of a person's height and midway from side to side and front to back. The center of mass can be made to shift by extending the limbs or by bending the torso.

20.1.2 Muscular Movement

Mechanical movement results from the contraction of muscles that are attached at each end to bones that can move relative to each other. The arrangement of this combination is commonly known as a class 3 lever (Figure 20.2), where one joint acts as the fulcrum (Figure 20.3), the other bone acts as the load, and the muscle provides the force interposed between the fulcrum and the load. This arrangement requires that the muscle force be greater than the load, sometimes by a very large amount, but the distance through which the muscle moves is made very small. These characteristics match muscle

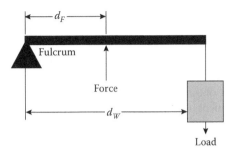

FIGURE 20.2 Class 3 lever is arranged with the applied force interposed between the fulcrum and the load. Most skeletal muscles are arranged in this fashion.

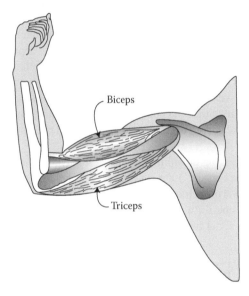

FIGURE 20.3 Biceps muscle of the arm is arranged as a class 3 lever. The load is located at the hand and the fulcrum is located at the elbow.

capabilities well (muscles can produce 7×10^5 N/m², but cannot move far). Since the distance is made smaller, the speed of shortening of the contracting muscle is also slower than it would be if the arrangement between the force and the load was different:

$$\frac{S_L}{S_M} = \frac{d_L}{d_M} \tag{20.3}$$

where S is the speed (m/s), d is the distance from the fulcrum (m), and L and M denote the load and the muscle, respectively.

20.1.3 Muscular Efficiency

Efficiency relates the external, or physical, work produced to the total chemical energy consumed:

$$\eta = \frac{\text{External work produced}}{\text{Chemical energy consumed}} \tag{20.4}$$

Muscular efficiencies range from close to zero to about 20–25%. The larger numbers would be obtained for leg exercises that involve lifting the body weight. In carpentry and foundry work, where both arms and legs are used, the average mechanical efficiency is approximately 10% (Johnson, 1991). For finer movements that require exquisite control, small muscles are often arranged in an antagonistic fashion, that is, the final movement is produced as a result of the difference between two or more muscles working against each other. In this case, efficiencies approach zero. Isometric muscular contraction, where a force is produced but no movement results, has an efficiency of zero (Johnson et al., 2002).

Generally, muscles are able to exert the greatest force when the velocity of muscle contraction is zero. The power produced by this muscle would be zero. When the velocity of muscle contraction is about 8 m/s, the force produced by the muscle becomes zero, and the power produced by this muscle again becomes zero. Somewhere in between the above conditions stated, the power produced and the efficiency become the maximum (Figure 20.4).

The isometric length–tension relationship of a muscle shows that the maximum force developed by a muscle is exerted at its resting length (the length of a slightly stretched muscle attached by its tendons to the skeleton) and decreases to zero at twice its resting length. The maximum force also decreases to zero at the shortest possible muscular length. Since the muscular contractile force depends on the length of the muscle and since the length changes during contraction, muscular efficiency is always changing (Figure 20.5).

Negative (eccentric) work is produced by a muscle when it maintains a force against an external force tending to stretch the muscle. An example of negative work is found in the action of the leg muscle during a descent of a flight of stairs. Since the body is being lowered, external work is less than zero. The muscles are using physiological energy to control the descent and prevent the body from accumulating kinetic energy as it descends.

Muscular efficiencies for walking downhill approach 120% (McMahon, 1984). Since heat produced by the muscle is the difference between 100% and the percent efficiency, the heat produced by muscles walking downhill is about 220% of their energy expenditure. The energy expenditure of muscles undergoing negative work is about one-sixth that of a muscle doing positive work (Johnson, 1991); so, a leg muscle going uphill produces about twice as much heat as a leg muscle going downhill.

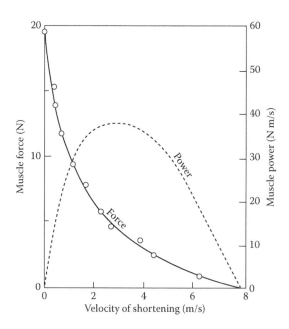

FIGURE 20.4   Force and power output of a muscle as a function of velocity. (Adapted and used with permission from Milsum, J. H. *Biological Control Systems Analysis*, McGraw-Hill, New York, 1966.)

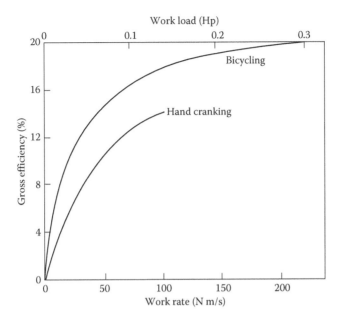

FIGURE 20.5 Gross efficiency for hand cranking or bicycling is a function of the rate of work. (From Goldman, R.F., 1978. *Safety in Manual Materials Handling*, National Institute for Occupational Safety and Health (NIOSH), Cincinnati, OH, pp. 110–116.)

20.1.4 Locomotion

The act of locomotion involves both positive and negative work. There are four successive stages of a walking stride. In the first stage, both feet are on the ground, with one foot ahead of the other. The trailing foot pushes forward and the front foot is pushing backward. In the second stage, the trailing foot leaves the ground and the front foot applies a braking force. The center of mass of the body begins to lift over the front foot. In the third stage, the trailing foot is brought forward and the supporting foot applies a vertical force. The center of mass of the body is at its highest point above the supporting foot. In the last stage, the body's center of mass is lowered and the trailing foot provides an acceleration force.

This alteration of the raising and lowering of the body's center of mass, along with the pushing and braking provided by the feet, makes walking a low-efficiency maneuver. Walking has been likened to alternatively applying the brakes and accelerator while driving a car. Just as the fuel efficiency of the car would suffer from this mode of propulsion, so does the energy efficiency of walking suffer from the way walking is performed.

There is an optimum speed of walking. If the walking speed is more than this optimum speed, additional muscular energy is required to propel the body forward. Moving slower than the optimal speed requires additional muscular energy to retard the leg movement. Thus, the optimal speed is related to the rate at which the leg can swing forward. A simple analysis of the leg as a physical pendulum shows that the optimal walking speed is related to the length of the leg:

$$S \propto \sqrt{L} \tag{20.5}$$

Unlike walking, there is a stage of running during which both feet leave the ground. The center of mass of the body does not rise and fall as much during running as during walking; so, the efficiency for running can be greater than for walking.

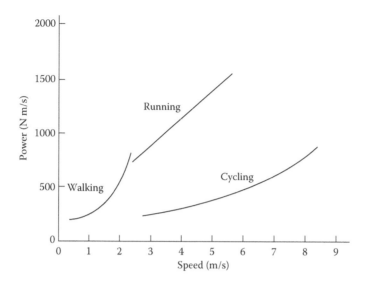

FIGURE 20.6 Power required for walking, running, and cycling by an adult male. The curves for walking and running interact at about 2.3 m/s and show that walking is more efficient below the intersection and running is more efficient above the intersection. (Redrawn with permission from Alexander, R.M. *Am. Sci.*, 72: 348, 1984.)

At a speed of about 2.5 m/s, running appears to be more energy efficient than walking, and the transition is usually made between these forms of locomotion (Figure 20.6). Unlike walking, there does not appear to be a functional relationship between speed and the length of the leg; so, running power expenditure is linearly related to speed alone.

Why would anyone want to propel the extra weight of a bicycle in addition to body weight? On the surface, it would appear that cycling would cost more energy than running or walking. However, the center of mass of the body does not move vertically as long as the cyclist sits on the seat. Without the positive and negative work associated with walking or running, cycling is a much more efficient form of locomotion than the other two (Figure 20.6), and the cost of moving the additional weight of the bicycle can be easily supplied.

Many sports or leisure activities have a biomechanical basis. An understanding of the underlying biomechanical processes can lead to improved performance. Yet, there are limits to performance that cause frustrations for competitive athletes. Hence, additional factors are sometimes employed to expand these limits. A brief discussion of some of these factors is given here.

20.1.4.1 Age

It is well established that structural and functional deterioration occurs to most physiological systems in the body with aging, independent of disease or inactivity (Juckett, 2010). There are both primary aging (i.e., age-dependent or normal aging) effects and secondary aging (i.e., temporally associated with age, but not necessarily due to the aging process) effects (Brody and Schneider, 1986). Both adversely influence the mechanical and physiological work performance. Aging effects on the cardiovascular, neuromuscular, and musculoskeletal systems have a particularly high impact on mechanical work capacity. Age-associated deterioration of these systems results in a decline in maximal oxygen consumption (aerobic capacity), and a loss of muscle mass, strength, power, fatigue resistance, and bone mineral density, as well as a gain in body fat, particularly in the abdominal region (Kyle et al., 2001; Kuk et al., 2009). These changes also lead to greater disease prevalence and a volitional decline in physical activity. For this reason, with advanced age, it is difficult to determine how much of the loss in work capacity can be attributed to primary aging versus inactivity.

Young athletes who continue to train to an older age maintain a large portion of their aerobic capacity with age, but still experience some losses due to both primary and secondary aging. Although the declines in aerobic capacity (Pollack et al., 1997) and skeletal muscle function (Kyle et al., 2001) with age can be considerable, regular exercise (training) results in substantial slowing of the age-associated declines in most systems. Many of the aging effects on both the cardiovascular (Bortz, 2010) and musculoskeletal (Lynch et al., 1999) systems can be at least partly reversed within the first couple of months of exercise training (Hurley and Kostek, 2001; Walts et al., 2008).

The loss of aerobic capacity with aging and inactivity is primarily due to losses in cardiac output, which in turn results from decreases in maximal heart rate, whereas the maximal capacity to extract oxygen from the peripheral blood does not change much with aging. Thus, aging results in a reduced blood flow to the active muscles during exercise as a result of a loss of cardiac output. Although inactivity can also result in loss of cardiac output, it appears to be largely the result of a loss in plasma volume, with reductions in heart volume and heart contractility playing a smaller role.

Maximal force production (muscular strength) is maintained for a much longer time period throughout aging than aerobic capacity. For example, significant declines in aerobic capacity (Fleg et al., 2005) is already observed in the thirties, whereas strength is maintained until the sixties (Lynch et al., 1999). Losses in aerobic capacity, though not linear, can be greater than 10% per decade (Buskirk and Hodgson, 1987), whereas age-associated strength losses occur at a rate of ~12–14% per decade (Lynch et al., 1999). Likewise, the loss of muscle mass occurs at a rate of ~6% per decade, again beginning in the sixties for men, but two decades earlier in women (Lynch et al., 1999). Muscle power has a faster rate of decline than strength (Kostka 2005) and appears to be more closely related to the functional abilities in the elderly than strength (Puthoff et al., 2008), presumably due to the relative importance of movement velocity in many activities of daily living.

20.1.4.2 Regular Exercise

For the purpose of this chapter, regular exercise will be divided into two training modalities: aerobic exercise training and resistance (strength) training. Aerobic training consists of regular muscular activities that use large amounts of oxygen for energy production. These include exercises such as walking, jogging, swimming, and cycling. Strength training (ST) refers to exercising regularly against an external load, such as during isotonic (same tension), isokinetic (same movement velocity), or isometric (same muscle length) ST. Isotonic and isokinetic ST can be divided into the shortening and lengthening phases (often incorrectly named concentric and eccentric phases) (Faulkner, 2003), and can be performed with free weights such as barbells and dumbbells, machines, or by just using one's body mass for resistance, such as is done with certain kinds of calisthenics.

20.1.4.2.1 Aerobic Exercise Training

When aerobic exercise is performed regularly, it stimulates many biochemical reactions that raise the critical threshold level of exercise intensity at which metabolic homeostasis (equilibrium) can be maintained. Many compensatory reactions allow the body to adapt to minor stresses, such as mild aerobic exercise, so that homeostasis (equilibrium) can be maintained. For example, the increased energy demands of aerobic exercise stimulate an increase in heart rate, respiration, blood flow, and many other cardiovascular and metabolic reactions that allow the body to maintain homeostasis. As the intensity of exercise increases, it becomes more difficult for compensatory mechanisms to maintain homeostasis. After exceeding about 80% of an untrained person's maximal exercise capacity, homeostasis can no longer be maintained for more than a few minutes before exhaustion results.

Regular aerobic exercise (training) elevates the threshold level that a single exercise session can be performed before disturbing and eventually losing homeostasis. It does this by elevating the maximal physiological capacity for homeostasis so that the same intensity of aerobic exercise may no longer disrupt homeostasis due to a lower percentage of maximal capacity. In addition, training produces specific adaptations during submaximal exercise that permit greater and longer amounts of work before losing homeostasis (Hurley and Hagberg, 1998). A good example of this is when blood lactate rises with increased intensity of exercise. Prior to training, blood lactate concentration rises substantially when the intensity of exercise exceeds ~75% of maximal oxygen consumption (VO_2max). Following training, the same intensity of exercise results in a lower concentration of blood lactate, resulting in a higher fraction of the untrained VO_2max before blood lactate reaches the same level as before training during exercise. This adaptation is so profound that blood lactate levels are often only slightly above the resting values after training, when performing submaximal exercise (e.g., <65% of VO_2max). Thus, exercise training allows an individual to perform a much greater amount of work during exercise before homeostasis is disturbed to the point at which fatigue ensues.

20.1.4.2.2 Strength Training

Muscular strength declines with age (Lindle et al., 1997; Lynch et al., 1999), disease, and as a consequence of the administration of some medications used for the treatment of the disease (Fiatarone-Singh, 2002; Hurley and Hanson, 2009). However, strength can be increased substantially in a relatively short time period with ST (Walts et al., 2008). Muscle power can also be increased with ST, but the magnitude of increase depends on the movement velocity of training used during the muscle shortening phase of exercise.

The typical training modalities of ~2 s during the shortening phase and ~4 s during the muscle lengthening phase of movement result in ~30% increase in strength (Lemmer et al., 2000) and ~25% increase in power (Jozsi et al., 1999; Delmonico et al., 2005). However, increases of almost 100% have been reported when high-velocity training has been incorporated (Fielding et al., 2002). Our group has reported increases in muscle mass of ~12% with ST, within the first couple of months of training, based on magnetic resonance imaging (MRI) measurements of the entire volume of the muscle being trained (Ivey et al., 2000) and about half that amount when the male sex hormone, testosterone, has been obliterated (Hanson and Hurley, unpublished data, 2010). The amount of force per unit of muscle volume, known as muscle quality, also increases substantially with ST (Tracey et al., 1999). We have shown that ~3 decades of age-related strength loss and two decades of age-related muscle mass loss can be recovered/reversed within the first couple of months of ST (Ivey et al., 2000; Lemmer et al., 2000).

20.1.4.3 Sex Differences

Cardiovascular fitness and muscular strength are substantially higher in men compared to women. The aerobic capacity in men is about 40–50% higher than women. In addition, the upper body strength is ~100% higher and the lower body strength is ~50% higher in men (Lynch et al., 1999). However, these differences are diminished substantially when body composition is taken into consideration. For example, when VO_2max is expressed with reference to body mass (mL/kg of body weight/min), this difference narrows to ~20% and to ~10% when differences in muscle mass are taken into consideration.

The differences in muscular strength between men and women are also narrowed when normalized for fat-free mass (Lynch et al., 1999). There does not appear to be any significant difference in responses to training between men and women when expressed on a relative basis (% change), but men appear to have greater muscle mass gains than women in response to ST when expressed in absolute terms (Ivey et al., 2000).

Women can be less fatigable than men for some muscle groups during isometric contractions, but sex differences vary substantially depending on the task, muscle groups involved, and age of the participant (Hunter, 2009). This conditional explanation is based on the fact that task differences are limited by different physiological systems.

20.1.4.4 Genetics

There appears to be evidence that genetic factors contribute significantly to whether one chooses to be sedentary or physically active, to aerobic capacity, and to muscular power, but the specific genes responsible for these influences are still not known (Rankinen et al., 2010). We have observed great interindividual variability in the loss of both muscle strength and mass with age (Lindle et al., 1997; Lynch et al., 1999), as well as the gain in muscle strength and muscle mass with exercise training (Ivey et al., 2000; Walts et al., 2008).

Seeman et al. (1996) reported that genetic factors accounted for 60–80% of the interindividual differences in lean body mass, whereas Huygens et al. (2004) reported the heritability of skeletal muscle mass of up to 90%. These data provide strong support that genetic factors may influence sarcopenia (i.e., alterations in strength and muscle mass with age), as well as strength and muscle mass response to ST. However, none of these studies assessed the effects of specific candidate genes or candidate gene variations (polymorphisms) on strength or muscle mass response to training.

The heritability of muscle mass and strength indicates that specific genes contribute to differences in muscle phenotype. More importantly, specific polymorphisms could at least partly explain the interindividual variability in sarcopenia and muscle response to ST. Moreover, our research group and others have explored the relationship of gene polymorphisms to muscle phenotypes in genes thought to have a plausible physiological connection to changes in strength and muscle mass. Unfortunately, however, this work has been largely unsuccessful in identifying either single genes or gene interactions that explain more than about 5% of training responses in these muscle phenotypes. Thus, despite the knowledge of important relationships between genetics and muscle function, little is known about the specific gene variations that may explain this genetic contribution (Rankinen et al., 2010).

References

Alexander, R.M. Walking and running. *Am. Sci.*, 72: 348, 1984.

Bortz, W. Disuse and aging. *J. Gerontol. A Biol. Sci. Med. Sci.*, 65(4): 382–385, 2010.

Brody, J. A., and Schneider, E. L. Diseases and disorders of aging: An hypothesis. *J. Chronic. Dis.*, 39: 871–876, 1986.

Buskirk, E. R., and Hodgson, J. L. Age and aerobic power: The rate of change in men and women. *Fed. Proc.*, 46: 1824–1829, 1987.

Delmonico, M. J., Kostek, M. C., Doldo, N. A., Hand, B. D., Bailey, J. A., Rabon-Stith, K. M., Conway, J. M., and Hurley, B. F. The effect of moderate velocity strength training on peak muscle power, velocity, and muscle power quality in older men and women. *J. Appl. Physiol.*, 99: 1712–1718, 2005.

Faulkner, J. A. Terminology for contractions of muscles during shortening, while isometric, and during lengthening. *J. Appl. Physiol.*, 95: 455–459, 2003.

Fiatarone-Singh, M. A. Exercise comes of age: Rationale and recommendations for a geriatric exercise prescription. *J. Geronto: Med. Sci.*, 57A: M262–M282, 2002.

Fielding R. A., LeBrasseur, N. K., Cuoco, A., Bean, J., Mizer, K., and Fiatarone-Singh, M. A. High-velocity resistance training increases skeletal muscle peak power in older women. *J. Am. Geriatr. Soc.*, 50: 655–662, 2002.

Fleg, J. L., Morrell, C. H., Bos, A. G., Brant, L. J., Talbot, L. A., Wright, J. G., and Lakatta, E. G. Accelerated longitudinal decline of aerobic capacity in healthy older adults. *Circulation*, 112(5): 674–682, 2005.

Hunter, S. K. Sex differences and mechanisms of task specific muscle fatigue. *Exerc. Sport Sci. Rev.*, 37: 113–122, 2009.

Hurley, B. F. and Hagberg, J.M. Optimizing health in older persons: Aerobic or strength training? In *Exerc. Sport Sci. Rev.*, 26: 61–89, Williams & Wilkins, Baltimore, MD, 1998.

Hurley, B. F. and Hanson, E. D. Can strength training reverse the side effects of cancer treatment? *J. Act. Aging*, Nov/Dec: 44–52, 2009.

Hurley, B. F. and Kostek, M. C. Exercise interventions for seniors. What training modality is best for health? *Orthop. Phys. Ther. Clin. North Am.*, 10: 213–225, 2001.

Huygens, W., Thomis, M. A., Peeters, M. W., Vlietinck, R. F., and Beunen, G. P. Determinants and upper-limit heritabilities of skeletal muscle mass and strength. *Can. J. Appl. Physiol.*, 29: 186–200, 2004.

Ivey, F. M., Tracy, B. L., Lemmer, J. T., Hurlbut, D. E., Martel, G. F., Roth, S. M., Fozard, J. L., Metter, E. J., and Hurley, B. F. The effects of age, gender and myostatin genotype on the hypertrophic response to heavy resistance strength training. *J Gerontol: Med. Sci.*, 55A: M641–M648, 2000.

Johnson, A. T. *Biomechanics and Exercise Physiology*, John Wiley, New York, 1991.

Johnson, A. T., Benjamin, M. B., and Silverman, N. Oxygen consumption, heat production, and muscular efficiency during uphill and downhill walking. *Appl. Ergon.*, 33: 485–491, 2002.

Jozsi, A. C., Campbell, W. W., Joseph, L., Davey, S. L., and Evans, W. J. Changes in power with resistance training in older and younger men and women. *J. Gerontol.*, 54A: M591–M596, 1999.

Juckett, D. A. What determines age-related disease: Do we know all the right questions? *Age (Dordr.)*, 32(2): 155–160, 2010.

Kostka, T. Quadriceps maximal power and optimal shortening velocity in 335 men aged 23–88 years. *Eur. J. Appl. Physiol.*, 95: 140–145, 2005.

Kuk, J. L., Saunders, T. J., Davidson, L. E., and Ross, R. Age-related changes in total and regional fat distribution. *Ageing Res. Rev.*, 8: 339–348, 2009.

Kyle, U. G., Genton, L., Hans, D., Karsegard, L., Slosman, D. O., and Pichard, C. Age-related differences in fat-free mass, skeletal muscle, body cell mass and fat mass between 18 and 94 years. *Eur. J. Clin. Nutr.*, 55: 663–672, 2001.

Lemmer, J. T., Hurbut, D. E., Martel, G. F., Tracy, B. L., Ivey, F. M., Metter, E. J., Fozard, J. L., Fleg, J. L., and Hurley, B. F. Age and gender responses to strength training and detraining. *Med. Sci. Sports Exerc.*, 32: 1505–1512, 2000.

Lindle, R., Metter, E., Lynch, N., Fleg, J., Fozard, J., Tobin, J., Roy, T., and Hurley, B. Age and gender comparisons of muscle strength in 654 women and men aged 20–93. *J. Appl. Physiol.*, 83: 1581–1587, 1997.

Lynch, N. A., Metter, E. J., Lindle, R. S., Fozard, J. L., Tobin, J. D., Roy, T. A., Fleg, J. L., and Hurley, B. F. Muscle quality I: Age-associated differences in arm vs. leg muscle groups. *J. Appl. Physiol.*, 86: 188–194, 1999.

McMahon, T. A. *Muscles, Reflexes, and Locomotion*, Princeton University Press, Princeton, NJ, 1984.

Milsum, J. H. *Biological Control Systems Analysis*, McGraw-Hill, New York, 1966.

Pollack, M. L., Mengelkoch, L. F., Graves, J. S., Lowenthal, D. T., Limacher, M. C., Foster, C., and Wilmore, J. H. Twenty year follow-up of aerobic power and body composition of older track athletes. *J. Appl. Physiol.*, 82: 1508–1516, 1997.

Puthoff, M. L., Janz, K. F., and Nielson, D. The relationship between lower extremity strength and power to everyday walking behaviors in older adults with functional limitations. *J. Geriatr. Phys. Ther.*, 31: 24–31, 2008.

Rankinen, T., Roth, S. M., Bray, M. S., Loos, R., Perusse, L., Wolfarth, B., Hagberg, J. M., and Bouchard, C. Advances in exercise, fitness, and performance genomics. *Med. Sci. Sports Exerc.*, 42: 835–846, 2010.

Seeman, E., Hopper, J., Young, N., Formica, C., Goss, P., and Tsalamandris, C. Do genetic factors explain associations between muscle strength, lean mass, and bone density? A twin study. *Am. J. Physiol.*, 270: E320–E327, 1996.

Tracy, B.L., Ivey, F.M., Hurlbut, D., Martel, G. F., Lemmer, J.T., Siegel, E. L., Metter, E. J., Fozard, J. L., Fleg, J. L., and Hurley, B. F. 1999. Muscle quality II: Effects of strength training in 65–75 year old men and women, *J. Appl. Physiol.* 86: 195–201.

Walts, C. T., Hanson, E. D., Delmonico, M. J., Yao, L., Wang, M. Q., and Hurley, B. F. Do sex or race differences influence strength training effects on muscle or fat? *Med. Sci. Sports Exerc.*, 40(4): 669–676, 2008.

Index